LIPPINCOTT'S REVIEW FOR

NCLEX-PN

4th EDITION

LIPPINCOTT'S REVIEW FOR

NCLEX-PN

4th EDITION

Barbara Kuhn Timby R.N.C., B.S.N., M.A.

Nursing Professor
Instructor, Medical–Surgical Nursing
Glen Oaks Community College
Centreville, Michigan

Jeanne C. Scherer R.N., B.S.N., M.S.

Formerly Assistant Director and Medical–Surgical Coordinator
Sisters of Charity Hospital
School of Nursing
Buffalo, New York

J. B. Lippincott Company Philadelphia

Acquisitions Editor: Donna L. Hilton, RN, BSN
Coordinating Editorial Assistant: Susan M. Keneally
Project Editors: Jim Slade and Sandra Cherrey
Design Coordinator: Kathy Kelley-Luedtke
Designer: Bill Donnelly
Production Manager: Helen Ewan
Production Coordinator: Maura C. Murphy
Compositor: Compset, Inc.
Printer/Binder: Courier Book Company/Kendallville

Fourth Edition

6 5 4 3 2 1

Library of Congress Cataloging-in-Publication Data

Timby, Barbara Kuhn.
    Lippincott's review for NCLEX-PN. — Ed. 4. / Barbara Kuhn Timby,
Jeanne C. Scherer.
        p.   cm.
    Rev. ed. of: Lippincott's state board review for NCLEX-PN /
LuVerne Wolff Lewis. Ed. 3. c1990.
    Includes bibliographical references.
    ISBN 0-397-55024-3
    1. Practical nursing—Examinations, questions, etc.   I. Scherer,
Jeanne C.   II. Lewis, LuVerne Wolff. Lippincott's state board
review for NCLEX-PN.   III. Title.   IV. Title: Review for NCLEX-PN.
    [DNLM: 1. Nursing—examination questions.   WY 18 T583L 1994]
RT62.T56   1994
610.73'076—dc20
DNLM/DLC
for Library of Congress   93-32988
                                                              CIP

Any procedure or practice described in this book should be applied by the health care practitioner under appropriate supervision in accordance with professional standards of care used with regard to the unique circumstances that apply in each practice situation. Care has been taken to confirm the accuracy of information presented and to describe generally accepted practices. However, the authors, editors, and publisher cannot accept any responsibility for errors or omissions or for any consequences from application of the information in this book and make no warranty, express or implied, with respect to the contents of the book.

Every effort has been made to ensure drug selections and dosages are in accordance with current recommendations and practice. Because of ongoing research, changes in government regulations, and the constant flow of information on drug therapy, reactions, and interactions, the reader is cautioned to check the package insert for each drug for indications, dosages, warnings, and precautions, particularly if the drug is new or infrequently used.

PREFACE

Most people would agree that the best way to prepare for a state licensing examination is to use good study habits while enrolled in an educational program for nursing. This includes keeping up to date in both clinical and classroom work. However, many candidates feel more secure and at ease when they plan for a period of concentrated review before taking their national licensing examination.

Lippincott's Review for NCLEX–PN, 4th edition, has been written to help students study during their educational program and candidates prepare for taking the practical nurse licensing examination. Features that make this review book especially helpful for persons preparing for the NCLEX examination or tests during school are summarized as follows:

The test plan adopted by the National Council of State Boards of Nursing for preparing the licensing examination for practical nurses was used as a guide to prepare this book. Even though the paper and pencil NCLEX–PN examination will be replaced by the computerized version, the National Council indicates that the test plan is the same for both and that they are parallel. Care was used so that the items in this book measure major abilities as described in the test plan. There is further discussion concerning the test plan and the preparation of the licensing examination in the introduction of this book.

There are four units containing review tests in this book:

Unit I.
The Nursing Care of Clients with Mental Health Needs (Unit I contains 1 review test)
Unit II.
The Nursing Care of Maternity Clients and Newborns (Unit II has 2 review tests)
Unit III.
The Nursing Care of Children (Unit III has 2 reviews tests)
Unit IV.
The Nursing Care of Adults with Medical–Surgical Disorders (Unit IV has 9 review tests)

It is hoped that this method of organization, according to clinical areas, will simplify reviewing by grouping items dealing with clinical content together.

The review tests are integrated in the same manner as the licensing examination. This means that the mental health, maternity, pediatric, and medical–surgical items incorporate information from all basic courses studied in nursing. This includes anatomy and physiology, pharmacology, diet therapy and nutrition, fundamentals of nursing, and psychosocial sciences that deal with legal and ethical issues, interpersonal relationships, communication, professional adjustments, human development (physical and psychosocial), and the like. The review tests provide client situations with a cluster of related questions.

There is a two-part comprehensive examination following the 14 review tests in this book. This examination, beginning on page 395, is as similar to the national licensing examination as possible. It contains a total of 240 items, 120 items in each of two parts. This equals the number on the two-part, pencil and paper licensing examination. It exceeds the maximum number of 180 questions that may be asked on the computerized version. Both parts of the comprehensive review test contain items that integrate all clinical areas, that is, mental health nursing, maternity nursing and the care of the newborn, nursing care of children, and medical–surgical nursing (adults). The comprehensive test in this text contains single-item questions. This reflects the pattern that will be followed in the computerized national examination. The Computerized Adaptive Testing–PN (CAT–PN) may ask questions that relate to client situations. However, there is only one question that applies to each scenario provided. If more than one question pertains to a situation, the situation is repeated with each question.

All of the items and client situations in this book resemble to the greatest degree possible the items and client situations used in the national licensing examination. The type of items and client situations used are described in the introduction of this book. Of course, it is unlikely that an item in this book will be identical to any appearing in the national licensing examination. However, the licensing examination uses common situations in which practical nurses work and items dealing with typical nursing measures required by clients described in those situations.

Principles of test construction were observed in the preparation of items for this book, just as they are by persons responsible for the final preparation of items used in the national licensing examination. Observing these principles helps to prepare items that are reliable and valid and that realistically resemble items appearing in the licensing examination.

Correct answers are given for all items in this book at the end of each review test and the comprehensive examinations. A rationale for the correct answer also is offered; that is, there are reasons given concerning why the correct answer is the best answer and why incorrect answers are wrong. Studying the rationale along with the items offers an excellent review of practical nursing. A textbook and a page in that textbook where correct answers can be verified are furnished for help when additional reviewing of content is necessary. People using this book may wish to determine in what area of nursing they need extra study because they have not done well in selecting correct answers for certain items. This review book has classified each item according to the step in the nursing process as well as client need category. By following directions for using the classification of test items following each review test and the comprehensive examinations, it is easy to identify areas of weakness where further study is indicated.

There are 1544 items in the 14 review tests in this book and 240 items in the two-part comprehensive examination for a total of 1784 items. An NCLEX Practice Test of 100 items on an accompanying computer disk is also provided. Most of the items in this edition are new. No review book or licensing examination can cover all aspects of nursing. Care was taken to avoid testing regional practices and policies.

You are urged to read the introduction of this book. The introduction, which begins on page xvii, offers many suggestions that will help candidates use this book and prepare for the national licensing examination for practical nursing. Omitting the introduction may well diminish the outcomes of the review and jeopardize the potential success on the licensing examination.

Although this book's primary purpose is to help candidates prepare for their national licensing examination, it can serve other purposes as well. For example, the book can be used to prepare for various types of achievement tests in nursing. Inactive practical nurses who wish to return to nursing will find the book useful for review and self-appraisal. People who will write challenge examinations for advanced school credit are encouraged to use the book for review purposes. Faculty members may find the book helpful for developing ideas for teaching and evaluation.

The ultimate goal of this book will have been achieved when its use helps nurses offer high quality care to their patients.

Barbara Kuhn Timby, RNC, BSN, MA and Jeanne C. Scherer, RN, BSN, MS

ACKNOWLEDGMENTS

The authors express sincere thanks for the expert review of test items presented in this book to Bill Lederman, RN, BSN, MA, Nursing Professor, Glen Oaks Community College, Centreville, Michigan and JoAnne Purlee, RN, BSN, MA, Nursing Professor, Glen Oaks Community College.

CONTENTS

INTRODUCTION

What Is NCLEX–PN and CAT–PN?

The acronym, NCLEX–PN, stands for the *N*ational *C*ouncil *L*icensure *E*xamination for *P*ractical *N*urses. CAT–PN are letters that represent the words *C*omputerized *A*daptive *T*esting for *P*ractical *N*ursing. The first is a paper and pencil test, and the second, as the name implies, is one that is taken at a computer. Regardless of the testing format, the content is parallel. This examination is used to assess the ability of graduates of practical and vocational nursing programs to provide safe and effective nursing care at the entry level. Entry level is defined as comparable to that expected of a newly licensed practical nurse who has been employed for 6 months or less. A passing score demonstrates that the test-taker can perform entry level nursing skills with at least a minimum level of competency.

The National Council of State Boards of Nursing, whose Examination Committee is responsible for developing the national licensing examination, is made up of representatives from all state boards of nursing. The member boards of nursing consist of all of this country's states, the District of Columbia, and United States territories (Guam, American Samoa, and the Virgin Islands).

All states use the examination prepared by the National Council of State Boards of Nursing. In some states, the terms vocational nurses and vocational nursing are used instead of practical nurses and practical nursing.

Practical and vocational student nurses have similar educational programs, and all candidates for licensure must take an examination. The paper and pencil version is identical in all states for each candidate. The computerized version is unique in that each test is individualized for each candidate, yet every test meets all of the test plan requirements. The computer selects questions randomly that are neither too difficult nor too easy for the candidate. It continues to make adjustments as each question is answered. There is such a vast number of questions stored in the computer's memory that no two tests are exactly alike. After sufficient questions are answered, the computer can determine with reliable certainty whether the candidate possesses the minimum knowledge to safely practice as a practical or vocational nurse.

What Is the Purpose for a National Licensing Examination?

The federal government gives to states the power and authority to ensure the health and safety of citizens. One example in which each state upholds this duty is by regulating the licensing and practice of individuals who provide services to the public. Each state's board of nursing is given the responsibility by its legislature to regulate licensure for practical nurses and practical nursing within its jurisdiction. Passing a licensing examination meets the criteria for state licensure. Licensure is both a legal and professional requirement that assures the public that a nurse is a valid practitioner and possesses appropriate job related skills. A license issued by the state indicates that the holder of the license has been judged to be a safe practitioner in practical nursing.

The examination prepared by the National Council helps state boards of nursing determine whether you are ready to give safe and effective nursing care. The examination includes questions that test the knowledge, skills, and abilities essential for an entry level practical nurse who will be applying the nursing process in order to meet the needs of clients with commonly occurring health problems having predictable outcomes.

How Is the National Licensing Examination Prepared?

The National Council of State Boards of Nursing is responsible for developing the NCLEX in both written and CAT formats. A test plan, discussed later, is prepared first. It must then be approved by representatives of the state boards of nursing. The states submit names of item writers who must themselves be licensed and meet a particular profile for expert nursing knowledge, clinical expertise, and geographical diversity.

After items are written, they are reviewed by a committee to ensure that they are not biased. State boards of nursing also are allowed to review the items that have been developed if they so choose. This privilege allows the boards of nursing to object to any item which conflicts with the spirit and law of its respective nurse practice act. If even one state legitimately challenges a test item, it is withdrawn.

All approved items are field tested before becoming an actual test question. To be trial tested, the item must meet criteria indicating that its content reflects the domain of nursing and represents what entry level practical nurses need to know to practice safely. So-called tryout items are placed throughout the licensing examination. The mix of answers to the trial items are then analyzed to determine whether they function well in helping to judge if a candidate knows nursing content sufficiently well to practice safe and effective nursing. Well-constructed items are used in later licensing examinations. Poorly constructed and ambiguous items are discarded. You will not know which items are tryout items but these items do *not* count in your final score.

What Is the Test Plan Used to Prepare the National Examination?

A specially-constructed test plan is used to guide people responsible for constructing the national licensing examination. To ensure test validity, the content of the items is based on data compiled in a study by M. Kane and D. Colton entitled *Job Analysis of Newly Licensed Practical/Vocational Nurses (1986–1987)*. The method of the study involved identifying the activities performed by entry level practical nurses along with the frequency with which the activities were performed.

The activities, the settings in which they were performed, and the range in client ages were further analyzed as to their impact on the safety to clients. Thus the results of the study provide an organizational pattern reflecting current nursing practice and pertinent content for test items.

Regardless of the clinical subject being tested, such as maternity nursing, each question includes two major components: A phase in the nursing process and a particular client need.

Phases of the Nursing Process

The phases of the nursing process that are tested on the practical nurse licensing examination include collecting data, planning, implementing, and evaluating nursing care. Not all phases of the nursing process are tested equally because some activities are shared between registered nurses and practical nurses in the clinical setting. Therefore, those phases, collecting data and implementing nursing care, that the practical nurse performs more often independently are tested in higher proportion.

Collecting data involves questions that reflect gathering information by observing the physiological, psychosocial, health, and safety needs of clients; acquiring facts from the client, his significant others, members of the health team, and client records; determining the need for additional information; and communicating the findings that were obtained. In addition, this phase of the nursing process includes participation in formulating nursing diagnoses.

Planning client care within the scope of practical nursing is reflected in items in which the nurse contributes to the development of nursing care plans by helping to formulate goals for nursing care; participating in identifying clients' needs and nursing interventions that will help achieve established goals; communicating changes that may necessitate altering the plan of care; and collaborating with the client, his or her significant others, and other health team members concerning the plan for nursing care.

Implementing care for clients is tested in items that ask questions concerning the performance of basic therapeutic and preventive nursing measures; ensuring a safe and effective environment; helping the client, his or her significant others, and other health care members understand the plan for care; and recording and reporting information to other members of the health team.

Evaluating client care involves questions whose content concerns participating in nursing activities that will determine the effectiveness of nursing care; documenting the responses that have been identified; determining if goals have been achieved, partially achieved, or remain unachieved; and lastly, assisting in making appropriate changes in the plan of care.

Client Needs

There are four broad categories referred to as *Client Needs* that involve nursing activities. They are safe, effective care environment; physiological integrity; psychosocial integrity; and health promotion and health maintenance. Test items are distributed in each of these categories with safe, effective care environment and physiological integrity tested in higher proportion.

Safe, effective care environment involves questions concerning nursing activities, such as participating in the coordination of client care, following standards of care, maintaining goal-oriented care, adhering to principles of environmental safety, preparing appropriately for treatments and procedures, and performing treatments and procedures safely and effectively. For example, the content in this area includes, but is not limited to: data gathering techniques; communication skills and appropriate alternatives for clients with special needs; infection control techniques; client rights, such as confidentiality; providing individualized care based on respect for clients' religious, cultural, and developmental differences; participating with the team in planning and evaluating care; and a knowledge of community health agencies.

Physiological integrity is a category of knowledge tested in questions involving nursing care that promotes physiological adaptation, reduces potential health risks, facilitates client mobility and comfort, and provides basic care. Questions in this category involve but are not limited to: knowledge of therapeutic and life-saving techniques, using specialized equipment, following principles of medication administration, maintaining body functioning and preventing complications, applying principles of body mechanics, correctly using assistive devices, implementing comfort measures, carrying out routine nursing measures, and reporting changes in a client's condition.

The category of *psychosocial integrity* concerns the nurse's ability to promote a client's psychosocial adaptation and meet his or her needs for coping and adjustment. Evidence of competence in this area involves knowledge, skills, and abilities that include but are not limited to: identifying signs of emotional and mental health problems, indications of the client's self-concept, characteristics of life crises, substance abuse, adaptive and maladaptive behavior, alterations in sensory perception, violent and suicidal behavior, understanding common therapeutic approaches, and knowledge of community referral agencies for clients with psychosocial needs.

The *health promotion and health maintenance* category refers to the nursing care involved in promoting the client's need for continued growth and development, self-care, maintenance of a support system, health promotion, and early diagnosis and treatment of illness. Success in this category, therefore, depends on being knowledgeable in areas that include but are not limited to: interactions among family members, wellness, methods of adapting to changes in health, sexuality and reproduction, current practices in birthing, parenting, growth and development across the life cycle, dying and death, routine immunization schedules, health teaching within the scope of practical nursing, and a knowledge of community resources.

The test plan used by the National Council and its item writers was followed while preparing review tests and the comprehensive examinations presented in this book. Each item has been coded to identify the phase of the nursing process and the category of client need it represents. People interested in more detailed information concerning the test plan are advised to write to the National Council of State Boards of Nursing, 676 North St. Clair, Suite 550, Chicago, IL, 60611.

What Type of Item is Used?

The items on the paper and pencil and computerized version are of the same type; that is, all items are objective, multiple choice questions. Some test items relate to a described client situation. Here is an example of a client situation:

John Kirk is hospitalized for treatment of pneumonia. His heart rate is 110 beats per minute, he has moist lung sounds, and he is short of breath.

The item that follows this situation relates to John's nursing care.

Regardless of whether a test question is related to a client situation or not, each test question consists of two parts, as follows:

The Stem. The stem presents a problem and is stated as an incomplete sentence or as a question. The example below illustrates.

The Options. The options present four alternatives from which you select one correct or best answer. The other three options are incorrect answers and are called distractors. The following examples illustrate:

Stem in the form of an incomplete sentence

The best position for promoting ventilation is

Options

1. supine.
2. Fowler's.
3. prone.
4. Sim's.

Option 2 is the correct answer. Options 1, 3, and 4 are incorrect answers, or distractors. This question reflects the test plan category for the implementation phase of the nursing process because it concerns the performance of a basic therapeutic nursing measure. It also tests the client need category for physiological integrity because it concerns promoting physiological adaptation. In order to select the correct answer, you need to know that a Fowler's position is one in which the head and the back of the client are elevated. This position lowers abdominal organs away from the diaphragm, allowing a larger volume of air to enter the lungs. More oxygen and carbon dioxide are able to diffuse through the alveolar capillary membrane.

Another example follows.

Stem in the form of a question

When a client is receiving oxygen, which one of the following nursing actions is most important?

Options

1. providing high caloric nourishment.
2. changing position every 2 hours.
3. enforcing the "No Smoking" policy.
4. limiting the number of visitors in the room.

Option 3 is the correct answer. Options 1, 2, and 4 are incorrect answers, or distractors. This question also reflects the test plan category for the implementation phase of the nursing process because it concerns the performance of a basic therapeutic nursing measure. It tests the client need category for a safe, effective care environment because it concerns a nursing activity that applies a principle of environmental safety. In order to select the correct answer, you need to know that oxygen supports combustion. Any open flame could endanger the client because it creates a fire hazard.

The items on the CAT–PN will not be paired strictly with a client situation reference. Some items will stand alone. Where a client situation does appear, perhaps only one of several questions stored within the computer's test bank memory will be asked of a particular candidate. The computer will randomly select an item that matches the person's test plan needs. It may be an item that tests the person's competence in a certain step of the nursing process or area of client need. The item that is chosen by the computer will be based on the person's level of skill demonstrated on previous questions and a particular test plan category. In order to assist you during this period of transition, the items in this review book have been written both as groups of questions relating to a situation and as single items.

There may be times when you believe the options do not offer the best possible response in a particular situation. Nevertheless, you are asked to select the best answer among the choices given. Also, remember that incorrect choices may be partially correct, but there is only *one* correct answer.

How Do I Indicate my Choice for a Correct Answer?

Until the NCLEX–PN is taken by computer, you will be asked to blacken a circle with a pencil in your test booklet directly in front of the option you have chosen for the correct or best answer. NCLEX–PN does *not* use answer sheets. This procedure helps eliminate errors because you may have lost your place on an answer sheet. Nevertheless, you should take care that you correctly blacken the proper circle.

This review book offers you practice in indicating your choice for the answer in the same manner as you would when taking the paper and pencil version of the national licensing exam, that is, by blackening a circle with a pencil in this book directly in front of the option you have chosen as the correct answer. This review book also offers you the option of using an answer sheet.

When the NCLEX–PN is administered using computerized adaptive testing (CAT), use of only two computer keys, the space bar and the enter key, are needed. To prevent keyboarding errors, all the other computer keys will be nonfunctional. At each computer there will be a description of the two keys and a written explanation on how to use them. Prior to taking the computerized version, each individual will receive a training session that will involve both verbal instruction and a practice exercise. Before the test can begin, the candidate must successfully pass a keyboard familiarity exercise. During trial tests, it did not appear that prior computer experience, or the lack of it, affected the performance of those who participated in the field testing.

When taking the paper and pencil NCLEX–PN it was possible to leave a question and go back and answer it later. That will not be the case with the CAT–PN. It will be impossible to skip questions, review previous questions and answers, or change an answer. In order for the test to progress, the candidate must enter an answer at the time each question is asked. The computer uses the pattern of the candidate's previous answer to select the next test item. To make sure that the answer selected is the one the candidate intended to make, it will be necessary to strike the enter key twice.

What Should I Do If I Don't Know the Answer?

Because you *must* answer every question on the CAT–PN in order to proceed, it will be impossible to leave an answer blank—the advice is the same as it was for the paper and pencil version: guess. However, you want to make an educated guess rather than selecting your answer at random. After studying the item, if you are still unsure, read the four options *carefully.* Rule out any option(s) you believe to be wrong. Then concentrate on the remaining options and try to select the correct answer. For example, if you believe two of the options are definitely wrong, you have a 50–50 chance of guessing which one of the remaining two options is correct. Even if you can find only one of the four options in the item that you believe is wrong, you still have a 1 in 3 chance of guessing the correct answer from the remaining three options. This is a better chance than haphazardly choosing one of the four options as your answer. Also, as you study an item's options to rule out the obviously incorrect answer(s), if you study the item carefully, you may well determine the correct answer by careful reasoning without having to guess. Be cautious, but chances are that your first instinct is generally correct.

How Long Is the National Examination and When Is It Offered?

The paper and pencil NCLEX–PN consists of two parts, each one containing 120 items. You are allowed two hours to complete each part. Testing involves responding to

240 real questions over a total time of 4 hours. Usual procedure is to take one part in the morning and one part in the afternoon on the day of the examination.

The number of items on the CAT version of the NCLEX–PN will vary depending on the person's ability and success in answering the items. The minimum number of questions that must be answered correctly in order to be successful is 75 items. The maximum number of real items (not including trial items) is 180. There will be between 15 and 25 tryout items on each examination. The test is terminated when the candidate answers enough questions to determine competence, 205 questions are asked, or the time limit of 5 hours expires. Because the test results for either passing or failing can be determined after at least 75 items are answered, finishing the test faster than others is no indication that the candidate passed the examination.

For most, the CAT examination will take less time than the paper and pencil version of the NCLEX–PN. If, however, after 2 hours of testing, there is insufficient data to determine if the individual has passed or failed, a 10-minute break will be provided. Ten minute breaks will be taken again after each additional 1½ hours of testing.

NCLEX–PN is offered presently twice a year, in April and October. All states offered NCLEX–PN on the same date in each of these two months. The last paper and pencil examination is scheduled for October 13, 1993 with tentative full implementation of the CAT–PN beginning in April 1994. This date may be amended if problems develop during beta testing (July 1993). Beta testing is a dry run of all the processes involved in administering the computerized test. This includes test security, the functioning of computer hardware and software, and so on.

Once there is a transition from the paper and pencil exam to CAT, each state can offer more frequent test administration. This will provide an opportunity to reduce the current shortage of qualified nurses by providing an ongoing supply of newly licensed practical nurses to the job market. Currently, the plan is that CAT–PN testing will be available 6 days a week, 15 hours a day, and on Sundays, when necessary.

What Will Computerized Testing Be Like?

Each testing facility will be able to accommodate up to 10 candidates at the same time. Its use will be solely for testing; no other activity will be taking place. No others than those with admission documents will be allowed in the testing area. Admission is further secured by requiring that each candidate provide two forms of identification, one of which contains their photographic likeness. The names on all pieces of information must match exactly.

Lockers will be available for personal belongings. At each work station there will be a computer, a lamp, and scratch paper. The work area will be modifiable for left- as well as right-handed people and will accommodate access by wheelchairs. Candidates will be observed directly by the test monitor and videotaped electronically.

How Will I Schedule Taking the National Licensing Examination?

The locations of test sites in your state and an application for the national licensing examination can be obtained from your state board of nursing. The director of your nursing program can provide you with a specific address. Deadlines for submitting the application vary by state. It is always advantageous to complete this requirement as soon as possible.

When the CAT–PN is available, and your eligibility is verified, you may make an appointment date for your test by calling an 800 phone number. Most will find that they can obtain a testing date within 30 days of their phone call. The candidate will be given the location and the phone number of the closest testing center, regardless of state.

Who Decides the Pass/Fail Score?

Each state has the responsibility of determining a passing score in its own jurisdiction. The National Council conducts a standard setting workshop every 3 years. At that time, the minimum standard (passing score) required to demonstrate minimal competence to practice nursing at the entry level is reviewed. Most states use the same pass/fail score, which is arrived at from a statistical analysis of all scores, as prepared by the National Council of State Boards of Nursing.

What Happens if I Fail?

Each candidate is notified as to whether they failed or passed the examination by the board of nursing in which they have applied for a nursing license. The results of paper and pencil testing often takes weeks to months to grade and tabulate. Results of the computerized examination will be much more efficient. Scores will be forwarded to the member boards within 48 hours after the candidate takes the examination. However, the board will decide when the candidates are informed.

Those candidates who fail are provided with a diagnostic profile so that they may know their particular areas of weaknesses as measured by the licensing examination. The primary purpose of the diagnostic profile is to help candidates who fail so that they can better prepare for taking the licensing examination again.

At the moment, the National Council is recommending that a candidate who fails retake the examination in no sooner than 3 months. They suggest that the number of retakes be limited to no more than four per year.

Can Foreign-educated Nurses Take the National Licensing Examination?

Yes, foreign-educated nurses can take NCLEX–PN and CAT–PN. However, before they can take the examination, they must first meet requirements set up in the state where they take the licensing examination. An example of such a requirement is that in most states, foreign-educated nurses are asked to present credentials describing the course of study in the country where they studied. When foreign-educated nurses meet eligibility requirements, this review book serves as an excellent resource, just as it does for graduates of nursing programs in the United States and its territories.

How Can I Best Use this Book?

Plan your review for the licensing examination well in advance. Use whatever techniques suit you best. This may include reviewing your texts and classroom notes. Then take the review tests in this book. Whichever way you choose to review, give yourself sufficient time.

Blacken the circle in front of the option you choose for your correct answer or use the perforated answer sheet provided at the back of the book. Avoid looking at the correct answers at the end of the test before completing each test. You will defeat your reason for reviewing if you begin by looking at the answers.

Do not look for clues to correct answers among the items in this book. Spend time understanding the information being tested. The correct answers are randomized, that is, they do not follow a pattern in which you can predict the sequence of correct answers.

Read *carefully,* think logically, and use only the information you are given. You can easily select a wrong answer when you have missed such words as "best," "least," "most," "contraindicated," and the like, when you have not thought out what knowledge the item is testing, or when you make assumptions.

Concentrate on understanding the knowledge on which each item is based and on understanding why wrong options are incorrect. Trying to memorize information is futile in helping you review.

For further review, ask yourself questions concerning each item, such as those that follow. Do you understand the knowledge on which the item is based? Do you understand why each wrong option is incorrect? Could you have answered the item correctly if the answer had been the stem and the stem had been stated as an option? Is there additional information about the client that was not sampled in these tests but which is important, in your opinion, and in need of further review?

Apply basic principles to new or unfamiliar health care situations when you have had little or no experience with the situation you are given. Unfamiliar situations will help call your attention to areas in which further study may be indicated.

Be prepared to find that some clients described in this book may have health problems not directly related to their present reason for seeking health care. For example, a client who requires the surgical removal of a diseased organ also may have diabetes mellitus. This book, like the national examination, is based on a philosophy that clients—not diseases—require care. It is hoped that the manner in which situations are presented will help you focus on a client in need of care that will help maintain health, cope with health problems, recover from the effects of illnesses or trauma, or meet death with comfort and dignity.

Pace yourself occasionally. If you are preparing for the paper and pencil version of the licensing examination, try to take no longer than 1 minute per test item. Drilling at this rate will provide practice at the same speed required on the NCLEX–PN. Progressing at this pace will allow you to take each of the 120 items in the allotted time of 2 hours. If you fall behind, practice working faster. If you are ahead, be sure you are proceeding carefully and consider slowing your pace somewhat.

Refer to the section on Correct Answers and Rationale *after* you have completed a test. The rationale for the correct answer is provided. In most cases there is also an explanation on why the distractors are incorrect.

Make a check mark next to the items that you answered incorrectly and return to them for more study. Consider if an incorrect answer was selected because you did not know the information. In that case, plan for a review of the subject matter. Use the cited sources for the correct answer as a resource for your review. If you answered incorrectly because you did not read the item carefully or because you carelessly blackened the wrong circle when choosing the answer, plan to practice reading and answering the items with greater care.

Study the rationale given for each item. They often contain information in addition to the specific knowledge being tested, and hence, will help you complete a more thorough review. Also, use the texts referred to at the end of each rationale for further study, as indicated.

Seriously practice taking the tests in this book, as though you were actually taking the licensing examination. This type of practice will familiarize you with taking a test like the national licensing examination—a skill that may be just as valuable as reviewing the subject content.

After you have completed the *14* review tests, plan to take Part I and Part II of the Comprehensive Examination, beginning on page 395. To help you prepare for the CAT-PN, take the NCLEX Practice Test on the computer disk provided in the sleeve at the back of the book. The NCLEX Practice Test consists of 100 integrated, single-item questions. The comprehensive examinations and the computerized practice test will serve as a final review to determine how well you do when confronted with an examination most nearly resembling the national licensing examination for practical nurses.

After Taking the Tests in this Book, How Can I Learn in Which Areas I Need Additional Review?

Suggestions given in the previous section on how to use this review book to your greatest advantage often will help you identify areas where you believe you need further review.

Also, following each of the review tests in this book, there is a classification of test items that shows the correct answer, the step of the nursing process, and the client need area for each item. Directions are given on how to calculate your score. After scoring your practice examinations, you can easily determine in which areas you most probably need further review before taking the national licensing examination.

When the computerized NCLEX Practice Test is completed, the computer will identify the number of items you answered correctly and their classification according to the step in the nursing process, client need, and clinical area. The incorrect items also are identified so that you can retake the practice test and analyze the options again.

How Can I Best Prepare for Taking the National Examination?

The following suggestions, some of which resemble those offered earlier on how to use this book, will help you prepare for taking the national licensing examination.

Follow instructions concerning the licensing examination in your state for completing application forms, submitting fees, and the like. Allow sufficient time for such requirements.

If you suspect a problem with your vision, schedule an eye examination. Make sure there will be enough time for obtaining prescription lenses, if they are required. Wear your corrective glasses or contact lenses while reviewing and when taking the examination.

Establish a schedule for long-term reviewing. A systematic plan for studying is *more* effective than last minute cramming. Cramming contributes to disorganized thinking. Facts and concepts are likely to be confused. With cramming, there is always an underlying fear of not being able to recall information. This will only compound your anxiety at the time of test-taking.

Study in an environment that provides adequate light, room temperature, and ventilation. Avoid studying on a bed. Subconsciously, the bed is associated with sleeping. It may be more difficult to stay awake and alert in this setting.

Select a time of day when you are most energetic and focused. Consider an interval when there will be few interruptions. Using a telephone answering machine to intercept calls can assist you in adhering to your plan.

Set aside realistic blocks of study time. Short, but frequent, review periods are usually more productive. Try to remain on task for a minimum of 30 minutes and no longer than 1½ hours at a time. Use a timer to provide a periodic break after each ½ hour of study or whenever your concentration diminishes.

Outline the content that you will cover during each review session. Try to focus on subjects or concepts that have been most difficult or confusing for you. To avoid wasting precious time, prepare appropriate references for the review material, such as textbooks, lecture notes, and so on, ahead of time.

Combine your personal examination preparation with a study group format. Peers tend to motivate one another. In addition, each member usually brings individual strengths to the group that tend to offset the weaknesses of others. If group study is not feasible, there are excellent review courses that are offered nationally. The most reliable are those that will guarantee a refund or free repetition of the review course if the examinee is not successful in passing the licensing examination.

Use the review tests, comprehensive examinations, and computer disk in this book either concurrently or at the completion of a comprehensive review of subject material.

As the day of the NCLEX–PN nears:

Know the location and room in which the examination is offered. Become familiar with transportation, parking, and eating facilities. Many persons recommend that you do a "dry run" so that you are thoroughly acquainted with how you will travel and how much time it takes.

If you are planning to spend the night, make hotel or motel reservations early. Although sharing a room with a friend reduces the expense, it can also interfere with restful sleep.

Plan some leisure-time activity the evening before the examination. This is healthful and also helps relieve tension and worry.

Get an adequate amount of sleep. Try to maintain a schedule that is similar to your usual bedtime hours. A tired person has more difficulty concentrating and tends to become more tense and confused than a rested person.

On the day of the NCLEX–PN:

Plan to awaken early. Rushing adds yet another source of stress. Give yourself enough time to eat a sensible light breakfast.

Dress up, but wear comfortable clothing. Feeling attractive and stylish improves self-esteem and self-confidence. This attitude can be transferred to the test-taking situation and enhance your performance. Dress in layers so that apparel can be worn or removed during the examination depending on the environment within the building.

Do not take any mind- or mood-altering drugs. Besides being an ineffective means of coping with stress, these medications can result in feeling tired, irritable, and distracted when they begin to wear off.

Bring all the identification papers that are required for admitting you to the testing room. Do not take books or notes to the licensing examination. You will not be allowed to take them into the testing area. Scrap paper and pencils are provided. You may wish to bring a snack which can be secured with your personal belongings if eating facilities are inconvenient or unsatisfactory.

Try getting some form of exercise, such as a brisk walk, immediately before the examination. This often helps one to relax.

Locate a water fountain and a restroom near the testing room. Empty your bladder shortly before the test begins. Listen for information on the procedure to follow if you must use the facilities while the test is in process.

Use relaxation exercises or meditation techniques when you feel anxious. The method you choose is an individual matter, but lowering your anxiety will help you to concentrate better during the examination.

Approach the examination with a feeling of confidence and a positive mental attitude. Worrying about the examination or having negative thoughts can stand in the way of sound thinking.

Listen carefully and follow all instructions given to you at the time of the examination. Be sure to give all identifying information accurately—your name, address, and school of nursing, for example.

Read each item carefully. Be aware of such words as "most," "best," and "contraindicated." Overlooking key words can result in giving a wrong answer, even when you know the information being tested.

Eliminate the obviously incorrect responses and then focus your attention on the other options. This avoids unnecessary and time-consuming reading as you concentrate on the best possible choice for the correct answer.

Use an educated guess if you are unsure of the correct answer. Do not read inferences into an item. Use only the information you are given without making assumptions or asking yourself, "What if . . ." Do not look for tricky interpretations and then proceed to miss the obvious.

Assume the nurses described in the client situations are practical nurses. You will be informed if a caretaker being described in an item is not a practical nurse.

Remember that correct answers are randomized throughout NCLEX–PN and do not follow a pattern.

What Editorial Policies Are Observed in this Book and in the Licensing Examination?

Certain policies are observed for consistency, clarity, and ease of reading, as follows:

The word *client* is used to refer to persons receiving services from healthcare personnel, although it is recognized that the term patient may be used in some health agencies.

Since men are joining their female colleagues in nursing programs, an effort has been made to avoid using feminine pronouns when referring to the nurse. Male pronouns are used when referring to a physician. This was done with no slight intended to the increasing ranks of female physicians.

The title *Mr.* is used when referring to men. The title *Ms.* is used when referring to women. Given names may be used for children, teenagers, and adults.

Generic names of drugs are used. Common brand, or trade, names are given in parentheses following the generic names when they first appear in a situation.

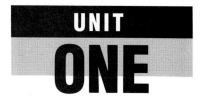

REVIEW TEST 1

The Nursing Care of Clients with
Mental Health Needs

REVIEW TEST 1

The Nursing Care of Clients with Mental Health Needs

Mental Health Needs During Infancy and Childhood
Mental Health Needs During Adolescence and Young Adulthood
Mental Health Needs During Middle Age
Mental Health Needs During Late Adulthood

Correct Answers and Rationale
Classification of Test Items

Directions: With a pencil, blacken the circle in front of the option you have chosen for your correct answer.

The Nursing Care of Clients with Mental Health Needs

MENTAL HEALTH NEEDS DURING INFANCY AND CHILDHOOD

A nurse working in a pediatrician's office is helping Ms. MacDonald prepare 4-year-old Timmy for his preschool physical examination. Ms. MacDonald also has brought her newborn son, Jason, for his first immunization.

1 Which one of the following statements indicates that Timmy is experiencing anxiety in relation to his new sibling?
   - ○ 1. Timmy wants to use his father's tools.
   - ○ 2. Timmy is taking shorter naps in the afternoon.
   - ○ 3. Timmy cries when his toys become broken.
   - ○ 4. Timmy has been wetting and soiling himself.

2 The nurse would be *most* correct in explaining that the behavior Timmy is demonstrating is based on a need to feel
   - ○ 1. powerful.
   - ○ 2. secure.
   - ○ 3. confident.
   - ○ 4. dependent.

3 The *best* advice the nurse can give Ms. MacDonald for relieving Timmy's current anxiety is to
   - ○ 1. give Timmy some old tools to play with.
   - ○ 2. let Timmy stay up later at night.
   - ○ 3. replace his broken toys right away.
   - ○ 4. spend more time alone with Timmy.

4 Ms. MacDonald asks the nurse what would be most helpful in preparing Timmy for kindergarten. Which one of the following would be the *most* beneficial?
   - ○ 1. Give him simple responsibilities to perform.
   - ○ 2. Teach him to print his first and last name.
   - ○ 3. Buy a set of children's encyclopedia books.
   - ○ 4. Have him watch daytime television programs.

5 Ms. MacDonald says that when Timmy asks her to buy candy at the grocery store and she refuses, he throws a temper tantrum. She resorts to buying the candy so Timmy will stop kicking and screaming. A useful suggestion for eliminating the tantrums when he doesn't get his way is to
   - ○ 1. give Timmy candy before entering the store.
   - ○ 2. ignore the unacceptable behavior.
   - ○ 3. explain to Timmy that his behavior is childish.
   - ○ 4. remind Timmy that he's a big boy now.

Marcia Nelson, a teenage mother, has brought Ashley, who is 6 months old, for a checkup. Marcia tells the nurse that her baby cries a lot, and she is concerned that the baby may be ill.

6 The *most important* information for the nurse to obtain at this time is
   - ○ 1. the infant's weight and length.
   - ○ 2. the infant's lung and heart sounds.
   - ○ 3. the infant's head and chest circumference.
   - ○ 4. the infant's sucking and grasp reflex.

7 No signs of illness are identified at this time. What information would be *most helpful* for the nurse to obtain next?
   ○ 1. Marcia's expectations of an infant's behavior
   ○ 2. How many more children Marcia would like to have
   ○ 3. Whether Marcia plans to finish high school
   ○ 4. The kind of toys Marcia has for the baby

8 Marcia says she doesn't want to spoil the baby, so she frequently puts her in the crib when she cries. The *best* advice the nurse can give Marcia is that
   ○ 1. holding will not result in spoiling.
   ○ 2. grandparents usually spoil babies.
   ○ 3. babies need to be spoiled.
   ○ 4. toddlers are more likely to be spoiled.

9 Which one of the following actions would be *most important* for the nurse to recommend to Marcia?
   ○ 1. Give the baby a pacifier whenever she cries.
   ○ 2. Turn on a radio in the room with the baby.
   ○ 3. Cuddle and talk to the baby frequently.
   ○ 4. Place a brightly colored mobile above the crib.

10 Marcia expresses that she feels inadequate in handling the responsibilities of caring for her baby. To meet Marcia's need for learning basic, childrearing skills, the nurse would be *most helpful* in recommending
   ○ 1. Project Head Start.
   ○ 2. Planned Parenthood.
   ○ 3. Parent-Teacher Association.
   ○ 4. parenting classes.

Ron and Michelle Hess are the parents of newborn Troy, who has been diagnosed as having Down syndrome.

11 When the nurse brings the baby to Michelle's room, Ron says, "These doctors don't know anything. We're going to take him to see specialists." The *best* response from the nurse would be,
   ○ 1. "The physicians here are experts in their field."
   ○ 2. "This diagnosis is very hard to accept."
   ○ 3. "Why do you feel you need a second opinion?"
   ○ 4. "It's not as bad as it may seem right now."

12 The nurse gathers all of the following information. Which is the *best* evidence that Michelle Hess is bonding with her infant?
   ○ 1. She smiles and talks to the infant.
   ○ 2. She asks questions about baby care.
   ○ 3. She wants to see visitors who come.
   ○ 4. She gets an adequate amount of rest.

13 The nurse observes that Michelle is nervous when Troy cries while she is bathing him. The *most helpful* nursing response would be to
   ○ 1. take over for Michelle momentarily.
   ○ 2. advise Michelle to discontinue the bath.

   ○ 3. give all future baths in the nursery.
   ○ 4. point out the good job she is doing.

It has been called to the attention of the school nurse that Jeremy Adams, age 9, frequently has been absent from school. Even when he attends school, he talks out of turn, fights with classmates, moves about in the classroom during a lesson, and does not complete his in-class assignments or homework. His current grades are not consistent with his past performance. The nurse plans to speak with Jeremy to determine if he has a health problem that has been causing these recent changes in school attendance and academic performance.

14 The school nurse watches for an opportunity to talk with Jeremy. Which one of the following would be *most appropriate* for this interaction?
   ○ 1. Sitting down at Jeremy's lunch table with him
   ○ 2. Arranging to see him in the nursing office before school
   ○ 3. Calling him aside in the hallway on the way to his classroom
   ○ 4. Meeting with him on the playground during recess

15 Jeremy tells the nurse all of the following. Which one is *most likely* to be affecting his recent behavior?
   ○ 1. His parents are involved in divorce proceedings.
   ○ 2. His pet dog just had a litter of puppies.
   ○ 3. He just acquired a neighborhood paper route.
   ○ 4. He plans to visit his out-of-state grandparents.

16 The nurse meets with Jeremy's teacher. Which one of the following approaches should the nurse recommend for helping Jeremy maintain acceptable behavior during class?
   ○ 1. Send him to the principal's office when he misbehaves.
   ○ 2. Suspend him until a family conference occurs.
   ○ 3. Have the school counselor see him on a daily basis.
   ○ 4. Enforce reasonable limits for behavior consistently.

The school nurse meets with Eric Sampson, age 7, and his parents. The purpose of the appointment is to follow up on Eric's progress since his hyperactivity was diagnosed as being attention deficit disorder.

17 The Sampsons relate that the drug methylphenidate hydrochloride (Ritalin) has been prescribed for Eric. They ask the nurse to tell them what kind of drug Eric is taking. The *best* response is that methylphenidate hydrochloride is a(n)
   ○ 1. central nervous system depressant.
   ○ 2. central nervous system stimulant.

     ○ 3. antidepressant.
     ○ 4. tranquilizer.

18 The nurse explains further that the *best* evidence that methylphenidate hydrochloride is achieving its desired action is that
     ○ 1. Eric is more alert and active.
     ○ 2. Eric is less easily distracted.
     ○ 3. Eric does not feel fatigued now.
     ○ 4. Eric's moods are more stable.

19 The Sampsons ask the nurse to identify the side effects associated with the drug methylphenidate hydrochloride. The nurse would be *most* accurate in listing the following cluster of signs and symptoms:
     ○ 1. Nausea, vomiting, and diarrhea
     ○ 2. Fatigue, drowsiness, and dry mouth
     ○ 3. Insomnia, tachycardia, and anorexia
     ○ 4. Hypotension, bradycardia, and constipation

20 The nurse tells the Sampsons that to avoid potentiating the effects of methlyphenidate hydrochloride, it would be best if Eric refrained from consuming
     ○ 1. dairy products.
     ○ 2. cola beverages.
     ○ 3. processed meats.
     ○ 4. saturated fats.

Mr. and Ms. Gaynor have been bringing their 3-year-old child Brent, who has infantile autism, to a mental health clinic on a regular basis. Today a care conference has been planned with the mental health team and the family.

21 While observing the Gaynors, the nurse should expect that the *most typical* characteristic of Brent's response to his parents will be one of
     ○ 1. indifference.
     ○ 2. friendliness.
     ○ 3. submissiveness.
     ○ 4. impatience.

22 Based on the nurse's knowledge of the common characteristics of autistic clients, which one of the following nursing diagnoses will *most likely* be a priority problem discussed at this conference?
     ○ 1. Altered Health Maintenance
     ○ 2. Chronic Low Self-Esteem
     ○ 3. High Risk for Activity Intolerance
     ○ 4. High Risk for Violence: Self-Directed

23 During the care conference Ms. Gaynor says that Brent helps dress himself, but he will not eat unless he is fed. The *best* suggestion that the nurse can offer is to
     ○ 1. continue to feed the child until he tries to pick up food.
     ○ 2. try giving the child finger foods while he is dressing.
     ○ 3. leave the food until he becomes hungry enough to eat it.

     ○ 4. demonstrate how to use a spoon every time it is time to eat.

24 The nurse should teach Brent's parents that the *best* home environment would be one that is
     ○ 1. stimulating, with a variety of sensory experiences.
     ○ 2. consistent, with a minimum amount of physical change.
     ○ 3. creative, with freedom to develop artistic talents.
     ○ 4. strict, with narrow limits for acceptable behavior.

25 Before the conference begins, the social worker, who has not had experience with autistic children, asks the nurse to identify *typical* characteristics of the disorder. One of these behaviors would be
     ○ 1. repetitive body movements.
     ○ 2. intense attachment to one parent.
     ○ 3. early sexual development.
     ○ 4. profound mental retardation.

26 The Gaynors express a desire to leave Brent with a responsible person for a few hours occasionally so they can have a respite from the constant care and supervision that is required. Which one of the following would be the *most appropriate* community resource for the nurse to recommend?
     ○ 1. Aid to Dependent Children
     ○ 2. Association on Mental Deficiency
     ○ 3. A children's day care facility
     ○ 4. A home health care agency

MENTAL HEALTH NEEDS DURING ADOLESCENCE AND YOUNG ADULTHOOD

Seventeen-year-old Kelly Shafer has been secretly dating a classmate because the relationship is a constant source of arguing in the Shafer household. Kelly has stopped attending church with her parents. She started smoking cigarettes, something her parents dislike, and has had sexual intercourse. Kelly has not had a menstrual period for 2 months.

27 Kelly makes an appointment at a birth control clinic. Which one of the following nursing qualities is *most important* for the nurse to communicate during this first meeting?
     ○ 1. Efficiency
     ○ 2. Intelligence
     ○ 3. Dexterity
     ○ 4. Acceptance

28 What is the *best* way to convey that the nurse is interested in Kelly?
     ○ 1. Make frequent eye contact with Kelly.
     ○ 2. Provide Kelly with free clinic literature.
     ○ 3. Write down information Kelly provides.
     ○ 4. Avoid long pauses between questions.

29 As Kelly talks with the nurse, she reveals how her parents disapprove of her friends, ideas, and actions. It would be *most helpful* for the nurse to share that adolescents generally test previously accepted values to establish their own
   ○ 1. ingenuity.
   ○ 2. identity.
   ○ 3. intuition.
   ○ 4. insight.

30 The nurse is called out of the room by the receptionist. She tells the nurse that Kelly's mother is on the phone and wants to know why Kelly has made an appointment there. The *best* advice for the receptionist is to inform Kelly's mother that
   ○ 1. the clinic cannot provide that information.
   ○ 2. Kelly will return her phone call shortly.
   ○ 3. she can call and talk to her in a few minutes.
   ○ 4. patients come to the clinic for birth control.

31 A pregnancy test is performed before a method of birth control will be provided. The test result is positive. Which one of the following will be *most essential* to Kelly at this time?
   ○ 1. A positive mothering instinct
   ○ 2. Making plans for marriage
   ○ 3. Financial support from her boyfriend
   ○ 4. Emotional support from her family

32 The question arises among the clinic nurses as to why Kelly came to the birth control clinic when she had missed two periods already. The nurse who was with Kelly is probably *most accurate* when stating that Kelly's behavior was probably a result of
   ○ 1. displacement.
   ○ 2. regression.
   ○ 3. denial.
   ○ 4. compensation.

Diana Billings, age 15, is brought to the emergency room after fainting in school. She is more than 25% below the normal weight for her height.

33 Which of the following should the nurse look for to support that Diana has an eating disorder?
   ○ 1. Growth of fine body hair
   ○ 2. Bruises over her upper torso
   ○ 3. Hyperactive bowel sounds
   ○ 4. Club-shaped finger tips

34 The nurse obtains a nursing history on admission of the client. Which of the following data *best* correlates with the profile of a person with anorexia nervosa?
   ○ 1. The client is the middle child of three siblings.
   ○ 2. The client is a high achiever in school and activities.
   ○ 3. The client thinks her classmates do not like her.

   ○ 4. The client experienced many illnesses during childhood.

35 The nursing team meets for a conference to plan Diana's care. Which of the following goals has the highest priority at this time?
   ○ 1. Improving her distorted body image
   ○ 2. Helping her use healthier coping techniques
   ○ 3. Restoring normal nutrition
   ○ 4. Developing assertiveness

36 Diana's mother visits at supper time. She is overheard to say, "Look at you, Diana, you're so thin. Please eat something." Which of the following would be *most* therapeutic for the nurse to say privately to Diana's mother?
   ○ 1. "All children know how to frustrate parents."
   ○ 2. "You need to stop pleading with her to eat."
   ○ 3. "You're concerned that she's starving herself."
   ○ 4. "I know how you're feeling; I'm a mother too."

37 The nursing assistant is frustrated and angry when she sees Diana rearranging the food on her tray but not eating any of it. The *best* advice the nurse can give the nursing assistant is to
   ○ 1. blend the food, and administer it by tube feeding.
   ○ 2. remind Diana that her intake is being recorded.
   ○ 3. review the treatment goals with Diana again.
   ○ 4. remove the food without making any comments.

38 Just before it is time for Diana to be weighed, the nursing assistant tells the nurse that she observed Diana drink a full pitcher of water. What is the *best* nursing action at this time?
   ○ 1. Postpone weighing Diana until later
   ○ 2. Confront Diana about what was observed
   ○ 3. Say nothing and weigh Diana as usual
   ○ 4. Subtract 2 lb from her weight

Janet Moser, age 20, is a client at an eating disorder clinic. Group therapy meetings are held every other day. A therapist is the group leader. A clinic nurse attends the meetings for purposes of continuity of care.

39 Janet Moser is being treated for bulimia. Which physical finding would the nurse find in *most* people with bulimia?
   ○ 1. Extremely low body weight
   ○ 2. Erosion of dental enamel
   ○ 3. Cessation of menstruation
   ○ 4. Patchy loss of hair

40 The nurse has been working with Janet at selecting measures to control her condition. All of the following are possibilities that have been suggested. Which one is likely to be *most effective*?

○ 1. Staying out of the bathroom after meals
○ 2. Taking a daily inventory of the unit's food
○ 3. Avoiding meals in fast food establishments
○ 4. Recording all the calories she consumes

41 Janet becomes verbally aggressive toward a very emaciated client at a group meeting. She says, "You're a real weirdo if you think you've got a weight problem." Which action would be *most appropriate*?
○ 1. Criticize the nature of her rude behavior.
○ 2. Support the person targeted by the remark.
○ 3. Let the clients respond to the situation.
○ 4. Embarrass her with a similar comment.

Justin Zales, age 16, has been selected to play on the junior varsity football team. He is extremely competitive. He hopes to be recruited eventually by a Big 10 college and attend school on a football scholarship. He spends several hours a day in a weight training facility.

42 Justin is approached one day by the owner of the gym and asked if he would like a drug to help him "bulk up." Which of the following factors will *most likely* influence Justin to accept?
○ 1. Several of his teammates are taking this drug.
○ 2. The team is currently having a winning season.
○ 3. His parents support his interest in football.
○ 4. He can afford to pay for a substantial supply.

43 Justin begins taking the anabolic steroid, oxymetholone (Anadrol). His weight increases dramatically, his muscles become more massive and well defined. Which other physical effect is associated with this group of drugs?
○ 1. Decreased lung capacity
○ 2. Bronzed skin
○ 3. Occurrence of or worsened acne
○ 4. Brittle nails

44 Ms. Zales mentions Justin's physical changes to her neighbor, who is a nurse. The nurse suspects that Justin is taking anabolic steroids. Based on this assumption, it would be correct for the nurse to recommend that Ms. Zales also observe her son for
○ 1. aggression and rage.
○ 2. confusion and doubt.
○ 3. friendliness and humor.
○ 4. elation and excitement.

Justin's coach discovers him taking the steroid drug. Justin is suspended from playing football for the rest of the season.

45 Ms. Zales tells her friend, the nurse, that Justin is now withdrawn, doesn't eat or sleep much, and has stopped going to school activities. He has said, "I might as well be dead. My football career is over." What advice is *most appropriate* to give Ms. Zales at this time?

○ 1. Disregard Justin's behavior; he's acting normal.
○ 2. Tell Justin to snap out of it; his life is not over.
○ 3. Inquire about transferring Justin to another school.
○ 4. Ask Justin if he is having any thoughts of suicide.

Alyse Foreman, age 18, lives at home with her parents. Six months ago she stopped attending classes. She was fired from her part-time job because she was not performing at the level expected. She says she hears voices telling her that she is a bad person. Her parents have brought her to the psychiatrist's office for evaluation.

46 The nurse who works in the psychiatrist's office explains to the Foremans that psychotic people are those who
○ 1. adjust poorly to new situations.
○ 2. have difficulty in relationships.
○ 3. cannot differentiate reality from fantasy.
○ 4. feel helpless in resolving problems.

47 The nurse proceeds to perform a brief assessment of the client's mental status. Which question is *most appropriate* for assessing the client's orientation?
○ 1. What is today's date?
○ 2. How did you get here?
○ 3. Where were you born?
○ 4. Who is the president?

48 Alyse becomes upset and demands to read the form on which the nurse has been writing. The *best* action would be to
○ 1. ask why she is so suspicious.
○ 2. put the clipboard away.
○ 3. hand her the form to read.
○ 4. tell her it is illegal.

49 Alyse tells the nurse that she refuses to be admitted to the psychiatric unit of the local hospital. The nurse tells her that she cannot be committed involuntarily unless she
○ 1. needs further assessment.
○ 2. may harm herself or others.
○ 3. will not keep office appointments.
○ 4. refuses to take medications.

50 The physician prescribes the antipsychotic drug haloperidol (Haldol) for Alyse. Which one of the following would be appropriate health teaching instructions for a client receiving this drug?
○ 1. Take the pills on an empty stomach.
○ 2. Don't skip meals while taking the drug.
○ 3. Stop taking the drug if sedation occurs.
○ 4. Rise slowly from a sitting position.

51 Which one of the following is the *best* indication that haloperidol is achieving a therapeutic effect?
○ 1. Alyse is no longer hearing voices.
○ 2. Alyse is sleeping more than before.

○ 3. Alyse thinks of herself as a good person.
○ 4. Alyse feels more energetic and rested.

52 Several weeks later Alyse calls the office nurse. The nurse should arrange for Alyse to be examined when she describes which one of the following adverse effects associated with her medication?
○ 1. Frequent diarrhea
○ 2. Severe sore throat
○ 3. Gradual weight loss
○ 4. Ringing of the ears

A nurse is asked about illegal drug use among teenagers.

53 When asked how to tell if someone has been smoking marijuana within the last few hours, the nurse would be *most accurate* in identifying a physical sign of recent use as
○ 1. shivering.
○ 2. inflamed eyes.
○ 3. rapid breathing.
○ 4. restlessness.

54 One of the students has been arrested several times for driving under the influence of alcohol. He tells everyone that he is not an alcoholic. The nurse informs the teacher that one of the signs of alcoholism is
○ 1. an inability to recall events that occurred while drinking.
○ 2. drinking that has occurred for 2 years or more.
○ 3. that hard liquor or wine, rather than beer, is consumed.
○ 4. that there is a preference for alcohol rather than soft drinks.

55 The nurse is asked to speak on drug abuse to a health class. One of the *most* life-threatening consequences of using highly potent forms of cocaine that would be essential for the nurse to identify is
○ 1. cardiac arrhythmia.
○ 2. depressed respiration.
○ 3. low blood pressure.
○ 4. elevated blood sugar.

MENTAL HEALTH NEEDS DURING MIDDLE AGE

Ms. Davis is being seen in the emergency department. She is very distressed about the chest discomfort she is experiencing. She is shaking and trembling. All data indicate that she is having a panic attack.

56 The nurse explains to the nursing assistant that a panic attack is a manifestation of severe anxiety. A common assessment finding that would be important for the nurse to identify is
○ 1. tachycardia.
○ 2. increased salivation.

○ 3. constricted pupils.
○ 4. hypotension.

57 During the interaction with Ms. Davis, which one of the following techniques will *best* reduce the anxiety that she is experiencing?
○ 1. Stand less than an arm's length from her.
○ 2. Wear a laboratory coat and name tag.
○ 3. Offer her a cup of coffee or tea.
○ 4. Explain all actions and procedures.

58 Ms. Davis begins crying and says, "I feel like I'm going to die." Which one of the following responses would be *most* therapeutic for the nurse to make?
○ 1. "Don't cry. It won't help matters right now."
○ 2. "You don't want the doctor to see you this way."
○ 3. "Everyone feels frightened in an emergency."
○ 4. "I'll stay with you until you feel better."

59 Ms. Davis is given a prescription for alprazolam (Xanax). While preparing discharge instructions, which of the following information should the nurse plan to tell the client about alprazolam?
○ 1. Avoid consuming alcohol while taking this drug.
○ 2. Long-term use will not cause drug dependency.
○ 3. This drug can cause insomnia in some people.
○ 4. A blood test will be required periodically.

Mr. Forsythe has been coming to the mental health clinic because he dreads leaving his home. His discomfort escalates when he is in crowds or public places. This feeling and his self-imposed isolation are interfering with his ability to lead a normal life.

60 Mr. Forsythe asks the nurse to repeat the name his therapist called his disorder. The nurse informs Mr. Forsythe that it is called
○ 1. claustrophobia.
○ 2. hydrophobia.
○ 3. photophobia.
○ 4. agoraphobia.

61 A nursing diagnosis of *Ineffective Individual Coping* has been identified on the clinic's nursing care plan. To assist in planning measures to resolve this problem, the nurse recalls that the coping mechanism used by *most* phobic individuals in an unhealthy manner is
○ 1. denial.
○ 2. compensation.
○ 3. avoidance.
○ 4. rationalization.

62 Nursing care efforts for Mr. Forsythe are *best* directed toward helping the client explore
○ 1. prior emotionally traumatic experiences.
○ 2. recent physical health changes.

○ 3. current abuse of chemical substances.
○ 4. present events causing stress.

Ms. Randall is being treated at the same clinic for a fear of spiders. Her treatment involves a form of behavior modification called desensitization.

63 When Ms. Randall finds herself in a situation in which she encounters a spider, the nurse would encourage her to
○ 1. spray it with insecticide.
○ 2. take some of her medication.
○ 3. move in the opposite direction.
○ 4. use relaxation techniques.

A nurse has been asked to be a member of a panel of mental health personnel for a community education program. The topic for this panel is post-traumatic stress disorder.

64 A person in the audience asks the nurse how to tell if someone has this condition. The nurse would be *most* correct in explaining that a common finding among people with this disorder is
○ 1. recurring nightmares.
○ 2. auditory hallucinations.
○ 3. angered easily by others.
○ 4. energy invested in worthy causes.

65 A military veteran with this disorder asks why he is startled and fearful when he attends fireworks displays on the fourth of July. The *best* explanation from the nurse is that
○ 1. he was frightened of them as a child.
○ 2. he has lost his spirit of patriotism.
○ 3. he associates the sound with gunfire.
○ 4. he is worried he may be drafted again.

66 Someone asks if anyone other than military veterans acquire this disorder. The *most accurate* statement by the nurse is that it can occur in anyone who
○ 1. has experienced multiple failures.
○ 2. has survived a catastrophic event.
○ 3. was abandoned or unloved as a child.
○ 4. has inherited a genetic tendency.

67 The question of how to help a person with post-traumatic stress disorder is asked. The *best* approach that the nurse could recommend would be to
○ 1. always act happy and enthusiastic around the victim.
○ 2. prevent him or her from becoming isolated.
○ 3. encourage the victim to talk about his or her feelings.
○ 4. plan frequent vacations or pleasurable activities.

Ms. Anne Foster has been hospitalized for diagnostic tests. She has multiple somatic complaints that have not resembled any specific disease.

68 Ms. Foster summons the nurse and says she feels weak and dizzy. The *most appropriate* nursing action would be to
○ 1. help Ms. Foster to relax.
○ 2. give Ms. Foster something to eat.
○ 3. administer oxygen by cannula.
○ 4. take Ms. Foster's vital signs.

69 Ms. Foster shares that she regrets never going to college or having children. The *best* explanation for Ms. Foster's statement is that during the middle years of life, adults generally
○ 1. assess their accomplishments.
○ 2. set unreasonable goals.
○ 3. envy others' achievements.
○ 4. doubt their own judgments.

70 One day Ms. Foster says to the nurse, "Do you think they'll ever be able to find out what's wrong with me?" It would be *best* for the nurse to reply
○ 1. "That's something to discuss with your doctor."
○ 2. "It sounds like you are feeling discouraged."
○ 3. "Let us worry about your lack of progress."
○ 4. "You need to practice a little more patience."

71 The nurse's coworker says, "Ms. Foster sounds just like any other hypochondriac to me." It would be important for the nurse to point out that the *most* damaging consequence of this type of attitude is that it
○ 1. violates the client's right to treatment.
○ 2. disregards a client's individuality.
○ 3. interferes with continuity of client care.
○ 4. disrupts good staff relationships.

72 Ms. Foster's pastor comes to see her and some of his other parishioners who have been hospitalized. He asks to see Ms. Foster's chart. The *most appropriate* nursing action would be to
○ 1. tell him to write his notes on the progress sheet.
○ 2. ask him if he is a hospital chaplain.
○ 3. inform him that he cannot read the chart.
○ 4. check with the nursing supervisor before doing so.

The nursing team holds a conference concerning Glen Sanders, who has been admitted with ulcerative colitis.

73 The nursing assistant hears ulcerative colitis referred to as a psychophysiologic disease. She asks if that means that Mr. Sanders isn't really physically sick. The *best* response from the nurse would be that a client with this type of illness
○ 1. pretends to be sick when he needs a rest.
○ 2. thinks he is sick, but tests are all negative.
○ 3. would rather be hospitalized than have to work.
○ 4. has an illness that is influenced by his emotions.

74 At the team conference the team leader helps the staff to identify the assessments that are important in the care of Mr. Sanders. Which one of the following would have the *highest* priority?
○ 1. The number and characteristics of his bowel movements
○ 2. How much Mr. Sanders knows about colostomy care
○ 3. What coping mechanisms he uses for handling stress
○ 4. The types of relationships he has with others his age

75 The discussion turns toward exploring ways to maintain Mr. Sanders' self-esteem. One of the *best* approaches the team can use would be to
○ 1. clean Mr. Sanders of stool in a nonjudgmental manner.
○ 2. ask Mr. Sanders' mother to help clean him when possible.
○ 3. hold Mr. Sanders responsible for all of his hygiene.
○ 4. assign only male nurses to care for Mr. Sanders.

Thirty-five-year-old Mr. Biddle is scheduled for a hemorrhoidectomy. He also is a chronic alcoholic, but he has not identified this problem to his physician or the nurse.

76 Which of the following postoperative observations is *common* among alcoholic people?
○ 1. Blood pressure is generally lower than normal.
○ 2. Pain is unrelieved with usual dosages of analgesics.
○ 3. Level of consciousness is likely to be lethargic.
○ 4. Pulse rates are slow, weak, and irregular.

77 Approximately 24 hours after his admission, Mr. Biddle becomes very restless and shouts that he must "kill all the bugs" in his room. In this situation it is *essential* for the nurse to
○ 1. place restraints on his arms and legs.
○ 2. reassure him that he is not seeing bugs.
○ 3. remain at the bedside with the client.
○ 4. close his door so others are not alarmed.

78 Based on the change in Mr. Biddle's condition, which of the following nursing actions should be performed next?
○ 1. Schedule a team conference.
○ 2. Call the supervisor.
○ 3. Notify the physician.
○ 4. Chart the assessed data.

79 The nurse should continue to monitor Mr. Biddle for which one of the following complications associated with alcohol withdrawal?
○ 1. Hypothermia
○ 2. Seizures
○ 3. Bleeding
○ 4. Jaundice

80 At the beginning of the shift a team member says in reference to Mr. Biddle, "Don't expect me to take care of that good-for-nothing." It is generally agreed that the first step in understanding and accepting the behavior of clients is
○ 1. understanding one's own behavior.
○ 2. analyzing what motivates clients' behavior.
○ 3. becoming familiar with abnormal behavior.
○ 4. taking courses in counseling.

Ms. Cordova, 49 years old, is admitted to a hospital's psychiatric unit with symptoms of depression.

81 If all of the following rooms are available for Ms. Cordova on admission, in which one would it be *best* for the nurse to place her?
○ 1. A room in which environmental stimuli are reduced
○ 2. A room with a cheerful and talkative roommate
○ 3. An empty room at the end of the unit's hall
○ 4. A room within view of the nursing station

82 When interviewing Ms. Cordova, which one of the following questions or statements made by the nurse is likely to generate the *most* information?
○ 1. "Tell me about your family."
○ 2. "Are you currently married?"
○ 3. "Who is your nearest relative?"
○ 4. "Give me a list of your family."

83 The nurse works to develop trust with Ms. Cordova. Trust is *best* promoted when the nurse demonstrates
○ 1. authority.
○ 2. sympathy.
○ 3. friendliness.
○ 4. consistency.

84 The nurse gathers all of the following data. Which one indicates the *highest risk* for suicide? The client
○ 1. feels hopeless about the future.
○ 2. has a plan in mind for suicide.
○ 3. states that she'd be better off dead.
○ 4. prefers to be alone in her room.

85 Amitriptyline hydrochloride (Elavil) is prescribed for Ms. Cordova. The nurse reviews the client's medical history. Which one of the following conditions would contraindicate the administration of this drug?
○ 1. Glaucoma
○ 2. Psoriasis
○ 3. Diabetes mellitus
○ 4. Pernicious anemia

86 A nursing assistant is assigned to care for Ms. Cordova. The nurse explains to a team member that the client should be observed very closely because the time during which a depressed client is *most likely* to make a suicide attempt is
- ○ 1. when first admitted to the unit.
- ○ 2. after being assessed by the treatment team.
- ○ 3. when it seems the depression is lifting.
- ○ 4. before psychotherapy has been initiated.

The nurse cares for other depressed clients on the unit.

87 Frank Simmons attempted suicide using a gun. He still is actively suicidal. Electroshock therapy is planned. Which one of the following is *most* essential for the nurse to carry out prior to this treatment?
- ○ 1. Obtaining the client's informed consent
- ○ 2. Administering an anesthetic drug
- ○ 3. Loosening all constrictive clothing
- ○ 4. Restricting the client's intake of food

88 A nursing assistant asks about the immediate effects of electroshock therapy. The nurse is *most* accurate in identifying that the client will experience
- ○ 1. brief episodes of anger and hostility.
- ○ 2. transient headaches and double vision.
- ○ 3. temporary memory loss and confusion.
- ○ 4. occasional periods of fear and anxiety.

89 A female student nurse asks how she should interact with her assigned client who is depressed. The *best* advice from the coassigned nurse is to demonstrate an attitude that is
- ○ 1. cheerful.
- ○ 2. reassuring.
- ○ 3. unemotional.
- ○ 4. caring.

90 A monoamine oxidase inhibitor (MAOI) antidepressant drug is ordered for a client who has not responded to the tricyclic antidepressants. The nurse determines that the client needs more teaching when he says he is permitted to have
- ○ 1. chicken liver.
- ○ 2. ice cream.
- ○ 3. orange juice.
- ○ 4. yellow apples.

The nurse cares for several clients who have thought disorders, such as schizophrenia.

91 A client on the unit sits in the day room and does not participate in any group activity. While helping to develop a plan of care, the *most* therapeutic nursing approach for this person would be to
- ○ 1. sit with the client, but don't urge participation.
- ○ 2. pull the client's arm, and ask that he join in.

- ○ 3. remove all the chairs so that there is nowhere to sit.
- ○ 4. plan a group activity that can be done while sitting.

92 A schizophrenic client says, "Wing ding, the world is a ring." The *best* response by the nurse would be
- ○ 1. "How clever, you've made up a poem."
- ○ 2. "I don't understand what you mean."
- ○ 3. "Earth does orbit in a circle."
- ○ 4. "Tell me more about the world."

93 A male client tells everyone that a famous country singer has asked him to make a record with him. At a team conference the nurse suggests that the *best* approach to follow is to
- ○ 1. challenge the client for proof.
- ○ 2. ask him to sign an autograph.
- ○ 3. repeat what the client says.
- ○ 4. disagree with what he says.

94 Which of the following would suggest to the nurse that a client is experiencing auditory hallucinations?
- ○ 1. The client sings a song as he or she walks down the hall.
- ○ 2. The client quickly changes the topic of conversation.
- ○ 3. The client repeats a sentence over and over again.
- ○ 4. The client cocks his or her head as if listening to someone.

95 A client asks a nurse if he or she hears the voice of God talking about destroying the world. The *best* response from the nurse would be
- ○ 1. "Nonsense! God couldn't be talking to you."
- ○ 2. "No. Hearing voices is part of the illness."
- ○ 3. "Does he say when or how it will happen?"
- ○ 4. "You'd better not tell the doctor about it."

96 A schizophrenic client has been taking chlorpromazine hydrochloride (Thorazine) for many years. What would indicate to the nurse that the client is manifesting tardive dyskinesia, a symptom associated with long-term antipsychotic drug therapy?
- ○ 1. The client makes chewing motions with his or her mouth.
- ○ 2. The client is lethargic and falls asleep easily.
- ○ 3. The client has difficulty initiating urination.
- ○ 4. The client experiences ringing in the ears.

The nurse cares for people with bipolar disorder (mixed and manic types).

97 While assessing an individual with bipolar disorder, the nurse should expect that the client will *most likely* display
- ○ 1. ritualistic behavior.
- ○ 2. symbolic aggressiveness.

○ 3.   exaggerated mood swings.
○ 4.   intermittent amnesia.

98   On admission, a male client says to a female nurse, "My goodness, you're a good looking babe. How about spending the night with me." Of the following possible responses the nurse could make, which one would be *best* in this situation?
○ 1.   "Don't say that. Someone may get the wrong idea."
○ 2.   "I am uncomfortable. Please stop speaking that way."
○ 3.   "That kind of relationship is better outside the hospital."
○ 4.   "The others are going on a walk. Let's join them."

99   Which of the following nursing activities would *most probably* be therapeutic for the client who is restless and physically very active?
○ 1.   Interest the client in a jigsaw puzzle.
○ 2.   Play a game of table tennis with him or her.
○ 3.   Join others who are watching television.
○ 4.   Recommend that the client read a magazine.

100   A client with bipolar disorder is receiving lithium carbonate (Lithane). Which one should the nurse monitor to determine the safe administration of this drug?
○ 1.   Vital signs
○ 2.   Urine volumes
○ 3.   Blood levels
○ 4.   Brain scans

101   The team leader has identified that a client with bipolar disorder has a nursing diagnosis of *Altered Nutrition: Less than Body Requirements related to restlessness.* The nurse caring for the client is asked to suggest some measures for resolving the problem. The *best* approach would be to
○ 1.   provide the client with finger foods every hour.
○ 2.   serve extra large portions on the dietary tray.
○ 3.   take him or her to the hospital coffee shop twice a day.
○ 4.   involve the client in preparing food on the unit.

102   A female client with bipolar disorder sees a table of four men playing pinochle in the day room. She says in a most provocative way, "Hey, let's play strip poker." She then begins to remove her clothing. The *most* therapeutic nursing response would be to
○ 1.   observe the response of the others.
○ 2.   terminate all further card playing.
○ 3.   reprimand her inappropriate behavior.
○ 4.   escort the client to her own room.

MENTAL HEALTH NEEDS DURING LATE ADULTHOOD

A nurse has accepted a position in a long-term care facility for the aging and infirmed. The questions that follow relate to clients for whom this nurse provides care, their family members, and coworkers.

103   To assist in planning care at the facility, the nurse reviews the health records of the clients. The data generally will reveal that a *common* problem among people in this age group is
○ 1.   dealing with losses.
○ 2.   memory development.
○ 3.   establishing relationships.
○ 4.   effective parenting.

104   Mr. Shorham, a client at the care facility, has had a stroke. He struggles to manage his own grooming and hygiene. He often comes to meals with soap on his face or an unbuttoned shirt. The *best* course of action for the nurse is to
○ 1.   send him back to his room to finish.
○ 2.   bathe, shave, and dress him daily.
○ 3.   schedule his hygiene for after meals.
○ 4.   comment on how self-reliant he is.

105   Ms. Carlisle, age 78, has been losing weight. Most of her food is still on her plate when the other clients have finished. Which one of the following courses of action is *best* for the nurse to follow at this time?
○ 1.   Have a nursing assistant observe her during mealtime.
○ 2.   Serve all the client's future meals in her room.
○ 3.   Tell her that she may end up going to the hospital.
○ 4.   Point out the dangers of excess weight loss to her.

106   Ms. Riley, age 78, says, "If I had to do it all over again, I wouldn't change a thing." The nurse interprets this to mean that Ms. Riley has acquired which one of the following characteristics associated with this stage in the life cycle?
○ 1.   Trust
○ 2.   Integrity
○ 3.   Intimacy
○ 4.   Autonomy

107   Documentation is discussed at an in-service meeting. The education director asks the group of nurses to critique the following example of an entry in a client's record: "States, 'I feel unwanted.' Appears to be confused." Which of the following statements *best* describes why this entry is unsatisfactory? The nurse failed to
○ 1.   interpret the meaning of "unwanted."
○ 2.   indicate the importance of the client's statement.
○ 3.   substantiate that the quote was made by the client.
○ 4.   describe the confused behavior.

108 The nurse assesses a new client being admitted to the facility. Which of the following questions is the *best* method for assessing long-term memory?
   ○ 1. "What is your current age?"
   ○ 2. "What is today's date?"
   ○ 3. "What is your date of birth?"
   ○ 4. "What occurred last January?"

109 A client responds inappropriately to several questions that are asked during an interview conducted by the nurse. Which of the following methods would be *most helpful* in determining if the problem is miscommunication or impaired cognition?
   ○ 1. Ask the client to repeat the question before answering it.
   ○ 2. Ask questions that require only a "yes" or "no" response.
   ○ 3. Ask the client's next of kin for answers to the questions.
   ○ 4. Ask questions to which the client is sure to know the answers.

110 Mr. Washington, a fairly new client, has a pattern of awakening during the night with a need to urinate. He wanders about the room looking for the toilet. Occasionally the nurse finds him relieving himself in the drawer of the bedside stand. The *best* addition to the care plan would be to
   ○ 1. leave a night-light on in room when the client retires.
   ○ 2. apply a jacket restraint when the client is put to bed.
   ○ 3. place a urinal between legs after preparing for sleep.
   ○ 4. attach an external catheter to the penis during nighttime.

111 Emma Moss has advancing dementia due to Alzheimer's disease. She seems confused about how to use items like a toothbrush, a comb, a fork, and a spoon. Which of the following techniques may prolong her self-care in relation to eating?
   ○ 1. Ask the physician to order a liquid diet.
   ○ 2. Position her so she can mimic other clients.
   ○ 3. Serve her first so she has more time to eat.
   ○ 4. Seat her alone so no one will notice her.

112 A client complains to the nurse that Ms. Johnson, one of the other residents, can never find her room after meals and activities. Several clients are becoming angry because she has even gone through their personal belongings. What is the *best* approach for the nursing team to use?
   ○ 1. Place a large sign with Ms. Johnson's name on the door.
   ○ 2. Keep the room doors on the unit locked at all times.
   ○ 3. Detain Ms. Johnson until all the others have left.

   ○ 4. Speak to Ms. Johnson about how the others are feeling.

113 Ms. Velmer's daughter is quite distraught. She says to the nurse, "I'm not sure mother knows who I am." The *best* response on the part of the nurse would be
   ○ 1. "This is probably the beginning of the end for her."
   ○ 2. "You're distressed that she does not respond to you."
   ○ 3. "Don't worry. We're taking very good care of her here."
   ○ 4. "Behind every cloud there's a silver lining."

114 Bertha Parks is a client who is always complaining about a variety of physical ailments. There are no changes in the nurse's physical assessment findings. Which approach may reduce Ms. Parks focus on her somatic complaints?
   ○ 1. Reassure her that she's just having another bad day.
   ○ 2. Administer a prescribed analgesic for her vague discomfort.
   ○ 3. Spend more time interacting with her on a daily basis.
   ○ 4. Notify the attending physician that she needs evaluating.

115 Mr. Brooks is experiencing more and more memory impairment. His attention span is short, and he forgets information quickly. At a team conference, the nurses explore ways to help him understand and respond appropriately. The *best* recommendation would be to
   ○ 1. speak loudly to get his attention.
   ○ 2. use short sentences when speaking.
   ○ 3. use written forms of communication.
   ○ 4. let him listen to news programs.

116 Mr. Baker, a client with terminal cancer, is alert but will not likely live through the night. He has discussed with his physician that he does not want any heroic measures used to prolong his life. What is the *most important* nursing action for the client at this time?
   ○ 1. Sit quietly and hold the dying client's hand.
   ○ 2. Move him into the hall where he can be observed.
   ○ 3. Place him in a room by himself near the nurse.
   ○ 4. Tell him to use his signal if he needs anything.

117 Following the death of a client, the nursing assistant is visibly shaken and begins to sob loudly. What approach would the assistant find *most helpful*?
   ○ 1. Being sent home for the rest of the shift
   ○ 2. Being terminated from this type of work
   ○ 3. Being allowed to express how he or she feels
   ○ 4. Being asked to perform postmortem care

118 Ms. Rogers visits her husband daily. She arrives before lunch and leaves only briefly in the late afternoon. She returns in the evening and helps prepare him for bed. The nurse observes that she is thin, pale, walks slowly, and has fallen asleep in a chair at the bedside several times. Based on the nurse's observations, what would be the *most* therapeutic nursing action?

○ 1. Suggest that Ms. Rogers make an appointment for a physical examination.

○ 2. Discuss modifying the amount of time she is devoting to caretaking.

○ 3. Remind Ms. Rogers of the scheduled times for agency visiting hours.

○ 4. Inform Ms. Rogers that there are sufficient trained staff at the facility.

119 The family of John Bowers, who has Alzheimer's disease, wants to take him home for a day. Which of the following is essential to determine at this time? The caregiver's understanding of

○ 1. what symptoms he manifests.

○ 2. when the client must return.

○ 3. when to administer medications.

○ 4. how to provide hygiene measures.

120 Ms. Reardon tells the nurse that she no longer wants to take the drug fluoxetine (Prozac), which has been ordered daily. The *most appropriate* nursing action to take at this time is to

○ 1. disguise the drug in food.

○ 2. withhold administering the drug.

○ 3. mix the drug into a beverage.

○ 4. give the drug later in the day.

Correct Answers and Rationale

Two numbers appear in parentheses following each rationale. The first number identifies the textbook listed in the references, page 451, and the second number identifies the page(s) in that textbook on which the correct answer can be verified. Occasionally, two textbooks are given to verify the correct answer.

Mental Health Needs During Infancy and Childhood

1 4. A toddler who is not accustomed to sharing attention may feel that the new child is taking his place. He may behave similarly to the infant in an attempt to regain attention or resort to behavior manifested during an earlier period of development to feel more secure. It is normal for a 4-year-old to begin identifying with and imitating the same-sexed parent at this age. Preschoolers begin to need less daytime sleep. At this age, crying is a natural emotional response to disappointing events. (9:46, 71)
   Nursing Process—Collecting data
   Client Need—Psychosocial integrity

2 2. Anxiety occurs when a person perceives himself or herself in a threatening situation. The perceived threat creates a feeling of insecurity. Mental mechanisms, like regression, are unconsciously or subconsciously used to eliminate or reduce conflict, protect one's self-image, and resolve an emotional dilemma. (1:38, 52)
   Nursing Process—Implementation
   Client Need—Health promotion/maintenance

3 4. Anxiety that results from competing for attention can be diminished if some time is spent just with him. The other choices in this item are not inappropriate, but they will not necessarily relieve the child's anxiety. (9:47)
   Nursing Process—Implementation
   Client Need—Health promotion/maintenance

4 1. A school-aged child must learn to follow directions and carry out a task. Providing the preschooler with activities that are within his level of accomplishment promotes success and a positive feeling about his own competence. Children may become confused and frustrated if a parent's instructions are different than the teacher's. A preschooler would have no immediate use for a children's encyclopedia. Daytime television programs are not necessarily educational. (9:51)
   Nursing Process—Implementation
   Client Need—Health promotion/maintenance

5 2. Children learn how to manipulate others through certain types of behavior. When a child realizes that a tantrum will not obtain the desired result, the behavior likely will be extinguished. Giving candy beforehand does not support the principle that candy is not allowed at this time. A young child is more likely to behave based on his emotions rather than intellectual logic. Therefore, the toddler is not likely to accept an explanation about the inappropriateness of his behavior or the plea that he act differently. (12:44, 83)
   Nursing Process—Implementation
   Client Need—Health promotion/maintenance

6 1. Infantile anxiety can be manifested by excessive crying. Severe anxiety can lead to weight loss and stunted growth, commonly referred to as a failure to thrive. Listening to the lung and heart sounds and measuring the head and chest are appropriate, but they will not indicate as readily how this child's growth compares to norms for infants her age. Assessing the sucking and grasp reflex is more appropriate for a newborn infant. (9:44)
   Nursing Process—Collecting data
   Client Need—Safe, effective care environment

7 1. A certain amount of crying is normal for an infant. It is the only means a baby has for communicating distress. Finding out her expectations helps the nurse determine if the mother's perception of her infant's behavior is realistic. The other selections would not provide significant additional data needed to analyze the basis for the young mother's observation. (9:42)
   Nursing Process—Collecting data
   Client Need—Health promotion/maintenance

8 1. Neglecting and isolating an infant promotes stress and affects normal development. Babies, like anyone else, cannot develop negative effects from being held and touched in an affectionate manner. Infants are extremely sensitive to the attitudes and actions of those caring for them. All humans, not just babies or toddlers, need physical and social contact with other humans for adequate nurturing. (9:41–42)
   Nursing Process—Implementation
   Client Need—Psychosocial integrity

9 3. Touching and hearing a parent's voice are essential for optimal emotional growth during infancy. When an infant receives affectionate, sensory stimulation, it helps promote a feeling of trust, the major developmental task during infancy. Inanimate sensory stimulation is appropriate, but physical human interaction is a priority. (9:42)
Nursing Process—Planning
Client Need—Health promotion/maintenance

10 4. Parenting classes are taught by one or more people who have expertise in successful childrearing techniques. Participants learn by imitating the modeled behavior of others in the group. Members of the group support one another by sharing common experiences. Project Headstart is for preschool children. Planned Parenthood is concerned with family planning. The Parent-Teacher Association is for parents of school children. (19:193)
Nursing Process—Implementation
Client Need—Health promotion/maintenance

11 2. Identifying the emotional reaction underlying the statement conveys empathy. Empathy involves experiencing what another person feels. Empathy communicates a caring attitude and facilitates further therapeutic interaction. Defending, the first example, is a nontherapeutic technique that implies to the clients that their feelings or actions are unnecessary and foolish. Asking a question using the word "why" is referred to as "demanding an explanation." It, too, is nontherapeutic because most people may not be able to verbalize their rationale. The last choice is another example of a nontherapeutic communication technique called disagreeing. Disagreeing with the client indicates that the clients have no right to feel as they do. (9:149–150, 139)
Nursing Process—Implementation
Client Need—Psychosocial integrity

12 1. Evidence of bonding includes eye contact, skin contact, smiling and talking to the infant, and cuddling. The other behaviors are normal and appropriate, but they are not the best evidence of bonding. (9:174)
Nursing Process—Evaluating
Client Need—Health promotion/maintenance

13 4. Allowing the mother to provide basic care promotes bonding. A mother's self-concept and self-confidence can be increased when the nurse offers supportive encouragement. Interfering with parenting skills will contribute to the mother's feelings of insecurity. (9:174)
Nursing Process—Implementation
Client Need—Psychosocial integrity

14 2. Privacy is an essential component of a therapeutic environment. Selecting a location where the person cannot be observed or overheard by others facilitates open communication and a therapeutic relationship. (12:259)
Nursing Process—Planning
Client Need—Safe, effective care environment

15 1. Besides the death of a parent, divorce is one of the most disruptive events a child can experience. Changes in family structure jeopardize a child's sense of security. Acting out is a behavioral manifestation of conflict. Even positive experiences, such as a dog having puppies, acquiring a paper route, and visiting grandparents, can be stressful. However, they do not have as intense an emotional impact as parental divorce. (1:133, 12:503)
Nursing Process—Collecting data
Client Need—Health promotion/maintenance

16 4. Discipline that is delivered immediately, fairly, and consistently helps a child understand the limits of acceptable and unacceptable behavior. Anxious people need reassurance that someone will enforce limitations if they are unable to remain in control. Sending the child to the principal indicates that the teacher is evading personal responsibility for controlling classroom behavior. Suspension isolates the child from any resource for help and is likely to contribute to continued low academic performance. Sending the child to the counselor on a daily basis is premature and severe for the behavior manifested at this time. (17:376)
Nursing Process—Planning
Client Need—Psychosocial integrity

17 2. Methylphenidate hydrochloride is a central nervous system stimulant that acts primarily on the cerebral cortex. Its action appears to be similar to amphetamines. (15:134)
Nursing Process—Implementation
Client Need—Health promotion/maintenance

18 2. Some of the chief characteristics of attention deficit disorder include distractibility, difficulty following directions, remaining focused on a task, and sustaining attention. Relief of these symptoms would indicate a therapeutic response. Despite the fact that methylphenidate hydrochloride is a central nervous system stimulant, it should not cause a child to be more alert, active, or less fatigued than he was prior to being treated with the drug. In fact overstimulation indicates a nontherapeutic or adverse response to the drug. Methylphenidate may cause a child to be less irritable and aggressive, but the primary

reason for administering this drug is not to alter a child's moods. (1:160)
Nursing Process—Evaluation
Client Need—Physiological Integrity

19 3. Because methylphenidate hydrochloride is a central nervous system stimulant, side effects reflect overstimulation. Some people experience an intense degree of these symptoms even with low dosages. The remaining choices are not associated with this particular drug. (15:135)
Nursing Process—Implementation
Client Need—Health promotion/maintenance

20 2. Caffeine is present in three fourths of all soft drinks. It is an ingredient in all cola products unless they are labeled caffeine free. Caffeine is a stimulating drug that could contribute to overstimulating effects in a child taking methylphenidate hydrochloride. (4:228–229)
Nursing Process—Implementation
Client Need—Health promotion/maintenance

21 1. Autistic children tend to show little or no ability to relate to other humans, including their parents. All the remaining examples require that the individual interact with and respond to one or more people. This is not a characteristic of a person with autism. (17:373)
Nursing Process—Collecting data
Client Need—Health promotion/maintenance

22 4. One of the common behaviors among autistic people is a tendency to cause self-harm by head banging, biting, and pulling out hair and fingernails. The autistic client would not be capable or responsible for maintaining his own health. Self-esteem is established on the basis of receiving approval or disapproval from others. Because an autistic client is indifferent to not only the physical presence, but the opinion, of others, low self-esteem is not likely to be a problem. An autistic person's physical health should not be affected by his mental disorder. Therefore, if the client cannot tolerate activity, it would be due to another unrelated condition. (17:373)
Nursing Process—Planning
Client Need—Safe, effective care environment

23 1. People with autism have varying levels of impairment and may require full assistance with some or all activities of daily living. When the child demonstrates an attempt at self-feeding, it would be appropriate to encourage him to participate in this aspect of his own self-care. Learning takes place when a person is ready. Until an autistic child demonstrates some interest, attempts to gain his cooperation are likely to be frustrating. (1:158)
Nursing Process—Planning
Client Need—Physiological integrity

24 2. If autistic individuals' possessions, routines, or environment are altered, they are likely to become very upset and combative toward others or themselves. A stimulating environment would create chaos and distress a person with autism. Autistic people often have limited artistic potential. Limit-setting is important, but a rigid, inflexible atmosphere can be distressing. (17:373)
Nursing Process—Planning
Client Need—Psychosocial integrity

25 1. Autistic children tend to display bizarre body movements. For example they rock their body or touch their hands to their face in peculiar mannerisms. None of the other items describes characteristics of autism. (1:158)
Nursing Process—Implementation
Client Need—Safe, effective care environment

26 4. Private home health care agencies employ various levels of health practitioners. An agency of this type would select the surrogate caregiver most appropriate for the type of client and level of care that is needed. Aid to Dependent Children is a social welfare agency that provides economic assistance to a parent who is unable to support financially the care of one or more children. The Association on Mental Deficiency is concerned with people who are mentally retarded, not mentally ill. Most day care facilities would not provide evening care and perhaps would not accept a child with special needs. (10:214–215)
Nursing Process—Implementation
Client Need—Safe, effective care environment

MENTAL HEALTH NEEDS DURING ADOLESCENCE AND YOUNG ADULTHOOD

27 4. The basis for developing a therapeutic relationship is acceptance. This attitude indicates that the client is unique and worthy of respect. Trust develops once a client feels accepted. All of the other qualities are desirable but are not as likely to facilitate building trust. (17:78)
Nursing Process—Planning
Client Need—Safe, effective care environment

28 1. Eye contact communicates that the nurse is paying attention. Giving away free literature does not communicate a sincere, personal regard for the client. Writing information is a job-related

task. Avoiding pauses could be interpreted as disinterest. (9:148)
Nursing Process—Implementation
Client Need—Psychosocial integrity

29 2. It is normal for teenagers to go through a period during which they reject the standards and ideals of their parents and other adults. By experimenting with new behaviors, often opposite those of the parents, the adolescent emerges with a unique identity and a lasting set of values. Adolescent rebellion is not likely to facilitate ingenuity, intuition, or insight. (1:33)
Nursing Process—Implementation
Client Need—Health promotion/maintenance

30 1. Treatment of a client is a confidential matter. Neither the nurse nor any other clinic personnel may reveal the identity of a client or the purpose for their treatment without the client's consent. All the other actions would overtly or covertly divulge a relationship between the clinic and the client and violate the principle of confidentiality. (1:308)
Nursing Process—Implementation
Client Need—Safe, effective care environment

31 4. One of the most important elements in resolving a crisis is the emotional support of significant others. The client's mothering instinct, marriage plans, and financial support are not as beneficial as a family's unconditional love and encouragement. (1:129)
Nursing Process—Evaluation
Client Need—Psychosocial integrity

32 3. Denial is a form of behavior used to protect one's consciousness from dealing with a catastrophic situation. By denying a situation exists, anxiety is kept to an acceptable level. Displacement involves discharging angry feelings onto an unrelated person or object. Regression occurs when a person resorts to behavior associated with a younger age. Compensation is characterized by pursuing an activity that ensures success to make up for feeling inadequate. (17:171)
Nursing Process—Evaluation
Client Need—Psychosocial integrity

33 1. People with anorexia nervosa manifest lanugo, a growth of fine downy hair, similar to that seen on newborn infants. It is thought that this occurs to promote or maintain normal body temperature on people who have little or no body fat. Bruises may indicate a vitamin deficiency, but they would not be limited to the upper torso. Generally, bowel sounds would be normal in anorectic people. Clubbing of the fingers is char-

acteristic of conditions causing chronic hypoxia. (17:379)
Nursing Process—Collecting data
Client Need—Safe, effective care environment

34 2. Generally, anorectics have been characterized as being perfect children with above average scholastic achievement, perhaps owing to a fear of failure. None of the other characteristics listed is unique to clients with anorexia nervosa. (17:380)
Nursing Process—Evaluation
Client Need—Health promotion/maintenance

35 3. Initial treatment of a client with anorexia nervosa focuses on meeting physiological needs. Once nutrients, fluids, vitamins, and electrolytes are administered, attention will shift to the client's psychosocial problems. (16:527)
Nursing Process—Planning
Client Need—Physiological integrity

36 3. Validation is a therapeutic communication technique in which the nurse interprets what he or she perceives to be the underlying meaning of the words. If the interpretation is correct, it increases rapport and forms a basis for future collaboration. The techniques of generalizing, giving advice, and responding with a stereotypical statement are all examples of nontherapeutic communication techniques. (12:264; 9:139)
Nursing Process—Implementation
Client Need—Psychosocial integrity

37 4. Controlling the desire to eat is a nonverbal technique the client with anorexia nervosa uses to demonstrate power and control. Getting attention as a result of this behavior reinforces its effectiveness. Until a client's malnutrition becomes life-threatening, force feeding would be unethical and inappropriate. Recording intake is not likely to be an incentive for eating. The fear of becoming fat often is greater than a prior commitment to collaborated goals. (4:297)
Nursing Process—Implementation
Client Need—Psychosocial integrity

38 2. Confrontation is a therapeutic communication technique that is useful in pointing out differences between an expected behavior and the actual action. Postponing weighing is likely to result in more accurate assessment data. However, this choice of action, as well as saying nothing or subtracting 2 lb, avoids the greater issue of dealing with the inappropriate behavior. (9:154)
Nursing Process—Implementation
Client Need—Safe, effective care environment

39 2. Bulimics usually are of normal weight. They manifest a cycle of eating binges followed by purging. A common form of purging is self-induced vomiting. Repeated contact between gastric acid and teeth results in deterioration of dental structures. Anorectics are more likely to cease menstruating when their body fat is depleted. Loss of hair also is correlated more with the malnutrition of anorexia nervosa. (9:274–275)

> Nursing Process—Collecting data
> Client Need—Safe, effective care environment

40 1. Binging and purging take place privately. If the client stays out of the bathroom following a meal, it interferes with the opportunity to induce vomiting and use laxatives or enemas to stimulate bowel elimination. Taking an inventory of food may precipitate an uncontrollable urge to go on an eating binge. The bulimic food binges are not isolated to fast-food establishments. Recording calories may only increase the anxiety bulimics experience when their eating is out of control. (4:298)

> Nursing Process—Planning
> Client Need—Psychosocial integrity

41 3. Peer censure is much more therapeutic. If the therapist or members of the treatment team react positively or negatively to the individuals involved in the conflict, it is likely to divide the group members and jeopardize group work. (12:318)

> Nursing Process—Implementation
> Client Need—Psychosocial integrity

42 1. The peer group becomes more influential than parents in determining how adolescents behave. Peer behavior is used as a model for establishing what activities are acceptable or nonacceptable. The fact that the team is winning is no more a motivation for taking controlled substances than if the team was losing. Affordability is not necessarily a factor in compromising values. (17:156)

> Nursing Process—Evaluation
> Client Need—Health promotion/maintenance

43 3. Acne occurs frequently in all age groups and both sexes who take anabolic steroids. The other physical changes are not related to the use of anabolic steroids. (15:210)

> Nursing Process—Collecting data
> Client Need—Physiological integrity

44 1. Anabolic steroids are synthetic drugs chemically related to androgens like testosterone. Androgens and anabolic steroids are associated with aggressive behavior. Severe mental changes, such as uncontrolled rage ("'roid rage") and personality changes, are not uncommon. The other

emotional changes would be due to some secondary cause unrelated to steroid use. (15:210)

> Nursing Process—Planning
> Client Need—Physiological integrity

45 4. The signs described indicate depression. Adolescents are likely to attempt suicide impulsively when they are unable to cope with a significant loss. It is appropriate to ask overtly about suicidal feelings. Talking or asking about suicide will not make a person more likely to act on his feelings; in fact, just the opposite is true. A dramatic change in behavior should never be disregarded. When dealing with crises, adolescents lack the perspective of a lifetime of experience to believe that their problem will ever be resolved. Establishing new peer relationships at another school may be equally traumatic for a depressed adolescent. (9:57)

> Nursing Process—Planning
> Client Need—Psychosocial integrity

46 3. People who are psychotic generally have thoughts that are unrealistic and irrational. Yet these thoughts seem real and logical to the psychotic person. Many people who are mentally healthy experience difficulty in relationships, have problems adjusting to new situations, and feel helpless in resolving some problems. (1:201)

> Nursing Process—Implementation
> Client Need—Psychosocial integrity

47 1. Orientation is the person's ability to identify who and where she is and the day, month, and year. Asking how the client arrived assesses short-term memory. Identifying one's place of birth assesses long-term memory. Knowing the current president assesses the client's fund of knowledge. (1:85)

> Nursing Process—Collecting data
> Client Need—Safe, effective care environment

48 3. The Mental Health Systems Act, passed by the United States Congress in 1980, contains a model for the mental health client's bill of rights. It states that a client has the right to access his or her own mental health care records, except for information provided by third parties and information deemed by a mental health professional to be detrimental to the client's health. Asking a "why" question is a nontherapeutic communication technique called demanding an explanation. Putting the clipboard away is a nonverbal method of denying her request. It is not illegal for clients to read their own medical records. (17:24)

> Nursing Process—Implementation
> Client Need—Safe, effective care environment

49 2. The most essential criterion for an involuntary commitment is that the person is a "clear and present" danger to herself or to others. Commitment criteria have been established to protect the right of the client to appropriate treatment in the least restrictive setting. There are other methods for assessing a client other than involuntary commitment. Failure to keep office appointments is not a criterion for commitment. All competent adults have the right to refuse treatment, which includes taking unwanted medications. (17:20)

   Nursing Process—Evaluation
   Client Need—Safe, effective care environment

50 4. Postural hypotension is a side-effect associated with this category of drugs. Cautioning a client to rise slowly would help moderate the drop in blood pressure, thus minimizing the potential for dizziness, fainting, or falling. Taking the medications on an empty stomach or skipping meals will not affect the drug's therapeutic action. This category of drugs is likely to make the client feel drowsy when treatment is first initiated. The client should never omit or discontinue a drug without collaborating with her physician. (15:257)

   Nursing Process—Implementation
   Client Need—Health promotion/maintenance

51 1. Antipsychotics are likely to reduce or eliminate psychotic symptoms, such as delusions and hallucinations. However, they do not generally relieve symptoms of apathy or withdrawal. Increased drowsiness is an undesirable side-effect. It is doubtful that the client will feel more energetic and rested because a common side effect is sedation. The drug will not alter the client's established self-concept. (15:255)

   Nursing Process—Evaluation
   Client Need—Physiological integrity

52 2. Antipsychotic drugs can depress the bone marrow's production of blood cells. A severe sore throat suggests that the client may not have sufficient white blood cells to fight off microorganisms. A complete blood count is needed to assess the possibility of this adverse effect. This drug is likely to cause constipation and weight gain. Tinnitus is not associated with haloperidol. (1:267)

   Nursing Process—Planning
   Client Need—Physiological integrity

53 2. Inflammation of the eyes is almost always present after smoking marijuana. The pulse rate is likely to be rapid. Other signs include euphoria, drowsiness, light-headedness, and hunger. Shivering may accompany opiate withdrawal. Rapid breathing and restlessness may be observed in abrupt alcohol withdrawal or use of a central nervous system stimulant. (15:84)

   Nursing Process—Collecting data
   Client Need—Psychosocial integrity

54 1. The criteria for alcohol abuse include "black-outs," a form of amnesia of actions and events that occurred during a period of intoxication. The onset of alcohol dependence is not related to the amount of time over which it has been consumed. Those who abuse alcohol consume it in any form. A preference for alcohol is just that, a personal choice. The consequence of consuming alcohol is the substantial criterion for alcoholism. (1:188)

   Nursing Process—Collecting data
   Client Need—Psychosocial integrity

55 1. Acute toxicity can result in dysrhythmias and death. Toxicity can occur any time and with any dose. Cocaine is a central nervous system stimulant. As such, it would increase respirations and raise blood pressure. Blood sugar may be lowered owing to the use of calories during periods of hyperactivity. (15:83)

   Nursing Process—Planning
   Client Need—Physiological integrity

MENTAL HEALTH NEEDS DURING MIDDLE AGE

56 1. Symptoms of anxiety are a result of sympathetic nervous system stimulation. The release of adrenalin causes an increase in the heart rate. Clients may even describe that they feel their heart racing or palpating. Sympathetic nervous system stimulation also is associated with a dry mouth, dilated pupils, and hypertension. (1:233)

   Nursing Process—Collecting data
   Client Need—Physiological integrity

57 4. Anxiety is heightened during situations in which there have been no prior experiences. Providing explanations and instructions diminishes insecurity. Standing within an arm's length invades a client's personal space and heightens anxiety. Wearing a laboratory coat may nonverbally upset a client, depending on what it represents from past experiences. Wearing a name tag and introducing oneself are always appropriate. Coffee and tea contain stimulating chemicals. (12:281)

   Nursing Process—Planning
   Client Need—Physiological integrity

58 4. Staying with a frightened client communicates genuine concern. The presence of a caring person tends to reduce anxiety. The first choice is an example of giving advice, which is a nontherapeutic communication technique. Trying to shame the client with the possibility that the out-of-control behavior may be seen by the phy-

sician is inappropriate. The third nontherapeutic example is one of generalizing. It disregards this client's right to be considered unique. (17:69)
　Nursing Process—Implementation
　Client Need—Psychosocial integrity

59　1.　Antianxiety drugs produce a calming effect. If alcohol is consumed with this medication, it is likely to potentiate the drug's action and endanger the client's safety owing to profound sedation. Drug dependency is related to this drug's dosage and length of administration. The drug will cause sedation. Treatment with lithium carbonate, not the benzodiazepines, is monitored through a blood test. (15:259)
　Nursing Process—Planning
　Client Need—Physiological integrity

60　4.　Agoraphobia is the term for a fear of being in public places, in open places, or alone where escape is difficult or help is unavailable. Claustrophobia is a fear of closed spaces. Hydrophobia is a fear of water. It also is a very old term for rabies. Photophobia is a sensitivity to light. (1:233)
　Nursing Process—Implementation
　Client Need—Health promotion/maintenance

61　3.　Phobic people avoid what they perceive as the cause of their discomfort. Denial is a coping mechanism characterized by a person's disbelief in what others know is obviously true. Compensation is characterized by pursuing an activity that ensures success to make up for feeling inadequate. Rationalization is a face-saving mechanism. It involves making an acceptable excuse for some failure, shortcoming, or disappointment. (12:198)
　Nursing Process—Planning
　Client Need—Psychosocial integrity

62　1.　The real cause of a phobia often is associated with an earlier developmental trauma that has been repressed and is now influencing the manifestation of the present problem. Phobias are unrelated to changes in physical health, substance abuse, or current situations. (1:233)
　Nursing Process—Planning
　Client Need—Psychosocial integrity

63　4.　By using relaxation techniques the client learns to control independently the uncomfortable feelings and symptoms that result from the phobic stimulus. Even spraying an insect will be accompanied by anxiety in a phobic person. Behavioral modification generally is not accompanied by the use of medications. Its goal is to restore the person with an active locus of con-

trol. Avoidance is an unhealthy coping mechanism that most phobic people overuse. (1:284)
　Nursing Process—Implementation
　Client Need—Psychosocial integrity

64　1.　The person with post-traumatic stress disorder has unresolved conflict concerning a traumatic event. He tries to suppress his feelings and memory of the experience. However, the stressful ordeal is relived during sleep in the form of terrorizing nightmares. Post-traumatic stress disorder is not characterized by hallucinations or investing energy in worthy causes. People with this condition tend to be apathetic and withdraw from investing in relationships. (1:235)
　Nursing Process—Collecting data
　Client Need—Psychosocial integrity

65　3.　A stimulus that simulates the original traumatic event can trigger the anxiety from the prior experience. If the person had been frightened of fireworks as a child, he probably would have manifested a continued fear response prior to his military experience. The startle response is not associated with a loss of patriotism or a fear of being drafted. (1:235)
　Nursing Process—Implementation
　Client Need—Psychosocial integrity

66　2.　Post-traumatic stress disorder can occur in anyone who has been involved in an uncommon event outside the realm of usual human experience. This can involve natural disasters like earthquakes or situational disasters like being raped. None of the other situations plays a role in developing post-traumatic stress disorder. (1:234)
　Nursing Process—Implementation
　Client Need—Health promotion/maintenance

67　3.　Withdrawal and nonverbalization are used to avoid dealing with the conflict of the precipitating event. These individuals tend to shut down their emotions to avoid feeling anything. Talking helps the victim work through the conflict and reduces the underlying anxiety. Acting happy and trying to make life pleasant will not relieve the symptoms of this condition. There is no legal or ethical way to prevent a person from isolating himself or herself. (12:197)
　Nursing Process—Planning
　Client Need—Psychosocial integrity

68　4.　Vital signs are useful in detecting changes in a patient's condition. Assessment is the first step in the nursing process. It should take place before any further action is implemented. (10:90)
　Nursing Process—Collecting data
　Client Need—Safe, effective care environment

69　1.　Middle adulthood is characterized as a period of generativity or stagnation. It is common for people during this stage in the life cycle to evaluate their contributions to society. People who do not see themselves as counting for much can experience what is known as a midlife crisis. Goals generally are established at an earlier age. Middle-aged people may regret their judgments, but they do not doubt them. (9:63)

> Nursing Process—Evaluation
> Client Need—Health promotion/maintenance

70 2. Therapeutic communication requires that the nurse be perceptive to hidden meanings within a client's statements or questions. It is then appropriate for the nurse to verbalize the feeling tone that was communicated back to the client for validation. Deferring discussion to the physician is a form of scapegoating in which the nurse chooses to remain uninvolved. Telling the client to let the staff worry and needing to practice more patience are forms of giving advice. Giving advice is a nontherapeutic form of communication. (12:249)

> Nursing Process—Implementation
> Client Need—Psychosocial integrity

71 2. Emotional care involves a sincere respect, interest, and concern for people. Nurses demonstrate emotional care when they accept individual differences in people and treat each client as a unique person. Although all of the other outcomes can occur, the most detrimental effect is to the client. A health worker's biases and prejudices, if unchallenged, can interfere with objective care. (18:18–19)

> Nursing Process—Evaluation
> Client Need—Safe, effective care environment

72 3. Only people who are immediately involved in the care of a client have the right to access the health record. The nurse must take all necessary measures to safeguard information about his or her clients. (12:330)

> Nursing Process—Implementation
> Client Need—Safe, effective care environment

73 4. The client with ulcerative colitis has an inflamed bowel and experiences severe diarrhea. Endoscopic examinations and x-rays confirm the presence of pathology. The exact cause of the disease is unknown, but emotional stress is one of many possible causes. Most clients with psychophysiologic diseases would rather work than experience their symptoms. (16:560)

> Nursing Process—Implementation
> Client Need—Safe, effective care environment

74 1. Meeting physiological needs always takes precedence over other needs, such as security, love and belonging, and so forth. The most important information needed at this time concerns his diarrhea and the impact it is having on his fluid status, nutrition, and electrolyte balance. (16:561)

> Nursing Process—Planning
> Client Need—Physiological integrity

75 1. A nonjudgmental attitude conveys to the client that help is being provided without morally judging his behavior. Cleaning stool is never pleasant, but the nurse can avoid making the client feel that he is an offensive person. When a client is treated with dignity, it sustains his self-esteem. It would not promote this client's self-esteem if he were cleaned by his mother or male nurses or if he were held totally responsible for that task himself. (17:79)

> Nursing Process—Planning
> Client Need—Psychosocial integrity

76 2. A consequence of alcohol abuse is a tolerance to all sedative drugs. Tolerance is a need to increase the dose or frequency of use to obtain the desired effect. A need for a higher dosage or more frequent administration can indicate that the client abuses alcohol or some other central nervous system depressant drug. An alcoholic's blood pressure and pulse become abnormally high, and he will become restless rather than lethargic during withdrawal. (15:81)

> Nursing Process—Collecting data
> Client Need—Psychosocial integrity

77 3. Visual hallucinations occur as a client withdraws from alcohol. These are real and terrifying experiences for the alcoholic. To maintain safety and reduce the client's fear and anxiety, it is essential that a nurse remain with the client. Restraints should never be used unless there is no other alternative for maintaining the client's or staff's safety. In the client's mind the hallucination is real. Telling him that he is not seeing it is illogical and untrue. Closing the client's door is unsafe and likely to heighten his fear. (17:305)

> Nursing Process—Implementation
> Client Need—Safe, effective care environment

78 3. Hallucinations occur during advanced withdrawal, known as delirium tremens. To restore normal sensory perception the client should receive one of the minor tranquilizers, such as chlordiazepoxide (Librium), or a central nervous system depressant, such as phenobarbital. The nurse must call the physician because a drug cannot be administered without a physician's order. (15:256)

> Nursing Process—Implementation
> Client Need—Physiological integrity

79 2. Seizures occur from rebound central nervous system stimulation as the depressant drug, alco-

hol, is metabolized from the client's system. Seizures may occur in some people as early as the first 24 hours of withdrawal. Bleeding and jaundice are the results of liver damage from alcohol abuse. Hyperthermia can occur during alcohol withdrawal. (15:85)
　　Nursing Process—Collecting data
　　Client Need—Physiological integrity

80 1. Staff members are better able to understand client behavior by increasing their own self-understanding. Nurses who are generalists are not academically prepared to analyze a client's motivation or provide psychotherapy. A knowledge of abnormal behavior is important, but it is not the first step in understanding the behavior of others. (1:98)
　　Nursing Process—Implementation
　　Client Need—Safe, effective care environment

81 4. Depression generally is accompanied by feelings of hopelessness, helplessness, guilt, and low self-esteem. These feelings can cause depressed clients to feel suicidal. In the interests of client safety, the client should be admitted to a location that facilitates frequent and close observation by the nursing staff. Being in a room with a cheerful and talkative person and being placed in a nonstimulating environment are not considered therapeutic modalities for relieving depression. (9:281)
　　Nursing Process—Planning
　　Client Need—Psychosocial integrity

82 1. An indirect leading statement or open-ended question is purposely general and nonspecific. It allows the client to give as much information as she wants. Close-ended questions or statements, exemplified in the other three options, provide facts or sometimes one-word replies. (1:104)
　　Nursing Process—Planning
　　Client Need—Psychosocial integrity

83 4. Consistency promotes trust and security. The client learns that she can expect the same response from the nurse and will not experience uncertainty in predicting the type of reaction she will receive. None of the other nonverbal behaviors is as effective in promoting trust. (1: 98–99)
　　Nursing Process—Planning
　　Client Need—Psychosocial integrity

84 2. A plan for suicide indicates that the client has given serious thought to ending her life. Once a plan has been developed, the client is much more likely to act on her feelings. The remaining examples are characteristic of passive suicide

ideation, which is not associated with as much lethal risk as an active suicide plan. (1:225)
　　Nursing Process—Evaluation
　　Client Need—Psychosocial integrity

85 1. Amitriptyline hydrochloride is a tricyclic antidepressant. Tricyclics produce anticholinergic effects similar to atropine sulfate, such as urinary retention, dry mouth, and dilated pupils. A person with glaucoma should not receive drugs that dilate the pupil. When the iris enlarges, resulting in dilation of the pupil, the canal through which aqueous humor drains narrows or occludes. This action raises intraocular pressure. Tricyclics are not contraindicated for clients with the other listed diseases. (1:270)
　　Nursing Process—Collecting data
　　Client Need—Safe, effective care environment

86 3. When the client demonstrates relief of symptoms, it can mean that the person is responding to treatment, has made the actual decision to commit suicide, or now has the energy to do it. During the period of deepest depression, a suicidal person often lacks the energy to carry out her death wish. (14:678)
　　Nursing Process—Planning
　　Client Need—Psychosocial integrity

87 1. It is essential to obtain written permission from the client prior to performing any act that will affect his body. One criterion for a valid consent is that the client be given the information necessary to weigh the advantages and disadvantages of the proposed treatment. All of the other nursing actions would take place if and when written consent has been obtained. (1:309)
　　Nursing Process—Implementation
　　Client Need—Safe, effective care environment

88 3. Confusion and memory loss regarding recent events are the two most common changes in mental state that result from electroshock therapy. The other described experiences are not associated with electroshock therapy. (1:263)
　　Nursing Process—Planning
　　Client Need—Safe, effective care environment

89 4. Depressed people often feel helpless and hopeless. They may believe that no one cares. Genuine caring and making the client feel worthwhile can improve self-concept and decrease feelings of alienation. A cheerful attitude often causes a depressed client to feel even more unworthy than ever. It often is difficult for the depressed client to feel optimistic despite reassurance from the nurse. The nurse should not restrict an expression of mood or affect. (17:241)
　　Nursing Process—Planning
　　Client Need—Psychosocial integrity

90 1. Substances such as chicken liver, which contain tyramine, a neurostimulating chemical, must be avoided. When the enzyme monoamine oxidase is inhibited, the body cannot break down and metabolize this stimulating compound. To ensure safety the client must be able to identify accurately the restricted substances. The other substances listed are not restricted when a client takes an MAOI. (15:257)

> Nursing Process—Evaluation
> Client Need—Health promotion/maintenance

91 1. Schizophrenia is characterized by marked social isolation and withdrawal. Group activities are likely to heighten anxiety. Sitting quietly is a nonthreatening approach that helps the client to develop trust in one person within the therapeutic environment. The other choices involve forcing the withdrawn client to interact, which would be nontherapeutic at this time. (1:209)

> Nursing Process—Planning
> Client Need—Psychosocial integrity

92 3. As a result of the schizophrenic's disordered thoughts, he or she has difficulty putting thoughts into words. The nurse should never pretend to understand the meaning of a client's illogical statement. (1:201)

> Nursing Process—Implementation
> Client Need—Psychosocial integrity

93 2. It is never therapeutic to agree, disagree, challenge, or enter in any way into the delusions of a schizophrenic client. Listening to, but not commenting on, the content is appropriate. Simply repeating the client's words indicates that the message was heard. (1:209; 17:218)

> Nursing Process—Planning
> Client Need—Psychosocial integrity

94 4. Hallucinations are sensory experiences outside of anyone other than the client's awareness. An auditory hallucination involves hearing a voice or sound that no one else perceives. The person rarely volunteers his or her altered perceptions. The observant nurse can draw inferences based on the client's nonverbal cues. The first three examples are not associated with the behavior of a hallucinating client. (17:214)

> Nursing Process—Collecting data
> Client Need—Psychosocial integrity

95 2. The honest answer on the part of the nurse presents the client with reality. It reinforces that the symptom he or she is experiencing is real to him or her but is caused by the disease process and not a paranormal experience. The first choice is an example of a nontherapeutic response called belittling. Belittling makes light of what the client believes. By entering into the bizarre

thinking of the schizophrenic in the third example, the nurse adds credibility to the client's distorted sense of reality. The fourth choice is another example of giving advice, a nontherapeutic technique for communication. (17:219)

> Nursing Process—Implementation
> Client Need—Psychosocial integrity

96 1. Tardive dyskinesia is characterized by rhythmic, involuntary movements of the tongue, the face, the mouth, the jaw, and sometimes the extremities. None of the other choices is a manifestation of tardive dyskinesia. (15:257)

> Nursing Process—Collecting data
> Client Need—Physiological integrity

97 3. All normal people can express a range of moods that parallels situations they are experiencing. However, people with bipolar disorder have cycles during which they display periods of extreme euphoria for weeks or months at a time. The exaggerated mood is followed or preceded by an interval of normal moods. Some forms of this disorder also include a span of deep depression. None of the other behaviors is symptomatic of bipolar disorder. (1:220)

> Nursing Process—Collecting data
> Client Need—Safe, effective care environment

98 2. The best response to inappropriate advances is to set limits on the behavior. It is therapeutic to accept a client's feelings, but limits must be drawn to contain his behavior. The nurse projects an assertive manner by telling the client how she feels in relation to his remark. Assertiveness is open, honest, direct communication that expresses a person's real feelings, wishes, wants, and needs. The response in the first choice, on the surface, resembles the nontherapeutic technique called giving advice. Depending on the tone of voice and body language, it also could be taken as a flirtatious response. The third choice of responses definitely implies that something more than a professional relationship is a possibility. In the last choice the nurse uses a nontherapeutic technique called changing the subject. Its use is a more passive way of indicating to the client that there will be no further discussion on the subject of his comment. (1:99; 12:71)

> Nursing Process—Implementation
> Client Need—Psychosocial integrity

99 2. A hyperactive client needs to discharge his or her energies. More energy is expended using large muscles than small muscles. An activity that requires concentration or inactivity, like piecing a puzzle together, watching television, or reading, may be too difficult a task for the client with bipolar disorder to accomplish. He or she may become distracted, or the frustration could lead to a violent outburst. (17:251)

Nursing Process—Implementation
Client Need—Health promotion/maintenance

100 3. Toxic reactions can occur during lithium carbonate therapy when blood levels more than 1.5 mEq/L are reached. Blood levels usually are drawn during therapy and the dosage of lithium adjusted according to the results. The client who takes lithium may develop polyuria, but the volume of urine eliminated is not used to monitor the lithium level. Neither vital signs nor brain scans are used to evaluate the client's ability to metabolize his lithium dose. (15:257)

Nursing Process—Evaluation
Client Need—Physiological integrity

101 1. A client with bipolar disorder finds it almost impossible to sit or stand in one location for more than a few minutes. He or she may not be able to concentrate long enough to eat or drink. Finger foods can be carried and eaten during the course of physical activity. None of the other approaches will be as effective in meeting this type of client's nutritional needs. (17:243, 248)

Nursing Process—Planning
Client Need—Safe, effective care environment

102 4. Clients with bipolar disorder do not demonstrate good judgment. The nurse intervenes to protect the client's dignity at a time when the client cannot control her exhibitionism. Avoiding criticism indicates that the nurse understands that the illness is responsible for the behavior. The client should not be depended on to set limits. It would not be fair to deprive the card players to control the bipolar client's behavior. A public reprimand is damaging to anyone's self-esteem. (17:256)

Nursing Process—Implementation
Client Need—Psychosocial integrity

103 1. The elderly must cope with a multitude of losses, for example, loss of health, loss of a spouse and friends, loss of employment, loss of income, loss of independence, and so on. Retaining memory is more of a problem than its development. Geriatric clients must deal with the loss of relationships. The effectiveness of parenting already has been established. (9:64–65)

Nursing Process—Collecting data
Client Need—Health promotion/maintenance

104 4. Self-worth is maintained by experiencing satisfaction in accomplishments. Giving genuine praise promotes a positive self-concept. The longer a person can maintain independence, the less likely that physical deterioration will occur. All of the other choices would communicate to the client that he is not able to manage his self-care satisfactorily. (17:361; 12:379)

Nursing Process—Planning
Client Need—Health promotion/maintenance

105 1. Assessment is the first step in the nursing process. Assessment involves gathering all the information needed to identify a problem and its cause. More data are needed in this case before determining the cause for her lack of food intake. Once a cause has been identified, the nursing team will be in a better position to select appropriate interventions for resolving the problem. Assigning a nursing assistant to make pertinent observations is an appropriate use of staff for the purpose of gathering more information. Serving the client in her room may be appropriate if the cause of her dawdling is distraction. Threatening her with hospitalization is a form of coercion. Intellectualizing the dangers of weight loss is not very effective in actually getting a client to eat. (9:204)

Nursing Process—Collecting data
Client Need—Physiological integrity

106 2. During senescence it is common for people to review their life experiences. If the analysis results in the belief that their existence has been satisfying and worthwhile, they acquire integrity. If the analysis results in regrets, they close their life with a feeling of despair. Trust is acquired during infancy. Intimacy is established during young adulthood. The toddler stage in the life cycle is associated with autonomy. (1:34;17:350)

Nursing Process—Evaluation
Client Need—Health promotion/maintenance

107 4. Words may not mean the same to all people. Reporting what was actually observed is a much more accurate and objective method for documenting behavior. None of the other critiques identified the vague and subjective quality of the charting. (18:65)

Nursing Process—Evaluation
Client Need—Safe, effective care environment

108 3. Asking the client to identify his or her birthdate is a standard technique for assessing long-term memory. The nurse should know the answer to the question that is asked to evaluate the client's response. Asking the client his or her current age and today's date would help in the assessment of short-term memory and orientation. Asking what occurred in January is too vague a question for a valid assessment. (17:115; 9:196)

Nursing Process—Collecting data
Client Need—Safe, effective care environment

109 1. Geriatric clients generally experience a decline in hearing acuity. Impaired sensory perception of this nature may cause the client to misinterpret what has been asked and respond in an unexpected manner. Asking a client to repeat the question helps to rule out a hearing deficit or possible dementia. A client has a 50% chance of being right when having to respond only with a "yes" or "no." Asking the next of kin is appropriate if the client is not a reliable historian. Asking questions only the client can answer will not provide comprehensive data. (9:204; 14:1027)
Nursing Process—Collecting data
Client Need—Safe, effective care environment

110 1. Geriatric clients tend to become confused and disoriented in unfamiliar surroundings. Using a nightlight can help to provide enough illumination in the room for the client to orient himself to his environment and locate the toilet independently. Using a restraint without justification is considered a form of battery. As long as the client senses a need to urinate, placing a urinal or attaching a catheter is inappropriate care. (7:630)
Nursing Process—Planning
Client Need—Safe, effective care environment

111 2. Confusion can be relieved by providing a client with environmental cues. Repetitious reminders can help the confused person maintain or relearn how to function. A liquid diet is unappetizing and unnecessary as long as the client can chew, swallow, and digest food naturally. Serving this client early will not eliminate her confusion. Seating her alone deprives her of any role models to imitate. It also shows disregard for this client's dignity. (9:206; 14:1099)
Nursing Process—Implementation
Client Need—Health promotion/maintenance

112 1. Labeling rooms with easily identifiable words or pictures promotes environmental awareness. Sensory cues can restore the confused client's ability to reorient herself. Locking the unit deprives all of the clients of a certain amount of freedom and privacy. If detaining the client involves threats or if unnecessary physical restraint is used, it could be considered assault or battery. A confused client may not be able to process the information about her behavior and the reaction of others. (9:207)
Nursing Process—Planning
Client Need—Health promotion/maintenance

113 2. Reflection is a therapeutic communication technique in which the receiver conveys to the sender her expressed thoughts and related feelings. One of the greatest stressors for family members of clients with dementia is that they are physically present but emotionally absent. The first and fourth responses are clichés. They probably will not encourage the client's daughter to talk more about her feelings. The third response combines giving advice and a defensive statement, both of which are nontherapeutic techniques of communication. (12:262; 14:1009)
Nursing Process—Implementation
Client Need—Psychosocial integrity

114 3. Elderly people often are lonely. They sometimes exaggerate or invent physical symptoms to receive attention. If the nurse provides unsolicited attention other than in response to her physical complaints, the client may not use somatizing as a mechanism for gaining attention. Giving an analgesic without justification is inappropriate nursing care. Telling the client this is just another bad day dismisses the client's underlying need for attention. If there are no physical changes, the physician would feel that a medical examination is unnecessary. (17:281, 351)
Nursing Process—Planning
Client Need—Psychosocial integrity

115 2. To facilitate attention, concentration, and retention, all verbal communication should be brief and simple. Directions should be given in understandable language with a minimum of distracting stimuli in the environment. Speaking loudly will not improve memory. Writing some information down may help a client remember oral instructions, but overall it is not the best recommendation of the choices provided. Listening to a news program helps maintain reality orientation, but it will not promote memory. (16:445)
Nursing Process—Planning
Client Need—Safe, effective care environment

116 1. Dying clients tend to become isolated and deserted by staff. The primary objective in this case should be providing a physical presence to listen and support the client as death draws near. All of the other choices involve leaving the dying client essentially by himself. (16:151; 18:759)
Nursing Process—Implementation
Client Need—Psychosocial integrity

117 3. Expressing feelings to an understanding listener helps facilitate the grieving process. Communication helps people deal openly with their emotions and feelings, which is healthier than suppressing the emotional impact of the event. Being sent home or terminated would not help promote grieving. Asking the nursing assistant to perform postmortem care in this emotional state shows a disregard for the trauma he or she is experiencing. (16:151)

Nursing Process—Implementation
Client Need—Health promotion/maintenance

118 2. Nurses need to be alert to signs of burnout among family members. Some may fear that by meeting their own needs they may be accused of abandoning the institutionalized client. If a caring staff member encourages longer periods of separation, it can relieve the potential for feeling guilty. The client's wife may benefit from a physical examination, but that would not be the most therapeutic action in the list of choices. Clients in a long-term health care facility have a right to see visitors at any time within reason. Indicating that the staff is capable of caring for the client's husband may imply that she is not appreciated or that her presence is an inconvenience. (14:1007)

Nursing Process—Implementation
Client Need—Health promotion/maintenance

119 3. Drugs are potentially unsafe if they are not administered correctly. Information about drug administration must be explained verbally. It also would be helpful to accompany verbal instructions with written information. Before the client leaves, the nurse should determine that they have an accurate understanding of the instructions. The family would already be familiar with the other types of information. (14:1009)

Nursing Process—Evaluation
Client Need—Health promotion/maintenance

120 2. Clients have the right to information about all medications that are prescribed and the right to refuse them. Overtly or covertly administering medication against the consent of a client is illegal because it violates a citizen's constitutional rights. It also is unethical because it violates the client's autonomy and right to self-determination. (17:26–27; 1:311–312)

Nursing Process—Implementation
Client Need—Safe, effective care environment

Classification of Test Items

Unit I Review Test 1

Directions: After each question the correct answer is given as well as a classification of each test question. Compare the correct answer with your answer. If a question has been answered *incorrectly,* draw a line to the end of the four columns. When finished, add up your correct scores and place the results at the bottom of each column.
Score Calculation:

To determine the percentage of the number of questions you answered correctly, divide the **Number Correct** by the **Number Possible,** as example 96 (the number of questions answered correctly) divided by 120 (the number of questions in the test) = .80 or 80%.

NURSING PROCESS

C = Collecting data
P = Planning
I = Implementation
E = Evaluation

CLIENT NEEDS

S = Safe, effective care environment
P = Physiological integrity
M = Psychosocial integrity
H = Health promotion/maintenance

Question #	Answer #	Nursing Process				Client Needs			
		C	P	I	E	S	P	M	H
1	4	C						M	
2	2			I					H
3	4			I					H
4	1			I					H
5	2			I					H
6	1	C				S			
7	1	C							H
8	1			I				M	
9	3		P						H
10	4			I					H
11	2			I				M	
12	1				E				H
13	4			I				M	
14	2		P			S			
15	1	C							H
16	4		P					M	
17	2			I					H
18	2				E		P		

NURSING PROCESS

C = Collecting data
P = Planning
I = Implementation
E = Evaluation

CLIENT NEEDS

S = Safe, effective care environment
P = Physiological integrity
M = Psychosocial integrity
H = Health promotion/maintenance

Question #	Answer #	Nursing Process				Client Needs			
		C	P	I	E	S	P	M	H
19	3			I					H
20	2			I					H
21	1	C							H
22	4		P			S			
23	1		P				P		
24	2		P					M	
25	1			I		S			
26	4			I		S			
27	4		P			S			
28	1			I				M	
29	2			I					H
30	1			I		S			
31	4				E			M	
32	3				E			M	
33	1	C				S			
34	2				E				H
35	3		P				P		
36	3			I				M	
37	4			I				M	
38	2			I		S			
39	2	C				S			
40	1		P					M	
41	3			I				M	
42	1				E				H
43	3	C					P		
44	1		P				P		
45	4		P					M	
46	3			I				M	
47	1	C				S			
48	3			I		S			
49	2				E	S			
50	4			I					H

NURSING PROCESS

C = Collecting data
P = Planning
I = Implementation
E = Evaluation

CLIENT NEEDS

S = Safe, effective care environment
P = Physiological integrity
M = Psychosocial integrity
H = Health promotion/maintenance

Question #	Answer #	Nursing Process				Client Needs			
		C	P	I	E	S	P	M	H
51	1				E		P		
52	2		P				P		
53	2	C						M	
54	1	C						M	
55	1		P				P		
56	1	C					P		
57	4		P				P		
58	4			I				M	
59	1		P				P		
60	4			I					H
61	3		P					M	
62	1		P					M	
63	4			I				M	
64	1	C						M	
65	3			I				M	
66	2			I					H
67	3		P					M	
68	4	C				S			
69	1				E				H
70	2			I				M	
71	2				E	S			
72	3			I		S			
73	4			I		S			
74	1		P				P		
75	1		P					M	
76	2	C						M	
77	3			I		S			
78	3			I			P		
79	2	C					P		
80	1			I		S			
81	4		P					M	

NURSING PROCESS

C = Collecting data
P = Planning
I = Implementation
E = Evaluation

CLIENT NEEDS

S = Safe, effective care environment
P = Physiological integrity
M = Psychosocial integrity
H = Health promotion/maintenance

Question #	Answer #	Nursing Process				Client Needs			
		C	P	I	E	S	P	M	H
82	1		P					M	
83	4		P					M	
84	2				E			M	
85	1	C				S			
86	3		P					M	
87	1			I		S			
88	3		P			S			
89	4		P					M	
90	1				E				H
91	1		P					M	
92	3			I				M	
93	2		P					M	
94	4	C						M	
95	2			I				M	
96	1	C					P		
97	3	C				S			
98	2			I				M	
99	2			I					H
100	3				E		P		
101	1		P			S			
102	4			I				M	
103	1	C							H
104	4		P						H
105	1	C					P		
106	2				E				H
107	4				E	S			
108	3	C				S			
109	1	C				S			
110	1		P			S			
111	2			I					H
112	1		P						H

NURSING PROCESS

C = Collecting data
P = Planning
I = Implementation
E = Evaluation

CLIENT NEEDS

S = Safe, effective care environment
P = Physiological integrity
M = Psychosocial integrity
H = Health promotion/maintenance

Question #	Answer #	Nursing Process				Client Needs			
		C	P	I	E	S	P	M	H
113	2			I				M	
114	3		P					M	
115	2		P			S			
116	1			I				M	
117	3			I					H
118	2			I					H
119	3				E				H
120	2			I		S			
Number Correct									
Number Possible	120	24	34	46	16	30	17	43	30
Percentage Correct									

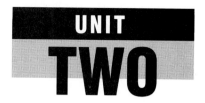

UNIT
TWO

REVIEW TESTS 2 AND 3

The Nursing Care of Maternity Clients and Newborns

REVIEW TEST 2

The Prenatal Period

Anatomy and Physiology of the Male and Female Reproductive Systems
Signs and Symptoms of Pregnancy; Tests for Pregnancy
Assessing the Pregnant Client
Common Discomforts of Pregnancy
High-Risk Factors and Pregnancy
Complications of Pregnancy
Nutrition During Pregnancy
Teaching the Pregnant Client
Elective Abortion
Individual Test Items

Correct Answers and Rationale
Classification of Test Items

Directions: With a pencil, blacken the circle in front of the option you have chosen for your correct answer.

The Prenatal Period

ANATOMY AND PHYSIOLOGY OF THE MALE AND FEMALE REPRODUCTIVE SYSTEMS

Ms. Betty Stevens is 29 years old, pregnant for the first time, and attending a prenatal clinic. Ms. Stevens appears interested in facts about pregnancy and human reproduction. During subsequent visits to the clinic, she asks many questions about this subject.

1 During a prenatal visit Ms. Stevens asks questions about female hormones and the ovaries. To develop a teaching plan and answer questions, the nurse should know that the ovaries normally secrete
   ○ 1. estrogen and progesterone.
   ○ 2. cortisone.
   ○ 3. estrogen only during pregnancy.
   ○ 4. luteinizing hormone.

2 Ms. Stevens also asks about ovulation. The nurse can plan to answer her questions about ovulation knowing that this phenomenon occurs when the anterior pituitary gland releases
   ○ 1. antidiuretic hormone.
   ○ 2. prolactin.
   ○ 3. oxytocin.
   ○ 4. luteinizing hormone.

3 Another question asked by Ms. Stevens concerns male hormones and their influence on her husband's sperm count. The nurse can plan to explain, in simple terms, the effect of hormones on the formation of sperm (spermatogenesis) by knowing that this process is under the *influence* of
   ○ 1. the posterior pituitary gland.
   ○ 2. testosterone.
   ○ 3. oxytocin.
   ○ 4. the anterior pituitary gland.

4 During a prenatal visit Ms. Stevens asks how the sex of the baby is determined. The correct explanation is based on the fact that the sex of a fetus is determined by a(n)
   ○ 1. gene in the sperm.
   ○ 2. gene in the ovum.
   ○ 3. X or Y chromosome in the sperm.
   ○ 4. Y chromosome in the ovum.

5 During a discussion of her pregnancy, Ms. Stevens asks about hormones and pregnancy. The nurse can develop a teaching plan for Ms. Stevens by knowing that the hormone that plays the *most* important role in preparing the uterus for pregnancy is
   ○ 1. prosecretin.
   ○ 2. progesterone.

○ 3. human growth hormone (HGH).

○ 4. follicle-stimulating hormone (FSH).

6 During a prenatal visit Ms. Stevens asks questions about human reproduction. To answer Ms. Stevens' questions a diagram can be used to display and describe the uterus. The nurse can label the *inner lining* of the uterus as the
○ 1. peritoneum.
○ 2. perimetrium.
○ 3. myometrium.
○ 4. endometrium.

7 Ms. Stevens asks how sperm travel. The nurse explains that after ejaculation of sperm into the vagina, sperm are propelled by
○ 1. cilia on their body.
○ 2. movements of their tail-like portions.
○ 3. peristalticlike cervical and uterine contractions.
○ 4. pressure differences in the uterus and fallopian tubes.

8 Part of the explanation about human reproduction given to Ms. Stevens concerns conception and includes a brief discussion of chromosomes. When planning the explanation the nurse will include the fact that the total number of chromosomes in each *mature* germ cell (ovum or sperm) is
○ 1. 23.
○ 2. 24.
○ 3. 46.
○ 4. 48.

9 When explaining conception to Ms. Stevens, the nurse plans to name the anatomic structure where the egg (ovum) normally unites with the sperm. This *structure* is called the
○ 1. ovary.
○ 2. cervix.
○ 3. uterus.
○ 4. fallopian tubes.

SIGNS AND SYMPTOMS OF PREGNANCY; TESTS FOR PREGNANCY

Ms. Mary Warner is 22 years old and makes an appointment to be seen in the prenatal clinic. She is not sure, but she thinks she may be pregnant. During the initial interview a history is taken.

10 Ms. Warner asks the nurse what signs or symptoms she will experience if she definitely is pregnant. The nurse can respond by stating that there are probable signs of pregnancy, but a *positive* sign of pregnancy is
○ 1. breast changes.
○ 2. weight gain.
○ 3. fetal movements.
○ 4. nausea and vomiting.

11 The nurse also explains that an example of a *probable* sign of pregnancy is
○ 1. quickening.
○ 2. morning sickness.
○ 3. enlargement of the uterus.
○ 4. tingling sensations in the breasts.

12 Ms. Warner was told by the physician that she has chloasma. She asks what this word means. *Chloasma* may be described as
○ 1. brown spots on the face.
○ 2. dark rings around the nipples.
○ 3. stretch marks on the abdomen.
○ 4. a dark vertical line on the abdomen.

The physician orders several blood tests for Ms. Warner.

13 In reviewing Ms. Warner's clinical record and planning for future teaching sessions, the nurse knows that the laboratory test capable of determining whether Ms. Warner is pregnant is
○ 1. blood for alpha-fetoprotein (AFP).
○ 2. blood for cortisol levels.
○ 3. blood or urine for human chorionic gonadotropin (HCG).
○ 4. urine for FSH.

Ms. Warner is scheduled to have an amniocentesis. Her physician has explained the reason for the test.

14 To correctly reinforce the physician's explanation, the nurse should know that an amniocentesis is *probably* performed to help determine
○ 1. the sex of the fetus.
○ 2. the maturity of the fetus.
○ 3. whether the amniotic fluid is excessive.
○ 4. whether a fetal abnormality is present.

15 Ms. Warner is scheduled to have a chorionic villus sampling. When preparing her for the procedure; and possibly answering some of her questions, the nurse should know that this procedure is performed to
○ 1. determine the levels of placental hormones.
○ 2. determine the presence of a fetal abnormality.
○ 3. identify the position of the umbilical cord.
○ 4. identify placement of the placenta.

ASSESSING THE PREGNANT CLIENT

Ms. Adele Gant makes an appointment to be seen in a prenatal clinic. It is determined that Ms. Gant is pregnant. She has three children, a son and twin daughters. She has no history of having had an abortion or a stillborn.

16 In terms of *gravida* and *para*, the nurse can make an entry on Ms. Gant's record as being
○ 1. gravida III, para II.
○ 2. gravida III, para III.

○ 3. gravida II, para II.

○ 4. gravida II, para III.

17 The nurse in charge of the prenatal clinic entered a nursing diagnosis of "anxiety related to emotional responses to pregnancy" on Ms. Gant's clinical record. When talking to Ms. Gant the nurse could ask

○ 1. if she wants this baby.

○ 2. how she feels about being pregnant.

○ 3. if her family has accepted her pregnancy.

○ 4. why she got pregnant.

18 During a prenatal visit Ms. Gant admits that during previous pregnancies she never saw a physician until she was ready to deliver her baby. Ms. Gant asks what the desired weight gain should be during pregnancy. The *most correct* reply is

○ 1. 25 to 30 lb.

○ 2. 10 to 20 lb.

○ 3. less than 15 lb.

○ 4. no more than 18 to 20 lb.

19 Ms. Gant asks when her baby will be due and states that her last menstrual period began on March 13. Using Nägele's rule, the nurse can tell Ms. Gant that her delivery date will be approximately

○ 1. November 13

○ 2. November 23

○ 3. December 3

○ 4. December 20

20 How many weeks can Ms. Gant be expected to be pregnant when the nurse can *first* hear fetal heart sounds?

○ 1. 7 to 8 weeks

○ 2. 10 to 12 weeks

○ 3. 13 to 15 weeks

○ 4. 18 to 20 weeks

21 Which of the following should the nurse do while listening with the fetoscope on the abdomen for fetal heart sounds?

○ 1. Have the mother lie on her left side.

○ 2. Obtain the mother's respiratory rate prior to listening for fetal heart sounds.

○ 3. Feel for the mother's radial pulse rate.

○ 4. Encourage the mother to take very deep breaths.

22 To evaluate the fetal heart rate the nurse should know that the normal fetal heart rate is

○ 1. 80 to 100 beats per minute.

○ 2. 80 to 160 beats per minute.

○ 3. 90 to 140 beats per minute.

○ 4. 120 to 160 beats per minute.

Ms. Alice Long is 3 months pregnant and is an insulin-dependent diabetic. This is her first pregnancy.

23 During a prenatal visit the nurse notes that Ms. Long appears anxious and somewhat nervous. When talking to Ms. Long the nurse should remember that

○ 1. diabetes may result in emotional instability during pregnancy.

○ 2. pregnancy causes substantial emotional stress on the diabetic and her family.

○ 3. her estrogen level may be low.

○ 4. she may be exhibiting signs that she is carrying a deformed fetus.

24 Ms. Long is to have an ultrasound examination. When explaining the purpose of this procedure, the nurse can describe it as an examination used to

○ 1. determine the size of the fetus.

○ 2. take a sample of amniotic fluid.

○ 3. determine the adequacy of hormone levels.

○ 4. estimate the fetal heart rate.

COMMON DISCOMFORTS OF PREGNANCY

Nurses working in a prenatal clinic or physician's office often are asked many questions about some of the minor problems that may occur during pregnancy.

25 Ms. Volare is 5 months pregnant and complains of constipation. The nurse can teach this client that constipation often can be controlled if pregnant women increase their

○ 1. periods of rest.

○ 2. exercise.

○ 3. caloric intake.

○ 4. vitamin intake.

26 Ms. Mueller has varicose veins and asks the nurse what can be done to relieve the discomfort associated with this problem. The nurse can advise the client to *avoid*

○ 1. crossing her legs, knees, or ankles.

○ 2. staying off her feet.

○ 3. eating foods high in fat.

○ 4. putting her feet higher than her hips.

27 Ms. Parker states that she has developed varicose veins. What advice regarding this problem should the nurse give Ms. Parker?

○ 1. Gently massage the affected areas several times a day.

○ 2. Apply an elastic bandage over the affected area.

○ 3. Sit in a chair with the feet flat on the floor for 20 minutes three to six times a day.

○ 4. Contact the physician if soreness, redness, or warmth develops in the veins.

28 Ms. Wiles also has varicose veins and has been following suggestions regarding situations to avoid. She states that the discomfort associated with her varicosities has markedly decreased. Which one of the following is the *most appropriate* entry on Ms. Wiles record?

○ 1. Varicosities have disappeared and require no further treatment.

    ○ 2. Arterial blood flow is decreased.
    ○ 3. Discomfort is controlled or minimized.
    ○ 4. Venous blood flow is decreased.

29 Ms. Young says, "My skin itches so much. What can I do about it?" The most appropriate suggestion the nurse can make is that this discomfort may be *relieved* by
    ○ 1. decreasing fluid intake.
    ○ 2. taking vitamin C.
    ○ 3. using a lotion on areas of dryness.
    ○ 4. taking frequent rest periods.

30 Ms. Gates, who has had no complications and is now approximately 8 months pregnant, has edema in her feet. The nurse should explain to Ms. Gates that edema late in pregnancy is believed to be *caused* primarily by
    ○ 1. a decrease in blood pressure.
    ○ 2. the pressure of an enlarged uterus on pelvic veins.
    ○ 3. the effect of hormones on the venous system.
    ○ 4. a change in pressure in the renal arteries.

31 The nurse can advise Ms. Gates that edema may *decrease* if she
    ○ 1. exercises for 45 minutes three times a day.
    ○ 2. lowers her daily intake of salt.
    ○ 3. eats more vegetables.
    ○ 4. takes extra vitamin C.

32 Another recommendation that the nurse can be give to Ms. Gates to *relieve* her edema is to
    ○ 1. elevate her legs and feet for short periods during the day.
    ○ 2. bathe her legs in warm water several times a day.
    ○ 3. massage her legs several times a day.
    ○ 4. eat a diet high in protein.

33 Ms. Booth complains of shortness of breath and occasional difficulty in breathing. To identify and evaluate this client's problem, the nurse should know that dyspnea often is a *normal* discomfort during the
    ○ 1. early part of the first trimester.
    ○ 2. late part of the first trimester.
    ○ 3. second trimester.
    ○ 4. third trimester.

34 The nurse in charge of a prenatal clinic charts a nursing diagnosis of "Anxiety related to the discomforts associated with normal physiological changes of pregnancy" on the record of a client who is pregnant for the first time. Based on this nursing diagnosis the nurse should plan to
    ○ 1. explain that discomfort is experienced by most pregnant women and therefore must be tolerated.
    ○ 2. give the client a list of books that may offer suggestions.

    ○ 3. tell the client to wait 2 weeks to see if the discomforts disappear.
    ○ 4. answer questions during prenatal visits.

35 Ms. Warren, who has been in good health during pregnancy, says she urinates frequently, "... just as I did early in pregnancy." The nurse should explain that the *most probable* cause of frequent urination late in pregnancy is that the
    ○ 1. mother has alkaline urine.
    ○ 2. mother is developing a urinary infection.
    ○ 3. enlarging uterus is causing pressure on the bladder.
    ○ 4. growing fetus is excreting increased amounts of wastes.

36 Ms. Harper is 2 months pregnant and complains of having to urinate at frequent intervals. The nurse should explain that frequent urination *early* in pregnancy usually subsides when the
    ○ 1. placenta is fully developed.
    ○ 2. fetal kidneys begin to function.
    ○ 3. uterus rises into the abdominal cavity.
    ○ 4. mother's kidneys adjust to the added load of fetal wastes.

37 Ms. Maples is 5 months pregnant and complains of a backache. To relieve this discomfort the nurse can advise her to
    ○ 1. avoid taking tub baths.
    ○ 2. decrease the amount of liquids in her diet.
    ○ 3. avoid coffee and spicy foods.
    ○ 4. wear low-heeled shoes.

38 Nausea is a common problem in the first trimester of pregnancy. Unless the nausea is severe the nurse may advise the client to
    ○ 1. drink extra water with meals.
    ○ 2. eat small, frequent meals.
    ○ 3. take an antacid after eating.
    ○ 4. eat only two large meals a day.

39 Ms. Allen has a history of blood clots and thrombophlebitis during past pregnancies. She is now pregnant again and asks what she can do to relieve leg cramps. Which of the following is the *most appropriate* response for this client?
    ○ 1. Stretch the leg by moving the foot so that the toes point toward the kneecap.
    ○ 2. Increase the fluid intake.
    ○ 3. Eat a diet high in proteins and vitamins C and E.
    ○ 4. Massage the muscles of the calf of the leg.

40 Ms. Kyle complains of heartburn and asks what may be done to relieve this problem. The nurse can suggest that the client
    ○ 1. drink one to three glasses of fluid with meals.
    ○ 2. eat her largest meal of the day after 7:00 PM.
    ○ 3. mix 1 teaspoon of sodium bicarbonate in a glass of water.
    ○ 4. eat frequent, small meals.

41 Ms. Leonard has a complaint for which the nurse recommends using the pelvic rock (pelvic tilt). For which of the following discomforts of pregnancy is the pelvic rock most often recommended?
○ 1. Backaches
○ 2. Heartburn
○ 3. Varicosities
○ 4. Constipation

HIGH-RISK FACTORS AND PREGNANCY

The nurse is asked to discuss high-risk factors with a small group of women attending a prenatal clinic

42 When planning for this discussion the nurse decides to bring up the topic of the consumption of alcohol by pregnant women, which is known to cause fetal alcohol syndrome (FAS). This disorder is evidenced in the newborn by problems such as mental deficiencies, flat facial features, and
○ 1. blindness.
○ 2. birth weight greater than 8 pounds.
○ 3. joint and limb abnormalities.
○ 4. an immature immune system.

43 Another topic the nurse can plan to discuss is the use of drugs. Newborns of mothers addicted to a narcotic such as heroin
○ 1. show no signs of narcotic addiction.
○ 2. rarely require treatment.
○ 3. suffer withdrawal symptoms.
○ 4. gain weight rapidly.

In the discussion of risk factors, the nurse plans to discuss smoking during pregnancy.

44 Smoking during pregnancy carries a risk of giving birth to a baby that
○ 1. is smaller than normal owing to intrauterine growth reduction.
○ 2. is 1 to 2 pounds overweight.
○ 3. has a higher than normal blood oxygen level.
○ 4. has a low carbon monoxide blood level.

COMPLICATIONS OF PREGNANCY

Ms. Laura Mitchell is a 25-year-old primigravida. Although she was sure she was pregnant, she waited 4 months before making an appointment to see a physician at the prenatal clinic sponsored by a hospital in her area.

45 In planning a teaching program for Ms. Mitchell, the nurse should include the importance of immediately contacting the physician
○ 1. the first time fetal movement is noted.
○ 2. if the breasts become tender or sore.
○ 3. if bleeding from the vagina occurs.
○ 4. if frequent urination is noted.

During her third prenatal visit, Ms. Mitchell complains of an abundant vaginal discharge, and the physician determines she has trichomoniasis.

46 When planning for questions this client may ask during prenatal visits, the nurse should know that this infection
○ 1. frequently occurs during the first trimester of pregnancy.
○ 2. is a sexually transmitted disease.
○ 3. usually disappears during the second trimester.
○ 4. poses no danger to the client or the developing fetus.

47 Ms. Mitchell calls her physician to say she has been vomiting at frequent intervals for almost 4 days. The nurse urges Ms. Mitchell to come to the office promptly, recognizing that this client may have
○ 1. reflex emesis.
○ 2. neurotic emesis.
○ 3. cyclic vomiting.
○ 4. hyperemesis gravidarum.

Ms. Camille Larson is a 31-year-old multipara. She has been seen regularly by a physician since she first noted that she may be pregnant.

48 Ms. Larson is told by the physician that she has an incompetent cervix. When explaining this term to Ms. Smith, the nurse should understand that an *incompetent cervix* means that the
○ 1. contents of the uterus force the cervix to close.
○ 2. cervix becomes short and thick.
○ 3. client will require a cesarean section.
○ 4. weight of the fetus causes the cervix to dilate.

49 To develop a plan of care for Ms. Larson, the nurse should know that *one* method of treating an incompetent cervix is by
○ 1. diet, moderate exercise, and long periods of rest.
○ 2. the Shirodkar procedure.
○ 3. the Keigel procedure.
○ 4. special exercises performed 3 to 4 times a day.

Ms. Marion Bradley is 21 years old and is told by her physician that she has pregnancy-induced hypertension (PIH), also called preeclampsia.

50 Ms. Bradley asks the nurse what caused this problem. The nurse should base her response on knowledge that the *cause* of PIH is
○ 1. unknown.
○ 2. related to the client's age.
○ 3. directly related to the number of pregnancies.
○ 4. the carrying of a malformed fetus.

Ms. Bradley now demonstrates typical signs and symptoms of PIH.

51 To collect pertinent data the nurse should know that the one sign or symptom *least* characteristic of PIH is
○ 1. fluid retention.
○ 2. albumin in the urine.
○ 3. an irregular pulse rate.
○ 4. an elevated blood pressure.

Ms. Bradley's symptoms become worse, and she is hospitalized. The physician orders her to be observed for signs of eclampsia.

52 Ms. Bradley will be considered to have developed *eclampsia* if she has
○ 1. convulsions.
○ 2. a dead fetus.
○ 3. renal failure.
○ 4. an irregular pulse.

53 To prepare for an emergency, which one of the following medications should the nurse make available for immediate administration if Ms. Bradley develops eclampsia?
○ 1. Morphine sulfate
○ 2. Oxytocin
○ 3. Ergonovine maleate (Ergotrate)
○ 4. Magnesium sulfate (MgSO$_4$)

54 If Ms. Bradley develops eclampsia, the care plan should include
○ 1. monitoring vital signs daily.
○ 2. hourly measurement of urine output.
○ 3. allowing the client to socialize with others.
○ 4. providing diversional therapy, such as reading material or television.

During a prenatal history Ms. Lottie Davis, who has four children, states that she had a previous ectopic pregnancy. The physician examining Ms. Davis suspects that she may have another ectopic pregnancy.

55 To develop an appropriate plan of care for Ms. Davis, the nurse should know that an ectopic pregnancy
○ 1. occurs outside of the uterus.
○ 2. causes rupture of the uterus.
○ 3. results in some form of fetal malformation.
○ 4. progresses even though the woman continues to menstruate.

56 When a client with an ectopic pregnancy is hospitalized, the *highest* priority stated in a care plan should be to observe her for signs of
○ 1. infection.
○ 2. hemorrhage.
○ 3. uterine relaxation.
○ 4. premature delivery.

Ms. Wyna Selkirk has a history of spontaneous abortion. She has delivered two live infants and has had one stillborn and two spontaneous abortions. Her physician decides to admit her to the hospital for evaluation of her present symptoms.

57 Two symptoms that may indicate to the nurse that Ms. Selkirk is very likely to abort are vaginal bleeding and
○ 1. ankle swelling.
○ 2. severe headaches.
○ 3. persistent nausea.
○ 4. abdominal cramping.

The physician decides that Ms. Selkirk should be observed closely for signs and symptoms of a spontaneous abortion.

58 When developing a care plan for Ms. Selkirk, the nurse should know that a spontaneous abortion
○ 1. rarely is associated with physical discomforts.
○ 2. occurs only during the first trimester of pregnancy.
○ 3. is the result of conditions that are not related to pregnancy.
○ 4. occurs without the client having done anything to cause it.

59 Assessment of Ms. Selkirk, who now has signs and symptoms of a threatened spontaneous abortion, should include
○ 1. monitoring vital signs every 8 hours.
○ 2. observing for uterine cramping and loss of amniotic fluid.
○ 3. observing for the presence of abdominal fluid.
○ 4. observing for an increase in uterine size.

Ms. Lottie Arnold is a 22-year-old diabetic patient who is pregnant for the first time. Ms. Arnold takes 24 U of NPH insulin daily and adheres to the diet prescribed by her physician. Now that she is pregnant, Ms. Arnold has many questions regarding pregnancy and diabetes.

60 The nurse is assigned to discuss pregnancy and diabetes with Ms. Arnold. The nurse should include in a teaching session
○ 1. the importance of avoiding episodes of hyperglycemia.
○ 2. a dietary plan that decreases protein intake.
○ 3. a chart for the mother to record movements of the fetus.
○ 4. the importance of eating a high calorie diet.

61 Ms. Arnold asks about the problems her baby may experience. When planning a teaching and discussion session the nurse should include the fact that diabetic clients are *most likely* to deliver an infant that
○ 1. has multiple birth defects.
○ 2. is a diabetic.

○ 3. cannot tolerate breast feeding.

○ 4. is larger than average.

62 One primary objective in the plan of care for the diabetic mother throughout her pregnancy is

○ 1. decreasing the mother's insulin needs.

○ 2. helping the mother to understand the changes that occur during pregnancy.

○ 3. keeping maternal blood glucose levels as close to normal as possible.

○ 4. explaining the need to decrease her calorie intake and increase her insulin dosage.

Ms. Marsha Jackson is a 26-year-old multigravida who is 8 months pregnant. She calls the prenatal clinic for an immediate appointment because she thinks she is having a problem.

63 During assessment of Ms. Jackson, the nurse in charge of a prenatal clinic tells the nurses that Ms. Jackson may have placenta previa because she complains of

○ 1. sudden, sharp abdominal pain.

○ 2. painless bleeding from the vagina.

○ 3. persistent headaches.

○ 4. continuous, painless uterine contractions.

64 To evaluate and act appropriately when Ms. Jackson tells the nurse about her symptoms, the nurse should know that placenta previa usually *first* becomes apparent during the

○ 1. first month of pregnancy.

○ 2. second or third month of pregnancy.

○ 3. the second trimester of pregnancy.

○ 4. the third trimester of pregnancy.

65 Ms. Jackson is admitted to the hospital. Which one of the following should the nurse obtain *first*?

○ 1. Weight

○ 2. Blood pressure and pulse rate

○ 3. A history of pregnancies

○ 4. A general health and drug history

66 To develop a care plan for Ms. Jackson, the nurse should know that placenta previa is due to a condition in which the placenta is

○ 1. invaded by polyps or myomas.

○ 2. degenerating on the maternal or the fetal side.

○ 3. covering the cervical os or implanted low in the uterus.

○ 4. failing in its ability to produce hormones or enzymes that act to maintain pregnancy.

Ms. Dolores Mason is in her last trimester and is diagnosed as having abruptio placentae.

67 To collect important data about Ms. Mason, the nurse should know that this condition is a

○ 1. form of premature labor.

○ 2. covering of the cervical os by the placenta.

○ 3. premature rupture of the membranes.

○ 4. premature separation of a normally implanted placenta.

68 A plan of care for the client with *severe* (complete) abruptio placentae should include

○ 1. asking the family to sign a surgical consent.

○ 2. observing the client for signs of shock.

○ 3. keeping the client in a sitting position.

○ 4. having the client lie on her left side.

NUTRITION DURING PREGNANCY

The physician determines that Ms. Chelsea Underwood, who is 4 months pregnant, has not been adhering to an adequate diet and requires counseling by the nurse.

69 Prior to counseling Ms. Underwood on the nutritional needs of pregnancy, the nurse needs to know

○ 1. if all family members are willing to adhere to a special diet regimen.

○ 2. what her diet is now.

○ 3. what foods the client likes to eat.

○ 4. if she can afford the special foods required during pregnancy.

70 When explaining the recommended diet to Ms. Underwood, the nurse should emphasize the importance of

○ 1. substituting animal proteins for plant proteins.

○ 2. eating foods that are low in iron and phosphorus.

○ 3. eating a well-balanced, nutritious diet.

○ 4. eating foods that are low in calories and folic acid.

71 It is determined that Ms. Underwood has not been eating a diet sufficiently high in calcium. In addition to milk and dairy products, which of the following foods or food types could the nurse recommend to Ms. Underwood?

○ 1. Fresh fruits

○ 2. White bread or rolls

○ 3. Green vegetables

○ 4. Gelatin

72 Ms. Underwood is told by her physician to "drink lots of milk." She asks the nurse how much milk she should drink every day. The most appropriate response to this question is

○ 1. 1 cup.

○ 2. 2 cups.

○ 3. 3 cups.

○ 4. 4 cups.

73 The nurse asks Ms. Underwood to bring in a list of foods that she has been eating during the past 2 weeks. The nurse must remember that it is important that Ms. Underwood's diet contains larger-than-

average amounts of the minerals calcium, phosphorus, and
- ○ 1. iron.
- ○ 2. sodium.
- ○ 3. potassium.
- ○ 4. chlorides.

TEACHING THE PREGNANT CLIENT

The nurse has been asked to develop a plan of instruction for women attending a prenatal clinic.

74 When planning an instructional program for pregnant women, the nurse plans to include a discussion about the importance of not taking any drug during pregnancy. When reviewing textbooks and references, the nurse notes the use of the word *teratogen*. This term refers to an agent or factor that is likely to cause
- ○ 1. premature labor.
- ○ 2. physical defects in the fetus.
- ○ 3. PIH.
- ○ 4. premature separation of the placenta.

75 During a discussion, one of the women in the class asks the nurse about sterilization procedures that will prevent further pregnancies. Which one of the following permanent sterilization procedures performed on the female can the nurse discuss with the class?
- ○ 1. Anterior colpopexy
- ○ 2. Vas ligation
- ○ 3. Unilateral oophorectomy
- ○ 4. Electrocoagulation of the fallopian tubes

76 Several women ask the nurse about the function of the placenta. In addition to carrying nourishment to the fetus and wastes from it, the *most correct* answer is based on the fact that the placenta also functions to
- ○ 1. store nutrients for the fetus.
- ○ 2. prevent certain fetal malformations.
- ○ 3. provide the body with several hormones.
- ○ 4. remove microorganisms from the maternal blood.

77 Another client in the prenatal class asks about amniotic fluid. The most correct answer is based on the fact that the purpose of amniotic fluid is to
- ○ 1. provide the fetus with antibodies.
- ○ 2. protect the fetus from external injury.
- ○ 3. provide oxygen for the fetus.
- ○ 4. help lower the body temperature of the mother.

78 One of the women in the prenatal class mentions that during her first prenatal visit, the physician stated that she had a positive Chadwick's sign and asks what this means. The nurse replies that a *positive* Chadwick's sign is a
- ○ 1. painless contraction.

- ○ 2. softening of the cervix.
- ○ 3. softening of the lower segment of the uterus.
- ○ 4. discoloration of the vulva and vagina during pregnancy.

79 The nurse plans to include a discussion of *TORCH*, which is
- ○ 1. the development of fetal distress in the third trimester.
- ○ 2. the development of fetal malformations.
- ○ 3. a group of diseases known to cause harm to the fetus in utero.
- ○ 4. the development of an immature placenta.

80 Another woman asks the nurse about the function of the umbilical cord. The most correct answer is based on the fact that *one* purpose of the umbilical cord is to
- ○ 1. provide oxygen to the fetus by means of the umbilical vein.
- ○ 2. remove waste products from maternal blood.
- ○ 3. deliver antibodies from the fetus to the mother.
- ○ 4. provide nourishment of the fetus by means of the umbilical artery.

ELECTIVE ABORTION

Ms. Grace Parker has discussed the possibility of terminating her pregnancy and has many questions and concerns regarding abortion.

81 Ms. Parker's first question is how many weeks a woman has to be pregnant before the fetus can live outside the uterus. The most correct answer is based on the fact that the legal threshold of viability usually is estimated to be
- ○ 1. 34 weeks.
- ○ 2. 10 to 15 weeks.
- ○ 3. 30 to 35 weeks.
- ○ 4. 20 to 24 weeks.

82 Ms. Parker decides to have an abortion and asks the nurse if there are any restrictions on this procedure. Being informed of legal issues allows the nurse to discuss the 1989 United States Supreme Court decision that a state cannot interfere with a client's right to have an abortion if she wants one and if she
- ○ 1. is not married.
- ○ 2. has had previous children.
- ○ 3. has the consent of the father.
- ○ 4. is not in violation of permissible state restrictions.

83 Ms. Parker, who is approximately 9 weeks pregnant, asks how the abortion will be performed. To answer the client's question the nurse should know that the preferred techniques for terminating a pregnancy of less than 3 months are dilatation and curettage and
- ○ 1. dilatation and aspiration.
- ○ 2. hysterotomy.

3. administration of intravenous progesterone.

4. injection of oxytocin into the amniotic sac.

INDIVIDUAL TEST ITEMS

84 Ms. Carnes makes her first visit to a prenatal clinic. She is pregnant for the first time. The term that will be entered in her clinical record that describes a first-time pregnancy is

1. multipara.

2. primipara.

3. primigravida.

4. multigravida.

85 When assessing a client with a history of PIH, the nurse should observe for

1. a decrease in urine proteins.

2. an increase in urine output.

3. a decrease in the pulse rate.

4. any sudden gain in weight.

86 Ms. Miller, who is 3 months pregnant, states that she recently had rubella (German measles). To collect important data about Ms. Miller's recent infection, the nurse should know that the *primary* danger of having had rubella early in pregnancy is

1. premature labor.

2. fetal deformities.

3. severe preeclampsia.

4. hydatidiform mole formation.

87 Ms. Johnson has a rubella screening test at the time of her first prenatal visit and asks why the test was performed. The nurse may answer the client's question by explaining that the purpose of this test is to determine the

1. mother's immunity to the rubella virus.

2. mother's ability to produce antibodies.

3. mother's need for a rubella virus vaccine.

4. fetus' immunity to the rubella virus.

88 When collecting data during Ms. Sharp's clinic visit the nurse should be aware of high-risk factors. Which one of the following should alert the nurse that the client may be in a high-risk group?

1. The client is pregnant for the third time.

2. The client has taken acetaminophen (Tylenol) occasionally for headaches prior to her pregnancy.

3. The client has a history of twins in the family.

4. The client has diabetes mellitus.

89 Ms. France, who is close to delivery, has herpes simplex virus type II (genital herpes). For which of the following related to Ms. France's delivery should the nurse prepare?

1. A forceps delivery

2. A cesarean delivery

3. A precipitate delivery

4. An artificial rupturing of the membranes

90 Ms. Hill, who has acquired immunodeficiency syndrome (AIDS), is 3 months pregnant. When preparing to answer her questions about AIDS and her newborn baby, the nurse must be aware that the virus may be transmitted from the mother to the newborn by means of

1. the placenta as it is expelled after delivery.

2. infant contact with infected maternal blood at birth.

3. handling the baby after birth.

4. Rh factors in the mother's blood.

91 Ms. Larkin has a *Chlamydia trachomatis* infection and is in her last trimester of pregnancy. When planning for her delivery, the nurse must be aware that this infection, *if untreated*,

1. can be transmitted to the newborn during delivery.

2. causes AIDS in the newborn.

3. results in an immature immune system in the newborn.

4. is not transmitted to the newborn.

Correct Answers and Rationale

Two numbers appear in parentheses following each rationale. The first number identifies the textbook listed in the references, page 451, and the second number identifies the page(s) in that textbook on which the correct answer can be verified. Occasionally, two textbooks are given for verifying the correct answer.

The Prenatal Period

ANATOMY AND PHYSIOLOGY OF THE MALE AND FEMALE REPRODUCTIVE SYSTEMS

1 1. Estrogens develop and maintain the female reproductive system. Increased estrogen levels during pregnancy are necessary for increasing the size of the uterus, the breasts, and glandular breast tissue. Progesterone and its derivatives (progestins) are necessary for the development of the placenta. Cortisone is a hormone produced by the adrenal gland of both sexes. (8:30; 15:214)
   Nursing Process—Planning
   Client Need—Health promotion/maintenance

2 4. The release of FSH stimulates the maturation of the ovarian follicle, followed by the release of luteinizing hormone, resulting in ovulation. Prolactin, when released by the pituitary gland, stimulates milk production in the breasts. Oxytocin is responsible for ejection of milk from the breasts. Luteinizing hormone is responsible for the maturation of the graafian follicle, ovulation, and the formation of the corpus luteum. Antidiuretic hormone prevents excessive water loss. (19:25)
   Nursing Process—Planning
   Client Need—Health promotion/maintenance

3 4. The anterior pituitary secretes FSH and luteinizing hormone, both of which are necessary for spermatogenesis (sperm production). The posterior pituitary gland secretes antidiuretic hormone and oxytocin. Testosterone, which is produced by the testes, is responsible for the development and maintenance of secondary male sex characteristics. (19:17–18)
   Nursing Process—Planning
   Client Need—Health promotion/maintenance

4 3. Each ovum has an X chromosome, but a sperm may carry an X or a Y chromosome. If a sperm carrying an X chromosome penetrates an ovum, the result is a female fetus. If a sperm carrying a Y chromosome penetrates an ovum, the result will be a male fetus. (13:80; 8:36)
   Nursing Process—Implementation
   Client Need—Health promotion/maintenance

5 2. Progesterone helps to prepare the uterus for pregnancy. It is produced by the corpus luteum. Prosecretin is a precursor of secretin, which is a hormone secreted by mucous membranes of the duodenum and jejunum. The human growth hormone, also called somatotropin, is concerned primarily with the growth of bones, muscles, and other organs. It is secreted by the anterior pituitary gland. FSH stimulates the development of ovarian follicles, the secretion of estrogen, the development of seminiferous tubules, and the maturation of spermatozoa. (13:54)
   Nursing Process—Planning
   Client Need—Health promotion/maintenance

6 4. The endometrium is the inner lining of the uterus. The myometrium is the middle muscular layer. The perimetrium is the outer layer and is continuous with the peritoneum, which lines the abdominal cavity. (8:24)
   Nursing Process—Planning
   Client Need—Health promotion/maintenance

7 2. Sperm are propelled by movements of their tail-like portion, called the flagellum. Sperm do not have cilia. They do not move in the female by contractions of the cervix or uterus or by pressure differences in the uterus and fallopian tubes. (13:67–69; 11:327)
   Nursing Process—Implementation
   Client Need—Health promotion/maintenance

8 1. Each cell in the human body contains 46 chromosomes, as do immature germ cells. By the process of meiosis the number of chromosomes decreases in each germ cell so that by maturity, each ovum and each sperm contains 23 chromosomes. When the sperm containing 23 chromosomes and the ovum containing 23 chromosomes unite, the new cell contains 46 chromosomes. (13:80; 11:350)

>Nursing Process—Planning
>Client Need—Health promotion/maintenance

9 4. Conception normally takes place in the outer half of a fallopian tube. The fertilized ovum then divides and subdivides many times (mitosis) while it journeys down the fallopian tube to the uterus, where it will implant. (19:21–22)

>Nursing Process—Planning
>Client Need—Health promotion/maintenance

SIGNS AND SYMPTOMS OF PREGNANCY; TESTS FOR PREGNANCY

10 3. Fetal movements usually are detectable by the trained examiner in the second trimester and are one of several positive signs of pregnancy. Other positive signs are fetal heartbeat and detection of a fetus by ultrasound. Breast changes, weight gain, and nausea and vomiting are presumptive signs of pregnancy because these symptoms may be due to other causes. (19:49)

>Nursing Process—Implementation
>Client Need—Health promotion/maintenance

11 3. An enlarged uterus is classified as a probable sign of pregnancy. Morning sickness, quickening, and tingling sensations in the breasts are classified as presumptive signs of pregnancy because they can be due to conditions other than pregnancy. (8:58; 14:541)

>Nursing Process—Collecting data
>Client Need—Health promotion/maintenance

12 1. Chloasma may be described as brown blotchy areas on the face. It often is called the mask of pregnancy. Pigmentation of the nipples and areolae also is typical during pregnancy. The dark vertical line on the abdomen is called linea nigra. Stretch marks on the abdomen, thighs, and breasts are called striae gravidarum. (14:540)

>Nursing Process—Implementation
>Client Need—Health promotion/maintenance

13 3. Levels of HCG rise significantly shortly after fertilization of the ovum. Blood or urine testing for HCG is the basis for most pregnancy tests. Alpha-fetoproteins can detect fetal neural tube malformations, which result in conditions such as hydrocephalus and spina bifida. (8:58–59; 5:219–220)

>Nursing Process—Planning
>Client Need—Health promotion/maintenance

14 4. Early in pregnancy, an amniocentesis usually is performed to help determine whether the fetus has a genetic abnormality. If one exists, the parents may decide to terminate the pregnancy. The fetal sex can be determined by amniocentesis but is not done primarily for this reason. In many cases, amniocentesis is performed to detect Down syndrome. Near-term and in high-isk pregnancies, an amniocentesis may be performed to determine fetal well-being. (14:536; 19:106–107)

>Nursing Process—Implementation
>Client Need—Safe, effective care environment

15 2. Some fetal abnormalities can be detected by chorionic villus sampling followed by DNA analysis or use of genetic markers. The physician must explain the procedure and why it is being performed, but the nurse must be aware that the client probably knows that a fetal abnormality is suspected and therefore must be prepared to give emotional support to the client. (8:324–325)

>Nursing Process—Implementation
>Client Need—Physiological integrity

ASSESSING THE PREGNANT CLIENT

16 1. Gravida is the term used to indicate that a woman is pregnant or has been pregnant. Gravida also may be described as the number of pregnancies a woman has had, regardless of whether she gave birth to a live infant, a stillborn infant, or an aborted fetus. The first time she is pregnant, she is gravida I. On subsequent pregnancies she is gravida II, III, and so forth. The client described is gravida III because she is pregnant for the third time. Her two pregnancies prior to this pregnancy resulted in three children—a son and twin daughters. Para is the term used to indicate the number of pregnancies a woman has completed that resulted in the delivery of a viable or potentially viable infant (an infant weighing more than 500 g or more than 20 weeks' gestation), regardless of whether the infant was born alive or was stillborn. Multiple births, such as twins, are counted as *one* para. The client described in this item is para 2. (8:63)

>Nursing Process—Collecting data
>Client Need—Health promotion/maintenance

17 2. Asking how a client feels about being pregnant may provide an opening for the client to discuss her feelings and emotions about this pregnancy. This, in turn, may reduce anxiety and allow the client an opportunity to explore her feelings. (8:81)

>Nursing Process—Implementation
>Client Need—Psychosocial integrity

18 1. Although references vary slightly, the approximate recommended average weight gain during pregnancy is 25 to 30 lb. (8:76–77; 19:57–58)
Nursing Process—Implementation
Client Need—Health promotion/maintenance

19 4. Nägele's rule requires adding 7 days to the first day of the woman's last menstrual period and then counting back 3 months. This means the client described in this item is due to deliver on December 20. (19:46; 8:66)
Nursing Process—Implementation
Client Need—Health promotion/maintenance

20 4. Using a fetoscope, fetal heart tones ordinarily are heard first after 18 to 20 weeks of pregnancy. They may be heard as early as 10 to 12 weeks by using ultrasound. (19:49)
Nursing Process—Collecting data
Client Need—Health promotion/maintenance

21 3. When using a fetoscope to auscultate for fetal heart sounds, the nurse must be careful not to confuse fetal sounds with pulsations in the mother's aorta. This can be avoided when the nurse feels for the mother's radial pulse while listening for fetal heart sounds. The fetal pulse usually is considerably faster than the mother's heartbeat. (13:217)
Nursing Process—Collecting data
Client Need—Health promotion/maintenance

22 4. The normal fetal heart rate is 120 to 160 beats per minute. Rates above or below these figures are reported to the physician immediately. (13:216–217)
Nursing Process—Evaluation
Client Need—Physiological integrity

23 2. Pregnancy places a great deal of stress on all women. The diabetic client may be faced with problems such as repeated tests, the added expense of these tests, and hospitalization to control her diabetes or correct problems associated with her diabetes *and* pregnancy. (19:76)
Nursing Process—Collecting data
Client Need—Psychosocial integrity

24 1. The size of the fetus can be determined by ultrasound examination, which is a painless, *noninvasive* procedure. This examination also may determine the sex of the fetus and the volume of amniotic fluid and estimate fetal growth rates. (8:171; 19:103)
Nursing Process—Planning
Client Need—Health promotion/maintenance

COMMON DISCOMFORTS OF PREGNANCY

25 2. Constipation often can be controlled during pregnancy when women observe an appropriate exercise program. Other measures that often relieve constipation include increasing roughage in the diet, increasing fluid intake, and observing regular habits of elimination. Pregnant women should be taught to avoid laxatives and enemas to relieve constipation, unless prescribed for them. In some difficult cases a stool softener may be prescribed or recommended by the physician. (19:63–64)
Nursing Process—Implementation
Client Need—Safe, effective care environment

26 1. Crossing the legs, knees, or ankles reduces venous return, resulting in a collection of blood in and distention of the veins of the legs. The discomfort of varicose veins can be prevented by avoiding crossing the legs, knees, or ankles. The client also can be instructed to avoid tight garments and stay off her feet as much as possible. Staying off her feet and putting her feet higher than her hips also may reduce discomfort. Foods high in fat should be avoided during pregnancy but would have no effect on relieving the discomfort associated with varicose veins. (13:123; 16:318–319)
Nursing Process—Implementation
Client Need—Safe, effective care environment

27 4. Varicose veins can result in thrombophlebitis, which is evidenced by soreness, redness, or warmth in the affected area. If varicosities occur, they should be examined by the physician during routine prenatal visits. The occurrence of thrombophlebitis requires immediate treatment by a physician. Varicose veins should never be rubbed or massaged, especially if signs and symptoms of thrombophlebitis are present. Sitting in a chair promotes venous stasis and may make the problem worse. The application of elastic stockings, only when recommended by the physician, usually is preferable to the application of an elastic bandage, which in the late stages of pregnancy may be difficult to apply. (13:123; 16:315–316)
Nursing Process—Implementation
Client Need—Safe, effective care environment

28 3. Elevating the legs; periodic rest periods; avoiding tight garments and crossing the legs, ankles, or feet; and avoiding prolonged standing are some of the measures that often help control or minimize the discomfort related to varicose veins during pregnancy. Evaluation of this client appropriately is aimed at determining if the symptoms appear to be decreased. Varicosities are not likely to disappear when the nurse's recommendations are used; most likely surgery may be required if the varicosities become worse. There should be an increase rather than a de-

crease in arterial blood flow and an increase rather than a decrease in venous blood flow if basic recommendations are followed. (8:165; 16:319–320)
Nursing Process—Evaluation
Client Need—Physiological integrity

29 3. Itching of the skin is not uncommon and is an annoying discomfort of pregnancy. There are several ways to help promote relief. Oiling the skin after bathing and increasing fluid intake may offer some relief. Soap probably should not be used, but if it is, it should be used sparingly and should be very mild. (13:123)
Nursing Process—Implementation
Client Need—Safe, effective care environment

30 2. Provided that no other medical complication or disorder is present, edema of the feet late in pregnancy usually is due to the pressure of the enlarged uterus on the veins of the pelvis. Blood flow returning by way of the venous system of the legs to the right side of the heart is slowed owing to pressure on the large veins by the enlarged uterus. The diminished blood flow increases the pressure in the veins of the legs, and fluids escape through the vein walls and into surrounding tissues. (14:548)
Nursing Process—Implementation
Client Need—Safe, effective care environment

31 2. Sodium is the electrolyte most responsible for controlling the amount of water that is present outside of body cells. Reducing the salt intake may help decrease edema. The client should be advised to not only limit her intake of table salt (*sodium* chloride), but also to read food labels carefully. If the word "sodium" combined with chloride or any other chemical name is found in the list of ingredients, the product may contribute to or cause edema. Clients with edema should be watched closely, and blood pressure should be monitored because PIH is a serious complication of pregnancy. (14:548)
Nursing Process—Implementation
Client Need—Safe, effective care environment

32 1. Elevating the legs and feet may help relieve edema. If the edema increases, the client is advised to bring this to the immediate attention of the physician because it may indicate a more serious problem. (13:123)
Nursing Process—Implementation
Client Need—Safe, effective care environment

33 4. As the uterus rises in the abdomen, pressure is exerted on the diaphragm, thus decreasing lung capacity. This decrease in lung capacity results in shortness of breath and difficulty in breathing (dyspnea). This problem usually is seen in the third trimester of pregnancy and usually is not abnormal. However, any client complaining of dyspnea should be examined by the physician to rule out any serious problem that may be occurring. (19:65)
Nursing Process—Collecting data
Client Need—Physiological integrity

34 4. Answering the client's questions reduces anxiety, especially when a client is pregnant for the first time. Many clients do not know what to expect or what discomforts are normal or abnormal. (19:53)
Nursing Process—Planning
Client Need—Psychosocial integrity

35 3. Frequent urination is common late in pregnancy because the enlarged uterus causes pressure on the bladder. Frequency is unrelated to having alkaline urine or increasing wastes from the fetus. A urinary tract infection could cause frequency, but this is not the most probable cause late in pregnancy, and it would be likely to cause additional symptoms, such as burning and painful urination. (19:47)
Nursing Process—Implementation
Client Need—Safe, effective care environment

36 3. Early in pregnancy frequent urination is common because the uterus causes pressure on the urinary bladder. When the uterus rises into the abdominal cavity, urinary frequency may subside. Urinary frequency recurs later in pregnancy when the uterus drops low in the abdomen. (19:53–54; 14:540)
Nursing Process—Implementation
Client Need—Safe, effective care environment

37 4. Low-heeled shoes place the back in a more proper alignment and therefore may relieve backache associated with pregnancy. The remaining suggestions in this question probably will be ineffective for relieving a backache. (19:64)
Nursing Process—Implementation
Client Need—Safe, effective care environment

38 2. Small, frequent meals prevent overdistention of the stomach and may relieve nausea. Drinking extra fluids with meals may overdistend the stomach and cause nausea. A pregnant woman should not take any drug, prescription or nonprescription, unless it has been prescribed or recommended by a physician. Eating two full meals a day may increase nausea. (19:64; 8:165–166)
Nursing Process—Implementation
Client Need—Safe, effective care environment

39 1. Dorsiflexion of the foot may help to relieve leg cramps. Because this client has a history of thrombophlebitis and blood clots, she should be instructed *not* to massage her legs when cramping occurs. Increasing the fluid intake or eating a diet high in proteins and vitamins C and E is not likely to relieve leg cramps. (13:123; 19:65)

Nursing Process—Implementation
Client Need—Safe, effective care environment

40 4. Heartburn often is seen in the last 6 weeks of pregnancy. As the fundus of the uterus rises, it presses against the stomach and the esophagus, thus causing a reflux of gastric acid into the esophagus. Eating small, frequent meals will avoid overdistention of the stomach and therefore may reduce heartburn. Avoiding spicy foods and foods that produce gas also may relieve heartburn. The use of any drug, including nonprescription drugs or household remedies, should be avoided when the client is pregnant. (13:122; 19:65)

Nursing Process—Implementation
Client Need—Physiological integrity

41 1. The pelvic rock (pelvic tilt), which involves moving the hips and pelvis back and forth, often helps relieve a backache. The exercise can be carried out while the woman is on her hands and knees, standing up, or lying down. The knee–chest position also is recommended for relieving lower backaches. (19:129)

Nursing Process—Implementation
Client Need—Physiological integrity

HIGH-RISK FACTORS AND PREGNANCY

42 3. Along with mental deficiencies and flat facial features, joint and limb abnormalities are the most prominent signs of FAS. Other signs include heart defects, growth retardation, mental retardation, microcephaly (small head size), and central nervous system abnormalities. There is no known safe amount of alcohol that can be consumed by the mother during pregnancy. All pregnant women should be encouraged to stop drinking any alcoholic beverage at any time during pregnancy. For those planning to become pregnant, it is recommended that the consumption of alcohol be stopped before conception occurs. (19:91–92)

Nursing Process—Planning
Client Need—Health promotion/maintenance

43 3. Infants born to mothers who are addicted to certain drugs, such as heroin, methadone, and cocaine, will go through drug withdrawal after birth. Some of the symptoms of withdrawal seen in newborns include tremors, irritability, sweating, yawning, and sneezing. (14:683–684)

Nursing Process—Planning
Client Need—Health promotion/maintenance

44 1. Women who smoke during pregnancy expose the developing fetus to serious health problems, including a low birth weight. Additional problems include fetal death and a higher incidence of placenta previa and abruptio placentae. (19:92)

Nursing Process—Planning
Client Need—Health promotion/maintenance

COMPLICATIONS OF PREGNANCY

45 3. Bleeding from the vagina may indicate a complication of pregnancy, such as abruptio placentae or placenta previa. This problem must be brought to the attention of the physician immediately. Breast tenderness, fetal movement, and frequent urination usually are normal occurrences during pregnancy and can be discussed with the physician at the time of a clinic visit. (8:67–68)

Nursing Process—Planning
Client Need—Health promotion/maintenance

46 2. Trichomoniasis is a sexually transmitted disease. The male partner may be asymptomatic. In the first trimester the physician may recommend gentle douching with warm water and vinegar. In the second or third trimester the physician may prescribe metronidazole (Flagyl). (19:88)

Nursing Process—Planning
Client Need—Health promotion/maintenance

47 4. Hyperemesis gravidarum is persistent vomiting, is serious, and can result in dehydration and electrolyte imbalances. Hospitalization may be required and the condition treated with intravenous fluids and electrolyte replacement. (8:166)

Nursing Process—Collecting data
Client Need—Physiological integrity

48 4. An incompetent cervix is unable to support a pregnancy and dilates because of the weight of the fetus. This problem may be seen at approximately the fifth or sixth month of pregnancy. If untreated, an incompetent cervix may result in a spontaneous abortion. (14:568)

Nursing Process—Implementation
Client Need—Physiological integrity

49 2. The Shirodkar procedure places a suture around the neck of the cervix at the level of the internal os. The suture is removed when the client begins labor. Additional measures may include bed rest. The MacDonald procedure is similar to the Shirodkar procedure. (14:568)

Nursing Process—Planning
Client Need—Physiological integrity

50 1. The cause of PIH is unknown. PIH is one of the three leading causes of maternal death. None of the other causes given in this question is known to be a direct cause of PIH. (13:140–143; 8:181–186)
  Nursing Process—Implementation
  Client Need—Physiological integrity

51 3. An irregular pulse is not associated with PIH. The three classic signs and symptoms of this condition are an elevated blood pressure, albuminuria, and fluid-retention edema. This condition is considered a serious complication of pregnancy. It is one of the chief causes of maternal mortality, and a surviving infant often suffers from intrauterine growth retardation. (13:140–143; 8:180–186)
  Nursing Process—Collecting data
  Client Need—Physiological integrity

52 1. The client with PIH is diagnosed as having eclampsia when she has convulsions and coma. Eclampsia may occur during the antepartum period, labor, delivery, or the postpartum period. When eclampsia occurs, precautions should continue after delivery for at least 48 hours because there is danger of convulsions occurring as long as irritability of the central nervous system exists. (13:142–143)
  Nursing Process—Collecting data
  Client Need—Physiological integrity

53 4. Intravenous or intramuscular magnesium sulfate may be used to prevent or control convulsions. (13:142)
  Nursing Process—Implementation
  Client Need—Physiological integrity

54 2. Urinary output is measured and recorded hourly. Any decrease in urine output is reported to the physician immediately. Measurement of the urinary output is especially important if the client receives magnesium sulfate because this drug is excreted in the urine. A decrease in urinary output would hinder the excretion of magnesium sulfate and therefore result in high levels of the drug in the bloodstream. Vital signs are monitored at frequent intervals, usually every 30 to 60 minutes; the frequency depends on the condition of the client. (13:142)
  Nursing Process—Collecting data
  Client Need—Physiological integrity

55 1. An ectopic pregnancy occurs somewhere outside the uterus. Most often, an ectopic pregnancy occurs in the fallopian tube, but it may occur in the abdomen, the ovary, or the cervix. If it occurs in the fallopian tube, the tube eventually will rupture or tear due to distention of the growing results of conception. (19:79–80)
  Nursing Process—Planning
  Client Need—Physiological integrity

56 2. An ectopic pregnancy often is associated with extremely serious hemorrhaging. If the fallopian tube ruptures, severe pain in the lower abdomen generally is present. Emergency surgical treatment and blood-loss replacement usually are necessary. (13:146; 8:177–178)
  Nursing Process—Collecting data
  Client Need—Physiological integrity

57 4. Vaginal bleeding and abdominal cramping or backaches are typical symptoms clients report with the threat of a spontaneous abortion. (19:78–79)
  Nursing Process—Collecting data
  Client Need—Physiological integrity

58 4. A spontaneous abortion occurs without having done anything to cause it. Induced abortion is the intentional termination of a pregnancy using medication or the dilatation and suctioning technique. (8:175–176)
  Nursing Process—Planning
  Client Need—Physiological integrity

59 2. The presence of uterine cramping, spotting, and the loss of amniotic fluid are symptoms of a threatened abortion. Assessment of the client should include close monitoring of any signs or symptoms that may occur, and the physician should be notified immediately if these occur. If blood loss and amniotic fluid loss are minimal, the threat of abortion may be relieved by conservative measures, such as bed rest. (8:177)
  Nursing Process—Collecting data
  Client Need—Physiological integrity

60 1. Maintaining normal glucose levels is an important aspect of managing the diabetic client. It may be necessary for the client to monitor her blood glucose levels with a glucometer to determine episodes of hyperglycemia. Frequent visits to the physician usually are required. (8:171; 19:76)
  Nursing Process—Planning
  Client Need—Health promotion/maintenance

61 4. Strict dietary control along with close monitoring of the client's diabetes may eliminate some of the problems seen with the pregnant diabetic, especially giving birth to a large baby. (19:169–172; 14:572)
  Nursing Process—Planning
  Client Need—Health promotion/maintenance

62 3. Keeping maternal blood glucose levels as close to normal as possible reduces the risk of com-

plications associated with pregnancy and diabetes. This involves a thorough explanation of the diet, insulin requirements, and frequent self-monitoring of blood glucose levels. (13:149–151; 19:170–171)
>   Nursing Process—Implementation
>   Client Need—Health promotion/maintenance

63 2. The most characteristic sign of placenta previa is painless bleeding from the vagina. It occurs late in pregnancy, usually after the 28th week of pregnancy, and is the most common cause of bleeding during the third trimester. Sharp abdominal pain, an elevated blood pressure, and continuous, painless contractions are not associated with placenta previa. (13:147–148)
>   Nursing Process—Collecting data
>   Client Need—Physiological integrity

64 4. Placenta previa becomes apparent during the last trimester of pregnancy and requires close medical supervision of the client and the fetus. (13:147–148)
>   Nursing Process—Evaluation
>   Client Need—Health promotion/maintenance

65 2. Clients with placenta previa have vaginal bleeding. A baseline blood pressure and pulse rate must be known so that further changes can be evaluated by the physician and those involved in the client's care. (8:180)
>   Nursing Process—Collecting data
>   Client Need—Physiological integrity

66 3. Placenta previa is a condition in which the placenta totally (complete or total placenta previa) or partially (partial placenta previa) covers the cervical os (opening), or the placenta may be implanted low in the uterus (marginal placenta previa) without covering any part of the os. The painless bleeding associated with placenta previa is due to a separation of the placenta from the uterus in the area that is near or covers the cervical os. The separation is caused by normal changes in the cervix that are occurring in preparation for labor. Placenta previa is unrelated to the development of polyps or myomas, degeneration of the placenta, or failure in the proper functioning of the placenta. (13:147–148; 8:178–179)
>   Nursing Process—Planning
>   Client Need—Physiological integrity

67 4. Abruptio placentae occurs late in pregnancy or during labor and may be a partial or complete separation of the placenta from the wall of the uterus. Complete abruptio placentae is an emergency because a delay can result in maternal hemorrhaging or fetal death. (13:148–149; 19:179)
>   Nursing Process—Collecting data
>   Client Need—Physiological integrity

68 2. A complete abruptio placentae requires emergency treatment. The client should not be left alone, and vital signs are taken frequently because shock may occur. Fetal monitoring also is necessary. (13:148–149; 19:179)
>   Nursing Process—Implementation
>   Client Need—Physiological integrity

NUTRITION DURING PREGNANCY

69 2. The present dietary habits of the client and her family must be known before a teaching plan can be formulated and implemented. Once basic dietary habits are known, the nurse can show the client and the family what foods must be added or subtracted from the diet. A printed example of a diet is most helpful when teaching clients. (13:121)
>   Nursing Process—Collecting data
>   Client Need—Health promotion/maintenance

70 3. A well-balanced, nutritious diet is essential for pregnant women. During pregnancy and lactation, calcium requirements are increased by almost 50%. The pregnant client should eat foods high in calcium, folic acid, and iron. The caloric intake may need to be increased. (19:59–60)
>   Nursing Process—Implementation
>   Client Need—Health promotion/maintenance

71 3. Of the foods listed in this question, green vegetables would contain the highest amount of calcium. (20:139)
>   Nursing Process—Implementation
>   Client Need—Health promotion/maintenance

72 4. One quart (4 cups) is the recommended intake of milk for pregnant women. Milk is an excellent source of calcium and protein, both of which are essential for the proper development of the fetus. A pregnancy of more than one fetus may require an supplement of calcium. (20:139)
>   Nursing Process—Implementation
>   Client Need—Health promotion/maintenance

73 1. A diet rich in iron is needed for a pregnant woman for the formation of hemoglobin and for transporting oxygen and carbon dioxide for the growing fetus. Anemia is relatively common during pregnancy because many women are not likely to include sufficient amounts in their diets, and as a result, iron may need to be prescribed by the physician as a dietary supplement. (20:139)
>   Nursing Process—Collecting data
>   Client Need—Health promotion/maintenance

TEACHING THE PREGNANT CLIENT

74 2. The term teratogen refers to an agent or a factor that has the potential to cause physical defects in the developing embryo or fetus. Prescription and nonprescription drugs may be teratogenic. These findings form the basis for teaching pregnant women not to use any medications without first consulting a physician. (14:915)
    Nursing Process—Planning
    Client Need—Health promotion/maintenance

75 4. Electrocoagulation of the fallopian tubes may be performed with a laparoscope introduced through a small incision below the umbilicus. This same procedure also may be used to place clips or rings on the fallopian tubes. Occlusion of the fallopian tubes by any method prevents sperm from fertilizing an ovum and results in permanent sterilization. A vas ligation is performed on the male for purposes of sterilization. (8:228–229)
    Nursing Process—Implementation
    Client Need—Health promotion/maintenance

76 3. The placenta provides the body with several hormones, including HCG, estrogen, progesterone, and various other hormones and enzymes. Certain microorganisms can cross the placental barrier and cause damage to the fetus. (11:337; 19:35–36)
    Nursing Process—Implementation
    Client Need—Health promotion/maintenance

77 2. The amniotic fluid protects the fetus, allows the fetus to move, keeps the environment for the fetus at a constant temperature, provides some nourishment for the fetus, serves as a reservoir for fetal urine, and prevents the amnion from adhering to the fetus. Providing the fetus with antibodies, providing oxygen for the fetus, and lowering the body temperature of the mother are not functions of amniotic fluid. (19:33–34)
    Nursing Process—Implementation
    Client Need—Health promotion/maintenance

78 4. Chadwick's sign is the discoloration of the vulva and the vagina during pregnancy. Hegar's sign is a softening of the lower segment of the uterus. Goodell's sign is a softening of the cervix, one of the first observable signs of pregnancy. These three are probable signs of pregnancy. Braxton Hicks contractions are painless uterine contractions that usually occur throughout pregnancy. They are believed to facilitate placental circulation. Ordinarily, a woman does not feel Braxton Hicks contractions until late in her pregnancy. (19:47)
    Nursing Process—Implementation
    Client Need—Health promotion/maintenance

79 3. TORCH (or TORCHES) includes *to*xoplasmosis, *r*ubella, *c*ytomegalovirus, *h*erpes, and *s*yphilis. These infections are known to cause harm to the fetus. Other infections also may cause harm to the developing fetus. (19:88; 8:396)
    Nursing Process—Planning
    Client Need—Health promotion/maintenance

80 1. Oxygen and nourishment are provided for the fetus by means of the umbilical *vein*. The umbilical *arteries* return the blood circulated through the fetus to the placenta. (19:38–39)
    Nursing Process—Implementation
    Client Need—Health promotion/maintenance

ELECTIVE ABORTION

81 4. Induced abortion for the purpose of terminating a pregnancy is legal in most areas up to the 16th to 20th week of gestation. After this time the fetus is *potentially* able to survive outside the uterus. Newborns of only 20 to 24 weeks' gestation rarely survive. (14:567; 8:61)
    Nursing Process—Implementation
    Client Need—Safe, effective care environment

82 4. In 1989 the United States Supreme Court upheld its 1973 decision that an abortion can be performed legally but ruled that states may set certain restrictions on abortions. An example is that a state may deny certain personnel from performing abortions and some agencies from being used for performing abortions. Another example is that a state may require that a test to determine fetal viability be conducted before an abortion is performed. If the fetus is not viable, an abortion may be performed, provided that no other of the state's restrictions are violated. There is a continuous effort to change abortion laws. The nurse must be familiar with recent changes, if any, in these laws. (13:304–305; 8:227–228)
    Nursing Process—Implementation
    Client Need—Safe, effective care environment

83 1. Dilatation and aspiration by the use of suction is the most preferred technique and has fewer complications. Dilatation and curretage also may be used to terminate a pregnancy but may result in more complications. (13:304–305; 8:227–228)
    Nursing Process—Implementation
    Client Need—Safe, effective care environment

INDIVIDUAL QUESTIONS

84 3. Primigravida describes a woman pregnant for the first time. A primipara describes a woman who has delivered her first viable infant. Multipara describes a woman who has delivered more than one viable infant. Multigravida describes a woman who has been pregnant before this pregnancy. (19:66)

> Nursing Process—Collecting data
> Client Need—Health promotion/maintenance

85 4. Any sudden weight gain brings suspicion of PIH. Other signs include proteinuria, a decrease in urine output, and a rise in blood pressure (over 140/90). (8:180–186; 14:569–572)

> Nursing Process—Collecting data
> Client Need—Health promotion/maintenance

86 2. The virus causing rubella (German measles) is believed to be responsible for many fetal deformities when a mother contracts the disease early in pregnancy, usually during the first trimester. The *time* during pregnancy when the mother has rubella is critical. The fetus is most susceptible during the first 2 months of pregnancy when cell differentiation is taking place, which is a time when some women do not even know they are pregnant. (8:306–307)

> Nursing Process—Collecting data
> Client Need—Health promotion/maintenance

87 1. A history of rubella (German measles) is not always reliable because having had rubella may not provide sufficient immunity. Pregnant women are not given the rubella virus vaccine. If the client does not have a sufficient immunity to rubella, the risks of fetal abnormalities are explained to the client. (13:113; 8:67)

> Nursing Process—Implementation
> Client Need—Health promotion/maintenance

88 4. The diabetic client is at risk during her pregnancy, especially if her diabetes is poorly con-trolled. Episodes of hyperglycemia (increase in blood glucose levels) can affect the fetus, resulting in problems such as abortion, fetal abnormalities, and intrauterine death (late in pregnancy). (8:176)

> Nursing Process—Collecting data
> Client Need—Health promotion/maintenance

89 2. When a pregnant woman has herpes simplex virus type II (genital herpes), a cesarean delivery is most often performed to prevent infecting the infant during vaginal delivery. The infant mortality rate is high, and surviving newborns often have neurologic damage when the virus is passed on to them during delivery. (13:85)

> Nursing Process—Planning
> Client Need—Health promotion/maintenance

90 2. Although the exact transmission of AIDS from the mother to the infant is not clear, it is believed that the disease may be transmitted by contact with maternal blood during passage through the birth canal. It also is possible that the disease may be transmitted to the fetus in utero. (13:87)

> Nursing Process—Planning
> Client Need—Health promotion/maintenance

91 1. The *Chlamydia* organism is passed from the mother to the fetus during vaginal delivery. Depending on the seriousness of the infection, as well as other factors, women with this type of infection are treated with antibiotics (usually erythromycin) prior to delivery to prevent transmission of the infection to the newborn. (13:87)

> Nursing Process—Planning
> Client Need—Health promotion/maintenance

Classification of Test Items

Unit II Review Test 2

Directions: After each question the correct answer is given as well as a classification of each test question. Compare the correct answer with your answer. If a question has been answered *incorrectly*, draw a line to the end of the four columns. When finished, add up your correct scores and place the results at the bottom of each column.

Score Calculation:

To determine the percentage of the number of questions you answered correctly, divide the **Number Correct** by the **Number Possible**, as example 76 (the number of questions answered correctly) divided by 91 (the number of questions in the test) = .835 or 84%.

NURSING PROCESS

C = Collecting data
P = Planning
I = Implementation
E = Evaluation

CLIENT NEEDS

S = Safe, effective care environment
P = Physiological integrity
M = Psychosocial integrity
H = Health promotion/maintenance

Question #	Answer #	Nursing Process C	Nursing Process P	Nursing Process I	Nursing Process E	Client Needs S	Client Needs P	Client Needs M	Client Needs H
1	1		P						H
2	4		P						H
3	4		P						H
4	3			I					H
5	2		P						H
6	4		P						H
7	2			I					H
8	1		P						H
9	4		P						H
10	3			I					H
11	3	C							H
12	1			I					H
13	3		P						H
14	4			I		S			
15	2			I			P		
16	1	C							H
17	2			I				M	
18	1			I					H

NURSING PROCESS

C = Collecting data
P = Planning
I = Implementation
E = Evaluation

CLIENT NEEDS

S = Safe, effective care environment
P = Physiological integrity
M = Psychosocial integrity
H = Health promotion/maintenance

Question #	Answer #	\multicolumn{4}{c}{Nursing Process}	\multicolumn{4}{c}{Client Needs}
		C	P	I	E	S	P	M	H
19	4			I					H
20	4	C							H
21	3	C							H
22	4				E		P		
23	2	C						M	
24	1		P						H
25	2			I		S			
26	1			I		S			
27	4			I		S			
28	3				E		P		
29	3			I		S			
30	2			I		S			
31	2			I		S			
32	1			I		S			
33	4	C					P		
34	4		P					M	
35	3			I		S			
36	3			I		S			
37	4			I		S			
38	2			I		S			
39	1			I		S			
40	4			I			P		
41	1			I			P		
42	3		P						H
43	3		P						H
44	1		P						H
45	3		P						H
46	2		P						H
47	4	C					P		
48	4			I			P		
49	2		P				P		

NURSING PROCESS

C = Collecting data
P = Planning
I = Implementation
E = Evaluation

CLIENT NEEDS

S = Safe, effective care environment
P = Physiological integrity
M = Psychosocial integrity
H = Health promotion/maintenance

Question #	Answer #	Nursing Process				Client Needs			
		C	P	I	E	S	P	M	H
50	1			I			P		
51	3	C					P		
52	1	C					P		
53	4			I			P		
54	2	C					P		
55	1		P				P		
56	2	C					P		
57	4	C					P		
58	4		P				P		
59	2	C					P		
60	1		P						H
61	4		P						H
62	3			I					H
63	2	C					P		
64	4				E				H
65	2	C					P		
66	3		P				P		
67	4	C					P		
68	2			I			P		
69	2	C							H
70	3			I					H
71	3			I					H
72	4			I					H
73	1	C							H
74	2		P						H
75	4			I					H
76	3			I					H
77	2			I					H
78	4			I					H
79	3		P						H
80	1			I					H

NURSING PROCESS

C = Collecting data
P = Planning
I = Implementation
E = Evaluation

CLIENT NEEDS

S = Safe, effective care environment
P = Physiological integrity
M = Psychosocial integrity
H = Health promotion/maintenance

Question #	Answer #	Nursing Process				Client Needs			
		C	P	I	E	S	P	M	H
81	4			I		S			
82	4			I		S			
83	1			I		S			
84	3	C							H
85	4	C							H
86	2	C							H
87	1			I					H
88	4	C							H
89	2		P						H
90	2		P						H
91	1		P						H
Number Correct									
Number Possible	91	22	26	40	3	16	24	3	48
Percentage Correct									

REVIEW TEST 3

Nursing Care of Clients During Labor, Delivery, and Postpartum
Admission of the Client to a Labor and Delivery Facility
Nursing Care of Clients During the First Stage of Labor
Nursing Care of Clients During the Second Stage of Labor
Nursing Care of Clients During the Third Stage of Labor
Nursing Care of Clients During the Fourth Stage of Labor
Nursing Care of Clients During the Postpartum Period
Nursing Care of Clients Having a Cesarean Delivery
Nursing Care of Clients Having an Emergency Delivery

Nursing Care of the Newborn Client
Nursing Care of the Normal Newborn Client
Nursing Care of Clients Having a Stillborn or a Newborn with Congenital Abnormalities
Nursing Care of Clients Considering Family Planning
Individual Test Items

Correct Answers and Rationale
Classification of Test Items

Directions: With a pencil, blacken the circle in front of the option you have chosen for your correct answer.

Nursing Care of Clients During Labor, Delivery, and Postpartum

ADMISSION OF THE CLIENT TO A LABOR AND DELIVERY FACILITY

Ms. Susan Dash, age 25, is admitted to the hospital for the delivery of her first child.

1 When the nurse is obtaining an admission history, Ms. Dash mentions that she felt contractions for the past several weeks, but they were not painful. When entering this fact in the client's history the nurse can use the term
○ 1. Hegar sign.
○ 2. Chadwick's sign.
○ 3. Braxton Hicks contractions.
○ 4. Goodell's sign.

2 Ms. Dash is having uterine contractions. Which one of the following questions that the nurse asks on admission is *least* pertinent?
○ 1. "When did you last eat?"
○ 2. "Have you ever had an enema?"
○ 3. "Have your membranes (bag of water) ruptured?"
○ 4. "When did your contractions start?"

3 A thorough admission history is important. Which one of the following procedures or examinations is *contraindicated* if Ms. Dash were to give a history of vaginal bleeding during the last trimester?
○ 1. Vaginal examination
○ 2. Monitoring of fetal heart rate (FHR)
○ 3. A nitrazine test
○ 4. Drawing blood for laboratory examination

NURSING CARE OF CLIENTS DURING THE FIRST STAGE OF LABOR

Ms. Pat Keppler is a primipara and is admitted to the labor and delivery department of a hospital.

4 On Ms. Keppler's admission record the physician writes that she is in the early first stage of labor. To develop a plan of care the nurse must know that the first stage of labor may be described as the

○ 1. onset of irregular and mild contractions.
○ 2. beginning of Braxton Hicks contractions.
○ 3. dilatation of the cervix to 8 to 10 cm and cervical effacement.
○ 4. movement of the fetus toward the pelvic inlet.

5 When reviewing Ms. Keppler's admission record, the nurse notes that the physician has determined the station of the fetus as minus two. To develop a plan of care the nurse should know that this term describes the
○ 1. anatomic position of the fetus.
○ 2. degree of descent of the fetal head or presenting part.
○ 3. height of the uterus.
○ 4. placement of the uterine fundus.

6 Early in labor the preferred position for Ms. Keppler if she is resting in bed is the
○ 1. back-lying position.
○ 2. semisitting position.
○ 3. left side-lying position.
○ 4. right side-lying position.

Eight hours after admission the nurse in charge performs a vaginal examination on Ms. Keppler and records that the cervix is dilated 4 cm.

7 The interpretation of this finding is correct when the nurse judges that in terms of cervical dilatation, the client is
○ 1. at a very early stage of dilatation.
○ 2. approaching half of the total amount of dilatation.
○ 3. nearing total dilatation.
○ 4. in labor but will most likely require a drug to become fully dilated.

8 Ms. Keppler requires fetal monitoring. To evaluate and correctly report the results of this procedure, the nurse should know that the FHR normally
○ 1. slows at the onset of a contraction.
○ 2. slows at the peak of the contraction.
○ 3. remains unchanged during a contraction.
○ 4. slows immediately after a contraction.

9 During which of the following stages of labor should the nurse anticipate that Ms. Keppler will ordinarily need the most encouragement and support?
○ 1. During the early part of stage one
○ 2. During the transition part of stage one
○ 3. During stage two
○ 4. During stage three

Ms. Keppler is nearing the end of the first stage of labor.

10 Which of the following nursing measures is *least* appropriate at the end of the first stage of labor?
○ 1. Encouraging the client to void
○ 2. Urging the client to breathe deeply

○ 3. Helping the client lie on her left side
○ 4. Having the client push with each contraction

Ms. Beth Williams is a 21-year-old primigravida who is admitted to labor and delivery. She tells the nurse that this is her first pregnancy and that there are many things she doesn't understand.

11 Ms. Williams thinks her membranes have ruptured, but she is not sure. The nurse in charge performs a nitrazine test. The primary purpose of this test is to
○ 1. differentiate between urine and amniotic fluid.
○ 2. differentiate between amniotic fluid and vaginal mucus.
○ 3. determine whether there is blood in the amniotic fluid.
○ 4. determine whether there is meconium in the amniotic fluid.

12 The nurse plans to check Ms. Williams' bladder. The rationale for this action is that the urinary bladder should *not* be allowed to become distended primarily because a full bladder tends to
○ 1. increase the risk of urinary incontinence.
○ 2. predispose to a prolapse of the umbilical cord.
○ 3. interfere with observations of uterine contractions.
○ 4. prevent the descent of the fetus into the birth canal.

13 The physician orders Ms. Williams on bed rest. To prevent bladder distention in Ms. Williams the nurse can
○ 1. limit Ms. Williams' fluid intake.
○ 2. decrease the rate of flow of intravenous fluids.
○ 3. suggest that Ms. Williams eat solid foods instead of drinking liquids.
○ 4. offer the bedpan at frequent intervals.

14 Ms. Williams asks if she will have to have an enema before she delivers her baby and why one is necessary. To relieve apprehension the nurse can explain to the client that an enema may be necessary to
○ 1. prevent contamination if feces is expelled during delivery.
○ 2. ease the discomfort of contractions.
○ 3. prevent constipation after delivery.
○ 4. relieve pressure in an area where an episiotomy may be performed.

15 Accurate recording of Ms. Williams' progress during labor is essential. The term used to describe the period when the uterus begins a contraction until the contraction ends is called the
○ 1. interval.
○ 2. duration.
○ 3. intensity.
○ 4. frequency.

16 Where on Ms. Williams' abdomen should the nurse's hand be placed when feeling a contraction?
  ○ 1. Just above the pubis
  ○ 2. Just above the umbilicus
  ○ 3. In the middle of the abdomen, halfway between the umbilicus and the pubis
  ○ 4. On either side of the abdomen, halfway between the umbilicus and the pubis

17 The nurse should check the FHR during the time when Ms. Williams has a contraction and again
  ○ 1. when she shows signs of becoming fully dilated.
  ○ 2. immediately after a contraction.
  ○ 3. immediately before the next contraction.
  ○ 4. as near to the end of the contraction as possible.

18 The nurse judges the FHR to be normal when the rate per minute is between
  ○ 1. 80 and 100 beats.
  ○ 2. 100 and 120 beats.
  ○ 3. 120 and 160 beats.
  ○ 4. 160 and 200 beats.

Ms. Ann Barnes, a 29-year-old multipara, is admitted to labor and delivery.

19 On the admission record the nurse reads that Ms. Barnes' contractions are irregular, they do not increase in intensity or duration, they decrease when she is ambulating, and there are no changes in the cervix. This information alerts the nurse that
  ○ 1. the client is in false labor.
  ○ 2. fetal distress is present.
  ○ 3. the client is in the third stage of labor.
  ○ 4. the size of the fetus is larger than normal.

Shortly after admission the physician decides to perform a vaginal examination on Ms. Barnes to determine cervical dilatation.

20 The nurse can help prepare for a vaginal examination by
  ○ 1. having clean gloves available.
  ○ 2. teaching the client to hold her breath during the examination.
  ○ 3. placing the client in a left lateral recumbent position.
  ○ 4. cleansing of the vulva.

21 Ms. Barnes is in true labor when
  ○ 1. her uterine contractions are regular.
  ○ 2. her membranes fail to rupture spontaneously.
  ○ 3. the fetus drops into the brim of the pelvis.
  ○ 4. a mucous plug in the cervical canal is expelled.

Ms. Helen Geary, a 26-year-old primipara, is admitted to labor and delivery. Her physician has determined that she is in the early stages of labor.

22 Knowing that Ms. Geary is in the very early stages of labor, the nurse can plan to offer water or clear fluids because the ingestion of solid or certain types of fluids may
  ○ 1. slow labor contractions.
  ○ 2. interfere with the medications given for pain and discomfort.
  ○ 3. cause fetal distress.
  ○ 4. result in vomiting.

23 When reviewing the physician's notations on Ms. Geary's progress record, the nurse reads that the position of the fetus is described as ROA. The position of the fetus refers to the presenting fetal body part in relation to the
  ○ 1. anterior abdominal wall.
  ○ 2. cervix.
  ○ 3. fundus of the uterus.
  ○ 4. mother's pelvis.

During the first stage of labor the physician explains to Ms. Geary that she may require an episiotomy. Ms. Geary is upset and asks many questions.

24 To reduce anxiety and correctly reinforce the physician's explanation, the nurse should know that the primary reason for an episiotomy is to help prevent
  ○ 1. uterine rupture.
  ○ 2. postpartum infection.
  ○ 3. prolonged pressure on the fetal head.
  ○ 4. undue trauma to the bowel.

25 When evaluating clients in the first stage of labor, the nurse must report any contractions that
  ○ 1. are more frequent than every 8 minutes.
  ○ 2. are 2 minutes or longer.
  ○ 3. start in the front of the abdomen.
  ○ 4. are accompanied by pain.

26 When evaluating the client in labor the nurse must know that primiparas normally are not taken to the delivery room until
  ○ 1. the cervix is dilated to 6 to 8 cm.
  ○ 2. contractions are 3 to 5 minutes apart.
  ○ 3. the intensity of contractions is decreased.
  ○ 4. the perineum is bulging.

NURSING CARE OF CLIENTS DURING THE SECOND STAGE OF LABOR

Ms. Laura Birch, a 30-year-old multipara, is admitted to labor and delivery. Her last three pregnancies resulted in a short stage one of labor. Her caretakers decide to observe her closely. The physician determines that Ms. Birch is in the late part of the first stage of labor because her cervix is dilated to 6 cm.

27 Ms. Birch states that she is extremely uncomfortable and has a great deal of pain. To effectively approach this client problem, the nurse should know that narcotic analgesics given late in the first stage of labor may

○ 1. increase the frequency of labor contractions.
○ 2. result in uterine rupture.
○ 3. result in respiratory depression of the newborn.
○ 4. increase fetal activity and movement.

28   To lessen Ms. Birch's discomfort the nurse can advise her to

○ 1. lie face down.
○ 2. not drink fluids.
○ 3. practice holding her breath between contractions.
○ 4. assume a Sims' position.

29   To effectively plan nursing care for Ms. Birch the nurse should know that the second stage of labor begins when

○ 1. the cervix is fully dilated.
○ 2. contractions are 2 to 5 minutes apart.
○ 3. the uterus is at the level of the umbilicus.
○ 4. the fetus has dropped into the pelvis.

30   During the second stage of labor Ms. Birch is encouraged to

○ 1. push down.
○ 2. drink extra fluids to avoid dehydration.
○ 3. relax and try to take short naps.
○ 4. conserve her energy.

31   Ms. Birch is encouraged to pant between contractions and should be observed for signs of hyperventilation, which include

○ 1. flushing of the face and decreased pulse rate.
○ 2. blurred vision and tingling of the extremities.
○ 3. increased blood pressure and bradycardia.
○ 4. dry mucous membranes and nausea.

32   Ms. Birch shows signs of hyperventilation. When detected early, the nurse can have Ms. Birch

○ 1. breathe into a small paper bag.
○ 2. inhale five to six quick, short breaths.
○ 3. lie on her left side.
○ 4. take sips of water between breaths.

Ms. Birch is transferred to the delivery room. The obstetric anesthesia planned for Ms. Birch is a saddle block (subarachnoid block).

33   To prepare Ms. Birch for administration of saddle block analgesia, the nurse can explain that the anesthetic will take effect

○ 1. almost immediately.
○ 2. in 10 to 20 minutes.
○ 3. in 30 to 40 minutes.
○ 4. in approximately 1 hour.

NURSING CARE OF CLIENTS DURING THE THIRD STAGE OF LABOR

Ms. Mary Packard is in the third stage of labor, which begins with the delivery of the newborn and ends with the delivery of the placenta and membranes.

34   Ms. Packard delivers a baby girl. The nurse working in the delivery room must prepare for the delivery of the placenta by encouraging Ms. Packard to

○ 1. turn on her side.
○ 2. take short, quick breaths for 3 minutes.
○ 3. breathe slowly and deeply.
○ 4. push with a contraction.

35   When working in the delivery room the nurse is responsible for having equipment available for the physician's use. Before Baby Girl Packard takes her first breath, the physician ordinarily will need equipment to

○ 1. repair the episiotomy.
○ 2. clamp and cut the umbilical cord.
○ 3. do an Apgar evaluation on the newborn.
○ 4. clean the newborn's airway of mucus and debris.

36   The nurse also must have clamps available for clamping the umbilical cord. This maneuver is performed

○ 1. after the cord stops pulsating.
○ 2. immediately after the placenta is delivered.
○ 3. within 1 hour of birth.
○ 4. when the newborn takes its first breath.

The physician orders an oxytocic agent to be given to Ms. Packard immediately after the delivery of the placenta.

37   The purpose of this type of drug is to

○ 1. decrease the blood pressure.
○ 2. prevent the uterus from inverting.
○ 3. strengthen contractions of the uterus.
○ 4. decrease the likelihood of uterine spasms.

The physician instructs the nurse to place Baby Girl Packard on her mother's abdomen so she and Baby Girl Packard's father can see, hear, touch, and feel their new baby girl.

38   When after birth is it believed best to begin a bonding relationship between the newborn and the parents?

○ 1. During the first hour after delivery
○ 2. Immediately after initial care is given to the newborn in the nursery
○ 3. Immediately after the mother is permitted to ambulate after delivery
○ 4. During the day, when the mother and the newborn are discharged from the hospital

39   The physician instructs the nurse to care for Baby Girl Packard. Unless an emergency situation exists,

the first step taken by the nurse is to prevent the loss of body heat by

- ○ 1. wrapping her in wet towels.
- ○ 2. holding her.
- ○ 3. placing her under a radiant heat source.
- ○ 4. immersing her in 80°F water.

40 The nurse prepares to instill 1% silver nitrate into the eyes of Baby Girl Packard. The correct procedure for administration of eye drops requires that the drug be instilled

- ○ 1. into the lower conjunctival sac.
- ○ 2. at a dose of 2 drops every 5 minutes for 30 minutes.
- ○ 3. into the inner canthus.
- ○ 4. directly on the cornea.

41 The nurse performs an Apgar scoring, which is

- ○ 1. an assessment of the mother's condition.
- ○ 2. an assessment of the physical condition of the newborn.
- ○ 3. a description of the placenta.
- ○ 4. the length of time required to deliver the newborn.

NURSING CARE OF CLIENTS DURING THE FOURTH STAGE OF LABOR

Ms. Tricia Adams has just delivered a boy. She is considered in the fourth stage of labor, which is the time when the placenta is delivered and up to 2 to 4 hours after delivery of the placenta.

42 During the fourth stage of labor the nurse plans to check Ms. Adams' fundus. Shortly after delivery of the placenta, the fundus should be

- ○ 1. soft and pliable.
- ○ 2. firmly contracted.
- ○ 3. at the level of the symphysis pubis.
- ○ 4. at the level of the umbilicus.

43 Ms. Adams is transferred to the recovery room. When assessing Ms. Adams the nurse looks for possible danger signs, such as

- ○ 1. a pulse rate between 70 and 80.
- ○ 2. saturation of one perineal pad over 4 hours.
- ○ 3. heavy bleeding.
- ○ 4. a systolic blood pressure above 100 mm Hg.

44 Ms. Adams' fundus is checked every 15 minutes for the first hour after delivery. The fundus should be massaged if it

- ○ 1. is firm and hard.
- ○ 2. is lower than midway between the umbilicus and symphysis pubis.
- ○ 3. begins to decrease in size.
- ○ 4. feels soft and boggy.

45 The nurse can massage the fundus by placing one hand on the fundus and the other hand

- ○ 1. just over the pubic bone.
- ○ 2. to the side of the abdomen.
- ○ 3. immediately below the rib cage.
- ○ 4. on the upper thigh.

NURSING CARE OF CLIENTS DURING THE POSTPARTUM PERIOD

The postpartum period extends from delivery of the newborn to approximately 6 weeks after birth. Ms. Kay Riley delivered a boy 6 hours ago and has been returned to her room. Her condition following 1 hour in the recovery room is reported as stable.

46 The nurse plans to check the color and amount of lochia (vaginal drainage). Shortly after delivery the color of Ms. Riley's lochia should be

- ○ 1. pink.
- ○ 2. dark or bright red.
- ○ 3. brown.
- ○ 4. yellow.

47 Thirty minutes after delivery the nurse changes Ms. Riley's perineal pad and notes that the lochia consists of several large clots and the perineal pad is saturated. The nurse should document that the amount of Ms. Riley's lochia is

- ○ 1. scant.
- ○ 2. light.
- ○ 3. moderate.
- ○ 4. heavy.

48 When changing Ms. Riley's perineal pads, the nurse checks Ms. Riley's perineum for a hematoma, the most common signs of which are

- ○ 1. heavy and foul-smelling lochia.
- ○ 2. swelling and discoloration of the skin around the perineum.
- ○ 3. irritated perineum and bloody vaginal discharge.
- ○ 4. separation of and purulent drainage from the episiotomy.

49 The nurse should know the symptoms of a perineal hematoma to identify and evaluate this problem. If Ms. Riley develops a hematoma, she is most likely to complain of

- ○ 1. discomfort when voiding.
- ○ 2. pain in the perineal area.
- ○ 3. itching of the vaginal meatus.
- ○ 4. a feeling of fullness in the vagina.

50 Ms. Riley's lochia is normal, and the physician allows her to ambulate. The nurse should encourage ambulation because this type of activity is especially beneficial to help prevent problems associated with the client's

- ○ 1. circulatory system.
- ○ 2. fluid balance.
- ○ 3. milk-producing ability.
- ○ 4. return to sexual activity.

The nurse uses measures to help Ms. Riley void after delivery. Ms. Riley voids frequently and in small amounts.

51   If Ms. Riley is allowed to have an overdistended bladder, she is at risk for developing
   ○ 1. a hematoma.
   ○ 2. thrombophlebitis.
   ○ 3. herniation of the bladder wall.
   ○ 4. a bladder infection.

One day after delivery Ms. Riley, who had been voiding small amounts of urine, is now unable to void. The physician orders the client to be catheterized.

52   When compared with techniques used to catheterize any female client, what technique, if any, is different when catheterizing a postpartum client?
   ○ 1. The meatal area is cleaned with normal saline rather than with an antiseptic.
   ○ 2. The catheter is not lubricated.
   ○ 3. The catheter is inserted farther for the postpartum client.
   ○ 4. The same techniques are used for the postpartum client that are used for other women.

53   Ms. Riley has had an episiotomy and complains of discomfort. The physician orders dry heat therapy with a heat lamp. When performing this procedure the nurse places the heat lamp
   ○ 1. 10 to 12 inches from the perineum.
   ○ 2. 18 to 24 inches from the perineum.
   ○ 3. directly over the lower back.
   ○ 4. directly over the abdomen.

54   Ms. Riley asks her physician what measures she may use to relieve discomfort from an episiotomy after she is home. To prepare discharge teaching, the nurse knows that a common method of relieving discomfort from an episiotomy is to
   ○ 1. take sitz baths.
   ○ 2. ambulate frequently.
   ○ 3. lie on the abdomen in bed.
   ○ 4. elevate the hips while in bed.

55   Propoxyphene hydrochloride (Darvon) is prescribed for Ms. Riley. The nurse judges that the desired effect has been met after administering this medication when Ms. Riley
   ○ 1. has a firm uterus.
   ○ 2. is producing more milk.
   ○ 3. has been relieved of nausea.
   ○ 4. no longer complains of discomfort.

56   The nurse plans to teach Ms. Riley about perineal care. The correct method of cleansing the perineum with soft wipes is to cleanse the area gently
   ○ 1. in a circular motion.
   ○ 2. from front to back.
   ○ 3. from side to side.
   ○ 4. from back to front.

57   Two days after delivery, the nurse notes that Ms. Riley is crying. Until now she has appeared happy and excited. In this situation it would be best for the nurse to
   ○ 1. ask the client why she is crying.
   ○ 2. offer the client any help she may need.
   ○ 3. volunteer to telephone the client's husband.
   ○ 4. explain to the client that crying delays recovery.

58   Before delivery Ms. Riley expressed a desire to breastfeed her baby. When planning a breastfeeding teaching program the nurse plans to include information regarding breast engorgement, which usually occurs
   ○ 1. immediately after delivery of the placenta.
   ○ 2. when estrogen is secreted by the ovaries.
   ○ 3. on approximately the third postpartum day.
   ○ 4. in approximately 1 week.

NURSING CARE OF CLIENTS HAVING A CESAREAN DELIVERY

Ms. Lorna Clark is admitted to the hospital. The physician has determined that she has placenta previa, and a cesarean delivery is planned. The physician orders immediate fetal monitoring.

59   Before placing the fetal transducer on Ms. Clark's abdomen, the nurse applies a gel to the transducer's surface primarily to
   ○ 1. improve the conduction of sound.
   ○ 2. prevent the transducer from sliding.
   ○ 3. prevent an electric shock from reaching the client.
   ○ 4. decrease the irritating effect of the transducer on the client's skin.

60   The physician orders an indwelling catheter to be inserted in Ms. Clark's bladder before surgery. The nurse can briefly explain to Ms. Clark that the purpose of the catheter is to
   ○ 1. make her more comfortable after surgery.
   ○ 2. keep her bladder empty during the surgical procedure.
   ○ 3. prevent a bladder infection.
   ○ 4. provide a safe way to collect urine specimens.

61   While preparing Ms. Clark for surgery, the nurse notes that an informed consent form has not been signed. In this situation the nurse should
   ○ 1. tell the nurse in charge that an informed consent has not been signed.
   ○ 2. ask Ms. Clark if she has signed an informed consent that the nurse has not seen.
   ○ 3. tell Ms. Clark that she will need to sign an informed consent after surgery.
   ○ 4. do nothing because an informed consent is unnecessary for a cesarean delivery.

The nurse develops a care plan for Ms. Clark.

62 The nursing care of Ms. Clark after the cesarean delivery will most nearly resemble the care of a client who has undergone
   ○ 1. a cystoscopy.
   ○ 2. chcst surgery.
   ○ 3. abdominal surgery.
   ○ 4. a dilatation and curettage.

63 Ms. Clark has returned from surgery and is receiving intravenous therapy. The nurse is assigned to care for Ms. Clark during the immediate postoperative period. Which one of the following would indicate Ms. Clark may be in shock?
   ○ 1. A drop in the pulse rate and a rise in the blood pressure
   ○ 2. A decrease in the amount of lochia
   ○ 3. A rise in the pulse rate and a drop in the blood pressure
   ○ 4. An increase in the urinary output

64 The nurse notes that the intravenous solution is labeled as containing an oxytocic drug. When assessing Ms. Clark, the nurse should know that the purpose of this drug is to
   ○ 1. increase the amount of lochia.
   ○ 2. keep the blood pressure stable.
   ○ 3. help the uterus contract.
   ○ 4. aid in healing of the incision.

65 Ms. Clark will require a narcotic analgesic for pain. The physician orders patient-controlled analgesia. When giving an explanation of the device to Ms. Clark, the nurse should tell her that
   ○ 1. pain relief should occur shortly after pushing the button.
   ○ 2. the button can be pushed only once every 6 hours.
   ○ 3. this device gives a larger than normal dose of the drug to provide instant pain relief.
   ○ 4. there is a danger in trying to push the button too often.

On the second postoperative day the physician orders the intravenous therapy to be discontinued and Ms. Clarke to be out of bed.

66 Which one of the following measures may be used to relieve pain or discomfort associated with postoperative abdominal distention?
   ○ 1. Increase her fluid intake to 3000 mL/d.
   ○ 2. Have her take all fluids through a straw.
   ○ 3. Have her periodically lie on her abdomen.
   ○ 4. Have her ambulate.

NURSING CARE OF CLIENTS HAVING AN EMERGENCY DELIVERY

Ms. Ellen Barker is a multigravida who is admitted as an emergency to the labor department. She gives a history of strong contractions 3 to 4 minutes apart for the past 2 hours. Ms. Wagner also states that her "last two babies came fast." Her physician is notified immediately, and a nurse is assigned to stay with her until the physician arrives.

67 Ms. Barker has several strong contractions and says to the nurse "The baby is coming!" If possible, the nurse's first course of action when Ms. Barker's delivery appears imminent should be to
   ○ 1. obtain the FHR.
   ○ 2. instruct the mother not to bear down.
   ○ 3. provide a clean field for delivery.
   ○ 4. assure the mother that help will arrive in time.

68 The nurse notes that the baby's head continues to crown at Ms. Barker's vaginal opening. In this situation it would be best for the nurse to
   ○ 1. allow the head to emerge slowly and deliver it between contractions.
   ○ 2. push back firmly on the head and place pressure on the vaginal meatus.
   ○ 3. place a sterile towel over the perineal area and have the client bring her legs close together.
   ○ 4. slide a finger into the vagina and enlarge its exit while delivering the head during a contraction.

Nursing Care of the Newborn Client

NURSING CARE OF THE NORMAL NEWBORN CLIENT

Baby Boy Morris is 45 minutes old. Ms. Morris experienced a normal delivery. Baby Boy Morris is transferred to the newborn nursery.

69 Baby Boy Morris is given vitamin K after birth. When administering this drug the nurse knows that Vitamin K primarily helps
   ○ 1. stimulate respiration.
   ○ 2. start peristaltic movements.
   ○ 3. promote blood coagulation.
   ○ 4. increase calcium absorption.

70 When giving vitamin K intramuscularly to Baby Boy Morris it is best for the nurse to inject the drug into the
   ○ 1. biceps brachii muscle.
   ○ 2. biceps femoris muscle.
   ○ 3. rectus femoris muscle.
   ○ 4. gluteus maximus muscle.

71 The nurse working in the newborn nursery plans to check Baby Boy Morris' umbilical cord frequently during the first few hours after his birth for signs of
   ○ 1. infection.
   ○ 2. herniation.

○ 3. prolonged pulsation.
○ 4. excessive bleeding.

72 When observing Baby Boy Morris' skin, the nurse notes a white cheesy substance on his body, which is called
○ 1. lanugo.
○ 2. petechiae.
○ 3. miliaria rubra.
○ 4. vernix caseosa.

73 When assessing Baby Boy Morris the nurse carefully looks for any abnormality. Which one of the following signs are abnormal and should be reported promptly to the nurse in charge?
○ 1. The scrotum appears swollen.
○ 2. The skin appears jaundiced a few hours after birth.
○ 3. Voiding is not seen until about 6 hours after birth.
○ 4. Mucus is vomited shortly after admission to the nursery.

74 If Baby Boy Morris has the following signs several hours after birth, which one should the nurse report promptly?
○ 1. His hands are bluish.
○ 2. His pulse rate is 140 per minute.
○ 3. He regurgitates after his first feeding since birth.
○ 4. His sternum moves inward with inspirations.

75 Baby Boy Morris is to be weighed. If the nurse uses the following techniques in the order given below, which one is *in error*?
○ 1. Placing a clean paper on the scale
○ 2. Balancing the scale
○ 3. Placing the undressed newborn on the scale
○ 4. Holding the baby's hands while obtaining a weight

76 The nurse is assigned to take the temperature on Baby Boy Morris. Within how many hours or days after birth can the nurse expect Baby Boy Morris' body temperature to stabilize?
○ 1. Within approximately 4 hours
○ 2. Within approximately 8 hours
○ 3. In 1 to 2 days
○ 4. After 1 week

Baby Girl Levy is admitted to the newborn nursery. When she is 3 days old her skin takes on a yellow appearance.

77 When recording and reporting this observation of Baby Girl Levy, the nurse can use the term(s)
○ 1. hepatitis.
○ 2. jaundice.
○ 3. erythroblastosis fetalis.
○ 4. biliary atresia.

The physician orders phototherapy, which is exposure to fluorescent light, for Baby Girl Levy to reduce jaundice.

78 When preparing Baby Girl Levy for this procedure, the nurse should
○ 1. cover her eyes.
○ 2. feed her only after she has had 6 hours of phototherapy.
○ 3. keep her on her abdomen.
○ 4. place a cap on her head and a shirt on the upper part of her body.

Baby Boy Martin is admitted to the newborn nursery. His parents have requested that he be circumcised.

79 When caring for Baby Boy Martin the nurse should plan to
○ 1. inspect his skin for drying and peeling.
○ 2. leave most of his body exposed as often as possible to reduce his body temperature.
○ 3. apply alcohol to areas that appear infected.
○ 4. inspect and change his diaper every 8 hours.

80 Following the circumcision Baby Boy Martin should be observed for signs of
○ 1. blood in his urine.
○ 2. swelling of his scrotum.
○ 3. profuse urine production.
○ 4. bleeding at the site of the circumcision.

Ms. Sally Pruett has a boy. This is her first child. Baby Boy Pruett is given to his mother for the first time while she is still in the delivery room. Ms. Pruett wishes to breastfeed her baby and is instructed to begin nursing her baby while she is still in the delivery room.

81 The nurse can explain to Ms. Pruett that breastfeeding shortly after delivery
○ 1. promotes the immediate flow of rich breast milk.
○ 2. increases the secretion of estrogen.
○ 3. promotes retraction of the breast nipples.
○ 4. helps her uterus to contract.

82 The nurse can explain to Ms. Pruett that the first secretion from the breasts after the birth of her baby is called colostrum and is especially beneficial for her neonate because colostrum contains
○ 1. estrogen.
○ 2. antibodies.
○ 3. predigested fats.
○ 4. digestive enzymes.

Baby Boy Pruett is taken to the newborn nursery and Ms. Pruett to the recovery room and then her hospital room. The nurse is responsible for assessing and evaluating the newborn.

83 After several days of breastfeeding, Baby Boy Pruett's stools will be considered normal in color if they are

○ 1. brown.
○ 2. yellow-orange.
○ 3. light green.
○ 4. black.

The nurse places the newborn next to Ms. Pruett and demonstrates that touching the baby's cheek encourages Baby Boy Pruett to turn his head toward Ms. Pruett's finger.

84 The nurse can explain that the reason Baby Boy Pruett responds to his mother's touch on his cheek is that the newborn is
○ 1. reacting to fear.
○ 2. looking for food.
○ 3. demonstrating a need for love.
○ 4. startled at being disturbed.

85 Following this demonstration, the nurse plans to teach Ms. Pruett how to breastfeed her baby by instructing her to brush the baby's cheek with her breast nipple to elicit the
○ 1. rooting reflex.
○ 2. startle reflex.
○ 3. swallowing response.
○ 4. grasp reflex.

86 Two days after breastfeeding begins Ms. Pruett complains of sore, cracked nipples. The nurse can advise Ms. Pruett to
○ 1. vigorously massage her nipples before breast-feeding.
○ 2. apply a lotion to the nipples before breast-feeding.
○ 3. start the baby feeding on the less tender breast.
○ 4. start the baby feeding on the most tender breast.

87 The nurse teaches Ms. Pruett that when she wishes to remove her baby from the nipple, she should put gentle downward pressure on her baby's
○ 1. lip.
○ 2. nose.
○ 3. chin.
○ 4. forehead.

88 Baby Boy Pruett is finished nursing. The nurse should explain to Ms. Pruett how to help him get rid of air he has swallowed while nursing. Which one of the following is the correct method for removing swallowed air from Baby Boy Pruett?
○ 1. Give water from a bottle and place him on his side.
○ 2. Hold him over the shoulder and rub his back.
○ 3. Give him a pacifier and hold him in a face-down position.
○ 4. Hold him with his head slightly elevated and rub his stomach.

89 Ms. Pruett tells the nurse that she wonders if her baby is getting enough milk. Which one of the following may indicate to the nurse that Baby Boy Pruett is *not* getting enough breast milk?
○ 1. Crying when hungry
○ 2. Failing to gain weight
○ 3. Sleeping well
○ 4. Appearing satisfied after breastfeeding

90 The nurse should teach Ms. Pruett that the best way to ensure her baby of an adequate milk supply from her breasts is for her to
○ 1. follow a daily exercise program.
○ 2. eat a diet high in fat content.
○ 3. empty the breasts with each feeding.
○ 4. include a generous amount of leafy green vegetables in her diet.

The type of foods eaten by the mother when breastfeeding is discussed with Ms. Pruett.

91 The nurse can explain to Ms. Pruett that the food she eats
○ 1. may change the taste of the breast milk or cause the baby to have gas.
○ 2. should be low in calories because the baby may gain too much weight.
○ 3. will have no affect on the nursing newborn.
○ 4. should be high in fat to help the newborn gain weight.

Ms. Ellen Dawson has delivered a baby girl. When admitted to the hospital for the birth of her first baby, she expressed a desire to not breastfeed her newborn. The nurse in charge of postpartum care enters the nursing diagnosis of potential altered health maintenance related to lack of knowledge of infant formula preparation.

92 When explaining feeding formulas to Ms. Dawson, the nurse should emphasize the importance of
○ 1. feeding a formula that is low in iron.
○ 2. not feeding the newborn cow's milk during the first year of life.
○ 3. avoiding commercially prepared formulas.
○ 4. feeding at least 5 oz of formula per feeding during the first week of life.

93 The nurse develops a teaching plan for preparing infant formulas. Which one of the following is an *incorrect* entry in this teaching plan?
○ 1. Milk is an ideal medium for the growth of microorganisms.
○ 2. Clean technique usually is sufficient unless several bottles of formula are prepared in advance.
○ 3. Sterile, distilled water must be used for powdered formulas.
○ 4. Most formulas try to duplicate breast milk.

94 The nurse plans to show Ms. Dawson that the bottle is held so that the nipple is always full of formula. This prevents the baby from
○ 1. getting too much formula at once.
○ 2. having to suck vigorously.
○ 3. regurgitating formula.
○ 4. swallowing air.

95 Ms. Dawson also is instructed in how to position her baby after feeding and burping and is told to lay Baby Girl Dawson on her right side or stomach to
○ 1. prevent soiling of her diapers.
○ 2. encourage a bowel movement shortly after feeding.
○ 3. prevent aspiration.
○ 4. encourage sleep.

NURSING CARE OF CLIENTS HAVING A STILLBORN OR A NEWBORN WITH CONGENITAL ABNORMALITIES

Ms. Helena Renaldo has given birth to a stillborn baby. The physician has stated that the parents can see the baby if they wish.

96 Ms. Renaldo wishes to see her baby. The nurse should
○ 1. show her the baby but not allow her to touch it.
○ 2. wash and clean the baby and wrap it in a colorful blanket before allowing Ms. Renaldo to hold or see it.
○ 3. request that only the mother see the baby.
○ 4. not allow her to remove the blanket from the baby.

97 The nurse in charge has selected a private postpartum room for Ms. Renaldo in a section adjacent to the maternity wing. To answer questions concerning this matter the nurse should know that most mothers of stillborn babies
○ 1. often prefer not to be with new mothers with healthy babies.
○ 2. must have time to be with clients with medical or surgical disorders.
○ 3. do not require the same physical care as those having delivered a live newborn.
○ 4. are not subject to infection and therefore can be transferred to a regular hospital unit.

98 The nurse plans to talk to the father of Baby Renaldo. When preparing for this the nurse should understand that
○ 1. fathers tend to grieve for a longer period than mothers.
○ 2. mothers should be allowed to grieve alone.
○ 3. the father should be advised to remove all objects from the area of the home to be used as a newborn nursery.

○ 4. the father should join the mother in mourning the loss of the baby.

Ms. Donna Weems gave birth 1 day ago to a baby girl with spina bifida. This is her first child.

99 When planning nursing care of Ms. Weems, the nurse should remember that the parents of a child with a birth defect
○ 1. are coping with a lifelong disability and chronic grief.
○ 2. must learn to accept this problem before the newborn goes home.
○ 3. do not go through stages of grief and mourning.
○ 4. should not be allowed to see the newborn's disability until they are ready to take the newborn home.

100 One method the nurse may use to help the parents of Baby Girl Weems respond in a positive manner to the newborn is to
○ 1. explain how surgery will most probably eliminate the defect and its consequences.
○ 2. act as a role model, and feed, hold, and change the newborn.
○ 3. assure the family that social agencies will most likely assume full care of the newborn.
○ 4. mention the importance of parents ignoring the defect when the child is older.

NURSING CARE OF CLIENTS CONSIDERING FAMILY PLANNING

The nurse is assigned to discuss family planning and various methods of contraception with a group of women who have expressed interest in this topic.

101 Ms. George asks how "the pill" prevents pregnancy. The most correct explanation is based on the fact that estrogen in an oral contraceptive will prevent a woman from becoming pregnant by
○ 1. preventing ovulation.
○ 2. depressing progesterone secretion.
○ 3. depressing corpus luteum formation.
○ 4. preventing sperm from reaching the ovum.

102 Ms. George asks what problems could occur if she takes an oral contraceptive. The most correct answer is based on the fact that the system of the body most likely to be affected is the
○ 1. urinary system.
○ 2. respiratory system.
○ 3. cardiovascular system.
○ 4. musculoskeletal system.

103 Ms. George asks if there are any precautions she should take to prevent serious side effects if she decides to take an oral contraceptive. The most cor-

rect answer is based on the fact that individuals taking an oral contraceptive should not
- ○ 1. take vitamin pills.
- ○ 2. smoke.
- ○ 3. exercise.
- ○ 4. increase their sexual activity.

104 Ms. Brown asks about intrauterine devices (IUDs). The *most correct* answer is based on the fact that these devices appear to
- ○ 1. interfere with ovulation.
- ○ 2. promote contraction of the fallopian tubes, thus preventing descent of the fertilized egg.
- ○ 3. change the character of cervical mucus.
- ○ 4. appear to interfere with fertilization of the egg or implantation of the fertilized egg.

105 Ms. Brown asks if the use of a condom with a spermicidal agent really is effective. The most correct answer is based on the fact that this method of contraception is
- ○ 1. not recommended.
- ○ 2. reliable.
- ○ 3. less reliable than an aerosol vaginal foam.
- ○ 4. not very reliable.

106 Ms. Lang asks about the use of a diaphragm or a cervical cap. The most correct answer is based on the fact that these two contraceptive devices
- ○ 1. are rarely effective as a contraceptive.
- ○ 2. must be fitted by a physician and require detailed instruction in their use.
- ○ 3. must be used along with an oral contraceptive.
- ○ 4. cannot be used by women who have never been pregnant.

INDIVIDUAL TEST ITEMS

107 All postpartum clients are observed for complications. Which of the following signs and symptoms indicates cystitis and would alert the nurse to notify the physician?
- ○ 1. Concentrated urine and pain in the upper abdomen
- ○ 2. Dysuria and hematuria

- ○ 3. Urinary retention and swelling of the extremities
- ○ 4. Thirst and voiding large amounts of urine

108 Ms. Banko has had a history of mastitis after her last two pregnancies. During discharge teaching the nurse should include measures that may help prevent mastitis. Which one of the following should the nurse include in discharge teaching?
- ○ 1. Only use one breast for breastfeeding.
- ○ 2. Wear a breast binder between breastfeedings.
- ○ 3. Apply petroleum jelly to the nipples before breastfeeding.
- ○ 4. Use a breast shield over the nipple when it becomes painful.

109 Ms. Garfield has been diagnosed as having postpartum psychosis. When Ms. Garfield comes to her physician's office, the nurse should observe her for behavior changes that may include
- ○ 1. talkativeness.
- ○ 2. anxiety.
- ○ 3. signs of withdrawal.
- ○ 4. sadness.

110 Ms. Taylor has had a temperature of 101°F for 3 days. Her physician suspects a puerperal (postpartum) infection, and she is readmitted to the hospital. Which one of the following observations made by the nurse is considered an additional sign of a puerperal infection?
- ○ 1. Bradycardia
- ○ 2. Abdominal tenderness and pain
- ○ 3. A decrease in the size of the uterus
- ○ 4. An absence of lochia

111 Ms. Fields developed thrombophlebitis 6 days after delivery of her baby and is readmitted to the hospital. Ms. Fields asks if the nurse could massage her leg to relieve the discomfort. The nurse must refuse to perform this task because massage
- ○ 1. would decrease the blood supply to the area.
- ○ 2. can be done only after applying heat to the leg.
- ○ 3. could loosen the blood clot (thrombus).
- ○ 4. will not reduce pain and tenderness.

Correct Answers and Rationale

Two numbers appear in parentheses following each rationale. The first number identifies the textbook listed in the references, page 451, and the second number identifies the page(s) in that textbook on which the correct answer can be verified. Occasionally, two textbooks are given for verifying the correct answer.

Nursing Care of Clients During Labor, Delivery, and Postpartum

ADMISSION OF THE CLIENT TO A LABOR AND DELIVERY FACILITY

1 3. Braxton Hicks contractions may be described as a tightening of the abdomen. They usually are not painful and occur at irregular intervals hours, days, or weeks before true labor begins. Hegar's sign is a softening of the lower uterine segment. Chadwick's sign is a bluish or purplish change in the coloration of the vulva, the vagina, and the cervix. Goodell's sign is a softening of the cervix and the vagina. (13:186)
Nursing Process—Collecting data
Client Need—Physiological integrity

2 2. Pertinent questions to ask a woman having uterine contractions when she is being admitted to the hospital include questions related to whether membranes have ruptured, when contractions started, and when the client last ate. The anesthesiologist is especially interested in knowing when the client last ate. Least pertinent of the questions given in this item deals with the administration of an enema. Not all clients have enemas. The appropriate time to ask a client if she has ever had one is shortly before administering the enema. (19:99; 8:110–111)
Nursing Process—Collecting data
Client need—Physiological integrity

3 1. A vaginal examination is contraindicated if there has been bleeding during the last trimester or if excessive bleeding is present at the time of admission to the hospital. The nitrazine test and drawing blood for laboratory examination would have no effect on the fetus and would not be contraindicated if there is vaginal bleeding. Fetal monitoring may be indicated, especially if there are signs or suspicion of fetal distress. (19:99)
Nursing Process—Collecting data
Client Need—Physiological integrity

NURSING CARE OF CLIENTS DURING THE FIRST STAGE OF LABOR

4 3. Full dilatation (8 to 10 cm) and effacement of the cervix represents the first stage of labor. This stage may be divided into three phases, early, midlabor, and transition. Various references may use other terminology, such as latent and active for the first two phases. Braxton Hicks contractions normally occur at irregular intervals after the first trimester and exercise the uterine muscle in preparation for labor. They may become more uncomfortable 12 to 24 hours before true labor begins. Movement of the fetus into the pelvic inlet (lightening) usually occurs 2 to 3 days before true labor begins. (14:552; 8:123–124)
Nursing Process—Planning
Client Need—Health promotion/maintenance

5 2. When the fetal head or presenting part, such as a shoulder or buttocks, is above the ischial spines, the distance is measured as minus one, two, three, and so on. At station zero the presenting part is at the level of the ischial spines and is described as being engaged. When the presenting part is below the ischial spines, it is descending into the birth canal (vagina). (14:553)
Nursing Process—Planning
Client Need—Health promotion/maintenance

6 3. If the client is in early labor and not ambulating, she is encouraged to rest in bed in the left side-lying position. This position interferes least with circulation in the mother and the baby and promotes urinary functioning and uterine efficiency. During assessments such as a vaginal examination, the client temporarily uses the back-lying position for the convenience of the examiner. Later in labor, especially during transition and while the mother is pushing, a low Fowler's position usually is used. (14:556)
Nursing Process—Implementation
Client Need—Health promotion/maintenance

7 2. When the cervix is dilated between 0 and 4 cm, the woman is considered to be active in the beginning of the first stage of labor. At approxi-

mately 4 cm the client is approaching half of the total amount of cervical dilatation. During the transition stage the cervix normally is dilated between 8 and 10 cm. (13:189–192)
   Nursing Process—Evaluation
   Client Need—Health promotion/maintenance

8 1. Normally, the FHR slows at the onset of a contraction. At the height of the contraction the FHR is at the slowest rate. An unchanged FHR during a contraction or a slow return to the original FHR after a contraction are danger signs and must be reported immediately. (14:558)
   Nursing Process—Evaluation
   Client Need—Health promotion/maintenance

9 2. The transition part of stage one is ordinarily the most difficult period of labor. It is a time when the mother often loses control of herself. The client requires the most encouragement and support from the nurse during this stage. This is a time when the nurse should stay with the client. The mother often suffers fatigue, may be nauseated, and has very forceful contractions. (13:227)
   Nursing Process—Implementation
   Client Need—Health promotion/maintenance

10 4. It is inappropriate to have the client push with contractions until she is in the second stage of labor. Until then, pushing will be ineffective and tiring. Helping the client onto her left side, urging her to void, and encouraging her to breathe deeply are appropriate nursing measures late in the first stage of labor. (14:556–557)
   Nursing Process—Implementation
   Client Need—Health promotion/maintenance

11 1. When there is a question concerning whether membranes have ruptured, a nitrazine test helps to determine if the client has amniotic fluid leaving the vagina or if she is leaking urine. The test strips used in this examination determine alkalinity or acidity. Urine is normally acid, and amniotic fluid is alkaline. If the nitrazine strips turn blue, the client is probably leaking amniotic fluid. If the strip remains yellow, she is probably leaking urine and the membranes are likely intact. (8:126–127)
   Nursing Process—Collecting data
   Client Need—Health promotion/maintenance

12 4. A full urinary bladder during labor tends to prevent the descent of the neonate into the birth canal by imposing on the canal. Also, it interferes with uterine contractions but not necessarily on the observations of contractions. It predisposes

the bladder to injury, and a full bladder is uncomfortable for the client in labor. (13:224)
   Nursing Process—Planning
   Client Need—Health promotion/maintenance

13 4. Offering the bedpan at frequent intervals for the client on bed rest or helping the ambulatory client to the bathroom will help keep the bladder empty. Limiting oral or intravenous fluid intake is not done because the client should not be allowed to become dehydrated. (13:224)
   Nursing Process—Implementation
   Client Need—Health promotion/maintenance

14 1. Contamination of the perineum may occur if feces are expelled during delivery of the baby. Although some physicians feel an enema may not be necessary, others order one routinely. A suppository or small disposable enema may be used to empty the contents of the rectum. An enema does not ease the discomfort of contractions, prevent constipation after delivery, or relieve pressure in an area where an episiotomy may be performed. (13:223)
   Nursing Process—Implementation
   Client Need—Health promotion/maintenance

15 2. The length of a contraction from its beginning to its end is called its duration. The degree of hardness or firmness when the uterus contracts is called intensity. The time from the beginning of one contraction to the beginning of the next contraction is called the frequency. Frequency refers to how often contractions occur and is described in minutes and seconds. (13:192)
   Nursing Process—Implementation
   Client Need—Health promotion/maintenance

16 2. The hand should be placed just above the client's umbilicus on the fundus, or top, of the uterus. This is where the strongest muscular contractions can be felt most easily. (8:112–113)
   Nursing Process—Collecting data
   Client Need—Health promotion/maintenance

17 2. It is recommended that the FHR be checked immediately after and during a contraction. This procedure helps to detect late deceleration of the heartbeat, which may be due to fetal distress. Fetal distress is very likely to be caused by placental insufficiency. Continuous, recorded monitoring of the FHR is preferred by many, but equipment to monitor is not available in all agencies. (8:114)
   Nursing Process—Collecting data
   Client Need—Health promotion/maintenance

18 3. The normal FHR is between 120 and 160 beats per minute. (8:116; 14:557)

Nursing Process—Evaluation
Client Need—Health promotion/maintenance

19 1. False labor is evidenced by irregular contractions that do not increase in frequency, duration, and intensity. The client may note that the contractions decrease when ambulating and that the contractions are located primarily in the abdomen rather than starting in the back and radiating to the abdomen. (14:551)

Nursing Process—Evaluation
Client Need—Health promotion/maintenance

20 4. A vaginal examination to determine how much cervical dilatation has occurred is performed under conditions of strictest cleanliness. The nurse should clean the client's vulva before the examination. The examiner should wash his or her hands well and then put on a sterile glove. A sterile lubricant is used. In some agencies a disinfectant may be poured over the gloved hand and the vulva. Vaginal examinations of women in labor ordinarily are performed by a registered nurse, a midwife, or a physician. (8:127)

Nursing Process—Implementation
Client Need—Health promotion/maintenance

21 1. True labor may be described as starting when uterine contractions occur regularly. During true labor the cervical canal is completely effaced, and the cervix dilates. Expelling the mucous plug from the cervical canal, called show (due to a softening of the cervix and effacement), is a sign that labor is about to start. Usually, the fetus drops into the brim of the pelvis approximately 1 to 2 weeks before delivery in mothers having their first baby. This phenomenon is called lightening. (13:186)

Nursing Process—Evaluation
Client Need—Health promotion/maintenance

22 4. Water or clear liquids such as tea are given in the early stages of labor. Vomiting may occur if solid foods or liquids such as milk are given. In addition the client may be scheduled for a possible general anesthetic, which cannot be given if she has recently had solid food. (14:557)

Nursing Process—Planning
Client Need—Health promotion/maintenance

23 4. ROA describes the fetal head as *right occipital anterior*. The first letter of the position is either L or R (eg, left or right). The second letter describes the fetal presenting part, such as the sacrum, the face, the occiput, or the shoulder. The third letter describes the relationship to the mother's pelvis (eg, anterior, posterior, or transverse). Examples of other normal fetal positions are ROP (right occipital posterior) and LOT (left occipital transverse). An example of a more complicated presentation is the breech position, examples of which are RSP (right sacral posterior) and RSA (right sacral anterior). (19:113; 14:553)

Nursing Process—Collecting data
Client Need—Health promotion/maintenance

24 3. An important reason for doing an episiotomy is to help prevent prolonged pressure on the fetal head. The incision also helps prevent undue stretching of perineal muscles and lacerations of the perineum. Mothers prepared for labor and delivery in childbirth classes are less likely to require an episiotomy than mothers who have not had this type of preparation. (14:554; 19:155–156)

Nursing Process—Implementation
Client Need—Health promotion/maintenance

25 2. Contractions lasting longer than 2 minutes can result in uterine rupture and therefore must be brought immediately to the attention of the physician or nurse in charge. Contractions that are 8 minutes apart, start in the front of the abdomen, or are accompanied by pain usually are normal events during the very early first stage of labor. (14:556)

Nursing Process—Evaluation
Client Need—Health promotion/maintenance

26 4. Bulging of the perineum and crowning of the fetal head indicate the primipara is ready for delivery. The multipara usually is taken to the delivery room when the cervix is dilated 6 to 8 cm because labor in the multipara often progresses at a faster rate than in the primipara. (14:558; 8:129)

Nursing Process—Evaluation
Client Need—Health promotion/maintenance

NURSING CARE OF CLIENTS DURING THE SECOND STAGE OF LABOR

27 3. All narcotic analgesics cross the placenta and therefore have an effect on the fetus. A baby born shortly after the administration of an analgesic may experience respiratory depression. Because this client has a history of rapid progression through stage one, analgesics would normally be withheld unless the physician determines that an analgesic is necessary. Analgesics also may slow the frequency and force of contractions. (19:134)

Nursing Process—Implementation
Client Need—Health promotion/maintenance

28 4. Unless there are complications, the Sims' position, the knee–chest position, or sitting on the

edge of the bed may help relieve discomfort. (19:133)
Nursing Process—Implementation
Client Need—Health promotion/maintenance

29 1. The second stage of labor begins with full dilatation of the cervix and ends with the birth of the baby. (13:193)
Nursing Process—Planning
Client need—Health promotion/maintenance

30 1. The mother must push in the second and third stage of labor for the delivery of the baby and the placenta. Pushing is the working stage of delivery, and the mother must focus her attention on this technique. Fluids may be withheld or limited during this stage, depending on the type of anesthetic (if any) the physician plans to administer. (19:132)
Nursing Process—Implementation
Client Need—Health promotion/maintenance

31 2. Hyperventilation is evidenced by blurred vision; tingling of the hands and feet, which can progress to muscle cramping or spasms; and numbness around the nose or mouth. (19:132)
Nursing Process—Collecting data
Client Need—Health promotion/maintenance

32 1. Additional methods of correcting hyperventilation include holding the breath, breathing slowly, breathing into cupped hands, and holding the breath a few seconds before exhaling. These maneuvers increase blood levels of carbon dioxide and therefore correct the condition. Lying on the left side, taking sips of water between breaths, and inhaling five to six short, quick breaths would not promote an increase of carbon dioxide in the blood. (19:132)
Nursing Process—Implementation
Client Need—Health promotion/maintenance

33 1. Analgesia (relief of pain) occurs almost immediately with this type of regional anesthetic. The abdomen, perineum, legs, and feet become numb. This type of anesthetic has no effect on the respirations of the newborn because it is given into subarachnoid space and not into the mother's bloodstream. (8:156)
Nursing Process—Implementation
Client Need—Health promotion/maintenance

NURSING CARE OF CLIENTS DURING THE THIRD STAGE OF LABOR

34 4. Pushing with a contraction aids in the delivery of the placenta. (8:118)
Nursing Process—Implementation
Client Need—Health promotion/maintenance

35 4. Before the newborn takes its first breath, the physician will ordinarily clear the airway of mucus and debris so that the baby will not inhale blood, mucus, or other liquid. A bulb syringe usually is used. The physician also first clears the airway after the birth of the baby's head before the body is delivered. Repairing an episiotomy, cutting the umbilical cord, and evaluating the newborn's condition (the Apgar) are done after the newborn's breathing is established. (14:559)
Nursing Process—Implementation
Client Need—Health promotion/maintenance

36 1. The physician waits until the cord stops pulsating and applies two clamps. The umbilical cord is then cut between the two clamps. (14:559)
Nursing Process—Implemention
Client Need—Health promotion/maintenance

37 3. An oxytocic may be administered after the delivery of the placenta to help strengthen contractions of the uterus and prevent excessive bleeding. This type of agent is not used to decrease blood pressure, prevent uterine inversion, or decrease uterine spasms. (15:224–225)
Nursing Process—Implementation
Client need—Health promotion/maintenance

38 1. It is best when parent–newborn bonding can be started within 1 hour after the birth of a newborn. Bonding means developing an attachment between the newborn and the parents. The senses are the means through which bonding develops, and therefore opportunities for the parents to see, touch, hear, and smell their newborn should be provided. (13:31–33)
Nursing Process—Implementation
Client Need—Health promotion/maintenance

39 3. Before birth the fetus was in an environment close to the mother's body temperature. After birth the neonate is in an environment cooler than the mother's body temperature. Placing Baby Girl Packard under a radiant heat source and quickly drying her reduces heat loss. Wet towels or water that is 80°F will still encourage heat loss because this temperature is below normal body temperature. Holding the newborn exposes its skin to room temperature air. (8:140)
Nursing Process—Implementation
Client Need—Health promotion/maintenance

40 1. The correct procedure for the instillation of any liquid ophthalmic medication is dropping the prescribed dose into the lower conjunctival sac. The dose for ophthalmic silver nitrate 1% is one drop in each eye, instilled in the lower conjunctival sac. (13:232–233)
Nursing Process—Implementation
Client Need—Health promotion/maintenance

41 2. The Apgar score is a method of assessing the physical condition of the newborn and determining whether additional assistance, resuscitation, or treatment is necessary. A score of 10 is the best possible score. Newborns with an Apgar below 5 are in danger. (14:586)
Nursing Process—Collecting data
Client Need—Health promotion/maintenance

NURSING CARE OF CLIENTS DURING THE FOURTH STAGE OF LABOR

42 2. Following delivery of the placenta the fundus should be firmly contracted and located approximately 2 cm *below* the umbilicus. (19:169)
Nursing Process—Collecting data
Client Need—Health promotion/maintenance

43 3. Heavy bleeding in the fourth stage may indicate a uterine problem, such as failure of the uterus to contract or retained placental tissue. Some blood loss will occur, but saturation of two perineal pads in ½ hour indicates hemorrhage. A systolic blood pressure below 90 mm Hg or a pulse rate above 100 also may indicate hemorrhage. (19:118–121)
Nursing Process—Collecting data
Client Need—Health promotion/maintenance

44 4. A soft and boggy fundus can lead to uterine bleeding. Normally, the fundus is firm and hard, begins to decrease in size, and is below the umbilicus. (19:169)
Nursing Process—Collecting data
Client Need—Health promotion/maintenance

45 1. Placing one hand on the fundus and the other hand just over the pubic bone prevents the uterus from being prolapsed or inverted. (8:210)
Nursing Process—Implementation
Client Need—Health promotion/maintenance

NURSING CARE OF CLIENTS DURING THE POSTPARTUM

46 2. Shortly after delivery, the lochia normally appears dark or bright red and should be moderate in amount. (8:201)
Nursing Process—Collecting data
Client Need—Health promotion/maintenance

47 4. The amount of lochia is described as being scant, light, moderate, or heavy. Lochia is considered to be heavy when perineal pads are quickly saturated, and the discharge contains blood clots. The occurrence of a heavy lochia is immediately reported to the physician. (19:170)
Nursing Process—Collecting data
Client Need—Health promotion/maintenance

48 2. A hematoma will cause a swelling on the perineum, and the skin will become bluish or purple. When this occurs a hematoma usually will be seen during the first few hours after delivery. (13:235–237)
Nursing Process—Collecting data
Client Need—Health promotion/maintenance

49 2. A client who develops a hematoma generally complains of a great deal of pain in the perineal area, especially when there are sutures following an episiotomy. The pain also may be felt in the rectum. The condition should be reported promptly. A hematoma is not associated with dysuria, itching in the perineal area, or a feeling of fullness in the vagina. (19:170–171)
Nursing Process—Collecting data
Client Need—Health promotion/maintenance

50 1. Early ambulation, when allowed, helps prevent problems with the circulatory, respiratory, gastrointestinal, urinary, and musculoskeletal systems. It is unlikely to help improve milk-producing ability, fluid balance, or returning to sexual activity. However, early ambulation with moderation should be encouraged to prevent fatigue. (19:182)
Nursing Process—Implementation
Client Need—Health promotion/maintenance

51 4. An overdistended urinary bladder is especially likely to predispose to the development of a bladder infection. Also, bladder muscle tonus decreases with overdistention. A full bladder also predisposes the client to increased uterine bleeding because it prevents the uterus from contracting properly. (19:171, 191–192)
Nursing Process—Implementation
Client Need—Health promotion/maintenance

52 4. The nurse should use essentially the same techniques for catheterizing a postpartum client as she uses for other women. The meatus is cleansed, the catheter is lubricated, and the catheter is introduced in the same manner as when catheterizing other women. (19:171–172)
Nursing Process—Implementation
Client Need—Physiological integrity

53 2. Heat lamps placed too close to the perineum can cause burns. If the lamp is too far away, the beneficial results of heat are lost. (18:497; 19:171)
Nursing Process—Implementation
Client Need—Safe, effective care environment

54 1. The physician often recommends Sitz baths to decrease the discomfort associated with an episiotomy. Ambulation, lying on the abdomen, and elevating the hips are not likely to relieve

the discomfort associated with an episiotomy. (19:171)

Nursing Process—Implementation
Client Need—Health promotion/maintenance

55 4. Propoxyphene hydrochloride (Darvon) is classified as a non-narcotic analgesic and may be prescribed to be taken every 3 to 4 hours as necessary for the relief of discomfort from afterpains, pain from sutures when an episiotomy has been performed, and breast engorgement. The drug does not act as an antiemetic or hypnotic, nor is it used to firm the uterus. The drug is a controlled substance, which means it cannot be obtained without a prescription. (15:62)

Nursing Process—Evaluation
Client Need—Physiological integrity

56 2. Cleansing from front to back (eg, from the vulva to the rectum) is necessary to prevent contamination of the perineum by microorganisms present in the feces and therefore present around the anal area. (19:182)

Nursing Process—Implementation
Client Need—Health promotion/maintenance

57 2. The "postpartum blues" are common. Most often a client cannot explain why she feels "down." In this situation it is best to stay with the client and offer any help she may need. If the client wishes to talk about her crying, the nurse should listen quietly and avoid trying to give advice. For some women it is helpful to explain that a "down" feeling *may* be related to the sudden drop in body hormones after delivery. (19:193)

Nursing Process—Implementation
Client Need—Psychosocial integrity

58 3. Breast engorgement usually occurs on approximately the third postpartum day, when milk production by the breasts comes under the influence of the hormone prolactin. (19:184)

Nursing Process—Planning
Client Need—Health promotion/maintenance

NURSING CARE OF CLIENTS HAVING A CESAREAN DELIVERY

59 1. A gel is placed on the transducer primarily to improve the conduction of sound. The gel is not used to prevent the transducer from slipping or to decrease irritating effects of the transducer on the skin. No electric current passes through the transducer to the client. (19:106–107)

Nursing Process—Implementation
Client Need—Health promotion/maintenance

60 2. The primary reason for placing an indwelling catheter in the client's bladder prior to abdominal surgery is to keep the bladder empty during the surgical procedure. An indwelling catheter also may be inserted in surgery, before the surgical procedure is performed and after the client is under anesthesia. A full bladder makes the handling of abdominal contents more difficult for the surgeon and poses a risk for puncturing the bladder with a surgical instrument. The indwelling catheter is not in place to prevent a bladder infection, prevent postoperative discomfort, or provide easy or safe access for obtaining urine specimens. (8:148–149)

Nursing Process—Implementation
Client Need—Physiological integrity

61 1. If a nurse notes that a consent form has not been signed prior to a surgical procedure, such as a cesarean delivery, the nurse should report this to the nurse in charge immediately. It is the physician's responsibility to inform a client about a surgical procedure, including the attending risks, benefits, and likely outcome. It is a nursing procedure to determine that a consent form is signed before the client is transferred to an operating room. (18:436; 8:148)

Nursing Process—Implementation
Client Need—Safe, effective care environment

62 3. The care of a client who has had a cesarean delivery most nearly resembles the care of one who has had abdominal surgery. The client is likely to develop complications and experience discomforts similar to those of any other client having abdominal surgery. In addition the client is subject to develop most of the complications and discomforts that other postpartum clients do. (8:214–215)

Nursing Process—Planning
Client Need—Physiological integrity

63 3. A rise in the pulse rate, a drop in blood pressure; pale skin, apprehension; a decrease in urinary output; and cool-to-cold, clammy skin are indications of shock. (8:234)

Nursing Process—Collecting data
Client Need—Physiological integrity

64 3. An oxytocic drug, such as oxytocin (Pitocin), may be administered to help the uterus contract and therefore prevent excessive bleeding or hemorrhage. Oxytocin does have a vasopressor effect and thus raises the blood pressure, but the drug is not used for this purpose. Oxytocic drugs have no effect on wound healing nor do

they directly increase the amount of lochia. (8:214; 15:224–225)

> Nursing Process—Collecting data
> Client Need—Physiological integrity

65 1. Relief from pain occurs quickly because the narcotic is given intravenously. The device regulates the dose of the drug and the interval between doses, and there is no danger of receiving too much of the drug. The dosage delivered by the device usually is less than the dosage required for oral or intramuscular administration on a 3- to 4-hour basis. (15:66)

> Nursing Process—Planning
> Client Need—Physiological integrity

66 4. Ambulation may increase peristalsis and help in the passage of flatus and the relief of abdominal distention. Increasing the fluid intake to 3000 mL will not relieve abdominal distention. Taking fluids through a straw may increase distention because the client may swallow air along with the fluid. Lying on the abdomen would cause discomfort or pain and may interfere with healing of the new incision. (8:215)

> Nursing Process—Implementation
> Client Need—Physiological integrity

NURSING CARE OF CLIENTS HAVING AN EMERGENCY DELIVERY

67 3. When a delivery appears imminent and the nurse is without help it is best, if possible, for him or her to prepare a clean field for delivery. This precaution helps prevent infection. Sometimes there is not time for this, but an attempt should be made without sacrificing efforts to control the birth. Assuring the mother that help will arrive offers false hope when the delivery is obviously imminent. A mother late in the first stage of labor and entering the second stage of labor is unable to avoid bearing down. Taking the FHR is less important in the situation described in this item. (8:146)

> Nursing Process—Implementation
> Client Need—Safe, effective care environment

68 1. When birth is imminent and no help is available, the nurse should gently control the delivery of the head, allow it to emerge, and deliver it between contractions. The nurse should *not* hold back the baby's head to prevent birth, nor should the nurse attempt to enter or enlarge the vaginal opening. (8:146–147)

> Nursing Process—Implementation
> Client Need—Physiological integrity

Nursing Care of the Newborn Client

NURSING CARE OF THE NORMAL NEWBORN CLIENT

69 3. A newborn has a very low level of blood prothrombin and therefore is prone to bleeding. Vitamin K is needed by the liver to manufacture prothrombin and various other factors involved with the clotting of blood. Vitamin K is given to many newborns to help improve blood clotting. After the newborn begins to take food, it takes about 2 weeks for normal intestinal bacteria, which synthesize vitamin K, to be present in the intestinal tract. Vitamin K does not stimulate respirations, start peristalsis, or increase calcium absorption. (19:180; 13:334)

> Nursing Process—Implementation
> Client Need—Health promotion/maintenance

70 3. It is recommended that intramuscular injections be given to the newborn in the rectus femoris, vastus lateralis, or deltoid muscles. The gluteus muscle should not be used because of the danger of injuring the sciatic nerve. The biceps brachii muscle, located in the arm, and the biceps femoris muscle, located in the back of the leg, are unsuitable sites for this age group. (18:611; 13:334)

> Nursing Process—Implementation
> Client Need—Physiological integrity

71 4. The umbilical cord should be checked frequently during the first few hours after birth for signs of bleeding. If an infection develops, it will appear later. Pulsation ceases soon after the cord is cut after delivery, and herniation, if it occurs, appears later. (19:175)

> Nursing Process—Collecting data
> Client Need—Health promotion/maintenance

72 4. The white substance on a newborn's skin is called vernix caseosa. It consists of old cutaneous cells and secretions from the skin's oil glands. Lanugo is the soft fine hair on the newborn's body. Petechiae are small blue or purple dots on the skin caused by capillary bleeding. Miliaria rubra is heat rash. (19:215)

> Nursing Process—Collecting data
> Client Need—Health promotion/maintenance

73 2. Jaundice appearing within a few hours after birth may be a sign of a pathologic condition and should be reported promptly. Jaundice 2 or 3 days after birth is not uncommon. Newborns void and pass stool within approximately 12 hours after birth; if these excretory functions do not occur within 12 hours after birth, the nurse in charge should be notified. It is normal for a newborn to spit up mucus shortly after birth.

The scrotum of the male newborn and the labia of the female newborn are likely to be swollen shortly after birth due to pressure on them during a vaginal delivery. (13:333–334)

    Nursing Process—Collecting data
    Client Need—Health promotion/maintenance

74 4. Normally, a newborn's abdomen rises and falls with respirations while the chest barely moves. This type of breathing is often called abdominal breathing. Sternal respirations are present when the sternum moves in (retracts) on inspiration; it is abnormal and should be reported promptly. The hands and feet and an area around the mouth may appear cyanotic (blue) for several hours after birth because of poor circulation to these areas. However, the remainder of the body should be pink shortly after birth. A pulse rate of 140 beats per minute is normal in a newborn. Regurgitating the first feeding or two after birth also is normal. (14:586–588)

    Nursing Process—Collecting data
    Client Need—Health promotion/maintenance

75 4. The nurse should have his or her hand *over* the baby and be ready to hold him or her if the newborn needs protection from injury while being weighed. The nurse's hand should be free of the newborn so that the hand does not interfere with an accurate weight. Placing a clean protective paper (a fresh one for each newborn) on the scale, balancing the scale, and weighing the baby without clothing describe proper techniques for weighing a newborn who is within the normal birth weight range. (14:592)

    Nursing Process—Implementation
    Client Need—Health promotion/maintenance

76 2. Normally, a newborn's temperature will stabilize within approximately 8 to 12 hours after birth. The heat-regulating mechanism of a newborn is still immature; therefore, a newborn responds readily to environmental temperatures. (8:241)

    Nursing Process—Implementation
    Client Need—Health promotion/maintenance

77 2. Jaundice (icterus), is a yellow cast of the skin. In newborns this also is called physiological jaundice. This is a normal phenomenon resulting from the breakdown of red blood cells. Serum bilirubin, which is a byproduct occurring when red blood cells are destroyed, is increased. The newborn's immature liver often is unable to handle the excretion of bilirubin, and jaundice occurs. Hepatitis is a viral infection of the liver, and biliary atresia is a narrowing of the biliary tree, which also may cause jaundice. Erythroblastosis fetalis refers to a formation and release of immature red blood cells seen in newborns and usually caused by Rh incompatibility. (8:240)

    Nursing Process—Collecting data
    Client Need—Health promotion/maintenance

78 1. To protect the retina the eyes are covered when the newborn requires phototherapy. The newborn is placed on an every-3-hour feeding schedule because this increases the excretion of bilirubin. The newborn is turned frequently to prevent overheating with resultant dehydration. The amount of clothing placed on the newborn varies with hospital policy. Some hospitals leave the newborn totally uncovered except for the eyes; others use a small diaper placed over the genitalia and a covering for the eyes. (14:603)

    Nursing Process—Implementation
    Client Need—Health promotion/maintenance

79 1. Normally the newborn's skin is dry and may peel (desquamate). Any abnormalities noted are recorded and reported to the nurse in charge or the physician. The newborn's temperature control center normally is immature. Leaving the skin exposed may lower body temperature. Alcohol would not be used on a newborn because this also can lower body temperature. The newborn's diaper is changed as needed. Newborns may void 12 to 18 times a day when they are 2 or 3 days old. When changing the diaper, the buttocks are thoroughly cleaned after a bowel movement. (14:592–593)

    Nursing Process—Planning
    Client Need—Health promotion/maintenance

80 4. After circumcision the baby should be observed for signs of bleeding at the circumcision site. If bleeding occurs, the condition should be reported. Urinary output should be observed because occasionally there is retention of urine following a circumcision owing to excessive swelling of the penis near the urinary meatus. Normally there should be no blood in the urine, but a urine-soaked diaper may be stained with blood because of slight oozing from the circumcision site. Swelling of the scrotum is not associated with circumcision. (14:594)

    Nursing Process—Collecting data
    Client Need—Health promotion/maintenance

81 4. Immediate breastfeeding promotes contraction of the uterus. Breast milk at this time is not rich but thin and yellowish in appearance. Estrogen inhibits milk production during pregnancy and is not involved in the production or flow of breast milk. Retracted breast nipples do not enhance the process of breastfeeding; raised breast nipples do enhance the ability of the newborn to breastfeed. (8:144)

> Nursing Process—Implementation
> Client Need—Health promotion/maintenance

82 2. Colostrum contains antibodies, vitamins A and E, and minerals. It also is rich in protein and acts as a mild laxative. Colostrum is replaced by breast milk on approximately the third or fourth day after birth. (19:183)

> Nursing Process—Implementation
> Client Need—Health promotion/maintenance

83 2. The normal stools of a breastfed newborn can be described as yellow-orange. They tend to be softer and more frequent for the first few weeks than stools of newborns receiving prepared formulas. The stools of formula-fed newborns tend to be more yellow and have a curdled appearance. There is a wide range of normal stool color and frequency of stool passage. (8:243)

> Nursing Process—Evaluation
> Client Need—Health promotion/maintenance

84 2. A newborn is in search of food when he or she turns the head toward an object that touches the cheek. The response is entirely normal. (8:186)

> Nursing Process—Implementation
> Client Need—Health promotion/maintenance

85 1. The rooting reflex is elicited by touching the newborn's cheek with the nipple or a finger. The newborn's head instinctively turns toward the breast, with his mouth open, searching for food. (8:186)

> Nursing Process—Implementation
> Client Need—Health promotion/maintenance

86 3. Starting the newborn to feed on the less tender breast may help relieve cracked and sore nipples because the most vigorous sucking occurs at the beginning of breastfeeding. A lotion or ointment may be recommended or prescribed by the physician for application between breastfeedings. Changing the baby's position frequently and air-drying the nipples after each feeding also may relieve the condition. (19:184–185)

> Nursing Process—Implementation
> Client Need—Health promotion/maintenance

87 3. Gentle downward pressure on the newborn's chin or at the corner of his mouth on the cheek usually will cause the baby to release the nipple. Also, the mother can carefully insert her finger into the neonate's mouth to break the suction if the newborn is reluctant to let go. If the mother has long fingernails, this technique of removal is not recommended because it may injure the delicate tissues of the baby's mouth. Nipples should

not be pulled from the newborn's mouth, because this is likely to injure the nipples. (8:260)

> Nursing Process—Implementation
> Client Need—Health promotion/maintenance

88 2. The best way to help an newborn get rid of air he has swallowed while nursing is to hold him over the shoulder and rub his back. A second technique that can be used includes laying the baby across the lap while supporting his head with a hand and gently patting the newborn's back. A third technique is sitting the newborn upright and patting or rubbing the back while supporting the newborn's chest and head with one hand. (19:187)

> Nursing Process—Implementation
> Client Need—Health promotion/maintenance

89 2. Failure to gain weight after several days of breastfeeding indicates the baby may not be getting enough milk. Additional signs may include failure to be satisfied after breastfeeding, failure to sleep well (especially after breastfeeding), and crying shortly after breastfeeding. (19:182)

> Nursing Process—Collecting data
> Client Need—Health promotion/maintenance

90 3. It has been found that emptying the breasts completely is the best way to ensure a good milk supply. If the newborn does not empty the breasts, the mother should empty them manually. A nourishing diet and a generous intake of milk are important, but to best ensure a good milk supply, the breasts should be emptied regularly. The mother can drink skim or low-fat milk to increase the calcium and protein intake, which is necessary when breastfeeding a newborn. (8:260)

> Nursing Process—Implementation
> Client Need—Health promotion/maintenance

91 1. Certain foods may change the taste of breast milk. The breastfeeding mother should increase her caloric intake because milk production requires energy. A high-fat diet or a low-calorie diet for the breastfeeding mother will not affect the newborn's weight gain. (20:147–148; 19:185)

> Nursing Process—Implementation
> Client Need—Physiological integrity

92 2. Cow's milk is not recommended for newborns younger than 1 year because it may cause gastrointestinal bleeding and kidney problems. Prepackaged formulas, when prepared according to the manufacturer's directions, meet the nutritional needs of the newborn. During the first few weeks of life the newborn may consume only 2 to 3 oz of formula. Iron is added to commercial formulas because it is needed for manufacturing red blood cells. (19:188–189; 8:263–265; 20:155, 159)

Nursing Process—Implementation
Client Need—Health promotion/maintenance

93 3. The use of sterile, distilled water is not necessary. Tap water may be used with powdered formulas. If the water source is questionable, the tap water should be boiled before use. (8:261)

Nursing Process—Planning
Client Need—Health promotion/maintenance

94 4. If the neck of the bottle and nipple is not filled with formula, the neonate swallows air. Air in the newborn's stomach causes discomfort or pain and decreases the amount of formula taken at any one time. (19:189)

Nursing Process—Planning
Client Need—Health promotion/maintenance

95 3. Newborns can regurgitate their formula. Laying the newborn on its back could result in aspiration of milk or vomitus into the lungs. Laying the newborn on its right side promotes digestion. Normally, newborns sleep after being fed, despite how they are positioned. Some newborns may have a bowel movement during or shortly after feeding. Lying on the right side does not necessarily encourage a bowel movement. (19:189)

Nursing Process—Implementation
Client Need—Health promotion/maintenance

NURSING CARE OF CLIENTS HAVING A STILLBORN OR A NEWBORN WITH CONGENITAL ABNORMALITIES

96 2. When the mother wishes to see her stillborn, the baby can be cleaned and wrapped in a colorful blanket. She and the father of the baby should be allowed to see, touch, and hold their baby. Although some parents may not wish to view the baby, doing so allows them to close the cycle of birth and death and accept the fact that their baby is dead. (13:321)

Nursing Process—Implementation
Client Need—Psychosocial integrity

97 1. Most mothers find it difficult to room with or be in the same area as mothers with live, healthy babies. The cry of newborns; the conversations of mothers, fathers, and family members; and the nurses carrying newborns to their mothers for breastfeedings or bottle feedings may intensify the loss. These mothers require frequent contact and emotional support from their family and their caregivers. In some hospitals the postpartum caregiver to those giving birth to a stillborn baby is a nurse from labor and delivery or postpartum who is skilled in the psychosocial aspects of grieving and loss. Mothers having a stillborn baby require the same type of care as those giving birth to a live newborn and are just as prone to postpartum complications as mothers who have had a live newborn. (13:321–322)

Nursing Process—Implementation
Client Need—Psychosocial integrity

98 4. The father should join the mother in the grieving process. As a rule, fathers grieve for a shorter period than mothers. The objects in the home related to the newborn should remain. Usually, the mother will put them away when she is ready and begins to resolve her grief. (13:322)

Nursing Process—Planning
Client Need—Psychosocial integrity

99 1. Parents with a baby born with one or more congenital anomalies or defects are coping, in many instances, with a lifelong disability and chronic grief. Even when the defect can be corrected, there still is some reminder that the defect was present at birth. They cannot be expected to accept this problem fully; they do move through the stages of grief and mourning and should view the defect or disability before the newborn is discharged. (13:322–323)

Nursing Process—Planning
Client Need—Psychosocial integrity

100 2. The nurse can act as a role model and encourage the parents to interact with the newborn. This establishes an early bond between the newborn and the parents. Surgery may correct spina bifida but may not correct the neurologic deficit that accompanies this condition. In this case the neurologic deficit cannot be ignored because it will most likely be permanent. While social agencies may be a source of help, they do not necessarily assume all care of the newborn. (13:323)

Nursing Process—Implementation
Client Need—Psychosocial integrity

NURSING CARE OF CLIENTS CONSIDERING FAMILY PLANNING

101 1. Oral contraceptives contain estrogen or progestin, or both. Natural or synthetic progesterones are collectively called progestins. It is theorized that estrogen suppresses ovulation to prevent pregnancy. Progestins appear to inhibit the secretion of pituitary gonadotropins and therefore prevent maturation of the ovarian follicle and consequent ovulation. (14:924; 15:214)

Nursing Process—Implementation
Client Need—Health promotion/maintenance

102 3. Adverse effects related to the use of oral contraceptives may affect the cardiovascular system with complications such as thrombophlebitis, strokes, heart attacks, and hypertension. Gastrointestinal symptoms, such as abdominal cramps, nausea, and vomiting, also are reported. However, "the pill" is a very reliable contraceptive and is used by many without serious untoward effects. These drugs do not affect the respiratory, urinary, or musculoskeletal systems. (15:214, 216)
      Nursing Process—Implementation
      Client Need—Health promotion/maintenance

103 2. Smoking has been reported as increasing the risk of adverse effects occurring in those taking an oral contraceptive. Vitamin pills, exercise, and increased sexual activity have no known effect on these drugs. (8:224)
      Nursing Process—Implementation
      Client Need—Health promotion/maintenance

104 4. An IUD appears to interfere with fertilization of the egg, implantation of the fertilized egg, or the ability of the inner lining of the uterus to accept the fertilized egg. An IUD has no apparent effect on ovulation, the fallopian tubes, or the character of the cervical mucus. (8:225)
      Nursing Process—Implementation
      Client Need—Health promotion/maintenance

105 2. The *correct* use of a condom along with a spermicidal agent is considered a reliable method of contraception. Aerosol vaginal foams, when used without other contraceptive measures, are only moderately reliable. (8:226–227)
      Nursing Process—Implementation
      Client Need—Health promotion/maintenance

106 2. A diaphragm or cervical cap requires fitting by a physician and is available in several sizes. They are considered a reliable method of contraception if they are fitted and then used properly. Many women who cannot tolerate oral contraceptives may decide to use a diaphragm or a cervical cap. The use of these devices is not limited to those who have already been pregnant. (8:223–224)
      Nursing Process—Implementation
      Client Need—Health promotion/maintenance

INDIVIDUAL TEST ITEMS

107 2. Dysuria (pain on urination) and hematuria are signs and symptoms of cystitis. Low abdominal pain, fever, malaise, and urgency and frequency of urination also may be seen. (14:583)
      Nursing Process—Collecting data
      Client Need—Physiological integrity

108 4. Using a breast shield, inspecting the nipples for cracks, treating cracked nipples with prescribed or recommended ointments, starting breastfeeding with the less tender breast, and avoiding prolonged periods at the breast may reduce the incidence of mastitis. The use of petroleum jelly before breastfeeding would coat the newborn's mouth and could be dangerous. Wearing a breast binder or using only one breast for feeding would not prevent mastitis. (14:583)
      Nursing Process—Implementation
      Client Need—Health promotion/maintenance

109 3. Disinterest and withdrawal are two prominent signs of a postpartum psychosis. The client also may appear belligerent and suspicious. In severe cases these individuals can be dangerous to themselves or others. (8:216)
      Nursing Process—Collecting data
      Client Need—Psychosocial integrity

110 2. The symptoms of a puerperal infection include fever, an increase in the pulse rate, abdominal tenderness and pain, foul-smelling lochia, an abnormally large uterus, and chills. (8:216)
      Nursing Process—Collecting data
      Client Need—Health promotion/maintenance

111 3. The extremity affected by thrombophlebitis must *never* be massaged because this may cause the thrombus to break loose and travel to vital organs, such as the brain, the heart, and the lungs. (13:317)
      Nursing Process—Implementation
      Client Need—Health promotion/maintenance

Classification of Test Items

Unit II Review Test 3

Directions: After each question the correct answer is given as well as a classification of each test question. Compare the correct answer with your answer. If a question has been answered *incorrectly*, draw a line to the end of the four columns. When finished, add up your correct scores and place the results at the bottom of each column.

Score Calculation:

To determine the percentage of the number of questions you answered correctly, divide the **Number Correct** by the **Number Possible**, as example 102 (the number of questions answered correctly) divided by 111 (the number of questions in the test) = .918 or 92%.

NURSING PROCESS

C = Collecting data
P = Planning
I = Implementation
E = Evaluation

CLIENT NEEDS

S = Safe, effective care environment
P = Physiological integrity
M = Psychosocial integrity
H = Health promotion/maintenance

Question #	Answer #	Nursing Process C	Nursing Process P	Nursing Process I	Nursing Process E	Client Needs S	Client Needs P	Client Needs M	Client Needs H
1	3	C					P		
2	2	C					P		
3	1	C					P		
4	3		P						H
5	2		P						H
6	3			I					H
7	2				E				H
8	1				E				H
9	2			I					H
10	4			I					H
11	1	C							H
12	4		P						H
13	4			I					H
14	1			I					H
15	2			I					H
16	2	C							H
17	2	C							H
18	3				E				H
19	1				E				H

NURSING PROCESS

C = Collecting data
P = Planning
I = Implementation
E = Evaluation

CLIENT NEEDS

S = Safe, effective care environment
P = Physiological integrity
M = Psychosocial integrity
H = Health promotion/maintenance

Question #	Answer #	Nursing Process				Client Needs			
		C	P	I	E	S	P	M	H
20	4			I					H
21	1				E				H
22	4		P						H
23	4	C							H
24	3			I					H
25	2				E				H
26	4				E				H
27	3			I					H
28	4			I					H
29	1		P						H
30	1			I					H
31	2	C							H
32	1			I					H
33	1			I					H
34	4			I					H
35	4			I					H
36	1			I					H
37	3			I					H
38	1			I					H
39	3			I					H
40	1			I					H
41	2	C							H
42	2	C							H
43	3	C							H
44	4	C							H
45	1			I					H
46	2	C							H
47	4	C							H
48	2	C							H
49	2	C							H
50	1			I					H
51	4			I					H

NURSING PROCESS

C = Collecting data
P = Planning
I = Implementation
E = Evaluation

CLIENT NEEDS

S = Safe, effective care environment
P = Physiological integrity
M = Psychosocial integrity
H = Health promotion/maintenance

Question #	Answer #	Nursing Process				Client Needs			
		C	P	I	E	S	P	M	H
52	4			I			P		
53	2			I		S			
54	1			I					H
55	4				E		P		
56	2			I					H
57	2			I				M	
58	3		P						H
59	1			I					H
60	2			I			P		
61	1			I		S			
62	3		P				P		
63	3	C					P		
64	3	C					P		
65	1		P				P		
66	4			I			P		
67	3			I		S			
68	1			I			P		
69	3			I					H
70	3			I			P		
71	4	C							H
72	4	C							H
73	2	C							H
74	4	C							H
75	4			I					H
76	2			I					H
77	2	C							H
78	1			I					H
79	1		P						H
80	4	C							H
81	4			I					H
82	2			I					H
83	2				E				H

NURSING PROCESS

C = Collecting data
P = Planning
I = Implementation
E = Evaluation

CLIENT NEEDS

S = Safe, effective care environment
P = Physiological integrity
M = Psychosocial integrity
H = Health promotion/maintenance

Question #	Answer #	Nursing Process				Client Needs			
		C	P	I	E	S	P	M	H
84	2			I					H
85	1			I					H
86	3			I					H
87	3			I					H
88	2			I					H
89	2	C							H
90	3			I					H
91	1			I			P		
92	2			I					H
93	3		P						H
94	4		P						H
95	3			I					H
96	2			I				M	
97	1			I				M	
98	4		P					M	
99	1		P					M	
100	2			I				M	
101	1			I					H
102	3			I					H
103	2			I					H
104	4			I					H
105	2			I					H
106	2			I					H
107	2	C					P		
108	4			I					H
109	3	C						M	
110	2	C							H
111	3			I					H
Number Correct									
Number Possible	111	28	13	61	9	3	15	7	86
Percentage Correct									

82

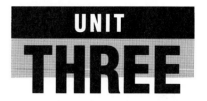

UNIT
THREE

REVIEW TESTS 4 AND 5

The Nursing Care of Children

REVIEW TEST 4

Normal Growth and Development of Infants and Toddlers

Nursing Care of Toddlers

Nursing Care of Preschool Children

Correct Answers and Rationale
Classification of Test Items

Directions: With a pencil, blacken the circle in front of the option you have chosen for your correct answer.

Normal Growth and Development of Infants and Toddlers

The nurse is assigned to a well-baby clinic. Each time an infant or toddler comes to the clinic, the nurse looks for signs of normal or abnormal development of each child.

1 Pattie Evans is 3 months old. Which one of the following would the nurse consider *abnormal* for this age?
○ 1. Engages in diffuse and random physical activity
○ 2. Holds rattle
○ 3. Attempts to roll over
○ 4. Unable to raise her head off of a flat surface

2 Jeffrey Baynes is 5 months old. Which one of the following tasks would the nurse consider *abnormal* for this age?
- ○ 1. Rolls from abdomen to back
- ○ 2. Cannot reach for object
- ○ 3. Smiles
- ○ 4. Purposely turns from side to side

3 Sean Abbott is 11 months old. Which one of the following would the nurse consider *abnormal* for this age?
- ○ 1. Has been creeping for 2 months
- ○ 2. Cannot sit without support
- ○ 3. Pulls himself to stand
- ○ 4. Picks up small objects using thumb and finger

4 Beth Garvey is 18 months old. Which one of the following would the nurse consider *abnormal* for this age?
- ○ 1. Has a vocabulary of approximately 6 words
- ○ 2. Uses a spoon
- ○ 3. Needs support to walk
- ○ 4. Shows signs of readiness for toilet training

Nursing Care of Infants

NURSING CARE OF AN INFANT WHO IS BORN PREMATURELY

Baby Boy Adler is born prematurely and remains hospitalized for care, which includes oxygen therapy. His mother has been discharged, and the parents of Baby Boy Adler visit him frequently.

5 Baby Boy Adler is monitored closely. The nurse should understand that if oxygen is administered in excess of ordered amounts and the concentration of oxygen becomes too high, there is risk of damage to the infant's
- ○ 1. eyes.
- ○ 2. heart.
- ○ 3. liver.
- ○ 4. kidneys.

6 When feeding Baby Boy Adler the nurse must remember that premature infants
- ○ 1. require feeding every hour.
- ○ 2. usually take 3 to 4 oz each feeding.
- ○ 3. have weak or absent sucking and swallowing reflexes.
- ○ 4. are given only glucose for the first 4 weeks of life.

7 When caring for Baby Boy Adler the nurse must remember that premature infants
- ○ 1. have not received antibody protection from their mothers and are subject to infection.
- ○ 2. are able to manufacture their own antibodies.

- ○ 3. rarely can breathe on their own and require respiratory assistance with a ventilator.
- ○ 4. almost always develop cerebral palsy.

8 Baby Boy Adler's parents ask why his respirations are closely monitored by his caregivers. The nurse can explain that Baby Boy Adler is monitored carefully because he is likely to lack a sufficient amount of pulmonary surfactant, which predisposes him to
- ○ 1. cystic fibrosis.
- ○ 2. tracheobronchitis.
- ○ 3. hyaline membrane disease.
- ○ 4. sudden infant death syndrome.

NURSING CARE OF AN INFANT WITH HEMOLYTIC DISEASE

Ms. Phillips, whose blood type is Rh negative, is in her 38th week of pregnancy when she delivers a boy. Ms. Phillips tells the nurse that this is her second pregnancy, and she had not seen a physician until she came to the hospital emergency room in active labor. Baby Boy Phillips is Rh positive. The physician states that the infant has congenital hemolytic disease caused by Rh incompatibility.

9 To answer Ms. Phillips' questions and concerns, the nurse should know that Baby Boy Phillips' congenital hemolytic disease is called
- ○ 1. thalassemia.
- ○ 2. sickle cell disease.
- ○ 3. megaloblastic anemia.
- ○ 4. erythroblastosis fetalis.

10 Which one of the following might the nurse observe if Baby Boy Phillips has congenital hemolytic disease?
- ○ 1. Slowed respiratory rate
- ○ 2. Absence of reflexes
- ○ 3. Limited movement in his lower extremities
- ○ 4. Jaundice within 24 to 36 hours after birth

11 A direct Coombs' test is ordered to confirm the diagnosis of hemolytic disease. The nurse should be prepared to assist with the collection of a blood specimen taken from Baby Boy Phillips'
- ○ 1. fingertip.
- ○ 2. jugular vein.
- ○ 3. femoral vein.
- ○ 4. umbilical cord.

12 After Baby Boy Phillips receives an exchange transfusion, the nurse observes him for signs of neurologic damage. All of the following signs suggest neurologic damage *except* having
- ○ 1. poor muscle tonus.
- ○ 2. poor sucking ability.
- ○ 3. decreased urine production.
- ○ 4. decreased responsiveness to stimuli.

NURSING CARE OF AN INFANT WITH SPINA BIFIDA

Andy Jones is 1 day old and was born with spina bifida with a myelomeningocele high in the spinal column. Andy is scheduled to have immediate surgical repair of the spina bifida and myelomeningocele.

13 Which of the following nursing measures is most important for the nurse to include in Andy's preoperative care?
- ○ 1. Prevent skin breakdown by placing a sheepskin under his head.
- ○ 2. Position him so that there is no pressure on the myelomeningocele.
- ○ 3. Keep his myelomeningocele clean by washing it with antiseptic soap.
- ○ 4. Support his bottle of formula on a rolled towel for ease in feeding him.

14 The physician explains the importance of immediate surgery for Andy. To answer the parents' questions and reinforce the surgeon's recommendations, the nurse should know that surgery for this disorder is performed as soon as possible to
- ○ 1. prevent paralysis of the upper extremities.
- ○ 2. restore bowel function.
- ○ 3. prevent infection.
- ○ 4. restore respiratory function.

15 Unless the physician orders otherwise, what position should the nurse use for Andy during the postoperative period and until the operative site heals?
- ○ 1. The supine position (back-lying position)
- ○ 2. The prone position (face-lying position)
- ○ 3. Either the right or left side-lying position
- ○ 4. The position in which the infant appears most comfortable

Andy's caretakers discuss the infant's prognosis in a conference in which his home care is considered.

16 To assist in developing a plan for Andy's home care the nurse should know that
- ○ 1. it is unlikely that Andy will be able to walk without crutches or braces.
- ○ 2. Andy has approximately a 50% chance of eventually walking alone if he has good health care.
- ○ 3. Andy has approximately a 95% chance of eventually walking alone if he has good health care.
- ○ 4. Andy will someday be able to walk without having to use crutches or braces.

17 When planning discharge teaching for Andy's parents the nurse should be aware of the many needs Andy will require now and in the future. Which one of the following neurologic disturbances usually is seen in those with spina bifida with a myelomeningocele?
- ○ 1. Respiratory difficulties
- ○ 2. Paralysis of the muscles of the head and neck
- ○ 3. Paralysis of the arms
- ○ 4. Urinary and bowel control problems

NURSING CARE OF AN INFANT WITH HYDROCEPHALUS

Baby Girl Lyons is born with hydrocephalus. Her parents have named her Jenny. She is now 1 week old and is scheduled for surgery.

18 To understand and plan for Jenny's care, the nurse should know that the most prominent symptom of hydrocephalus is
- ○ 1. an increase in head size.
- ○ 2. paralysis of the lower extremities.
- ○ 3. an absence of the sucking reflex.
- ○ 4. a marked depression of the anterior fontanel.

19 To reinforce the physician's explanation of Jenny's congenital malformation and allow the family to talk about Jenny's problem, the nurse should know that hydrocephalus is probably due to
- ○ 1. an absence of the dura mater.
- ○ 2. a blockage that prevents proper circulation of cerebrospinal fluid.
- ○ 3. an increased amount of cerebrospinal fluid proteins.
- ○ 4. a blockage in the cerebral arteries.

20 During the preoperative period the nurse should plan to
- ○ 1. weigh Jenny every week.
- ○ 2. change Jenny's position every 2 hours.
- ○ 3. feed Jenny a low-fat formula to decrease the formation of cerebrospinal fluid.
- ○ 4. observe Jenny for signs of decreased intracranial pressure.

21 The position of choice for Jenny *after* feeding her is the
- ○ 1. sitting position.
- ○ 2. back-lying position.
- ○ 3. face-lying position.
- ○ 4. side-lying position.

22 The nurse places a sheepskin under Jenny's head and shoulders; the primary purpose is to
- ○ 1. keep the infant's head higher than her trunk.
- ○ 2. prevent strain on the infant's neck and shoulders.
- ○ 3. relieve areas of pressure on the infant's head and ears.
- ○ 4. allow the infant to remain undisturbed for longer periods.

A shunting device is placed through an incision on the right side of Jenny's head.

23 The postoperative position of choice is on Jenny's
  ○ 1. right side to increase absorption of cerebrospinal fluid.
  ○ 2. abdomen to prevent obstruction in the shunt catheter.
  ○ 3. left side to avoid pressure on the operative site.
  ○ 4. back to promote ventricular drainage.

24 Postoperatively, the nurse should observe Jenny closely for signs of increased intracranial pressure; one sign is
  ○ 1. depression of the fontanels.
  ○ 2. a decrease in the pulse and respiratory rate.
  ○ 3. changes in the number of bowel movements.
  ○ 4. a sudden gain in weight.

NURSING CARE OF AN INFANT WITH A CLEFT LIP

Billy Keeler, 3 weeks old, is admitted to a children's hospital. He is being readied for surgical repair of a unilateral cleft lip.

25 When developing a care plan the nurse should expect that, until repaired, Billy's anomaly most likely will make him unable to
  ○ 1. suck.
  ○ 2. salivate.
  ○ 3. breathe.
  ○ 4. swallow.

26 Which of the following utensils is best for the nurse to use preoperatively and postoperatively when feeding Billy his formula?
  ○ 1. A gavage tube
  ○ 2. A plastic spoon
  ○ 3. An Asepto syringe with a rubber tip
  ○ 4. A firm rubber nipple

27 Postoperatively, the nurse should plan to
  ○ 1. position Billy on his abdomen.
  ○ 2. hold Billy as little as possible.
  ○ 3. feed Billy with a regular bottle.
  ○ 4. apply arm restraints as ordered by the physician.

NURSING CARE OF AN INFANT WITH PYLORIC STENOSIS

Three-week-old Joseph Morgan, who has pyloric stenosis, is admitted to a hospital for surgery to correct the defect.

28 To develop a care plan for Joseph, the nurse should understand that pyloric stenosis prevents food from moving normally in the gastrointestinal tract from his

  ○ 1. jejunum into his ileum.
  ○ 2. esophagus into his stomach.
  ○ 3. duodenum into his jejunum.
  ○ 4. stomach into his duodenum.

29 Intravenous therapy to correct fluid and electrolyte imbalances is to be started on Joseph. To obtain the necessary materials for assisting with starting an intravenous infusion, the nurse should know that the vein most frequently used for an infant is a vein located in the
  ○ 1. neck.
  ○ 2. scalp.
  ○ 3. upper extremity.
  ○ 4. lower extremity.

Joseph has a surgical repair of his pyloric stenosis.

30 What is the position of choice for Joseph once he is allowed oral glucose water?
  ○ 1. A back-lying position
  ○ 2. A semi-sitting position
  ○ 3. A normal left side-lying position
  ○ 4. An exaggerated right side-lying position

NURSING CARE OF AN INFANT WITH CONGENITAL HIP DISLOCATION

Six-month-old Cindy Connors has congenital dislocation of the hip (CDH) and is scheduled for the application of a bilateral hip spica cast for correction of the disorder.

31 The nurse is assigned to collect materials necessary for application of the cast. To help eliminate skin irritation from the edges of Cindy's cast, the physician usually
  ○ 1. trims the cast edges with sandpaper.
  ○ 2. covers the cast edges with plastic.
  ○ 3. petals the cast edges with strips of adhesive.
  ○ 4. protects the cast edges with a disposable diaper.

32 Following application of the cast the nurse should observe Cindy for signs of complications. Which one of the following might indicate that a neurovascular problem is occurring?
  ○ 1. She cries 4 hours after her last feeding.
  ○ 2. She wiggles her toes.
  ○ 3. Her toes are pale and cold.
  ○ 4. Her pulse rate is 110.

NURSING CARE OF AN INFANT WITH BILATERAL CLUBFOOT

Nicky Harris is born after 36 weeks of gestation by breech presentation. He has the talipes equinovarus form of bilateral clubfoot. The physician has recommended immediate treatment for this congenital disorder.

33 To answer questions raised by Ms. Harris, the nurse should know that early treatment of clubfoot is necessary because
- ○ 1. later treatment is more expensive.
- ○ 2. early treatment may prevent the need for surgery.
- ○ 3. if not treated, the bones and muscles continue to develop abnormally.
- ○ 4. it is easier on the infant.

34 At a nursing conference, the nurse assistant asks the nurse why Nicky's legs and feet are to be elevated on pillows after the cast has been applied. The *most correct* answer is based on the fact that this position
- ○ 1. hastens drying of the cast.
- ○ 2. keeps his hips and lower back off the bedding.
- ○ 3. helps avoid postoperative shock.
- ○ 4. prevents his feet from swelling.

35 Of the following techniques, the best one for the nurse to use when moving Nicky's wet casts is to handle them with
- ○ 1. the fingers.
- ○ 2. gloved hands.
- ○ 3. slings made of gauze.
- ○ 4. the palms of the hands.

36 Nicky is 8 weeks old, and his cast is to be changed. Which of the following types of amusement can the nurse use to determine if Nicky appears to be following a normal growth and development pattern?
- ○ 1. Encourage the infant to crawl about in his crib.
- ○ 2. Play peek-a-boo with his favorite blanket.
- ○ 3. Permit him to reach for cuddly toys.
- ○ 4. Place a brightly colored mobile over his crib.

37 During discharge teaching, Nicky's mother says to the nurse, "I can barely feel the soft spot in the back part of Nicky's head. My daughter's soft spot did not close until about 3 months of age. Is there anything wrong?" The *most correct* response is based on the fact that the amount of closure of the posterior fontanel for 8-week-old Nicky is judged to be
- ○ 1. normal because the posterior fontanel usually closes at approximately 2 months of age.
- ○ 2. abnormal because the posterior fontanel usually closes in male children later than in female children.
- ○ 3. abnormal because the posterior fontanel usually does not close until about 6 to 8 months of age.
- ○ 4. normal because the posterior fontanel usually closes early in children with any type of congenital skeletal defects.

NURSING CARE OF AN INFANT WITH OTITIS MEDIA

Ms. Hale brings 6-month-old Ricky to the clinic because he has an elevated temperature. She states that Ricky has been irritable and crying frequently. Ricky is examined by a physician and found to have otitis media.

38 The physician asks the nurse to weigh Ricky. Ricky's weight probably will be used to help
- ○ 1. determine the nutritional needs of the infant.
- ○ 2. determine dosages for drugs to be prescribed for the infant.
- ○ 3. calculate whether the infant needs to receive parenteral fluids.
- ○ 4. calculate whether the infant is suffering from an electrolyte imbalance.

39 The nurse observes Ricky. Which one of the following would most likely indicate he has pain in his ear?
- ○ 1. Lying on his unaffected ear
- ○ 2. Pulling on his unaffected ear
- ○ 3. Rolling his head from side to side
- ○ 4. Tipping his head toward the affected ear

The physician prescribes an antibiotic to be given to Ricky for 10 days.

40 Which one of the following should the nurse emphasize when explaining the prescribed antibiotic treatment to Ms. Hale?
- ○ 1. Stop the drug if Ricky feels better.
- ○ 2. Limit Ricky's fluid intake during the time he is given the drug.
- ○ 3. Do not allow Ricky to lie on his unaffected ear.
- ○ 4. Stopping the drug too soon may result in a return of the infection.

NURSING CARE OF AN INFANT WITH AN INFECTIOUS DISEASE

Jeff Baker, age 3 months, has chickenpox and is taken by his mother to the emergency room. Following examination by a physician, Jeff is admitted to the hospital because he also has a congenital heart defect with possible congestive heart failure. He is placed on strict isolation.

41 The nurse is assigned to prepare Jeff's room. Which one of the following is instituted for strict isolation?
- ○ 1. Used gowns may be discarded with the general linen.
- ○ 2. Clothing and articles in the room must be decontaminated before reuse.
- ○ 3. Gloves are not required for caretakers.
- ○ 4. The door to the room may be left open.

42 The nurse wears a mask when caring for Jeff. Which one of the following actions is *incorrect?*
- ○ 1. The nurse's fingers and hands should not touch the mask.
- ○ 2. A supply of unused, disposable masks is kept outside the client's room.
- ○ 3. The mask should be changed every hour.
- ○ 4. The used mask is discarded outside the room.

43 The nurse prepares to leave Jeff's room after giving morning care. Which one of the following is *incorrect?*
- ○ 1. The gown is removed before the gloves are removed.
- ○ 2. Clean hands are used to unfasten the gown for removal.
- ○ 3. When removing the gown, touching the front of the gown is avoided.
- ○ 4. Clean paper towels are used to open the door of the room.

44 To prepare Jeff for intravenous therapy, the nurse should withhold fluids and food immediately prior to starting the therapy because
- ○ 1. fluids and calories will be supplied by intravenous fluid therapy.
- ○ 2. vomiting and aspiration may occur.
- ○ 3. oral food and fluids may interfere with the absorption of intravenous fluids.
- ○ 4. intravenous fluids must be given on an empty stomach.

45 When an infant requires intravenous therapy, the nurse should
- ○ 1. request that the parents not see the infant until intravenous therapy is completed.
- ○ 2. encourage the family to continue providing tactile and verbal stimulation to the infant.
- ○ 3. warn the parents not to touch the infant until intravenous therapy is completed.
- ○ 4. ask the parents to disturb the infant as little as possible.

46 The nurse is assigned to closely monitor Jeff while he is receiving intravenous therapy. Which one of the following should the nurse report to the nurse in charge?
- ○ 1. Jeff sleeps for short intervals during the day.
- ○ 2. An increase in the frequency and amount of urine voided.
- ○ 3. Jeff occasionally cries when he is disturbed by noise.
- ○ 4. An increase in the rate of flow of the intravenous infusion.

47 If the intravenous solution infuses too rapidly, the nurse should closely observe Jeff for signs of
- ○ 1. heart failure.
- ○ 2. renal failure.
- ○ 3. excessive voiding.
- ○ 4. diarrhea.

NURSING CARE OF AN INFANT WITH ATOPIC DERMATITIS

Ms. Scott brings 2-year-old Timmy to the clinic because the skin on his face and neck is inflamed and covered with tiny vesicle-type lesions. Timmy is diagnosed as having atopic dermatitis (acute infantile eczema). Ms. Scott shows concern and asks many questions about Timmy's problem.

48 The nurse explains to Ms. Scott that when the vesicles on Timmy's skin break, they typically release a fluid containing
- ○ 1. pus.
- ○ 2. blood.
- ○ 3. lymph.
- ○ 4. serum.

49 Ms. Scott asks what caused Timmy's skin condition and why the physician asked many questions about Timmy's home environment. The nurse explains that it is believed that the probable cause of atopic dermatitis is thought to be
- ○ 1. poor nutrition.
- ○ 2. a premature birth.
- ○ 3. an allergic reaction.
- ○ 4. a hormone imbalance.

50 The nurse should be prepared to give Ms. Scott suggestions concerning care measures that will help relieve Timmy's
- ○ 1. nausea.
- ○ 2. vomiting.
- ○ 3. severe itching.
- ○ 4. prolonged drowsiness.

51 Ms. Scott is instructed to use hydrocortisone ointment on Timmy's skin lesions. On a subsequent visit the nurse judges that the ointment has accomplished its intended purpose for Timmy when
- ○ 1. weeping of the infant's skin has subsided.
- ○ 2. there is no spread of the infant's skin disease.
- ○ 3. inflammation of the infant's skin has decreased.
- ○ 4. there has been an increase in the infant's white blood cell count.

52 The physician advises Timmy's mother to use colloid baths for Timmy. The nurse explains to Ms. Scott that a typical colloid bath consists of tepid water to which has been added
- ○ 1. cornstarch or baking soda.
- ○ 2. a little mineral, olive, or bath oil.
- ○ 3. unperfumed, liquid glycerine soap.
- ○ 4. salt, to make a normal saline solution.

The Nursing Care of Toddlers

NURSING CARE OF A TODDLER WITH SICKLE CELL CRISIS

Acutely ill, 21-month-old Hank Douglas is admitted to the hospital with sickle cell crisis. He has a brother who is 6 years old and also has sickle cell disease.

53 During Hank's admission the nurse should be prepared to use nursing measures appropriate for the relief of Hank's
○ 1. pain.
○ 2. diarrhea.
○ 3. hemorrhaging.
○ 4. bradycardia.

54 The nurse also should anticipate and develop a plan of care that will most likely
○ 1. include transfusions of plasma.
○ 2. be directed toward decreasing hemoglobin levels.
○ 3. include large doses of iron.
○ 4. be supportive.

55 Which of the following might indicate that Hank is dehydrated?
○ 1. Diaphoresis and increased urinary output
○ 2. Dry skin and decreased urinary output
○ 3. Low body temperature and flushed skin
○ 4. Edema of the extremities and anxiety

NURSING CARE OF A TODDLER WITH CYSTIC FIBROSIS

Stephanie Reed was diagnosed as having cystic fibrosis when she was 3 months old. At 18 months she is admitted to the hospital because of increasing respiratory difficulty and repeated respiratory infections.

56 The nurse should judge that Stephanie has a typical sign of cystic fibrosis when assessment includes noting that Stephanie has
○ 1. a poor appetite.
○ 2. excessive perspiration.
○ 3. low urine output.
○ 4. sticky, foul-smelling stools.

57 If Stephanie's mother makes the following comments, which one should the nurse recognize as describing a typical finding in a child with cystic fibrosis?
○ 1. "Stephanie rarely cries."
○ 2. "Stephanie has gained a lot of weight."
○ 3. "Stephanie tastes salty when I kiss her."
○ 4. "Stephanie does not care for her formula."

58 To develop a plan of care for Stephanie, the nurse should know that maximum therapeutic efforts are directed to the
○ 1. lungs.
○ 2. liver.

○ 3. spleen.
○ 4. kidneys.

59 The nurse must be familiar with the rationale for drug therapy for all clients. Stephanie is given pancreatic enzyme (Pancrease), which is a pancreatic enzyme, because in those with cystic fibrosis
○ 1. enzymes in the stomach are unable to digest carbohydrates.
○ 2. the small intestine cannot absorb minerals.
○ 3. supplemental vitamins are part of the treatment regimen.
○ 4. fats and proteins are not digested and absorbed.

It has been determined that Stephanie's parents have not been feeding her the diet recommended for those with cystic fibrosis.

60 The nurse should stress that the nutrient in Stephanie's diet that should be offered only in *limited* to *moderate* amounts is
○ 1. fats.
○ 2. salt.
○ 3. proteins.
○ 4. carbohydrates.

61 The parents ask about including exercise in Stephanie's activities of daily living. In addition to improving Stephanie's well-being, the nurse can explain that exercise is particularly important for Stephanie to help
○ 1. stimulate excretory functioning.
○ 2. rid the pulmonary system of secretions.
○ 3. absorb calcium from the digestive tract.
○ 4. enhance digestion and absorption of nutrients.

62 A bronchodilator is prescribed for Stephanie. The nurse can evaluate the successful effects of therapy with this type of drug when
○ 1. there is decreased mucus in the stool.
○ 2. serum sodium levels decrease.
○ 3. breathing is improved.
○ 4. excess fat is lost from body tissues.

63 When discussing home care, the nurse plans to emphasize the importance of increasing Stephanie's fluid intake because extra fluids
○ 1. prevent kidney failure.
○ 2. increase cardiac action.
○ 3. help reduce pain and discomfort.
○ 4. help liquify secretions in the lungs.

64 Because of Stephanie's increased risk for complications, the nurse should plan to instruct the parents to guard against exposing Stephanie to
○ 1. airborne pollens.
○ 2. infections.
○ 3. pet dander.
○ 4. bright sunlight.

NURSING CARE OF A TODDLER WITH ASTHMA

Brandon Parks is 2½ years old and has been diagnosed as having asthma. The physician has determined that Brandon has allergic (extrinsic) asthma. At present he has an upper respiratory infection.

65 The nurse is assigned to develop a plan of care for Brandon. The nurse should know that asthma is characterized by difficulty in breathing that occurs because of
  ○ 1. spasm of the bronchi.
  ○ 2. thinning of bronchial secretions.
  ○ 3. narrowing of the trachea.
  ○ 4. a congenital malformation of the epiglottis.

66 Which of the following can the nurse use to help ease Brandon's respiratory difficulty?
  ○ 1. Have Brandon lie on his left side.
  ○ 2. Raise the foot gatch and place two pillows under his head.
  ○ 3. Elevate the head of the bed to a near sitting position.
  ○ 4. Have Brandon lie prone.

67 Brandon responds to treatment and is scheduled for discharge. The nurse should discuss with the parents the importance of
  ○ 1. keeping Brandon quiet until he no longer has attacks of asthma.
  ○ 2. eliminating vegetables from his diet.
  ○ 3. keeping Brandon's fluid intake low to decrease mucus production.
  ○ 4. eliminating factors from the environment that may trigger a future asthma attack.

68 Brandon's parents ask questions about his bedroom. Which one of the following can the nurse suggest be *removed* from this area?
  ○ 1. Foam rubber pillow
  ○ 2. Cotton blanket
  ○ 3. Rugs
  ○ 4. Alarm clock

NURSING CARE OF A TODDLER WHO HAS SWALLOWED A TOXIC SUBSTANCE

Johnny Lane, a 2½-year-old boy, is brought to a hospital emergency department by his mother, who says that Johnny just swallowed at least 10 children's aspirin.

69 When Johnny is seen in the emergency department, the nurse's responsibilities include assessing for signs of salicylate poisoning, one of which is
  ○ 1. a skin rash.
  ○ 2. a slow pulse rate.
  ○ 3. an inflamed throat.
  ○ 4. a rapid respiratory rate.

70 With which of the following procedures should the nurse be prepared to assist on Johnny's admission?
  ○ 1. Gastroscopy
  ○ 2. Throat culture
  ○ 3. Gastric lavage
  ○ 4. Gastrostomy

Following an initial examination, the physician decides to admit Johnny to the hospital for observation.

71 Which of the following safety measures is most appropriate for the nurse to take when Johnny is well enough to go to the hospital's playroom?
  ○ 1. Tell him not to touch anything in the room.
  ○ 2. Show him which substances he should not eat.
  ○ 3. Remove harmful substances or objects from areas within his reach.
  ○ 4. Post warnings in the playroom about poisonous substances.

The nurse plans a teaching program for Ms. Lane concerning the ingestion of toxic substances by small children.

72 Which of the following medications should Ms. Lane be advised to keep in a locked cupboard at home and use as an antidote if Johnny eats or drinks a toxic substance?
  ○ 1. Metamucil
  ○ 2. Kaopectate
  ○ 3. Syrup of ipecac
  ○ 4. Milk of magnesia

NURSING CARE OF A TODDLER WITH LEAD POISONING

Amy Pierce is 3 years old and is brought to the clinic because of weakness, weight loss, anorexia, and periodic episodes of vomiting. After a thorough physical examination and laboratory studies, it is found that Amy has lead poisoning. After thorough questioning it is learned that the Pierce family has been living in a very old home for the last 4 years. They are now in the process of renovating this home.

73 When preparing to talk to Ms. Pierce, the nurse should ask questions concerning
  ○ 1. Amy's possible ingestion of paint.
  ○ 2. the type of heating system presently being used.
  ○ 3. the type of flooring in the house.
  ○ 4. Amy's possible exposure to new paint fumes.

74 The physician explains the treatment regimen to the Pierces. To reinforce the physician's explanations, the nurse should know that lead poisoning is treated
  ○ 1. conservatively.
  ○ 2. with analgesics and antiemetics.

○ 3. with antibiotics.

○ 4. with a heavy metal antagonist.

75 Mr. Pierce asks the nurse if they should apply new paint over all walls, furniture, and trim, such as windowsills. The correct reply is

○ 1. yes, providing that the new paint is lead-free.

○ 2. no, a coat of varnish applied over the old paint will prevent exposure to lead.

○ 3. no, the old paint first must be completely removed.

○ 4. yes, providing that you apply two coats of a darker color.

NURSING CARE OF A TODDLER WITH CROUP

Ms. York brings 2¹/₂-year-old Laura to a physician's office because, Ms. York says, "Amy had croup last night and was very sick." The physician makes a diagnosis of croup, which also is called laryngotracheobronchitis (LTB).

76 The nurse plans to explain the cause of LTB to Ms. York. The *most correct* explanation is based on the fact that this disorder is

○ 1. most often caused by a virus.

○ 2. an upper respiratory infection in those with asthma.

○ 3. related to whooping cough.

○ 4. primarily due to inadequate development of the lungs.

77 The nurse asks Ms. York to describe Laura's cough. The typical cough of a child with LTB sounds

○ 1. moist.

○ 2. hoarse.

○ 3. muffled.

○ 4. high-pitched.

78 The nurse should explain to Ms. York that laryngeal spasms often can be relieved if Laura is in a room with air that is

○ 1. dry.

○ 2. hot.

○ 3. humid.

○ 4. dust-free.

79 The nurse should explain to Ms. York that the physician should be contacted immediately if Laura

○ 1. raises thin, clear mucus.

○ 2. develops difficulty in inhaling and exhaling.

○ 3. coughs during the night.

○ 4. refuses to play with her toys.

80 Ms. York asks if she can give Laura aspirin if she has a fever. Based on recent studies the nurse should tell Ms. York that aspirin use in young children with a fever

○ 1. has been associated with the development of Reye's syndrome.

○ 2. causes stomach ulcers.

○ 3. does not effectively reduce body temperature.

○ 4. produces severe diarrhea.

Laura continues to have difficulty breathing and is taken to the hospital emergency department. An emergency tracheostomy is performed.

81 The nurse should observe Laura for mucus accumulating in the respiratory tract, which is evidenced by

○ 1. a decrease in the pulse and respiratory rate.

○ 2. noisy, labored, moist respirations.

○ 3. crying and an attempt to talk.

○ 4. a decrease in the blood pressure.

82 Laura requires suctioning. Which one of the following is the most correct technique for this procedure?

○ 1. The suction catheter must be larger than the opening of the tracheostomy tube.

○ 2. The suction catheter is inserted for a minimum of 30 seconds.

○ 3. The vent on the suction tube is covered after the catheter is inserted and when it is being withdrawn.

○ 4. Between insertions the suction catheter is cleared with tap water.

NURSING CARE OF A TODDLER WITH PNEUMONIA

Manuel Garcia, a 3-year-old, is admitted to a hospital with pneumonia. He is acutely ill with an elevated temperature.

83 When performing an initial assessment on Manuel, the nurse should expect to see respirations that are

○ 1. slow and deep.

○ 2. intermittently shallow and deep.

○ 3. intermittently rapid and slow.

○ 4. rapid and shallow.

84 The best measure for the nurse to use to assist in determining Manuel's need for fluid is to

○ 1. test his urine *p*H.

○ 2. monitor his pulse rate.

○ 3. weigh his liquid feedings.

○ 4. record his urinary output.

85 Manuel's most recent rectal temperature is 103.8°F. Because of Manuel's age the nurse should be prepared

○ 1. to offer fluids every 4 hours.

○ 2. to measure intake and output every hour.

○ 3. for the occurrence of seizures.

○ 4. for prolonged episodes of coughing.

86 The physician orders a tepid water sponge bath to aid in reducing Manuel's temperature. Some textbooks recommend rubbing the child's skin with a dry washcloth before beginning a sponge bath to

reduce body temperature, because rubbing the skin helps to
- ○ 1. open the skin's pores.
- ○ 2. remove excess oil from the skin.
- ○ 3. remove excessive dirt and debris from the skin.
- ○ 4. stimulate the skin and prevent chilling.

87 An important nursing measure that should be carried out approximately 30 minutes *after* completing Manuel's sponge bath is to
- ○ 1. give him aspirin.
- ○ 2. obtain his vital signs.
- ○ 3. start him on oxygen therapy.
- ○ 4. offer him foods high in vitamin C.

The primary language of Martin's mother is Spanish. On the day of Manuel's discharge, Ms. Garcia receives written instructions about Manuel's diet, activity, and medications and instructions to schedule a clinic appointment for Manuel in 2 weeks.

88 The best action for the nurse to take to determine if Ms. Garcia understands the instructions is to
- ○ 1. read the written instructions to the mother.
- ○ 2. have the instructions written in Spanish for the mother.
- ○ 3. repeat the instructions in words that the mother can understand.
- ○ 4. ask the mother to repeat the instructions the way she understands them.

89 Prior to Manuel's discharge the nurse checks his admission history and notes that the immunizations he has received were diphtheria, tetanus, and pertussis (DPT) and trivalent oral polio vaccine (TOPV). Which of the following should the nurse tell Ms. Garcia that Manuel also needs?
- ○ 1. Meningococcal vaccine
- ○ 2. Measles, mumps, and rubella vaccines
- ○ 3. Bacille Calmette-Guérin (BCG) vaccine
- ○ 4. Hepatitis vaccine

Nursing Care of Preschool Children

NURSING CARE OF A CHILD WITH SEIZURE ACTIVITY

Susan Green, 4½ years old, has what her parents believe to be seizures. She is admitted to the hospital for diagnosis, observation, and treatment.

90 Which one of the following nursing tasks may aid the physician in establishing a diagnosis of a seizure disorder?
- ○ 1. Ask Susan what she felt when she had a seizure.
- ○ 2. Note how Susan responds to the nurse's questions.
- ○ 3. Ask the parents to describe Susan's body movements when she has had a seizure.
- ○ 4. Obtain vital signs if Susan has a seizure.

91 In anticipation of the possibility that Susan will have a seizure, the nurse prepares a crib that includes padding on the crib sides. Placing padding on the crib sides is primarily to help prevent
- ○ 1. injury to the child during seizure activity.
- ○ 2. attempts by the child to get out of the crib.
- ○ 3. unnecessary drafts reaching the child that may bring on seizure activity.
- ○ 4. undue environmental stimuli to the child that may bring on seizure activity.

92 Certain equipment should be kept at Susan's bedside for convenience when seizure activity occurs. Which one of the following equipment is *unnecessary*?
- ○ 1. Suction equipment
- ○ 2. A tracheostomy set
- ○ 3. An oral airway
- ○ 4. A good source of light

93 Susan has a tonic-clonic (grand mal) seizure while the nurse is at her beside. Which one of the following should be the *first* action taken by the nurse?
- ○ 1. Call for assistance.
- ○ 2. Turn Susan on her side.
- ○ 3. Insert a padded tongue blade into Susan's mouth.
- ○ 4. Administer oxygen.

94 The physician prescribes phenytoin (Dilantin). To help prevent adverse drug effects, what precautions should the nurse take when administering phenytoin to Susan?
- ○ 1. Give the medication when the child's stomach is empty.
- ○ 2. Administer the medication while assisting the child to eat.
- ○ 3. Avoid giving the child the medication with carbonated beverages.
- ○ 4. Withhold dairy products for 1 hour after giving the child the medication.

95 Which one of the following should the nurse include in a teaching plan for Susan's parents?
- ○ 1. Keep Susan out of preschool for several days after she has a seizure.
- ○ 2. Limit Susan's play activity.
- ○ 3. Limit Susan's fluid intake.
- ○ 4. Do not omit, increase, or decrease the prescribed dose of medication.

96 Susan will take phenytoin after discharge, and her parents should be taught the adverse effects of long-term use of this drug. One common adverse effect is
- ○ 1. a poor appetite.
- ○ 2. urinary incontinence.

○ 3. painful joints following exercise.

○ 4. an excessive growth of gum tissues.

NURSING CARE OF A CHILD WITH LEUKEMIA

Four-year-old Beth Norris, who is suspected of having leukemia, is admitted to a hospital for diagnosis and treatment.

97 The nurse is assigned to help develop a plan of care for Beth. The nurse should anticipate that the test most likely to be used to determine whether Beth has leukemia is

○ 1. a gastric analysis.

○ 2. an angiogram.

○ 3. a bone marrow aspiration.

○ 4. arterial blood gas analysis.

98 Tests confirm that Beth has acute lymphocytic leukemia. The nurse should recognize that the most probable reason for an order for bed rest for Beth is to relieve a common symptom of the disease, which is

○ 1. dizziness.

○ 2. palpitations.

○ 3. painful joints.

○ 4. blurred vision.

99 Because the white blood cells are not functioning normally, the nurse should be aware that

○ 1. the platelet count rises.

○ 2. ulcerations often develop in the mouth.

○ 3. the client has developed a resistance to infection.

○ 4. the red blood cell count rises.

100 The nurse plans to evaluate Beth's general condition daily. Which one of the following events is a complication associated with leukemia?

○ 1. Diuresis

○ 2. Weight gain

○ 3. Epistaxis

○ 4. Decrease in the size of the liver

Beth is started on vincristine sulfate (Oncovin) and prednisone (Meticorten) in an effort to place her in remission.

101 The nurse observes Beth for signs of infection because these drugs

○ 1. increase red blood cell production.

○ 2. suppress the bone marrow.

○ 3. destroy platelets.

○ 4. depress lymph production.

102 Beth receives a blood transfusion. If Beth makes the following comments after approximately half of the blood is transfused, which one should cause the nurse to suspect that Beth may be having a transfusion reaction?

○ 1. "I'm thirsty."

○ 2. "I feel cold."

○ 3. "I feel so tired."

○ 4. "I need to go to the bathroom."

103 Beth appears to be having a reaction to the blood. The nurse's *first* course of action should be to

○ 1. administer oxygen.

○ 2. discontinue the transfusion and remove the needle.

○ 3. clamp the tubing to stop the blood transfusion, and open the clamp to the normal saline.

○ 4. see to it that the nurse in charge and the blood bank are notified immediately.

104 One day Beth asks the nurse, "Am I going to die?" Which of the following responses is best for the nurse to make to Beth's question?

○ 1. "Are you feeling especially bad today? Tell me more about how you feel."

○ 2. "You shouldn't worry about things like that. You are only a little girl."

○ 3. "We are all going to die someday."

○ 4. "Let's talk about something else. What is your favorite television program?"

105 To deal with Beth's concept of death, the nurse must understand that the age at which children *first* recognize the phenomenon of death in a manner similar to adults is when children are between about ages

○ 1. 5 and 6 years.

○ 2. 7 and 8 years.

○ 3. 9 and 10 years.

○ 4. 12 and 14 years.

NURSING CARE OF A CHILD WITH STRABISMUS

Four-year-old Sally Cromwell is to be admitted to an ambulatory surgical center for the correction of strabismus (crossed eyes), a condition she has had since infancy.

106 In preparation for surgery the nurse tells Ms. Cromwell that Sally is to have nothing by mouth after midnight the evening before surgery. The primary reason for this preparation for surgery is to

○ 1. prevent aspiration of vomitus during surgery.

○ 2. enhance the effectiveness of preoperative sedation.

○ 3. dry the respiratory mucous membranes before surgery.

○ 4. reduce the need for the child to urinate prior to surgery.

107 To select materials to be applied in the recovery room, the nurse should know that the type of restraint usually required following this type of surgery on a 4-year-old child are

○ 1. full arm and leg restraints.
○ 2. elbow restraints.
○ 3. wrist restraints.
○ 4. full body (mummy) restraints.

108 Sally asks if she will hurt after surgery. The best response by the nurse would be to tell her
○ 1. not to think about that now.
○ 2. that she will not have pain.
○ 3. the pain may be severe, but the nurses will give her something for pain.
○ 4. that her eye may be sore after surgery.

109 Which of the following general care measures is *inappropriate* to teach the parents in relation to Sally's postoperative home care?
○ 1. Allow the child to be up and about.
○ 2. Offer the child a regular diet once nausea has ceased.
○ 3. Do not allow the child to play with toys for at least 4 weeks.
○ 4. Amuse the child by reading stories.

NURSING CARE OF A CHILD HAVING A TONSILLECTOMY AND ADENOIDECTOMY

Bob Donnelly, who is 5 years old, is admitted to a hospital for a tonsillectomy and adenoidectomy.

110 On the morning of the surgery, the nurse obtains Bob's vital signs. Which of the following should the nurse report immediately to the nurse in charge or the physician?
○ 1. Blood pressure, 96/60 mm Hg
○ 2. Temperature, 101°F (38.3°C)
○ 3. Respiratory rate, 20 per minute
○ 4. Pulse rate, 110 beats per minute

Bob's surgery is completed, and he is to have a clear liquid diet postoperatively.

111 The nurse should check Bob's meal tray to ensure that the prescribed diet is provided. Which of the following items is included in a clear liquid diet?
○ 1. Sherbet
○ 2. Ice cream
○ 3. Clear broth
○ 4. Milk shake

112 The nurse should report postoperative observations to the nurse in charge immediately when it is noted that Bob is
○ 1. vomiting a small amount of dark red blood.
○ 2. swallowing frequently.
○ 3. asking for fluids when awakening.
○ 4. breathing at a rate of 30 respirations per minute.

113 Bob is to be discharged from the hospital. To plan discharge teaching the nurse should know that home management usually includes
○ 1. keeping the child quiet for a few days.
○ 2. limiting fluid intake for the next 48 hours.
○ 3. giving aspirin if a fever occurs.
○ 4. starting the child on solid foods after 12 hours.

114 Which one of the following should the nurse also include in a discharge care plan for Bob?
○ 1. Bob will probably have a great deal of pain for the first 7 days.
○ 2. Bob will have difficulty swallowing for approximately 3 weeks.
○ 3. A large amount of bright red blood may be expectorated for approximately 1 week.
○ 4. A transient earache may occur for 1 to 3 days.

Correct Answers and Rationale

Two numbers appear in parentheses following each rationale. The first number identifies the textbook listed in the references, page 451, and the second number identifies the page(s) in that textbook on which the correct answer can be verified. Occasionally, two textbooks are given for verifying the correct answer.

Normal Growth and Development of Infants and Toddlers

1 4. This 3-month-old infant should be able to raise her head approximately 90 degrees off of a flat surface. The other observations in this question are normal for a 3-month-old infant. (8:346)
Nursing Process—Collecting data
Client Need—Health promotion/maintenance

2 2. Jeffrey, who is 5 months old, should be able to reach for an object placed in his line of vision. The other observations in this question are normal for an infant of this age. (8:348)
Nursing Process—Collecting data
Client Need—Health promotion/maintenance

3 2. The 11-month-old should be able to sit up without support. The other observations in this question are normal for an infant of this age. (8:350)
Nursing Process—Collecting data
Client Need—Health promotion/maintenance

4 3. The 18-month-old child should be able to walk without support and climb stairs while holding on to a railing. The other observations in this question are normal for a toddler of this age. (8:354–355)
Nursing Process—Collecting data
Client Need—Health promotion/maintenance

Nursing Care of Infants

NURSING CARE OF AN INFANT WHO IS BORN PREMATURELY

5 1. Oxygen given to a premature infant in high concentrations makes the infant especially vulnerable to developing blindness due to hemorrhage of the blood vessels of the eyes followed by a detachment of the retina. This is called retrolental fibroplasia. *Frequent* monitoring of the concentration of oxygen being administered is necessary to be sure excessive amounts are not being given. (8:274–275)
Nursing Process—Implementation
Client need—Safe, effective care environment

6 3. A weak or absent sucking and swallowing reflex may be seen in premature infants. These infants may require nasogastric feeding or feeding by an umbilical catheter or peripheral vein. The normal interval between feedings is 2 to 3 hours. The amount fed depends on the size of the infant but may be as small as 1 to 5 mL for each feeding. Glucose is given only the first few days. If the glucose is tolerated, the physician may order a formula similar to that fed to normal-sized newborns. (8:273–274)
Nursing Process—Implementation
Client Need—Physiological integrity

7 1. Premature infants are deprived of their mother's antibodies and therefore are subject to infection. They cannot manufacture their own antibodies at this time. Many premature infants do breathe on their own, although some may require ventilator assistance. Some children with cerebral palsy are born prematurely, but many premature infants do not develop this condition. (8:275)
Nursing Process—Implementation
Client Need—Safe, effective care environment

8 3. Hyaline membrane disease, also known as respiratory distress syndrome, occurs in infants who do not have enough surfactant in their lungs. In the absence of surfactant, a membrane forms around the alveoli and interferes with the exchange of oxygen across the alveolar membrane. Approximately half of the infants born preterm are affected by hyaline membrane disease. (8:275)
Nursing Process—Collecting data
Client Need—Physiological integrity

NURSING CARE OF AN INFANT WITH HEMOLYTIC DISEASE

9 4. Erythroblastosis fetalis is a congenital disease in which the infant's Rh-positive red blood cells are destroyed by the mother's Rh-positive antibodies. This disease is much less prevalent today than it once was because of the use of Rho immune globulin (RhoGAM). The manner in which a woman is sensitized to the Rh factor rarely results in problems for her first infant. Thalassemia is a congenital blood disorder characterized by the body's inability to manufacture sufficient hemoglobin. Sickle cell disease is characterized by improperly formed red blood cells. Megaloblastic anemia is due to an inadequate intake of vitamin C and folic acid, resulting in abnormal blood cell formation. (8:290–292)

   Nursing Process—Implementation
   Client Need—Health promotion/maintenance

10 4. Jaundice within 24 to 36 hours after birth indicates congenital hemolytic disease (erythroblastosis fetalis). Physiological jaundice, which occurs in some newborns, is seen 3 to 4 days after birth. (8:292)

   Nursing Process—Collecting data
   Client Need—Health promotion/maintenance

11 4. When an infant is born with hemolytic disease, the usual procedure is to collect blood from the infant's umbilical cord for the Coombs' test. A negative direct Coombs' test result indicates that there are no antibodies on the infant's red blood cells. A positive test result indicates the presence of antibodies. (19:263–264)

   Nursing Process—Implementation
   Client Need—Safe, effective care environment

12 3. Signs of neurologic damage in infants with hemolytic disease include lethargy, poor sucking ability, and poor muscle tone, which often are followed by spasticity and convulsions. Scanty urine production is not a sign of neurologic damage. (8:292)

   Nursing Process—Collecting data
   Client Need—Physiological integrity

NURSING CARE OF AN INFANT WITH SPINA BIFIDA

13 2. Important nursing measures to use while caring for a child with a meningocele or a myelomeningocele include avoiding pressure on and preventing injury to the sac. Some agencies use a Bradford frame to make handling of the infant safe and convenient. The frame should be well protected to prevent irritation of the infant's skin. Positioning the infant on his abdomen on a Bradford frame also helps to protect the defect. Direct pressure must not be exerted on the sac; thus, washing the area would not be appropriate. Supporting his formula bottle and preventing skin breakdown by placing a sheepskin under his head is not as important as preventing injury to the sac. (8:283–285)

   Nursing Process—Implementation
   Client Need—Physiological integrity

14 3. Infants with spina bifida and a myelomeningocele are prone to infection; thus, surgical repair

is performed as soon as possible. In some instances, and depending on the location (level of the spine), neurologic symptoms related to the lower extremities may be improved following a surgical repair. (19:249)

   Nursing Process—Implementation
   Client Need—Health promotion/maintenance

15 2. The prone position (lying on the abdomen) is used after surgical repair of a meningocele or myelomeningocele. These positions are maintained until the operative site heals. It is important to keep the operative area free of pressure and as clean as possible to prevent infection. (8:285)

   Nursing Process—Implementation
   Client Need—Physiological integrity

16 1. A child born with spina bifida with a myelomeningocele located high in the spinal column has a poor prognosis in terms of being able to walk alone. The child *may* be able to use a wheelchair or possibly braces and crutches. When the myelomingocele is located low in the spine, for example in or near the sacral area, only minimal weakness of the lower extremities may be seen. (8:283)

   Nursing Process—Planning
   Client Need—Safe, effective care environment

17 4. Urinary and bowel control problems usually are seen in those with spina bifida and a myelomeningocele. (8:283)

   Nursing Process—Planning
   Client Need—Physiological integrity

NURSING CARE OF AN INFANT WITH HYDROCEPHALUS

18 1. An increase in head size is the most prominent symptom of hydrocephalus. Paralysis of the lower extremities may or may not be present, depending on the degree of hydrocephalus. Some hydrocephalus infants also have spina bifida with a myelomeningocele and may have lower extremity paralysis, but this neurologic deficit is not a prominent symptom of hydrocephalus. The sucking reflex may or may not be present, but the presence or absence of this reflex is not considered a prominent sign. Usually there is a bulging of the fontanels. (19:246–249)

   Nursing Process—Implementation
   Client Need—Health promotion/maintenance

19 2. The cause of hydrocephalus in most infants is a blockage (obstruction) that prevents proper circulation of cerebrospinal fluid. This is known as the noncommunicating type of congenital hydrocephalus and is the most common type. Another type, less frequently observed, is the com municating type of hydrocephalus in which no obstruction exists, but cerebrospinal fluid is inadequately absorbed for excretion. Absence of the dura mater, increased spinal fluid proteins, and a blockage in the cerebral arteries are not known causes of hydrocephalus. (19:245)

    Nursing Process—Implementation
    Client Need—Psychosocial integrity

20 2. The infant's position must be changed every 2 hours to prevent skin breakdown. Daily weights, along with other measurements, may be used to determine the degree of mounting cerebrospinal fluid pressure. A low-fat formula would have no effect on the production of cerebrospinal fluid. Those with hydrocephalus have an increase in intracranial pressure. (19:248)

    Nursing Process—Planning
    Client Need—Safe, effective care environment

21 4. The side-lying position is the position of choice after feeding an infant with hydrocephalus. Infants with hydrocephalus tend to vomit easily, and by placing them on their side, vomitus can escape easily from the mouth, and the chance of aspiration of vomitus is reduced. (19:248)

    Nursing Process—Implementation
    Client Need—Safe, effective care environment

22 3. The head and ears of an infant with hydrocephalus are especially prone to pressure and the development of decubitus ulcers. The primary reason for using a sheepskin in this situation is to help relieve pressure on the head and ears. The client's position should be changed frequently to help prevent complications due to inactivity. (19:248)

    Nursing Process—Implementation
    Client Need—Safe, effective care environment

23 3. The position of choice after installing a shunting device in an infant with hydrocephalus is on the side *opposite* the site for the surgical entry. The infant described in this question should be placed on her left side postoperatively because the surgical site of entry was on the right side of the head. This position prevents damage to the shunt valve. (19:248)

    Nursing Process—Implementation
    Client Need—Safe, effective care environment

24 2. Signs of increased intracranial pressure in an infant include bulging or tense fontanels, a decrease in pulse and respiratory rate, irritability, lethargy, and poor eating often associated with vomiting. (19:248; 8:279)

    Nursing Process—Collecting data
    Client Need—Physiological integrity

NURSING CARE OF AN INFANT WITH A CLEFT LIP

25 1. An infant with a cleft lip is unable to form a vacuum in his mouth, and thus he us unable to suck. He will need to be fed by means that do not require normal sucking. The infant is able to swallow. The cleft lip does not hinder salivation. Infants with severe cleft lip tend to be mouth breathers. (19:251)

    Nursing Process—Planning
    Client Need—Physiological integrity

26 3. Of the four options, an Asepto syringe with a rubber tip attached is the best method of feeding the infant with a cleft lip. If the infant is small (eg, premature or less than 5 lb), a medicine dropper may be used initially to begin formula feedings. The decision to use an Asepto syringe or medicine dropper depends on how well the infant takes the formula and on the amount of formula given at each feeding. Infants with a cleft lip usually produce considerable saliva and mucus, which they often do not handle well. It is wise, both preoperatively and postoperatively, to have suction equipment readily available to help prevent the aspiration of mucus and saliva. (19:251)

    Nursing Process—Implementation
    Client Need—Physiological Integrity

27 4. Arm restraints are necessary to prevent the infant from injuring the operative site. The infant should never be turned onto the abdomen because this may injure the operative site. Feeding is accomplished with a dropper or a soft tube attached to an Asepto syringe. Cuddling, talking to the infant, and other measures of affection should be performed by caretakers and the parents. (19:252)

    Nursing Process—Implementation
    Client Need—Safe, effective care environment

NURSING CARE OF AN INFANT WITH PYLORIC STENOSIS

28 4. Pyloric stenosis is a congenital disorder involving narrowing of the pyloric sphincter, which prevents the normal passage of food from the stomach into the duodenum. The decrease in the size of the lumen is caused by hypertrophy of the circular muscles at the pyloric valve. (19:696)

    Nursing Process—Planning
    Client Need—Physiological integrity

29 2. The veins of an infant are small and difficult to locate and enter with a needle. Any number of veins can be used, but most often veins in the scalp are used for infants receiving intravenous therapy. (19:524)

> Nursing Process—Implementation
> Client Need—Safe, effective care environment

30 2. After the surgical repair of a pyloric stenosis, an infant is placed in a semisitting position after giving him fluids or formula. In this position gravity helps carry feedings to the lower end of the stomach and makes regurgitation less likely. An infant seat can be used to attain this position. Another position that may be used is placing the infant in a normal right-side position. The back should be supported with a firm object, such as a small, rolled towel. (19:698)

> Nursing Process—Implementation
> Client Need—Physiological integrity

NURSING CARE OF AN INFANT WITH CONGENITAL HIP DISLOCATION

31 3. The edges of casts should be petaled with adhesive to prevent the edges from irritating the infant's skin. The edges may be trimmed with a file or cutter before petaling. Sandpaper would not be used because the grains from the sandpaper could fall between the cast and the skin. Plastic squares often are used for infants with hip casts to protect the area of the cast left open around the perineal and rectal area, *after* petaling the edges. The insertion of a thick disposable diaper under cast edges could create excessive pressure on the skin beneath or near the cast edges. Trimming the cast edges with a file will not eliminate skin irritation unless something is applied over the cast edge. (8:568–569)

> Nursing Process—Implementation
> Client Need—Physiological integrity

32 3. Pale, cold extremities are signs of impaired circulation to the extremities caused by pressure of the cast. This problem must be reported and corrected *immediately*. Crying 4 hours after her last feeding is normal because the infant is most likely hungry, but unexplained crying may indicate pain or discomfort. Wiggling the toes is a sign that the nervous system has not been compromised by application of a cast. A pulse rate of 110 is normal. (8:568–570)

> Nursing Process—Collecting data
> Client Need—Safe, effective care environment

NURSING CARE OF AN INFANT WITH BILATERAL CLUBFOOT

33 3. Early treatment is necessary because growth and development of an infant's bones and muscles are rapid. Lack of early treatment may result in abnormal development of bones and muscles. Early treatment is not easier on the infant or less expensive, nor does it prevent the possible need for surgery at a later date. (19:253)

> Nursing Process—Implementation
> Client Need—Health promotion/maintenance

34 4. After a cast is applied to the lower extremities, the extremities are elevated on pillows to improve circulation and prevent swelling of the feet. The cast is changed occasionally until the correction is reached. Elevating the legs and feet has no effect on the drying of the cast. Surgery is normally not required to apply this type of cast. (19:254)

> Nursing Process—Implementation
> Client Need—Physiological integrity

35 4. Wet casts should be handled by the palms of the hands. Gloves are unnecessary. A wet cast should never be lifted with the fingers because this will cause indentations on the cast. Slings are inappropriate and may cut into a cast. Sturdy commercial slings made of heavy canvas-type material sometimes are used, especially for older children or adults. (19:254)

> Nursing Process—Implementation
> Client Need—Physiological integrity

36 4. An infant develops the ability to look at his surroundings during the first month of life. By 2 months he is able to follow an object with both eyes. The mobile is an appropriate amusement for a 2-month-old infant. By 4 months the infant can normally reach for objects, and by 7 to 9 months he is able to crawl and play peek-a-boo. (19:326–327)

> Nursing Process—Collecting data
> Client Need—Health promotion/maintenance

37 1. The posterior fontanelle normally closes at approximately 2 months of age. (19:326–327)

> Nursing Process—Implementation
> Client Need—Health promotion/maintenance

NURSING CARE OF AN INFANT WITH OTITIS MEDIA

38 2. Dosages for medications are determined on an individual basis after considering a child's weight and age. Weight is an unlikely basis for determining an infant's nutritional needs, except when the child is extremely overweight or underweight. An electrolyte imbalance or the need for parenteral fluids cannot be determined by weighing the child. (15:14)

> Nursing Process—Collecting data
> Client Need—Safe, effective care environment

39 3. Ricky probably will indicate that he has an earache by rolling or shaking his head from side

to side or, if he were older, by tugging at the affected ear. This usually is accompanied by crying. (19:553)
 Nursing Process—Collecting data
 Client Need—Physiological integrity

40 4. Stopping an antibiotic before the course of therapy is completed may result in a return of the infection. Extra fluids should be offered, especially if the infant has an elevated temperature. Lying on the unaffected side is allowed. (15:166)
 Nursing Process—Implementation
 Client Need—Health promotion/maintenance

NURSING CARE OF AN INFANT WITH AN INFECTIOUS DISEASE

41 2. All articles worn or used by the infant and caretakers must be discarded or decontaminated before re-use. These articles are not mixed with the linen from a regular hospital unit. Masks, gowns, and gloves normally are required, and the door to the room should be closed to prevent the spread of the infection to other areas of the hospital. (19:541–543)
 Nursing Process—Implementation
 Client Need—Safe, effective care environment

42 4. Used masks are discarded *inside* the room because the mask is contaminated, and the room is the contaminated area. (19:545)
 Nursing Process—Implementation
 Client Need—Safe, effective care environment

43 1. Gloves are removed *before* the gown is removed. (18:365)
 Nursing Process—Implementation
 Client Need—Safe, effective care environment

44 2. The excessive crying that normally occurs when an infant has a painful or uncomfortable treatment, such as starting intravenous fluid therapy, may cause vomiting. Because the infant is crying, aspiration of vomitus is possible. Oral fluids and food do not interfere with the absorption of intravenous fluids nor must intravenous fluids be given on an empty stomach. (19:526)
 Nursing Process—Implementation
 Client Need—Safe, effective care environment

45 2. An infant receiving intravenous therapy still requires tender, loving care by the parents and caretakers. Tactile and verbal stimulation is most important. (19:526)
 Nursing Process—Implementation
 Client Need—Safe, effective care environment

46 4. An increase in the rate of flow is reported to the nurse in charge or the team leader because other measures must be taken to control the infusion rate. Voiding frequently, sleeping, and crying can be considered normal events when an infant is receiving parenteral fluids. (19:524)
 Nursing Process—Collecting data
 Client Need—Safe, effective care environment

47 1. The rapid infusion of intravenous fluids may result in fluid overload and congestive heart failure, which is an extremely dangerous event. (19:524; 52:113–114)
 Nursing Process—Collecting data
 Client Need—Safe, effective care environment

NURSING CARE OF AN INFANT WITH ATOPIC DERMATITIS

48 4. A vesicle is defined as a small sac made up of an elevation of epidermis and filled with a serous liquid. The vesicles on an infant with atopic dermatitis (infantile eczema) are filled with a yellow, sticky serum. If blood and pus are present, the infant most likely has scratched the area, and it has become infected. (8:596)
 Nursing Process—Implementation
 Client Need—Health promotion/maintenance

49 3. Infantile eczema is thought to be caused, at least in part, by allergic reactions to some irritant(s), which is why the physician asked questions about the home environment. Also, it appears that hereditary factors may play a role. This skin disease is most often seen during the first year of life, after approximately 2 months of age. (8:596–597)
 Nursing Process—Implementation
 Client Need—Health promotion/maintenance

50 3. An infant with eczema experiences severe itching of his skin lesions. The nurse must be prepared to teach home caretakers about nursing measures that will help to relieve itching so that the child does not scratch his skin and introduce microorganisms into the lesions. Itching usually is so severe that if it is not relieved, the child may require restraints, such as elbow restraints, and face masks may be necessary to protect the face. (8:596–597)
 Nursing Process—Implementation
 Client Need—Health promotion/maintenance

51 3. Hydrocortisone is an antiinflammatory agent. It helps reduce inflammation and its symptoms, such as swelling, redness, heat, and discomfort. This drug does not influence weeping of lesions, the spread of the disease, or the white blood cell count. (8:596–597)
 Nursing Process—Evaluation
 Client Need—Health promotion/maintenance

52 1. Colloid baths have been found effective for their soothing effects on the irritated and itching skin of an infant with eczema. Baking soda and cornstarch added to tepid water is used most frequently. Cooked oatmeal or a commercial bath preparation of oatmeal also is effective for a colloid bath. The bath should last approximately 15 minutes, and then the child is patted dry. Soaps tend to irritate the skin. Normal saline is not particularly soothing. Oils should be avoided on the skin of a child with eczema. (8:598)

> Nursing Process—Implementation
> Client Need—Health promotion/maintenance

Nursing Care of Toddlers

NURSING CARE OF A TODDLER WITH SICKLE CELL CRISIS

53 1. The sickle-shaped cells tend to clump together in vessels and obstruct the normal blood flow. A thrombosis may form and cause death of tissues because of poor blood circulation. The characteristic symptom when tissue is denied normal blood circulation is severe pain in the affected parts of the body. Diarrhea, bradycardia, and hemorrhage usually are not associated with sickle cell crisis. (8:726–728)

> Nursing Process—Implementation
> Client Need—Physiological integrity

54 4. Nursing care of a child with sickle cell crisis is primarily supportive. Whole blood transfusions may be given to increase hemoglobin levels. Iron is of no value in the treatment of this blood disorder. (19:666–669; 14:640)

> Nursing Process—Planning
> Client Need—Physiological integrity

55 2. Dry skin; poor skin turgor; decreased urinary output; weight loss; elevated temperature; and a weak, rapid pulse indicate dehydration. (19:667)

> Nursing Process—Collecting data
> Client Need—Physiological integrity

NURSING CARE OF A TODDLER WITH CYSTIC FIBROSIS

56 4. Typically, the stools of a child with cystic fibrosis are large, sticky, and foul-smelling. The condition is due to a diminished or a lack of flow of pancreatic enzymes that leads to faulty absorption of nutrients, especially fat-soluble vitamins. Other signs include malnutrition despite a hearty appetite, chronic coughing, distended abdomen, and flabby muscles. (8:696)

> Nursing Process—Collecting data
> Client Need—Physiological integrity

57 3. Many times, caretakers of children with cystic fibrosis become aware of a typical sign of the illness when they report that a child tastes salty when they kiss the child. The perspiration, tears, and saliva contain abnormally high concentrations of salt. Sweat analysis is an important diagnostic tool when children are examined for cystic fibrosis. These children typically are underweight. (8:696)

> Nursing Process—Collecting data
> Client Need—Physiological integrity

58 1. The leading cause of death in those with cystic fibrosis usually is related to the lungs and the heart. (8:698)

> Nursing Process—Planning
> Client Need—Physiological integrity

59 4. The pancreas is unable to secrete a sufficient amount of pancreatic enzymes owing to blockage of the pancreatic duct by thickened secretions. Pancreatic enzymes are necessary for the digestion and absorption of food, particularly fats and proteins, and are given so that the digestion and absorption of these foods is enhanced. (19:649)

> Nursing Process—Implementation
> Client Need—Physiological integrity

60 1. Fats are poorly absorbed by those with cystic fibrosis and therefore are given in limited to moderate amounts. (20:288)

> Nursing Process—Implementation
> Client Need—Health promotion/maintenance

61 2. Exercise is important for well-being and general good health. For a person with cystic fibrosis, exercise is particularly important to help rid the pulmonary system of excessive respiratory secretions. (19:653)

> Nursing Process—Implementation
> Client Need—Health promotion/maintenance

62 3. The air passages of the lungs of those with cystic fibrosis become clogged with mucus, thus decreasing the amount of oxygen reaching the lungs. A bronchodilator increases the diameter of the bronchi, thereby allowing more air to enter the lungs, and breathing is improved. (19:648–649)

> Nursing Process—Evaluation
> Client Need—Physiological integrity

63 4. Children with cystic fibrosis lose fluid through frequent bowel movements and sweating. Increasing the fluid intake helps liquefy secretions in the lungs and aids in raising secretions, which ultimately may improve breathing. (19:651)

> Nursing Process—Planning
> Client Need—Physiological integrity

64 2. Children with cystic fibrosis are very susceptible to infections, especially infections of the respiratory tract. The parents should be taught to guard against exposing the child to infections to the greatest extent possible. Immunization against childhood diseases is highly recommended, especially those that may place the respiratory tract at risk. (19:651)

> Nursing Process—Planning
> Client Need—Safe, effective care environment

NURSING CARE OF A TODDLER WITH ASTHMA

65 1. The difficulty in breathing associated with asthma is due to thickened bronchial secretions, spasm of the bronchi, and edema of the lining of the bronchi. (19:644)

> Nursing Process—Planning
> Client Need—Physiological integrity

66 3. Medical (drug) therapy is necessary to relieve respiratory distress, but elevating the head of the bed may ease breathing. Another method is to place a pillow on the overbed stand and have the child lean forward and extend his arms over the pillow. Elevating the upper part of the body encourages the use of the accessory muscles of breathing. (19:647)

> Nursing Process—Implementation
> Client Need—Physiological integrity

67 4. When the client has asthma due to an allergy to one or more environmental factors, general control of the environment is necessary to reduce chances of future asthma attacks. A generous fluid intake is recommended because fluid is lost through sweating and an increased respiratory rate, especially when the client has periodic asthma attacks. A well-balanced diet is necessary, especially for the growing child. Asthma cannot be cured, but often it can be controlled. (19:647)

> Nursing Process—Implementation
> Client Need—Safe, effective care environment

68 3. Rugs collect dust and dirt (a common source of allergy) even when vacuumed and cleaned often. Cotton blankets and a foam-rubber pillow are recommended. An alarm clock usually is allowed. (19:647)

> Nursing Process—Implementation
> Client Need—Safe, effective care environment

NURSING CARE OF A TODDLER WHO HAS SWALLOWED A TOXIC SUBSTANCE

69 4. A common early sign of salicylate poisoning is rapid and deep breathing because aspirin stimulates the respiratory center. The pulse rate would increase when acidosis accompanies salicylate poisoning. Other signs of salicylate poisoning include electrolyte imbalance, restless-

ness, fever, profuse perspiration, bleeding, and finally, convulsions and coma. (19:713)

> Nursing Process—Collecting data
> Client Need—Physiological integrity

70 3. A goal in the emergency treatment for salicylate poisoning is to empty the stomach of the drug either by performing a gastric lavage or by inducing vomiting. This is done to prevent additional absorption of the ingested drug. Gastroscopy is likely to be used to retrieve nonsoluble objects from the stomach but would be useless in retrieving the dissolved aspirin. A gastrostomy is a surgically created opening in the stomach wall for the purpose of introducing food into the stomach. (19:713)

> Nursing Process—Planning
> Client Need—Physiological integrity

71 3. As can be expected of a toddler, the child in this item most likely will be naturally curious about his environment. Children between the ages of 1 and 4 years like to taste substances and cannot determine for themselves whether a substance is poisonous. Therefore, it is most appropriate to remove harmful substances from areas where children play. A 2½-year-old child is too young to understand a verbal warning that certain substances are poisonous or to read warning signs. Telling the child not to touch anything defeats the purpose of a playroom for recreational or diversional activity. (19:713)

> Nursing Process—Implementation
> Client Need—Safe, effective care environment

72 3. Parents of small children should be taught to keep syrup of ipecac in a locked cupboard in their homes for emergency use. This drug causes vomiting. However, parents should be taught *not* to use ipecac if the child has ingested a volatile or corrosive substance, such as lye or kerosene. Vomiting after ingestion of volatile or corrosive substances can make the situation worse by causing dangerous inhalation of petroleum fumes or by further irritating or damaging the upper gastrointestinal tract. Whenever there is the slightest doubt, parents should be advised to call their local poison control center for information. (19:876; 15:276)

> Nursing Process—Implementation
> Client Need—Safe, effective care environment

NURSING CARE OF A TODDLER WITH LEAD POISONING

73 1. Small children may chew on or give a history of chewing on old furniture, window sills, and other objects painted with lead-based paint. In this instance, Amy's parents lived in the house before Amy was born and have just begun renovations. Paint now being sold does not contain lead; therefore, exposure to new paint fumes would not cause lead poisoning. The heating system and floors of the house are unlikely sources of lead, although old plumbing also may be a source of lead. (19:713)

> Nursing Process—Collecting data
> Client Need—Safe, effective care environment

74 4. The heavy metal antagonist edetate calcium disodium (Calcium Disodium Versenate) usually is the drug of choice for lead poisoning. Treatment of this type of poisoning requires an intensive approach to rid the body of lead. Other drugs used during treatment are for symptoms rather than the removal of lead from the body. (15:284, 287)

> Nursing Process—Implementation
> Client Need—Safe, effective care environment

75 3. Lead from the old paint may leach through a new coat or coats of paint or varnish applied over the old paint. It is recommended that the old lead-based paint be completely removed before applying a new coat of paint. All paint sold today is lead-free. (15:289)

> Nursing Process—Implementation
> Client Need—Safe, effective care environment

NURSING CARE OF A TODDLER WITH CROUP

76 1. LTB most often is caused by a virus. It is not related to whooping cough or inadequate development of the lungs. LTB may occur in those with or without a history of asthma. (19:634; 8:701–702)

> Nursing Process—Planning
> Client Need—Safe, effective care environment

77 2. The child with LTB has a cough that sounds hoarse, much like a loud, barking, metallic sound. A high-pitched sound is typical of the child's breathing, not a cough. (8:701–702)

> Nursing Process—Collecting data
> Client Need—Safe, effective care environment

78 3. To help liquefy secretions and reduce laryngeal spasms, the child with croup should breathe air that is high in humidity. A croup tent or an electric vaporizer may be used. A dust-free environment would be required for children who need a sterile environment or for those who are allergic to dust. Dry or hot air provides no relief for a child with croup. (8:702)

> Nursing Process—Implementation
> Client Need—Safe, effective care environment

79 2. Respiratory difficulty may be a sign of more serious involvement of the trachea and bronchial tree, and the physician should be contacted immediately. Thin, clear mucus; coughing during the night; or refusal to play with toys would not be considered signs of a more serious involvement. (8:702)

> Nursing Process—Implementation
> Client Need—Physiological integrity

80 1. Aspirin, a salicylate, is contraindicated in young children with a fever, flu-like symptoms, or chickenpox because aspirin use has been associated with Reye's syndrome. This rare but life-threatening disorder is characterized by vomiting and lethargy, which may progress to coma and possibly death. (15:71)

> Nursing Process—Implementation
> Client Need—Health promotion/maintenance

81 2. Noisy, moist, and labored respirations indicate a problem with the patency of the tracheostomy tube. Often, the tube can become blocked by mucus and secretions, although other events can cause respiratory difficulty. The blood pressure, pulse, and respiratory rate rises. Crying and attempting to talk are normal events in children and do not indicate a problem with the tracheostomy tube. (18:718)

> Nursing Process—Collecting data
> Client Need—Safe, effective care environment

82 3. Suction is applied by covering the vent on the suction tube. Once the catheter has been inserted and is being withdrawn, suction is applied. Suction is not applied while the catheter is being inserted. The catheter size must be smaller than the tracheostomy tube opening and is inserted for approximately 15 seconds. More than one pass of the suction catheter may be necessary. Between insertions the suction catheter may be cleared with sterile water and not tap water because this is an aseptic procedure. (18:718; 19:533)

> Nursing Process—Implementation
> Client Need—Safe, effective care environment

NURSING CARE OF A TODDLER WITH PNEUMONIA

83 4. The respiratory rate in children with pneumonia is rapid and shallow. The rate seen in infants with pneumonia may become 40 to 80 per minute and in older children 30 to 50 per minute. The rapid respiratory rate is the body's way of compensating for the decreased ventilation in the lungs and, to a certain extent, helping the body rid itself of excess heat. When the temperature is elevated, the metabolic rate is increased, which also causes respirations to increase. (8:692–693)

> Nursing Process—Collecting data
> Client Need—Physiological integrity

84 4. Recording the child's urinary output will assist in determining fluid needs. Fluid loss because of high fever, vomiting, and diarrhea are common in pneumonia. As a result of fluid loss, urinary output is decreased. The urine appears dark amber and has a high specific gravity. The nurse should measure the fluid intake as well. (8:693; 18:644–646)

> Nursing Process—Collecting data
> Client Need—Physiological integrity

85 3. Seizures may occur in young children with a high temperature and are called febrile seizures. The cause of febrile seizures is not clear, but it may be related to their immature nervous systems. The nurse should take measures to institute seizure precautions in a child with an elevated temperature. Fluids should be offered at least hourly and the intake and output measured every 8 hours unless there is evidence of renal involvement or disease. (8:580, 693)

> Nursing Process—Implementation
> Client Need—Safe, effective care environment

86 4. Rubbing the skin before giving a tepid water sponge bath helps bring blood to the skin's surface, stimulates the skin, and prevents chilling. This assists with reducing the child's temperature. When cool, moist cloths are applied to the skin. Rubbing the skin should be done *briefly*. Prolonged rubbing causes heat by friction, which is contraindicated for those with an elevated temperature. (19:507)

> Nursing Process—Implementation
> Client Need—Physiological integrity

87 2. During a tepid water sponge bath to reduce body temperature, the nurse should observe the child carefully and check the vital signs regularly. Any untoward reactions to the bath should cause the nurse to stop the procedure. About 30 minutes after the bath, the nurse should check the child's vital signs to evaluate the effectiveness of the procedure in helping to reduce the temperature. If a child is not already on oxygen therapy, its use is unlikely to depend on the result of a tepid water sponge. Aspirin is never given to young children because it has been associated with Reye's syndrome. The administration of oxygen or giving foods high in vitamin C is not likely to reduce body temperature. (19:506)

> Nursing Process—Implementation
> Client Need—Safe, effective care environment

88 4. The nurse should have the mother repeat home-going instructions so that it can be determined if she has understood them correctly. It may become necessary to write, or have someone write, the instructions in Spanish for the mother described in this item if she does not understand. Reading the instructions again or repeating them in terms that the mother can understand does not ensure that she understands the material. Having someone translate the instructions into Spanish does not evaluate the mother's ability to understand the instructions given in English. (15:34; 18:28)

> Nursing Process—Evaluation
> Client Need—Health promotion/maintenance

89 2. A 3-year-old child should have received DPT, TOPV, measles, mumps, and rubella vaccines. BCG, hepatitis, and meningococcal vaccines are not indicated at this time. (15:303)

> Nursing Process—Implementation
> Client Need—Health promotion/maintenance

Nursing Care of Preschool Children

NURSING CARE OF A CHILD WITH SEIZURE ACTIVITY

90 3. When a seizure is not seen by medical personnel, family members or friends who do observe and then describe the seizure may give a clue as to the type of epilepsy (seizure disorder) the child has. The client who has had a seizure is unable to describe what the seizure felt like. The way in which Susan responds to questions and obtaining vital signs if Susan has a seizure will not identify the type of seizure. (19:577)

> Nursing Process—Collecting data
> Client Need—Physiological integrity

91 1. The sides of a crib should be padded to help prevent injury to a child during seizure activity. The padding serves no other therapeutic purpose. (14:645)

> Nursing Process—Implementation
> Client Need—Safe, effective care environment

92 2. It is not necessary to keep a tracheostomy set at the bedside of a child subject to seizure activity. Suction equipment may be required to remove mucus from the child's mouth as necessary. A good source of light is important for observations that should be made during a seizure, such as the child's color, respiratory rate, and eye movements. An oral airway can be inserted, whenever possible, to create a patent airway during a seizure. Force is never used to insert an oral airway. (8:662)

> Nursing Process—Implementation
> Client Need—Safe, effective care environment

93 2. Turning the child on her side establishes a patent airway and prevents aspiration of saliva. Inserting a padded tongue blade is no longer recommended because injury to the mouth and teeth may occur. Oxygen would be of no value because respirations cease during this type of seizure. Calling for assistance is not an appropriate first action because the prime function of the nurse is to maintain a patent airway; prevent injury; and record the events that occur before, during, and after the seizure. (8:662; 19:573)

Nursing Process—Implementation
Client Need—Safe, effective care environment

94 2. Phenytoin (Dilantin) should be given with food or immediately after a meal to reduce stomach irritation. (15:245)

Nursing Process—Implementation
Client Need—Physiological integrity

95 4. The dose of an anticonvulsant must not be increased, decreased, or omitted except on the advice of the physician. Omission of one or more doses may result in status epilepticus, which is a state of continuous seizures. It is not necessary to limit school time, play activity, or fluid intake. (15:245–246)

Nursing Process—Implementation
Client Need—Health promotion/maintenance

96 4. Phenytoin, when used over time, tends to cause an overgrowth of gum tissues. The condition is called gingival hyperplasia. Periodic visits to the dentist and good oral hygiene can help reduce the incidence of the condition. A poor appetite, urinary incontinence, and painful joints are not associated with the use of phenytoin. (15:246)

Nursing Process—Implementation
Client Need—Health promotion/maintenance

NURSING CARE OF A CHILD WITH LEUKEMIA

97 3. A commonly used test to help diagnose leukemia is a bone marrow aspiration. The bone marrow of the client with leukemia is characterized by being hypercellular, lacking fat globules, and having blast cells (immature white cells). The diagnosis also is based on the child's history, symptoms, and various other blood tests. (19:674)

Nursing Process—Planning
Client Need—Safe, effective care environment

98 3. Painful joints, a common symptom of leukemia, often are relieved by bed rest. Other signs and symptoms of leukemia include low-grade fever, pallor, listlessness, bruising, and swollen lymph glands. (19:673)

Nursing Process—Implementation
Client Need—Safe, effective care environment

99 2. Bacterial infections are common in those with leukemia. Ulcerations often develop in the mouth and around the anal area, and they may bleed. Good oral care is essential. The platelet count and red blood cell count usually are decreased. (19:674)

Nursing Process—Collecting data
Client Need—Safe, effective care environment

100 3. Epistaxis (nose bleed), petechiae, and bruising are complications associated with a decreased platelet count. Often the liver enlarges, and weight loss due to anorexia is not uncommon. Diuresis is not associated with leukemia. (19:677)

Nursing Process—Collecting data
Client Need—Physiological integrity

101 2. Drugs capable of suppressing bone marrow function are used in the treatment of leukemia in the hope that cancerous cells will be destroyed. These drugs suppress the normal function of the bone marrow; therefore, all blood cells produced by the bone marrow, normal and cancerous, are decreased in number. (19:676)

Nursing Process—Collecting data
Client Need—Safe, effective care environment

102 2. Signs of a transfusion reaction include feeling cold and having chills, fever, and a rapid pulse rate. The client also may complain of itching and low back pain. If feeling chilly occurs very early in a blood transfusion, it *may* be the result of the cold transfused blood entering the body. Nevertheless, a transfusion reaction should be suspected until proven otherwise. (19:678)

Nursing Process—Collecting data
Client Need—Physiological integrity

103 3. If a client is having a reaction to blood, the nurse should *first* clamp the tubing to stop the blood flow. The clamp on the second bottle (normal saline) should then be immediately opened. The needle should not be removed because it is important to keep an intravenous line for the administration of substances other than blood, such as fluids, electrolytes, and drugs. The nurse in charge should be notified promptly after the transfusion is stopped. (19:678)

Nursing Process—Implementation
Client Need—Physiological integrity

104 1. The question, "Am I going to die?" can be answered in many different ways. However, the nurse's response should encourage the child to vent her feelings about dying. The nurse should avoid responses that would either make the child guilty or discourage the child from talking about her anxieties. The nurse's response also should not reinforce denials and unrealistic perceptions of the client's prognosis. When dealing with children, it is important to answer questions honestly based on the child's level of understanding. (19:675)

Nursing Process—Implementation
Client Need—Psychosocial integrity

105 3. Children between the ages of 9 or 10 usually first recognize death in a manner similar to adults. This may vary and depend on the child's prior exposure to the death of a close family member and the explanation of death given by the parents. (19:832)

Nursing Process—Implementation
Client Need—Psychosocial integrity

NURSING CARE OF A CHILD WITH STRABISMUS

106 1. Foods and fluids generally are withheld for 6 to 12 hours before surgery to reduce the risk of aspirating vomitus when the client is under anesthesia and when recovering from anesthesia. For those who are hospitalized, it is recommended that all food and fluids be removed from the bedside. Also, a sign indicating that the child is to have nothing by mouth should be clearly posted at the bedside. (8:521; 16:156–157)

Nursing Process—Implementation
Client Need—Safe, effective care environment

107 2. If restraints are necessary and are ordered by the physician, elbow restraints usually are all that is necessary for this age group. This type of surgery is performed on structures outside the eyeball, and therefore restraints, if needed, may be necessary only for a short period and are applied only to the elbow. (19:559)

Nursing Process—Implementation
Client Need—Safe, effective care environment

108 4. Some soreness may occur after this type of eye surgery. Children need to be told the truth. (8:416)

Nursing Process—Implementation
Client Need—Psychosocial integrity

109 3. Unless the physician orders otherwise, a regular diet can be given once nausea has ceased and the child can be up and about. Unless both eyes are bandaged, the child can play with toys with adult supervision. Reading to a child of this age is appropriate. (19:559–560)

Nursing Process—Implementation
Client Need—Safe, effective care environment

NURSING CARE OF A CHILD HAVING A TONSILLECTOMY AND ADENOIDECTOMY

110 2. It is important to report promptly an elevated temperature of a preoperative client, along with any other signs of infection, such as a sore throat, cough, or excessive nasal discharge. Surgery will be cancelled if the child has an infection. The other vital signs in this question are normal for a child this age. (18:452)

Nursing Process—Collecting data
Client Need—Safe, effective care environment

111 3. Examples of clear liquids include clear broth, Jell-O, synthetic juices, water, and ice chips. Natural juices are irritating to the throat. When a full liquid diet can be tolerated, sherbet, milk shakes, ice cream, puddings, and custard may be added. (20:262–263)

Nursing Process—Implementation
Client Need—Physiological integrity

112 2. Signs of excessive bleeding following a tonsillectomy include frequent swallowing (which may be due to blood trickling down the back of the throat), a rapid pulse rate, restlessness, and vomiting of bright red blood. Vomiting dark old blood is to be expected unless it occurs in large amounts. Usually, children are eager for fluids when awakening despite throat soreness. A respiratory rate of 30 per minute is within normal range for a 5-year-old child. (19:643)

Nursing Process—Collecting data
Client Need—Physiological integrity

113 1. It is recommended the child be kept quiet for a few days to discourage bleeding in the operative site. Fluids and soft foods can be taken as desired, but solid food usually is not recommended for several days. Aspirin is contraindicated for a child of this age because its use has been associated with Reye's syndrome. Aspirin also may affect the ability of the blood to clot and therefore increase bleeding tendencies.(19:643–644)

Nursing Process—Planning
Client Need—Safe, effective care environment

114 4. A transient earache for 1 to 3 days following a tonsillectomy and adenoidectomy is common. The discomfort is due to pain referred from the throat to the ear. A nurse should advise parents of the possibility of the occurrence of an earache while giving discharge instructions. Difficulty swallowing for 3 weeks, severe pain for the first 7 days after surgery, and expectorating bright red blood for 1 week are not normal and should be brought to the attention of the physician. (19:643–644)

Nursing Process—Implementation
Client Need—Safe, effective care environment

Classification of Test Items

Unit III Review Test 4

Directions: After each question the correct answer is given as well as a classification of each test question. Compare the correct answer with your answer. If a question has been answered *incorrectly*, draw a line to the end of the four columns. When finished, add up your correct scores and place the results at the bottom of each column.
Score Calculation:
   To determine the percentage of the number of questions you answered correctly, divide the **Number Correct** by the **Number Possible**, as example 90 (the number of questions answered correctly) divided by 114 (the number of questions in the test) = .789 or 79%.

NURSING PROCESS
C = Collecting data
P = Planning
I = Implementation
E = Evaluation

CLIENT NEEDS
S = Safe, effective care environment
P = Physiological integrity
M = Psychosocial integrity
H = Health promotion/maintenance

Question #	Answer #	Nursing Process				Client Needs			
		C	P	I	E	S	P	M	H
1	4	C							H
2	2	C							H
3	2	C							H
4	3	C							H
5	1			I		S			
6	3			I			P		
7	1			I		S			
8	3	C					P		
9	4			I					H
10	4	C							H
11	4			I		S			
12	3	C					P		
13	2			I			P		
14	3			I					H
15	2			I			P		
16	1		P			S			
17	4		P				P		
18	1			I					H
19	2			I				M	
20	2		P			S			

NURSING PROCESS

C = Collecting data
P = Planning
I = Implementation
E = Evaluation

CLIENT NEEDS

S = Safe, effective care environment
P = Physiological integrity
M = Psychosocial integrity
H = Health promotion/maintenance

Question #	Answer #	Nursing Process				Client Needs			
		C	P	I	E	S	P	M	H
21	4			I		S			
22	3			I		S			
23	3			I		S			
24	2	C					P		
25	1		P				P		
26	3			I			P		
27	4			I		S			
28	4		P				P		
29	2			I		S			
30	2			I			P		
31	3			I			P		
32	3	C				S			
33	3			I					H
34	4			I			P		
35	4			I			P		
36	4	C							H
37	1			I					H
38	2	C				S			
39	3	C					P		
40	4			I					H
41	2			I		S			
42	4			I		S			
43	1			I		S			
44	2			I		S			
45	2			I		S			
46	4	C				S			
47	1	C				S			
48	4			I					H
49	3			I					H
50	3			I					H
51	3				E				H
52	1			I					H
53	1			I			P		

NURSING PROCESS
C = Collecting data
P = Planning
I = Implementation
E = Evaluation

CLIENT NEEDS
S = Safe, effective care environment
P = Physiological integrity
M = Psychosocial integrity
H = Health promotion/maintenance

Question #	Answer #	Nursing Process				Client Needs			
		C	P	I	E	S	P	M	H
54	4		P				P		
55	2	C					P		
56	4	C					P		
57	3	C					P		
58	1		P				P		
59	4			I			P		
60	1			I					H
61	2			I					H
62	3				E		P		
63	4		P				P		
64	2		P			S			
65	1		P				P		
66	3			I			P		
67	4			I		S			
68	3			I		S			
69	4	C					P		
70	3		P				P		
71	3			I		S			
72	3			I		S			
73	1	C				S			
74	4			I		S			
75	3			I		S			
76	1		P			S			
77	2	C				S			
78	3			I		S			
79	2			I		P			
80	1			I					H
81	2	C				S			
82	3			I		S			
83	4	C					P		
84	4	C					P		
85	3			I		S			
86	4			I			P		

NURSING PROCESS
C = Collecting data
P = Planning
I = Implementation
E = Evaluation

CLIENT NEEDS
S = Safe, effective care environment
P = Physiological integrity
M = Psychosocial integrity
H = Health promotion/maintenance

Question #	Answer #	Nursing Process				Client Needs			
		C	P	I	E	S	P	M	H
87	2			I		S			
88	4				E				H
89	2			I					H
90	3	C					P		
91	1			I		S			
92	2			I		S			
93	2			I		S			
94	2			I			P		
95	4			I					H
96	4			I					H
97	3		P			S			
98	3			I		S			
99	2	C				S			
100	3	C					P		
101	2	C				S			
102	2	C					P		
103	3			I			P		
104	1			I				M	
105	3			I				M	
106	1			I		S			
107	2			I		S			
108	4			I				M	
109	3			I		S			
110	2	C				S			
111	3			I			P		
112	2	C					P		
113	1		P			S			
114	4			I		S			
Number Correct									
Number Possible	114	30	14	67	3	48	38	4	24
Percentage Correct									

REVIEW TEST 5

Nursing Care of School-Aged Children
Nursing Care of a Child with Appendicitis
Nursing Care of a Child with Rheumatic Fever
Nursing Care of a Child with Diabetes Mellitus
Nursing Care of a Child with Second- and Third-Degree Burns
Nursing Care of a Child with Juvenile Rheumatoid Arthritis
Nursing Care of a Child with a Head Injury
Nursing Care of a Child with a Brain Tumor
Nursing Care of a Child in Traction

Nursing Care of Adolescents
Nursing Care of an Adolescent with Dysmenorrhea
Nursing Care of an Adolescent Who Is Abusing Drugs
Nursing Care of an Adolescent with a Sexually Transmitted Disease
Nursing Care of an Adolescent with Scoliosis
Individual Test Items

Correct Answers and Rationale
Classification of Test Items

Directions: With a pencil, blacken the circle in front of the option you have chosen for your correct answer.

Nursing Care of School-Aged Children

NURSING CARE OF A CHILD WITH APPENDICITIS

Jimmy Harkins, 6 years old, has an elevated temperature and complains of generalized abdominal pain. The physician suspects appendicitis, and Jimmy is hospitalized for observation and possible appendectomy.

1 Which of the following events should the nurse recognize as the *most significant* sign or symptom of appendicitis and should be reported to the nurse in charge or the physician?
   ○ 1. Jimmy's appetite is poor.
   ○ 2. Jimmy cried when his parents left the room.
   ○ 3. Jimmy lies on his side with his knees flexed toward his abdomen.
   ○ 4. Jimmy wants to be out of bed.

Surgery is performed on Jimmy, and he returns to his room with an intravenous line.

2 The physician's order reads that 200 mL of the intravenous solution is to be infused in 8 hours. The nurse should know that the amount of intravenous solution given each hour is
   ○ 1. 10 mL.
   ○ 2. 25 mL.
   ○ 3. 35 mL.
   ○ 4. 50 mL.

3 Which one of the following nursing tasks is performed during the *first 24 hours* after Jimmy's surgery?
   ○ 1. Asking Jimmy what foods he likes to eat
   ○ 2. Telling Jimmy that he will be getting out of bed in a few days
   ○ 3. Having Jimmy do postural drainage
   ○ 4. Encouraging Jimmy to take deep breaths and cough

4 The nurse plans to observe Jimmy for complications. Which of the following might indicate a postoperative complication during the first 24 to 48 postoperative hours and should be reported to the nurse in charge or the physician?
   ○ 1. Anxiety, crying
   ○ 2. Oral temperature of 99.4°F, respiratory rate of 28

112

○ 3. Nausea, pain in the incision
○ 4. Reluctance to move about in bed

NURSING CARE OF A CHILD WITH RHEUMATIC FEVER

Seven-year-old Martha King is admitted to a hospital with possible rheumatic fever. She appears to be acutely ill.

5 The nurse obtains a health history from Martha's parents. Which one of the following events might be significant with regard to the tentative diagnosis and should be brought to the attention of the physician?
○ 1. Exposure to measles within the last 4 weeks
○ 2. A recent severe sore throat
○ 3. A disinterest in school work
○ 4. A bump on the head while playing

6 When obtaining the health history the nurse should recognize the signs and symptoms of rheumatic fever, which include
○ 1. decreased pulse rate, diarrhea.
○ 2. aching in the legs and migrating joint tenderness.
○ 3. lower than normal body temperature and increased pulse rate.
○ 4. increased blood pressure and generalized erythema.

7 The nurse is assigned to develop a plan of care for Martha. Which one of the following would be included in a care plan for the *acute* phase of Martha's illness?
○ 1. Promote complete bed rest.
○ 2. Limit the fluid intake.
○ 3. Encourage short periods of sleep during daytime hours.
○ 4. Schedule ambulatory activity every 4 hours.

Martha is started on penicillin.

8 The nurse checks several references, which state that penicillin is given to those with rheumatic fever to
○ 1. eliminate any remaining probable causative microorganisms and prevent a reinfection.
○ 2. decrease joint size and prevent joint deformities.
○ 3. reduce inflammation and prevent spread of the disease to other joints.
○ 4. decrease pain and prevent renal damage.

9 Martha also is prescribed aspirin. The nurse, when checking nursing literature, notes that the *most probable* reason for giving this drug to those with rheumatic fever is to
○ 1. protect the body's immune system.
○ 2. prevent infection.

○ 3. relieve joint tenderness.
○ 4. prevent cardiac enlargement.

10 Martha responds to therapy and is to be discharged from the hospital. Which one of the following is the *most* important inclusion in a discharge teaching plan for Martha's parents? The importance of
○ 1. exercise.
○ 2. controlling behavioral problems.
○ 3. long-term penicillin therapy to prevent recurrences.
○ 4. avoiding mental stress.

NURSING CARE OF A CHILD WITH DIABETES MELLITUS

Paul Meyers, 8 years old, is admitted to a hospital in a coma. The tentative diagnosis is diabetic coma due to untreated insulin-dependent diabetes mellitus.

11 The nurse should be prepared to assist with establishing a diagnosis by testing Paul's urine for the presence of
○ 1. blood.
○ 2. sucrose.
○ 3. ammonia.
○ 4. ketones.

12 Paul has now been diagnosed as having diabetes mellitus. The physician reviews Paul's records and decides to prescribe regular insulin. If breakfast is normally served at 8:00 AM, regular insulin is given at
○ 1. 6:00 AM.
○ 2. 7:30 AM.
○ 3. 8:00 AM.
○ 4. 9:00 AM.

13 When Paul receives his insulin, the nurse is assigned to check Paul for signs of hypoglycemia (hyperinsulinism). Which of the following indicate that Paul may be developing this problem?
○ 1. Polyuria and glucosuria
○ 2. Confusion and diaphoresis
○ 3. Muscle cramps and thirst
○ 4. Dehydration and weight loss

14 If Paul were to develop hypoglycemia (hyperinsulinism) and it is recognized immediately, the nurse should first
○ 1. have Paul drink orange juice to which sugar is added.
○ 2. administer 10% IV glucose.
○ 3. notify Paul's physician.
○ 4. administer a second dose of insulin.

15 Paul is scheduled to receive regular insulin and an intermediate-acting insulin. When consulting references the nurse understands that two types of insulin are being given to

- ○ 1. allow Paul more flexibility in his diet.
- ○ 2. allow Paul to eat his favorite foods.
- ○ 3. provide immediate and long-lasting insulin coverage.
- ○ 4. prevent episodes of hypoglycemia.

16 Mr. Meyers asks why Paul has to be given injections and if he cannot be treated with diet or pills. Before answering Mr. Meyers, the nurse should know that juvenile diabetics cannot be treated by diet alone; they require insulin, and "pills" can be used only in the treatment of

- ○ 1. non–insulin-dependent diabetes mellitus.
- ○ 2. adolescents older than 14 years of age with diabetes mellitus.
- ○ 3. children whose fasting blood glucose is no higher than 150 mg/dL.
- ○ 4. those who have reduced blood levels of glucagon.

17 The nurse is assigned to develop a teaching plan for Paul and his family. Included in the teaching plan is the fact that insulin sites are rotated to

- ○ 1. slow the absorption of insulin.
- ○ 2. prevent insulin from being deposited in subcutaneous tissues.
- ○ 3. decrease the duration of insulin.
- ○ 4. prevent lipodystrophy of subcutaneous fat.

18 In preparing a teaching plan the nurse schedules a discussion of events that could increase or decrease Paul's insulin requirements. Of the following events, the one that may cause Paul to require *less* than his usual amounts of insulin is when Paul

- ○ 1. eats too much food.
- ○ 2. increases his activity.
- ○ 3. develops an infection.
- ○ 4. undergoes emotional stress.

19 Ms. Meyers asks how the physician determines the amount and type of insulin for Paul. The *most correct* response is based on the fact that insulin requirements often are based on

- ○ 1. the type of food Paul likes.
- ○ 2. when Paul prefers to take his insulin.
- ○ 3. Paul's caloric intake.
- ○ 4. the cheapest brand of insulin.

20 Paul and his parents are to be taught the techniques of blood glucose self-monitoring. The nurse should demonstrate the procedure and instruct Paul and his parents to perform this test

- ○ 1. 30 minutes before eating.
- ○ 2. 15 minutes after eating.
- ○ 3. at least 8 times a day.
- ○ 4. whenever a hypoglycemic reaction occurs.

21 The nurse can evaluate the effectiveness of a part of the teaching that has been presented by

- ○ 1. asking Paul to discuss how insulin helps metabolize glucose.
- ○ 2. having Paul administer his own insulin or a family member administer insulin to Paul.
- ○ 3. giving a written test to Paul or a family member.
- ○ 4. asking Ms. Meyers to discuss how Paul's food will be prepared.

NURSING CARE OF A CHILD WITH SECOND- AND THIRD-DEGREE BURNS

Eight-year-old Tommy Adams was trapped in his bedroom during a fire. He is hospitalized for treatment of extensive second- and third-degree burns on his face, neck, anterior chest, and left arm.

22 Which of the following isolation techniques should the nurse plan to carry out for Tommy?

- ○ 1. Enteric isolation
- ○ 2. Protective isolation
- ○ 3. Respiratory isolation
- ○ 4. Drainage or secretion isolation

23 To develop a plan of care and be prepared for emergencies, the nurse must be sure that which of the following is kept in Tommy's room?

- ○ 1. A bed board and footboard
- ○ 2. A tracheostomy set and endotracheal tube
- ○ 3. Equipment to administer pain medications
- ○ 4. Extra pillows and sheets

24 Of particular importance during Tommy's early postburn care is for the nurse to closely monitor his

- ○ 1. unburned skin areas.
- ○ 2. intestinal elimination.
- ○ 3. intravenous fluid therapy.
- ○ 4. pupillary responses to light.

The physician orders hourly measurement of Tommy's urinary output.

25 Which one of the following must be *immediately* reported to the nurse in charge or the physician?

- ○ 1. 12 mL/h
- ○ 2. 25 mL/h
- ○ 3. 30 mL/h
- ○ 4. 34 mL/h

26 Intravenous meperidine hydrochloride (Demerol) is given to Tommy by the nurse in charge. The nurse should evaluate the result of the medication because the primary reason for the use of this drug is to

- ○ 1. promote sleep.
- ○ 2. reduce anxiety.
- ○ 3. prevent nausea.
- ○ 4. relieve discomfort.

27 During a patient care conference one nurse brings up the problem of footdrop in patients such as

Tommy. Which one of the following measures could the nurse suggest be used to prevent footdrop?

○ 1. Apply braces to Tommy's feet and ankles.
○ 2. Keep Tommy on his side.
○ 3. Have Tommy rest his feet against a firm pillow.
○ 4. Have Tommy rest his feet upright against a footboard.

28 Tommy is watched carefully for complications. When he has a black, tarry stool, the nurse reports this finding promptly because a stool of this nature may be a sign of

○ 1. a stress ulcer.
○ 2. postburn shock.
○ 3. an electrolyte imbalance.
○ 4. an increase in blood plasma volume.

Four weeks after his accident, a diet high in protein is ordered for Tommy.

29 Of the following between-meal snacks that are likely to appeal to Tommy, which two can be selected by the nurse because they have the highest protein content?

○ 1. Custard or a milk shake
○ 2. An apple or an orange
○ 3. Flavored gelatin or a bread and jelly sandwich
○ 4. Candy or peanuts

30 Tommy's condition improves, and the nurse plans diversional activities for him. The most appropriate activity for an 8-year-old is

○ 1. reading the newspaper.
○ 2. coloring simple designs.
○ 3. playing with his car collection.
○ 4. playing solitaire.

NURSING CARE OF A CHILD WITH JUVENILE RHEUMATOID ARTHRITIS

Karen Fischer is a 10-year-old who has juvenile rheumatoid arthritis. She is being seen in a clinic specializing in joint disorders in children.

31 The physician has prescribed aspirin for Karen. To explain the purpose of the drug to Karen's parents the nurse should know that aspirin is primarily used to

○ 1. reduce joint inflammation.
○ 2. prevent muscle spasms.
○ 3. reduce fever.
○ 4. increase the prothrombin time.

32 The nurse plans to discuss with Karen's parents the possible adverse effects that may occur during aspirin therapy, primarily symptoms of salicylism, which may occur with prolonged use of large doses of aspirin. Which of the following signs and symp-

toms of salicylism would the nurse include in this explanation?

○ 1. Constipation, weight gain, fluid retention
○ 2. Ringing in the ears, nausea, difficulty in hearing
○ 3. Anorexia, weight loss, double vision
○ 4. Headache, dry mouth, dental cavities

33 The physician has suggested that Karen should be encouraged to move and exercise as much as can be tolerated. Which of the following activities could the nurse suggest as an exercise for Karen?

○ 1. Skipping rope for 15 minutes three times a day
○ 2. Participating in sports such as softball
○ 3. Joining a gymnastic team
○ 4. Swimming

Karen is to be discharged because the acute phase of her disorder has subsided.

34 Which one of the following suggestions could the nurse give to Karen's parents?

○ 1. Provide Karen with a high calorie diet to help her gain weight.
○ 2. Use a soft mattress on Karen's bed.
○ 3. Avoid weight gain.
○ 4. Karen should be told to stay in bed most of the day.

35 After the acute phase of the rheumatoid arthritis subsides, the nurse can best help Karen from developing contractures by demonstrating the prescribed

○ 1. ways of applying temporary splints to her joints
○ 2. method of restraining her ankles during sleep.
○ 3. ways of massaging her lower leg muscles.
○ 4. method of putting her joints through range-of-motion exercises.

NURSING CARE OF A CHILD WITH A HEAD INJURY

Brian Carter, age 9 years, is brought to the emergency room. He fell off his bicycle and struck his head on the pavement. Following examination by a physician, he is admitted to the hospital for observation.

36 The nurse is assigned to observe Brian for any change in his neurologic status. Which one of the following is a sign of increased intracranial pressure?

○ 1. A rapid response of the pupils to light
○ 2. A decrease in body temperature
○ 3. A rise in blood pressure
○ 4. An increase in awareness of his surroundings

37 The nurse is asked to check Brian's level of consciousness. Which one of the following questions would be most appropriate for this evaluation?
  ○ 1. "What is your name?"
  ○ 2. "What is the number of this hospital room?"
  ○ 3. "What is the name of this hospital?"
  ○ 4. "What time is it?"

38 The nurse is asked to use the Glasgow Coma Scale to determine Brian's level of consciousness. Which one of the following is a correct interpretation of the Glasgow coma scale?
  ○ 1. A total of 15 indicates a serious change in the level of consciousness.
  ○ 2. The lower the number, the deeper the coma.
  ○ 3. The higher the number, the deeper the coma.
  ○ 4. A positive response to painful stimuli indicates damage to the brain stem.

NURSING CARE OF A CHILD WITH A BRAIN TUMOR

David Foster, 11 years old, has a brain tumor and is admitted to the hospital for treatment.

39 The physician orders the osmotic diuretic mannitol (Osmitrol) to relieve increased intracranial pressure due to cerebral edema. To develop a care plan the nurse should know that the this type of drug will cause
  ○ 1. an increase in urinary output.
  ○ 2. an increase in cerebrospinal fluid pressure.
  ○ 3. a decrease in the pulse rate.
  ○ 4. a decrease in urinary output.

40 David is scheduled to have chemotherapy. Which one of the following statements would best help David cope with the effects of chemotherapy? "The medicine the doctor will give you
  ○ 1. will not make you sick."
  ○ 2. may make you feel better, but you may feel sicker at first."
  ○ 3. will make you well so that you can go back to school in a few weeks."
  ○ 4. will not hurt."

41 David experiences severe nausea and vomiting following chemotherapy. The nurse places David on his side when he is sleeping to
  ○ 1. prevent aspiration of vomitus.
  ○ 2. decrease intracranial pressure.
  ○ 3. prevent cardiac and respiratory complications.
  ○ 4. prevent bedsores.

42 David requires nasogastric tube feedings. When administering a tube-feeding the nurse should know that
  ○ 1. this method of feeding is never administered to unconscious clients.

  ○ 2. the height of the container holding the liquid feeding affects the rate of instillation.
  ○ 3. the feeding formula is followed by 250 mL of water.
  ○ 4. the feeding formula is introduced over a period of 2 to 3 minutes.

David's parents express their feelings of helplessness and anxiety to the nurse after they learn of the child's poor prognosis.

43 Which of the following statements would be best to help David's parents deal with their despair?
  ○ 1. "Perhaps you would feel better if you visited David for shorter periods of time."
  ○ 2. "This is a difficult time for you. How do you think you will feel if David dies?"
  ○ 3. "What are some of the things you usually do for David that make him feel good?"
  ○ 4. "It's sad that you feel helpless. What do you usually do to take your mind off your worries?"

NURSING CARE OF A CHILD IN TRACTION

Bobby Meade, age 9 years, fractured the femur in his right leg while playing football with his friends. He is placed in 90–90 degree skeletal traction to reduce his fractured femur.

44 When developing a plan of care, a major consideration that should be included in a care plan is
  ○ 1. keeping Bobby off his back.
  ○ 2. avoiding any sudden movement of the bed or traction setup.
  ○ 3. performing range-of-motion exercises to both lower extremities.
  ○ 4. encouraging Bobby to sit up when he eats his meals.

45 The nurse plans to check Bobby frequently for evidence of skin breakdown, which is most likely to develop
  ○ 1. over the calf muscles.
  ○ 2. over bony prominences.
  ○ 3. on the knee.
  ○ 4. on the buttocks.

46 Which one of the following events noted by the nurse would be considered a problem that requires the attention of the physician or registered nurse?
  ○ 1. Bobby asks for food between meals.
  ○ 2. The foot of the bed is elevated on blocks.
  ○ 3. The weights of the traction are hanging freely.
  ○ 4. A traction rope is out of a pulley groove.

47 Which one of the following nursing tasks should the nurse include in Bobby's care plan?
  ○ 1. Encourage a high fluid intake.
  ○ 2. Help Bobby select a diet that is low in fiber.

○ 3. Encourage Bobby to exercise and move his right leg.

○ 4. Turn Bobby on his side every hour.

48 Which one of the following events noted by the nurse must be immediately reported to the nurse in charge?

○ 1. Bobby's fails to eat his lunch.

○ 2. Bobby persists in moving his left leg.

○ 3. A change in the color of the toes of the right leg.

○ 4. Bobby appears to be angry and upset.

49 The nurse notes that Bobby's parents are concerned about his discomfort and are attempting to try to make him comfortable. Which one of the following warnings should the nurse give Bobby's parents?

○ 1. "Do not remove or touch the weights attached to the ropes."

○ 2. "Do not give toys to Bobby because he may hurt himself."

○ 3. "It is best if you do not give Bobby anything to drink. This should be done by the nurse."

○ 4. "Leave Bobby alone. He will be more comfortable in a few days."

Nursing Care of Adolescents

NURSING CARE OF AN ADOLESCENT WITH DYSMENORRHEA

Molly Loring, 16 years old, is brought by her mother to the pediatric clinic because Molly is complaining of dysmenorrhea. The physician has determined that Molly has primary dysmenorrhea and recommends the use of aspirin or ibuprofen (Advil, Nuprin) for discomfort. He also asks the nurse to discuss with Molly some of the actions she could take to reduce the pain and discomfort she is experiencing.

50 Which one of the following actions could the nurse suggest to Molly?

○ 1. Stay in bed until cramping is relieved, increase your fluid intake, and eat a low-fat diet.

○ 2. Drink plenty of cold liquids, add extra salt to your diet, and take a nap in the afternoon.

○ 3. Apply ice packs to the abdomen, eat a high-calorie diet, and eat your largest meal at noon.

○ 4. Get proper sleep, eat a good diet, and apply heat to the abdomen.

51 Which of the following explanations regarding the use of aspirin should the nurse discuss with Ms. Loring?

○ 1. Once the bottle is opened, aspirin has a shelf life of 2 years.

○ 2. Diarrhea is a common adverse effect of aspirin.

○ 3. If aspirin does not help, take one or two ibuprofen (Advil) tablets along with the aspirin.

○ 4. If nausea occurs, the drug may be taken with food.

52 Molly says to the nurse, "One of my classmates says she is scared because she has amenorrhea. What does the word mean?" The nurse should explain that amenorrhea means

○ 1. absence of menstruation.

○ 2. excessive vaginal bleeding.

○ 3. discomfort prior to menstruation.

○ 4. discomfort midway between menstrual periods.

NURSING CARE OF AN ADOLESCENT WHO IS ABUSING DRUGS

Ms. Norell calls for a pediatric clinic appointment because she has discovered amphetamine capsules in the room of her 14-year-old son, Barry.

53 The nurse should recognize that Barry is most likely abusing amphetamines when Ms. Norell describes Barry as having

○ 1. watery eyes.

○ 2. drowsiness.

○ 3. excessive nasal discharge.

○ 4. marked nervousness.

54 To answer questions asked by Ms. Norell, the nurse reviews drug references for information on amphetamine abuse. Which one of the following statements regarding amphetamine abuse is *incorrect*?

○ 1. Amphetamine abuse may be associated with the abuse of other substances.

○ 2. Amphetamines have addiction potential.

○ 3. Amphetamines are central nervous system stimulants.

○ 4. Amphetamines do not have addiction potential.

55 Ms. Norell asks "What made Barry take amphetamines? Why is he always with a gang that is known to get into trouble and abuse drugs?" To answer Ms. Norell's questions the nurse should be aware that Barry is most likely trying to meet his needs by wanting to be with a group of his peers. This psychosocial need is termed

○ 1. self-identity.

○ 2. intimacy.

○ 3. integrity.

○ 4. idealism.

56 The nurse reviews Barry's immunization record while Barry is talking to the physician. Which one

of the following infectious diseases requires booster immunization every 10 years?
- ○ 1. Tetanus
- ○ 2. Small pox
- ○ 3. Whooping cough (pertussis)
- ○ 4. Rubella (German measles)

57 Ms. Norell asks if Barry should be forced to enter a drug treatment program. The best response the nurse can make to Ms. Norell's question is
- ○ 1. "Barry should first discuss the dangers of drug abuse with a parent."
- ○ 2. "It will be necessary to first obtain a court order to place Barry in a drug rehabilitation center."
- ○ 3. "The success of a drug rehabilitation program depends on the person's desire to become drug-free."
- ○ 4. "It is best if Barry is forced to enter a drug free program because he cannot think clearly at this time."

NURSING CARE OF AN ADOLESCENT WITH A SEXUALLY TRANSMITTED DISEASE

Sixteen-year-old Ann Mills has learned that she has been exposed to gonorrhea. She visits the clinic for diagnosis and treatment.

58 The nurse can best assist with a common diagnostic measure when Ann learns of her exposure to gonorrhea by
- ○ 1. collecting a blood specimen.
- ○ 2. testing the client's urine for the presence of pus.
- ○ 3. assisting with the collection of a specimen of the client's vaginal discharge.
- ○ 4. determining when the client had her last menstrual period.

59 The nurse also assists with testing Ann for *Chlamydia trachomatis,* a sexually transmitted disease that
- ○ 1. is found only in females with gonorrhea.
- ○ 2. may coexist with other sexually transmitted diseases, primarily gonorrhea.
- ○ 3. is primarily found in teenagers.
- ○ 4. rarely causes symptoms.

Ann is given intramuscular aqueous penicillin G procaine for the treatment of gonorrhea and a prescription for oral erythromycin for the treatment of chlamydia.

60 Which one of the following regarding erythromycin therapy should the nurse include in the instructions for given to Ann?
- ○ 1. Therapy can be discontinued once symptoms have disappeared.
- ○ 2. Take the drug with milk.

- ○ 3. The drug is taken once daily in the morning.
- ○ 4. Take the drug on an empty stomach 1 hour before or 2 hours after a meal.

61 Before leaving the clinic, Ann asks the nurse, "When can I be certain that I am no longer infectious?" The nurse should explain to Ann that she will be considered noninfectious when
- ○ 1. her vaginal discharge has stopped.
- ○ 2. her next menstrual period is free of discomfort.
- ○ 3. she has negative follow-up examinations after completing therapy.
- ○ 4. she has received drug therapy for at least 24 hours without untoward adverse effects.

Seventeen-year-old Heather Walker has herpes genitalis (herpes simplex virus type II).

62 The nurse assists the physician while Heather is examined. Which one of the following can be entered on the client's record and best describes the appearance of the initial lesions of genital herpes?
- ○ 1. Keloid formation
- ○ 2. Fissure
- ○ 3. Fever blister
- ○ 4. Ulcerated macule

63 Acyclovir (Zovirax) is prescribed for Heather. The nurse should emphasize the importance of long-term, follow-up care because recent research suggests that there may be an association between genital herpes and the eventual development of
- ○ 1. cervical cancer.
- ○ 2. uterine fibroids.
- ○ 3. chronic vaginitis.
- ○ 4. premature menopause.

64 Heather states that she is sexually active. Which one of the following recommendations should the nurse give to Heather?
- ○ 1. "It is essential that a diaphragm be worn to prevent infecting the male partner."
- ○ 2. "The male partner should use a condom at all times, especially when there is a recurrence of the lesions."
- ○ 3. "Douching before and after sexual intercourse prevents infecting the male partner."
- ○ 4. "Taking acyclovir when the lesions are active prevents infecting the male partner."

65 Heather asks if she could get acquired immunodeficiency syndrome (AIDS) even though she knows her sexual partner, and he has no symptoms. The best response to this question is
- ○ 1. "Symptoms of AIDS may appear months and even years after the original infection."
- ○ 2. "If your partner has no symptoms then you need not worry."

○ 3. "If I were you I'd stop being sexually active."
○ 4. "The spread of AIDS can now be controlled with antiviral drugs."

66 Heather asks "What are the symptoms of AIDS?" The most correct response should include
○ 1. increased appetite, night sweats, and double vision.
○ 2. tachycardia, dyspnea, and constipation.
○ 3. malaise, fever, and opportunistic infections.
○ 4. weight gain, peripheral edema, and jaundice.

NURSING CARE OF AN ADOLESCENT WITH SCOLIOSIS

Linda Kraft, age 14 years, has thoracic scoliosis. Although this was brought to their attention by a physician when she was younger, Linda's parents did not seek medical evaluation and treatment of her problem until this past month.

67 Ms. Kraft knows that Linda has problems with her back and asks the nurse what the physician meant when the term scoliosis was used. The nurse can tell Ms. Kraft that scoliosis is
○ 1. an exaggerated curvature of the lumbar spine.
○ 2. a lateral or sideways curvature of the spine.
○ 3. another term for humpback.
○ 4. a condition that results from an injury.

68 Ms. Kraft asks if treatment is really necessary. The nurse can reinforce the physician's recommendations by telling Ms. Kraft that untreated scoliosis may ultimately
○ 1. correct itself.
○ 2. affect bladder control.
○ 3. affect bowel control.
○ 4. affect heart and lung function.

69 Treatment for Linda will consist of a spinal fusion and insertion of a Harrington rod. Which one of the following should be included in Linda's preoperative preparation?
○ 1. Demonstrate coughing and deep breathing exercises.
○ 2. Show Linda a Harrington rod.
○ 3. Tell Linda she will have pain after surgery.
○ 4. Demonstrate how to adjust the brace that will be applied during surgery.

70 Linda is given a regular diet a few days after surgery. The nurse assistant reports that Linda is eating poorly. Which one of the following might the nurse plan to use in an effort to improve Linda's appetite?
○ 1. Allow Linda to select foods with the aid of the dietitian.
○ 2. Ask Linda's parents or friends to bring in food.

○ 3. Select foods that the caretakers believe Linda will like.
○ 4. Promise Linda a reward if she eats.

71 Linda complains of constipation. Which one of the following measures can the nurse use in an effort to correct this problem?
○ 1. Encourage Linda to participate in recreational activities.
○ 2. Provide a low-residue diet.
○ 3. Encourage frequent ambulation.
○ 4. Encourage a liberal fluid intake.

72 Before changing Linda's position or turning her from side to side or back to side the nurse should
○ 1. place a pillow between her thighs.
○ 2. raise the head of the bed.
○ 3. elevate the foot of the bed.
○ 4. place a pillow in the lumbar area.

INDIVIDUAL TEST ITEMS

73 Darryl is 5 months old and is brought to the clinic for treatment of a rash. The physician's diagnosis is miliaria rubra (prickly heat, heat rash). What suggestions may the nurse give to Darryl's mother?
○ 1. Expose affected areas to sunlight, and apply baby oil.
○ 2. Avoid overdressing in warm weather, and dust the affected area with fine cornstarch.
○ 3. Apply baby lotion and baby powder to the affected area.
○ 4. Apply a dressing to the affected areas, and avoid bathing until the rash disappears.

74 It is determined that Steven Cooper has pulmonary tuberculosis. Long-term therapy with isoniazid and para-aminosalicylic acid is prescribed. The nurse should explain to Steven's mother that two drugs in combination are used in his therapy to help prevent
○ 1. tolerance to drug therapy.
○ 2. allergic reactions to drug therapy.
○ 3. adverse systemic reactions to drug therapy.
○ 4. resistance of the causative organisms to drug therapy.

75 Kevin has acne vulgaris and tetracycline hydrochloride is prescribed by the physician. The nurse should teach Kevin that this drug
○ 1. is taken with food.
○ 2. is taken on an empty stomach.
○ 3. interferes with the absorption of vegetables and meat.
○ 4. is taken with an antacid.

76 Bryan Wilson is 14 years old. At birth he was diagnosed as having Down syndrome. Which of the fol-

lowing signs and symptoms may the nurse detect in a client with Down syndrome?
- ○ 1. Large head and curved index finger
- ○ 2. Long fingers and protruding tongue
- ○ 3. Small head and upward-slanting eyes
- ○ 4. Protruding eyes and simian crease on the soles of the feet

77 Melanie Stark is 14 years old and has had diabetes mellitus since 5 years of age. During a visit to the clinic the nurse in charge states that Melanie appears to show concern over her sexual identity and body image because of her diabetes. The nurse could suggest that Melanie
- ○ 1. talk to her parents about her problem.
- ○ 2. read more information about diabetes.
- ○ 3. attend lectures given by the diabetes association.
- ○ 4. join a support group and meet other adolescents with diabetes.

78 Peggy Wade has acute lymphocytic leukemia (ALL) and is in remission. The physician has decided to perform a bone marrow transplantation. When reinforcing the physician's explanation the nurse can tell Peggy's parents that the purpose of this procedure is to provide Peggy with
- ○ 1. a source of immunity to viral and bacterial infections.
- ○ 2. antibodies to destroy leukemia cells.
- ○ 3. healthy bone marrow that can manufacture normal blood cells.
- ○ 4. antileukemic bone marrow cells that will place Peggy in remission.

79 Donald Hayes is 16 years old and is involved in school sports. He asks the nurse for suggestions in relieving muscle cramps, which he experiences during football practice. The nurse can advise him to
- ○ 1. not warm up before an athletic activity.
- ○ 2. drink plenty of water during and after athletic activities.
- ○ 3. wear heavy clothing on the upper part of his body.
- ○ 4. not eat for 12 hours before an athletic activity.

80 Paul Chandler has cerebral palsy and wears braces on his legs. The nursing assistant asks the nurse why Paul needs braces. The nurse can explain that Paul's braces
- ○ 1. encourage him to use unaffected muscles.
- ○ 2. prevent footdrop and muscle spasticity.
- ○ 3. strengthen and support weakened muscles.
- ○ 4. prevent muscle atrophy in the upper extremities.

81 Danny Watson is a hemophiliac who acquired AIDS by means of a blood transfusion. He is eating poorly because of thrush and herpes simplex infections of the oral cavity. Which one of the following diets could the nurse suggest to his parents?
- ○ 1. High-caloric bland diet
- ○ 2. Soft, high-vitamin, low-protein diet
- ○ 3. Low-residue, low-fat diet
- ○ 4. High-residue, low-cholesterol diet

82 Peggy Layne has a new brother who has been diagnosed as having phenylketonuria (PKU). She asks the nurse for information on this disorder so she can help her mother care for her brother. The nurse can tell Peggy that people with PKU must eat a diet that is low in phenylalanine, an amino acid found in
- ○ 1. vegetables.
- ○ 2. natural protein foods.
- ○ 3. whole grains.
- ○ 4. fruits.

83 Glenn Walters, age 14 years, visits the clinic after having had the mumps. To correctly instruct Glenn on the need for further or additional immunizations, the nurse should know that having mumps gives
- ○ 1. a naturally acquired active immunity to mumps.
- ○ 2. a naturally acquired passive immunity to mumps.
- ○ 3. no antibodies against mumps.
- ○ 4. no immunity to mumps and needs to be immunized.

84 Mary Beth has Tay-Sachs disease. The nurse correctly plans that the parents will need help and emotional support because the organ damaged by this disease is the child's
- ○ 1. lungs.
- ○ 2. heart.
- ○ 3. brain.
- ○ 4. kidneys.

85 A child who has had a mild head injury may be seen in a hospital emergency department and discharged to the care of the parents. To be sure that intracranial bleeding has not occurred, the nurse should tell the parents that the child
- ○ 1. must be seen by another physician in 3 to 5 days.
- ○ 2. is not to be given food or fluids for the next 12 hours.
- ○ 3. is to kept awake the first night.
- ○ 4. should be awakened at least once during the first night.

86 Laurie Case comes to the clinic because of scalp ringworm (tinea capitis). Her mother asks "What causes ringworm?" The most correct answer is based on the fact that ringworm is caused by a
- ○ 1. virus.
- ○ 2. fungus.

○ 3. rickettsia.
○ 4. *Staphylococcus.*

87 Larry Baxter is diagnosed as having pinworms. His mother has many questions about this problem. To answer questions correctly the nurse should know that pinworms are most often spread by children who
○ 1. share their bed with a pet.
○ 2. play in contaminated water.
○ 3. tend to eat nonfood substances.
○ 4. are careless about toilet hygiene.

88 A nurse is assigned to discuss communicable diseases with mothers bringing their children to a clinic. To develop an effective teaching plan the nurse should know that a common problem is the tendency of many people to
○ 1. think that communicable diseases are not preventable.
○ 2. believe that communicable diseases are never serious.
○ 3. neglect having their children immunized.
○ 4. refuse antibiotics for communicable diseases because of possible allergic reactions.

89 Ms. Grey states that her 6-year-old son occasionally develops hiccups and asks what she can do to stop them. The nurse can suggest Ms. Grey have him
○ 1. rebreathe in and out of a paper bag.
○ 2. chew gum.
○ 3. eat dry crackers.
○ 4. drink a carbonated beverage.

90 The nurse is assigned to give morning care to Jimmy Collins, age 2 years. When lowering the sides of the crib the nurse should
○ 1. restrain Jimmy with straps.
○ 2. keep a hand securely on Jimmy while the crib sides are lowered.
○ 3. ask another nurse to hold Jimmy when he is being bathed.
○ 4. give Jimmy a toy so he won't try to get out of his crib.

91 Kyle Thomas, age 4 months, is to be given an oral medication in the form of a liquid suspension. Which of the following is *incorrect* for the administration of a liquid drug to a 4-month-old infant?
○ 1. Add the medication to the formula.
○ 2. Use a rubber-tipped medicine dropper.
○ 3. Use a small medicine cup.
○ 4. Place the suspension in a nipple fitted with a standard ring from a ring-and-disk type baby bottle.

92 Jackie Strong has hemophilia. A teaching program for his parents should include explaining that they must avoid giving Jackie medications containing

○ 1. aspirin.
○ 2. caffeine.
○ 3. barbiturates.
○ 4. antacids.

93 Which one of the following restraints should the nurse plan to use for a child who has had a cleft lip repair?
○ 1. Papoose board
○ 2. Leg restraints
○ 3. Elbow restraints
○ 4. Posey belt or jacket

94 The nurse should plan to remove and reapply restraints
○ 1. daily.
○ 2. every 8 hours.
○ 3. every 4 hours.
○ 4. every 2 hours.

95 The nurse is assigned to observe Jeffrey Dowd for signs of hypokalemia. Which of the following are signs and symptoms of this electrolyte imbalance?
○ 1. Full bounding pulse, dyspnea, and thirst
○ 2. Weak irregular pulse, muscle weakness, and vomiting
○ 3. Hypertension, tetany, and nausea
○ 4. Constipation, clammy skin, and coma

96 Bob Stone requires parenteral nutrition, which is supplied by a multipurpose Hickman catheter. When assigned to give morning care to Bob, the nurse should check the catheter insertion site, which is normally located at the site of the
○ 1. carotid artery.
○ 2. jugular vein.
○ 3. femoral artery.
○ 4. brachial vein.

97 The nurse is assigned to assist the physician in performing a lumbar puncture. In which one of the following positions will the nurse place the child?
○ 1. Prone
○ 2. Lateral decubitus
○ 3. Supine
○ 4. Sims'

98 The nurse is assigned to discuss cerebral palsy with parents. Which one of the following statements is *correct*?
○ 1. Cerebral palsy is not a progressive disease.
○ 2. Brain surgery often can help or cure those with cerebral palsy.
○ 3. Physical therapy is of little value for those with this disorder.
○ 4. Injury to sensory areas of the brain causes cerebral palsy.

99 Sixteen-month-old Mary Gordon is being observed and treated for ricketts at a pediatric clinic. When reviewing the dietary habits of the family, the nurse

should know that the vitamin that has been lacking or deficient in Mary's diet is vitamin

○ 1. A.
○ 2. B$_{12}$.
○ 3. C.
○ 4. D.

100 Beth Jordan, age 4 years, has possible iron-deficiency anemia and is scheduled for laboratory tests. Which of the following signs and symptoms of anemia might the nurse observe when preparing Beth for laboratory studies?

○ 1. Weight gain, hypertension, and tetany
○ 2. Edema of the extremities, nervousness, and diarrhea
○ 3. Constipation, nausea, and vomiting
○ 4. Pallor, listlessness, and irritability

101 The physician examining Martha Hale, age 3 years, enters a diagnosis of oral moniliasis on her record. When explaining the prescribed treatment to Ms. Hale the nurse can use the more common name for this disorder, which is

○ 1. threadworm.
○ 2. thrush.
○ 3. Hirschsprung's disease.
○ 4. colic.

102 Bobby Michaels has pinworm, and the physician prescribes mebendazole (Vermox). Which one of the following should be included in the nurse's explanation of the treatment regimen?

○ 1. Bobby must wash his hands thoroughly after using the toilet.
○ 2. Bobby must be isolated from other family members for 7 days.
○ 3. Asymptomatic family members need not be examined or treated.
○ 4. Drug treatment will be necessary for 14 days.

103 Cathy Weaver, age 16 years, has been diagnosed as having nephrotic syndrome and is admitted to the hospital. Which one of the following obtained during an initial physical assessment would indicate Cathy has hypertension?

○ 1. A systolic pressure of 128 mm Hg
○ 2. A diastolic pressure of 94 mm Hg
○ 3. A pulse deficit of 6 per minute
○ 4. An irregular pulse

104 Francis Bartlett, age 12 years, sprained her ankle. Her mother asks the nurse if there is any danger in applying an ice bag to her ankle. The most correct reply is

○ 1. "ice can be applied and left on until the swelling is gone."
○ 2. "ice can be applied but must be removed every 30 to 45 minutes to observe the skin."
○ 3. "ice should not be used in treating sprains."

○ 4. "there is no danger associated with the application of an ice bag."

105 Kevin Wall has Duchenne's muscular dystrophy. His parents have had a difficult time accepting the diagnosis. Recognizing this the nurse could

○ 1. recommend Kevin be placed in a long-term health care agency.
○ 2. refer them to a social welfare agency.
○ 3. put them in contact with parents of children with muscular dystrophy.
○ 4. give them literature to read about the disorder.

106 Which one of the following is a main goal when caring for a child with a heart defect?

○ 1. Reducing the workload of the heart
○ 2. Finding ways to amuse the child
○ 3. Giving morning care as early as possible
○ 4. Allowing the parents to bring toys to the hospitalized child

107 Which one of the following 3- to 6-year-old children seen in an emergency department is *most likely* a victim of child abuse?

○ 1. Kenny, who has a small first-degree burn on the back of his hand
○ 2. Mark, who has several small bruises and appears frightened, turns his head away, and avoids his parents
○ 3. Millie, who has a sprained ankle
○ 4. Patty, who is crying and has a bump on her head

108 Which one of the following statements made by a parent might indicate their son or daughter may be abusing drugs?

○ 1. "Clayton's grades have dropped. He has gone from a 92 to a 90."
○ 2. "Tiffany seems to avoid some of her friends."
○ 3. "Barbara argues with her sisters."
○ 4. "Carl seems to be acting different, and his personality has changed."

109 Which one of the following suggestions to prevent accidents could the nurse give to the parents of a toddler?

○ 1. Never leave the child unattended on a sofa.
○ 2. Point out the importance of having fun without getting hurt.
○ 3. Use gates on stairways.
○ 4. Point out the importance of safe play.

110 Mary Willis, age 2 years, has been diagnosed as having a Wilms' tumor. Which one of the following nursing tasks must be *avoided* when giving care to Mary?

○ 1. Giving Mary a book to read
○ 2. Feeding Mary
○ 3. Combing Mary's hair
○ 4. Palpating Mary's abdomen

111 A nurse working at a children's summer camp receives a notice from the camp physician that a child has impetigo. Which one of the following measures should be instituted for this child?

○ 1. The child can play with others.

○ 2. Contact with other children should be avoided.

○ 3. Medication is not necessary because the infection is self-limiting.

○ 4. Continuous wet soaks will be necessary.

Correct Answers and Rationale

Two numbers appear in parentheses following each rationale. The first number identifies the textbook listed in the references, page 451, and the second number identifies the page(s) in that textbook on which the correct answer can be verified. Occasionally, two textbooks are given for verifying the correct answer.

Nursing Care of School-Aged Children

NURSING CARE OF A CHILD WITH APPENDICITIS

1 3. A frequently seen position of the child with appendicitis is lying on the side with the knees flexed. This position appears to reduce the pain of appendicitis. A poor appetite may indicate only an illness and is not specific for appendicitis. The remaining items in this question are normal activities of a child of this age. (19:705)
Nursing Process—Collecting data
Client Need—Physiological integrity

2 2. If a total of 200 mL is to be given over 8 hours, the amount to be given (200 mL) is divided by the total number of hours (8). 200 mL divided by 8 hours is 25 mL per hour. (18:658)
Nursing Process—Implementation
Client Need—Safe, effective care environment

3 4. Coughing and deep breathing help aerate the lungs and prevent postoperative complications, such as pneumonia. For this type of surgery the child usually is urged to get out of bed 12 to 24 hours after surgery. Postural drainage is not indicated for this type of surgery. (19:706)
Nursing Process—Implementation
Client Need—Safe, effective care environment

4 4. A reluctance to move about in bed could be a sign of infection or other postoperative complication. Although incisional pain is present, children often become active shortly after surgery and usually recover more quickly than an adult. Nausea may be of some concern, but vomiting, which could be a concern, has not occurred. The nausea may be due to normal factors, such as anxiety, separation from the parents, and the anesthetic. Pain in the incision 24 to 48 hours after surgery is normal. In a child of this age anxiety and crying would not be considered unusual during the immediate postoperative period unless other signs and symptoms were present. A slight elevation in the temperature

and respiratory rate is not abnormal after surgery. (19:706)
Nursing Process—Implementation
Client Need—Physiological integrity

NURSING CARE OF A CHILD WITH RHEUMATIC FEVER

5 2. The exact cause of rheumatic fever is not clearly understood. There is evidence that rheumatic fever may be seen in those with a recent bacterial infection caused by group A beta-hemolytic streptococci. Although not all sore throats are caused by this microorganism, some are, and therefore this is brought to the physician's attention. Measles is caused by a virus. A bump on the head and a disinterest in school work probably are not related to a diagnosis of rheumatic fever but should be recorded in the health history. (8:737)
Nursing Process—Collecting data
Client need—Safe, effective care environment

6 2. Migrating joint tenderness and aching in the lower extremities suggest signs of rheumatic fever. Hot, swollen, tender, and enlarged joints, fever, and fatigue may be seen in the acute stage of this disorder. (8:737)
Nursing Process—Collecting data
Client Need—Safe, effective care environment

7 1. Rheumatic fever may affect the heart (rheumatic carditis). During the acute phase of the illness it is important to reduce the workload of the heart by promoting complete bed rest. Limiting the fluid intake and ambulation usually are not included in a plan of care for a child with rheumatic fever. (8:739)
Nursing Process—Planning
Client Need—Physiological integrity

8 1. The probable causative microorganism is the *Streptococcus*. Penicillin is given to eliminate any remaining streptococcal microorganisms and to prevent reinfection. Penicillin does not

decrease joint size, prevent joint deformities, decrease pain, or prevent renal damage. (8:739)
Nursing Process—Implementation
Client Need—Safe, effective care environment

9 3. Aspirin is an analgesic, antipyretic, and antiinflammatory drug and therefore reduces pain, fever, and joint inflammation and tenderness. Aspirin has no effect on the body's immune system nor can it prevent cardiac enlargement or prevent an infection. (8:739)
Nursing Process—Implementation
Client Need—Safe, effective care environment

10 3. Oral or intramuscular long-acting penicillin therapy normally is prescribed for these clients. Parents should be made aware of the importance of preventing recurring streptococcal infections by means of constant penicillin blood levels. Failure to follow the physician's recommendations regarding penicillin therapy may result in a recurrence of the disorder and consequent damage to the valves of the heart. (8:739)
Nursing Process—Implementation
Client Need—Safe, effective care environment

NURSING CARE OF A CHILD WITH DIABETES MELLITUS

11 4. Urine specimens often are tested when establishing a diagnosis of diabetes mellitus. If the client is in a diabetic coma, glucose and ketones would be expected to be present in the urine. The body turns to fats and proteins as a source of energy in diabetes (sugar has been lost as a source of energy). These nutrients break down into ketones; when too many are present, acidosis will follow. This is called ketoacidosis. Other diagnostic tools include fasting blood glucose, postprandial blood glucose, glycosylated hemoglobin test, and the glucose tolerance test. The physician also may order testing of blood glucose using the capillary blood glucose method (glucometer). Sucrose (table sugar) would not be found in the blood or urine. Ammonia and blood in the urine are not characteristic findings of diabetes mellitus. (8:755)
Nursing Process—Implementation
Client need—Physiological integrity

12 2. Regular insulin is given ½ hour before a meal because the onset of this type of insulin is ½ to 1 hour. (15:139)
Nursing Process—Implementation
Client need—Physiological integrity

13 2. Confusion and diaphoresis are two of the most common signs and symptoms of hypoglycemia.

The remaining items in this question are signs and symptoms of hyperglycemia. (15:140)
Nursing Process—Collecting data
Client need—Physiological integrity

14 1. Hypoglycemia must be corrected immediately. If Paul is awake and *able to swallow*, he can be offered orange juice with sugar or dilute corn syrup added, or a lump of sugar that he can allow to dissolve in his mouth. Intravenous administration of glucose is reserved for those who have had a change in their level of consciousness and are unable to swallow. Insulin would not be given because Paul already has too much insulin (hyperinsulinism). The physician is contacted as soon as possible but *after* the problem is corrected. Some hospitals have a standard procedure to follow when a client receiving insulin develops hyperinsulinism (hypoglycemia). (15:142)
Nursing Process—Implementation
Client need—Physiological integrity

15 3. Once Paul has been stabilized it is most likely that the physician will order regular insulin plus an intermediate- or long-acting insulin. Future treatment of Paul may include only an intermediate- or long-acting insulin, or the physician may determine that regular insulin also may be required. The physician may advise blood glucose self-monitoring once Paul is home. Depending on circumstances, such as Paul's age and physical activity, the physician may advise the use of regular insulin, the dose and administration of which is based on the results of blood glucose levels. (15:139)
Nursing Process—Implementation
Client Need—Safe, effective care environment

16 1. Oral hypoglycemic agents, such as tolazamide (Tolinase) and glyburide (Micronase), stimulate the pancreas to produce insulin. For these agents to benefit the person, the pancreas must be able to produce some insulin. Those with insulin-dependent diabetes (once called juvenile diabetes) require insulin because their pancreas is unable to produce insulin. An oral hypoglycemic agent will be of no value for these people. Reduced blood levels of glucagon are seen in those with pancreatic disease or surgical removal of the pancreas. An adolescent older than 14 years most likely will require insulin. Fasting blood glucose levels are not used to determine if a child with diabetes mellitus should be treated with insulin or an oral hypoglycemic agent. A child developing diabetes almost always requires insulin. (15:145)
Nursing Process—Implementation
Client need—Health promotion/maintenance

17 4. If insulin sites are not rotated by use of a planned rotation schedule atrophy (lipodystrophy) of subcutaneous fat may occur. Lipodystrophy can interfere with the absorption of insulin if insulin is given in areas affected by this problem. (15:142)
  Nursing Process—Implementation
  Client Need—Health promotion/maintenance

18 2. Activity requires glucose for energy. Therefore, increasing activity uses up glucose, and the body then requires less-than-usual amounts of insulin. Eating too much, having an infection, and experiencing emotional stress are situations in which the client tends to require more, not less, insulin. (8:757)
  Nursing Process—Planning
  Client need—Physiological integrity

19 3. The amount and type of insulin is based on the caloric needs of a child of Paul's age. The daily caloric intake is determined and should supply sufficient calories to meet the needs of exercise, growth, and appetite of a child of this age. (8:757)
  Nursing Process—Implementation
  Client Need—Health promotion/maintenance

20 1. Unless the physician orders otherwise, the testing of blood glucose levels is performed at least twice daily. The test is performed 30 minutes before a meal. (8:761)
  Nursing Process—Implementation
  Client Need—Physiological integrity

21 2. Evaluation of a diabetic teaching program can be made by observing the administration of insulin by the client or a family member. Paul is most likely too young to understand or discuss the action of insulin in the body. It is more important to have Ms. Meyers discuss the various parts of Paul's special diet rather than how food is prepared. A written test is not appropriate. (15:144)
  Nursing Process—Evaluation
  Client Need—Physiological integrity

NURSING CARE OF A CHILD WITH SECOND- AND THIRD-DEGREE BURNS

22 2. Protective (reverse) isolation techniques are used when caring for a child with severe burns because the child is highly susceptible to infection. This type of isolation is used to help prevent a highly susceptible person, in this case a severely burned person, from acquiring an infection. A gown, a mask, and a cap are worn by staff and visitors when in the room of a client on protective isolation. The other types of isolation mentioned in this question have as their primary goal preventing a client's microorganisms from being spread to others. (19:768)
  Nursing Process—Planning
  Client Need—Safe, effective care environment

23 2. It is important for the nurse to know that respiratory distress from a blocked airway may occur following burns to the head, face, neck, and chest. A tracheostomy set and a endotracheal tube should be kept in the client's room. An oral airway also should be readily available. In this situation the other devices and equipment stated in the options would not be considered appropriate for treating an emergency, especially an emergency arising from respiratory distress. (8:603; 19:765)
  Nursing Process—Planning
  Client need—Physiological integrity

24 3. A burn victim requires very careful monitoring of intravenous therapy and an *accurate* record of all intake and output. Burn victims are subject to shock early in their care as a result of excess fluid loss. To help prevent shock, strict monitoring is required. This monitoring is among the nurse's most important responsibilities when helping with the care of a burn victim. (19:765)
  Nursing Process—Implementation
  Client Need—Physiological integrity

25 1. An average of 20 to 30 mL/h usually is considered adequate for a child older than 2 years; 12 mL would be considered dangerously low and might indicate the start of acute renal failure. (19:765)
  Nursing Process—Collecting data
  Client Need—Physiological integrity

26 4. There often is considerable pain associated with severe burns, and a narcotic is used. Either meperidine hydrochloride (Demerol) or morphine sulfate may be prescribed. Other analgesics also may be used. Meperidine may promote sleep or reduce anxiety, but this is not the *primary* reason for giving the drug. Meperidine does not prevent nausea; instead, nausea is one of the adverse effects of this drug. (19:774)
  Nursing Process—Evaluation
  Client Need—Physiological integrity

27 4. A footboard is a nursing measure that may be used to prevent footdrop. Braces cannot be used without a physician's order. Keeping Tommy on his side would not prevent footdrop because this problem can be prevented only when the feet are supported in a normal position. Having Tommy rest his feet against a firm pillow is satisfactory on a temporary basis, but this measure should not be used for long periods because sup-

port to the feet usually is not sufficiently adequate to prevent footdrop. (19:774)
Nursing Process—Implementation
Client Need—Physiological integrity

28 1. Stress ulcers, often called Curling's ulcers, frequently occur in the stomach or duodenum as a complication of burns. Symptoms resemble those of a peptic ulcer, but they may be vague. If the ulcer bleeds, the stools become black and tarry and have a foul odor. Postburn shock occurs early when body fluids fill burn areas; this phenomenon leads to marked dehydration and shock. Electrolyte imbalances are more common early after a burn but will normally not produce changes in the client's stools. After the initial phase, when dehydration and shock are likely to occur, the client typically experiences a phase in which fluid imbalance occurs with diuresis (excessive urinary output) or with hypervolemia (increase in normal blood volume). Hypervolemia may become sufficiently severe to cause pulmonary edema. (19:766; 8:604; 607)
Nursing Process—Collecting data
Client Need—Physiological integrity

29 1. Custard or a milk shake have high protein content. A diet rich in protein is essential for the body to rebuild tissue destroyed by burns. Apples, oranges, bread and jelly, and candy contain little or no protein. Gelatin is not a significant source of protein. (19:773–774; 20:44)
Nursing Process—Implementation
Client Need—Physiological integrity

30 3. Of the diversional activities described in this item, a child of 8 years is likely to enjoy playing with his car collection. Television also may provide diversion. Playing a solitary game of cards, reading the newspaper, or coloring simple designs would probably not appeal to a boy of this age. (19:775)
Nursing Process—Planning
Client Need—Safe, effective care environment

NURSING CARE OF A CHILD WITH JUVENILE RHEUMATOID ARTHRITIS

31 1. The primary reason for using aspirin in the treatment of juvenile rheumatoid arthritis is this drug's ability to reduce inflammation. Although aspirin does lower the body temperature, this is not the foremost reason for using this drug. Muscle spasms are not prevented by the administration of aspirin. Although aspirin does increase the prothrombin time, increasing the prothrom-

bin time is not a part of treatment for this disorder. (8:652; 19:600)
Nursing Process—Implementation
Client Need—Health promotion/maintenance

32 2. Salicylism is a condition that occurs when larger than normal doses of aspirin are taken daily. Symptoms of mild salicylism include tinnitus (ringing in the ears), nausea, vomiting, difficulty in hearing, lassitude, dizziness, diarrhea, and mental confusion. (15:71)
Nursing Process—Implementation
Client Need—Health promotion/maintenance

33 4. Of the four items in this question, swimming would most likely be the safest form of exercise. When exercise is recommended by the physician it is most important that this activity be of the type that would cause the least trauma to the affected joints. (19:601)
Nursing Process—Implementation
Client need—Health promotion/maintenance

34 3. Weight gain is to be avoided because extra weight places additional stress on the joints. A firm bed mattress helps prevent joint deformities. A continuous, planned exercise program provides exercise for the joints and may help prevent joint deformity. The child would not be required to stay in bed most of the day once the acute phase has subsided. (19:601; 8:652)
Nursing Process—Implementation
Client Need—Safe, effective care environment

35 4. After the acute phase subsides, a child with rheumatoid arthritis should resume activity gradually. Range-of-motion exercises should be performed with each joint to prevent disuse syndrome. Immobilization of the affected joint(s) by splinting or restraining may produce contractures. Massaging the lower leg muscles to prevent contractures is not as effective as range-of-motion exercises. (19:601)
Nursing Process—Implementation
Client Need—Safe, effective care environment

NURSING CARE OF A CHILD WITH A HEAD INJURY

36 3. The classic signs of increased intracranial pressure are a change in the level of consciousness, a rise in blood pressure, an increase in body temperature, a decrease in the pulse rate, and a widening of the pulse pressure. (19:602; 16:407–408)
Nursing Process—Collecting data
Client Need—Physiological integrity

37 1. Asking the client's name is the most appropriate question for a child of this age. Because the child

has had a head injury and may have lost consciousness, he might not know what hospital he is in, the time of day, or his room number. (19:603)

Nursing Process—Implementation
Client Need—Physiological integrity

38   2.   The Glasgow Coma Sale is divided into three parts: an evaluation of eye-opening ability, verbal response, and motor response. When the nurse uses the Glasgow Coma Scale any change is reported immediately. A normal (perfect) total is 15. The lower the number, the deeper the coma. (19:603)

Nursing Process—Implementation
Client Need—Physiological integrity

NURSING CARE OF A CHILD WITH A BRAIN TUMOR

39   1.   An osmotic diuretic, such as mannitol (Osmitrol), may be used to relieve increased intracranial pressure. Administration will result in an increase in urinary output. The increased excretion of urine helps dehydrate tissues in the body, including those in the brain. Osmotic diuretics do not increase spinal fluid pressure or decrease the pulse rate. (15:125)

Nursing Process—Planning
Client Need—Safe, effective care environment

40   2.   Children should be told the truth. Explaining to the child that he may be sick at first but that he may feel better later is the most honest answer. (19:571–572)

Nursing Process—Implementation
Client Need—Psychosocial integrity

41   1.   The primary reason for placing David on his side is to prevent the aspiration of vomitus. Placing David in this position will not decrease intracranial pressure or prevent cardiac or respiratory problems. Unless David is completely inactive, his daytime activity in or out of bed would prevent bedsores. (19:571)

Nursing Process—Implementation
Client Need—Safe, effective care environment

42   2.   The higher the container (Asepto syringe, syringe, or other type of container) is held, the faster the feeding formula enters the stomach. Tube feedings can be given to unconscious clients. Tube feedings are best given over a period of approximately 30 minutes. The nasogastric tube is flushed with approximately 30 mL of water after the formula has been administered. (18:141, 145)

Nursing Process—Implementation
Client Need—Physiological integrity

43   3.   The goal in helping parents through the stage of despair is to involve them in their dying child's care so that they can see their continuing importance to the child. The nurse is correct in exploring what the parents usually did for their child that made him feel good. The nurse can point out the importance of the child's relationship with his parents and suggest ways they can continue to bring him comfort. (18:763)

Nursing Process—Implementation
Client Need—Psychosocial integrity

NURSING CARE OF A CHILD IN TRACTION

44   2.   It is most important that any movement of the bed or traction setup is avoided because proper alignment of the fractured bone is of primary concern. Movement may result in a displacement of the two bone ends at the fracture site. The client must lay in a supine position for this type of traction. Range-of-motion exercises cannot be performed on the right leg, which is the site of the fracture. The physician will describe the amount of movement allowed. (8:556–557)

Nursing Process—Planning
Client Need—Safe, effective care environment

45   2.   Pressure areas and skin breakdown are most likely to first develop over bony prominences, such as the heels, elbows, sacrum, ankles, and scapulae. (8:556)

Nursing Process—Planning
Client Need—Physiological integrity

46   4.   A traction rope that has slipped out of a pulley groove requires placing the rope in the pulley groove. This should be performed by the physician or the registered nurse skilled in orthopedic care. Asking for food between meals, elevation of the foot of the bed, and traction weights that hang freely are normal events. (8:555; 19:590)

Nursing Process—Evaluation
Client Need—Physiological integrity

47   1.   A high fluid intake and a diet high in fiber are recommended to prevent constipation and other complications of immobilization, such as kidney stones. The right leg, which is in traction, is kept immobile. Turning is not done unless the physician allows this maneuver. (19:591)

Nursing Process—Planning
Client Need—Physiological integrity

48   3.   Cyanosis or blanching of the toes of the leg in traction might indicate a circulatory problem in the client's leg and therefore must be reported immediately. Failure to eat lunch and being angry or upset may require nursing intervention,

but these are not emergencies. Moving the un-affected leg is encouraged. (19:591)
>   Nursing Process—Collecting data
>   Client Need—Physiological integrity

49 1. Overzealous and concerned parents may attempt to adjust devices that they feel may be making their child uncomfortable. They should be warned, in a polite and understanding manner, not to touch any part of the traction apparatus. Bringing toys or games or offering fluids usually is allowed. Leaving Bobby alone or ignoring his complaints could make him feel rejected. (19:590)
>   Nursing Process—Implementation
>   Client Need—Safe, effective care environment

Nursing Care of Adolescents

NURSING CARE OF AN ADOLESCENT WITH DYSMENORRHEA

50 4. Proper sleep, a well-balanced diet, warm tub baths or the application of heat to the abdomen, drinking warm liquids, and moderate exercise are some of the recommendations that can be made by the nurse. The other items mentioned are not known to relieve menstrual cramps or pain. (19:739)
>   Nursing Process—Implementation
>   Client Need—Health promotion/maintenance

51 4. If gastrointestinal distress occurs, aspirin may be taken with food or milk. If gastrointestinal distress persists, the physician should be contacted. Once an aspirin bottle has been opened, it has a short shelf life. Diarrhea is not a common adverse effect of aspirin taken in normal doses. Aspirin should not be taken along with a nonsteroidal antiinflammatory agent such as ibuprofen. (15:74)
>   Nursing Process—Implementation
>   Client Need—Health promotion/maintenance

52 1. Amenorrhea means the absence of menstruation. The classmate described in this item may be frightened of pregnancy because amenorrhea is a presumptive sign of pregnancy. Excessive vaginal bleeding is called menorrhagia. Discomfort between menstrual periods is called mittelschmerz. Discomfort prior to menstruation is related to premenstrual tension. (8:31)
>   Nursing Process—Implementation
>   Client Need—Physiological integrity

NURSING CARE OF AN ADOLESCENT WHO IS ABUSING DRUGS

53 4. Symptoms of amphetamine abuse include marked nervousness, restlessness, excitability, talkativeness, and excessive perspiration. The remaining items in this question are not characteristic of amphetamine abuse. (8:406; 15:84)
>   Nursing Process—Collecting data
>   Client Need—Psychosocial integrity

54 4. Amphetamines, which are central nervous system stimulants, are potentially addicting. Whether addiction will occur depends on many factors, such as whether the drug is used for a prolonged period of time or used in high doses. Those abusing amphetamines also may be involved with the abuse of other drugs. (15:84)
>   Nursing Process—Implementation
>   Client Need—Safe, effective care environment

55 1. Adolescents normally try to develop self-identity. It is believed that one way the adolescent gains self-identity is through peer relationships. The search for intimate relationships occurs during the years between 18 and 40. Integrity is a need most often demonstrated by adults rather than adolescents. Idealism is the pursuit of one's ideas or attempting to achieve an idea and is most likely not related to amphetamine abuse. (1:33)
>   Nursing Process—Implementation
>   Client Need—Psychosocial integrity

56 1. Booster doses of tetanus toxoid are recommended every 10 years. Smallpox vaccination is no longer advised because it is believed that the disease has been essentially eradicated. There are vaccines to protect children from rubella and whooping cough, but ordinarily they are given earlier in life. Boosters are not usually recommended during adolescence. If this client were a female, rubella protection is not indicated, because if the girl is pregnant or becomes pregnant shortly after receiving the vaccine, she may deliver a malformed infant. If rubella protection is advised for an adolescent girl, she must be instructed *not* to become pregnant for at least 2 months after receiving the vaccine. (15:304–305)
>   Nursing Process—Collecting data
>   Client Need—Health promotion/maintenance

57 3. The successful treatment of substance abuse largely depends on the person's desire to become drug free. When forced to enter a drug rehabilitation program, there is less chance that the person will remain drug free. Normally, a court order is not necessary for participation in

a drug abuse program. Discussing the dangers of drug abuse with a parent is not likely to change Barry's pattern of substance abuse. (15:85–86)
Nursing Process—Implementation
Client Need—Psychosocial integrity

NURSING CARE OF AN ADOLESCENT WITH A SEXUALLY TRANSMITTED DISEASE

58 3. A diagnosis of gonorrhea is confirmed when the microorganism is found in the client's vaginal discharge. Diagnosis can be accomplished by microscopic examination of a smear of the vaginal discharge. Cultures of the discharge also may be taken. Blood and urine examinations and determining when the client last menstruated are not used to confirm a diagnosis of gonorrhea. (19:745)
Nursing Process—Implementation
Client Need—Safe, effective care environment

59 2. Chlamydia infection often is seen in those with other sexually transmitted diseases, primarily gonorrhea, and is considered to be one of the most common in the United States. It is found in men and women of all ages. Although some people may be asymptomatic, others experience symptoms. In the male, urethritis and epididymitis may be seen. In the female, a mucopurulent vaginal discharge may be seen. (16:85; 8:174)
Nursing Process—Implementation
Client Need—Safe, effective care environment

60 4. Erythromycin is taken on an empty stomach. These instructions normally are printed on the prescription label but should be reinforced during client teaching. The drug is normally taken four times per day or every 6 hours. The nurse should emphasize the importance of not stopping the medication even though symptoms are relieved. (15:165)
Nursing Process—Implementation
Client Need—Health promotion/maintenance

61 3. One or preferably two follow-up smears or cultures should be taken after completing therapy on people who have gonorrhea. If the cultures and smears are negative, the person is considered noninfectious. It is unsafe to assume that a client is no longer infectious when a vaginal discharge ceases, when menstrual periods are normal, or when drug therapy is free of adverse effects. (3:782–783)
Nursing Process—Implementation
Client Need—Health promotion/maintenance

62 3. The initial lesion of genital herpes (herpesvirus type II) most nearly resembles a fever blister. It

may become a pustule and then, in time, may become a crusted area. Healing of the initial lesion often occurs, but the condition typically recurs. The other terms in this question do not accurately describe herpes genitalis lesions. (8:174–175)
Nursing Process—Collecting data
Client Need—Physiological integrity

63 1. At the present time, evidence suggests that there is an association between genital herpes and the eventual development of cervical cancer. Because of these findings, it is recommended that women with the disease be urged to continue with long-term, follow-up care. (8:175)
Nursing Process—Implementation
Client Need—Health promotion/maintenance

64 2. Use of a condom by the male partner prevents infecting the male with herpes simplex virus type II. Infecting the male partner cannot be prevented by douching, use of a diaphragm, or taking acyclovir. (16:88)
Nursing Process—Implementation
Client Need—Health promotion/maintenance

65 1. Symptoms of AIDS may appear months or years after the original infection; therefore, the absence of symptoms is no assurance that a sexual partner does not have AIDS. AIDS cannot be cured nor can the spread of AIDS be controlled with antiviral drugs. The drugs presently in use today *may* slow the progression of the disease in some people. Telling the adolescent to cease sexual activity is rarely effective. (16:87)
Nursing Process—Implementation
Client Need—Health promotion/maintenance

66 3. Malaise, fever, and opportunistic infections are some of the common symptoms of AIDS. Opportunistic infections (eg, those that occur because of a breakdown of the body's immune system) are sometimes the first symptoms that make the client seek medical attention. Other symptoms may include anorexia (which may be severe), weight loss, sore throat, diarrhea, lymph node enlargement, and abdominal cramps. Some people have few or no early symptoms. (16:87)
Nursing Process—Implementation
Client Need—Health promotion/maintenance

NURSING CARE OF AN ADOLESCENT WITH SCOLIOSIS

67 2. Scoliosis is a lateral curvature of the spine, which may be congenital, idiopathic, or a result of paralysis. Kyphosis is also known by the lay term humpback or hunchback. An exaggerated curvature of the lumbar spine is lordosis. (8:655)

    Nursing Process—Implementation
    Client Need—Health promotion/maintenance

68 4. This client's scoliosis is at the level of the chest (thoracic); therefore, if untreated, heart and lung function may be compromised. Scoliosis is not likely to correct itself. Scoliosis of the thoracic region is not likely to affect bowel or bladder control. (8:656)

    Nursing Process—Implementation
    Client Need—Health promotion/maintenance

69 1. Demonstration of coughing and deep breathing exercises is essential. A body cast may be applied at the time of surgery, thus limiting movement of chest muscles. Showing the Harrington rod and telling Linda she will have pain (without explaining that the nurses will give her medication for pain) are inappropriate. If an external brace is applied, only the physician can adjust this apparatus. (19:608)

    Nursing Process—Implementation
    Client Need—Safe, effective care environment

70 1. Allowing this client to select foods that she likes gives the adolescent some control over her environment. Food selection should be made with the assistance of a dietitian so that a well-balanced diet is provided. (19:608)

    Nursing Process—Planning
    Client Need—Health promotion/maintenance

71 4. Encouraging fluids and foods high in bulk is the best method of correcting constipation. Linda is somewhat immobile owing to a body cast. Engaging in recreational activities that require little or no movement would probably not correct constipation. Because a body cast has been applied, ambulatory activity is most likely limited to getting out of bed and into a chair. Depending on the extent of the body cast, some clients may need to remain in bed until the cast is removed. (8:658)

    Nursing Process—Implementation
    Client Need—Physiological integrity

72 1. When changing this client's position, a pillow placed between the thighs prevents strain on the lumbar area and adduction of the top leg. The other tasks mentioned in this question would not be appropriate for this client. (8:659)

    Nursing Process—Implementation
    Client Need—Safe, effective care environment

Individual Test Items

73 2. Avoid overdressing in warm weather because this reduces perspiration in areas of the body that are covered with clothes. Fine cornstarch or baby powder applied to the affected areas may reduce perspiration. Exposing the affected areas to sunlight, applying baby oil *and* baby powder, and applying a dressing may increase rather than decrease the problem. (8:595)

    Nursing Process—Implementation
    Client Need—Health promotion/maintenance

74 4. The tubercle bacillus has a tendency to develop resistance to drugs used to treat tuberculosis. Giving two drugs in combination helps prevent resistance to develop in the causative microorganism. Combination drug therapy does not prevent tolerance to drug therapy, allergic reactions to drugs, or adverse systemic reactions to drug therapy. (15:173)

    Nursing Process—Implementation
    Client Need—Health promotion/maintenance

75 2. Tetracycline hydrochloride should be taken when the stomach is empty. If the medication is taken on an empty stomach, the person must wait 1 hour before eating. It also is important to avoid taking this drug with milk, milk products, or antacids because they interfere with the absorption of the tetracyclines. (15:165)

    Nursing Process—Implementation
    Client need—Health promotion/maintenance

76 3. A small head, upward-slanting eyes, protruding tongue, curved little finger, round face, flat nose, and a simian crease on the palms are outward signs of Down syndrome. (19:261)

    Nursing Process—Collecting data
    Client Need—Health promotion/maintenance

77 4. Although talking to parents and reading about or listening to information about diabetes may help to a certain extent, being with peers having the same problem would more likely help Melanie emotionally cope with her problems. (19:795)

    Nursing Process—Implementation
    Client Need—Health promotion/maintenance

78 3. Bone marrow transplantation supplies normal, healthy bone marrow from a compatible donor. It is anticipated that the new bone marrow will manufacture normal blood cells. Bone marrow transplantation does not provide antibodies to destroy leukemic cells, antileukemic cells that place the client in remission, or directly provide immunity to bacterial or viral infections. (19:675)

    Nursing Process—Implementation
    Client Need—Health promotion/maintenance

79 2. Muscle cramps occurring during or shortly after vigorous exercise may be relieved by drinking plenty of water and warming up before engaging in physical activity. Wearing heavy clothing or fasting for 12 hours may result in muscle cramps because these actions encourage excessive perspiration and deprive the body of electrolytes gained from food. (19:608)
Nursing Process—Implementation
Client Need—Health promotion/maintenance

80 3. Braces strengthen and support weakened muscles thereby providing some clients with cerebral palsy the ability to walk with or without assistance. Braces do not encourage the use of unaffected muscles or prevent muscle atrophy of the upper extremities. Muscle spasticity cannot be prevented because it is an inherent part of the disorder. (8:581)
Nursing Process—Implementation
Client Need—Health promotion/maintenance

81 1. A high-caloric bland diet serves two purposes. A bland diet will not irritate the client's sore mouth, and a high-caloric diet is indicated because the client is eating poorly. The diet is best served in small amounts and at frequent intervals in an attempt to prevent weight loss, a common occurrence in those with AIDS. The other diets in this question may contain foods that are irritating to the oral mucosa. (19:269)
Nursing Process—Implementation
Client Need—Health promotion/maintenance

82 2. PKU is a genetic disorder characterized by the person's inability to metabolize phenylalanine, an amino acid found in natural protein foods. Because phenylalanine cannot be converted to tyrosine, phenylketones are excreted in the urine (phenylketonuria). High blood levels of phenylalanine are seen. Mental retardation, skin problems, failure to thrive, and epileptic seizures are associated with PKU. (19:257–258)
Nursing Process—Implementation
Client Need—Health promotion/maintenance

83 1. An immunity acquired after having a disease is called a naturally acquired active immunity. A killed or attenuated organism that promotes an immunity is called an artificially acquired active immunity. Passive immunity provides the person with antibodies made by another human or by an animal. (15:302)
Nursing Process—Collecting data
Client Need—Health promotion/maintenance

84 3. Tay-Sachs disease is an inherited illness caused by a recessive gene that causes progressive brain damage. Because there is no treatment, and death within 3 to 5 years usually is inevitable, the parents need considerable support and help. Tay-Sachs disease occurs most frequently among eastern and central European Jews. (14:688)
Nursing Process—Planning
Client Need—Psychosocial integrity

85 4. The person sustaining a head injury should be observed for signs of intracranial bleeding, which can occur even after a "mild" or "slight" head injury. Because signs of bleeding are most likely to occur in the first 24 hours the client is awakened at least once during the night to determine the level of consciousness or other neurologic changes. Some hospitals may suggest that the client be awakened every 2 hours during the night. Examples of changes requiring prompt medical attention include slurred speech, headache, visual problems, or difficulty arousing the client from sleep. (19:601–602)
Nursing Process—Implementation
Client Need—Safe, effective care environment

86 2. Tinea is caused by a fungus, and an antifungal agent, such as griseofulvin (Grisactin), is commonly used to treat the condition. (8:599)
Nursing Process—Implementation
Client Need—Health promotion/maintenance

87 4. The pinworm ova hatch in feces. Pinworms are spread by people who are careless about washing their hands after a bowel movement or who scratch the worm-infested anal area and then fail to wash their hands. (19:692–693)
Nursing Process—Implementation
Client Need—Health promotion/maintenance

88 3. Some people may neglect having available immunizations for any number of reasons, including lack of knowledge, indifference, or carelessness. In some cases diseases that are preventable through immunization have been endemic because of this tendency. These findings point out the important work health personnel have in public educational programs to help in the prevention of communicable diseases for which immunization is available. (18:354–355)
Nursing Process—Implementation
Client Need—Health promotion/maintenance

89 1. Rebreathing in and out of a paper bag held tightly over the face may relieve hiccups. Chewing gum and eating dry crackers may be dangerous because these substances may be aspirated during a hiccup. Carbonated beverages can induce hiccups because they tend to cause abdominal distention, which is one cause of hiccups. (18:448)
Nursing Process—Implementation
Client Need—Health promotion/maintenance

90 2. Children of this age may try to get out of their crib when the side rails are lowered. Restraining or asking for assistance normally is not necessary. Giving a toy to the child will not prevent him from falling out of his crib. (18:236)
Nursing Process—Implementation
Client Need—Safe, effective care environment

91 1. When an oral medication is added to the infant's formula there is no guarantee that *all* of the medication will be taken if the infant does not drink all of the formula. With the infant in an upright position, a rubber-tipped medicine dropper or a small medicine cup may be used to administer a drug slowly in liquid form. The medication also can be placed in an empty nipple from a ring-and-disk type baby bottle. The infant is then allowed to suck on the nipple. Most liquid medications are flavored so that the infant or child is encouraged to drink the fluid. (8:487)
Nursing Process—Implementation
Client Need—Physiological integrity

92 1. The salicylates prolong bleeding time by interfering with blood platelet aggregation (eg, the ability of the blood to clot). Aspirin is a salicylate and is contraindicated for anyone with a bleeding disorder because it interferes with the ability of the blood to clot. This is especially important when a person has hemophilia or any other bleeding disorder because stopping bleeding often is extremely difficult, and a person can bleed to death from even a relatively small lesion. (15:70)
Nursing Process—Implementation
Client Need—Health promotion/maintenance

93 3. Elbow restraints prevent the child from touching the face. This type of restraint allows the child to move the arms. However, the nurse must be sure that no toy or object is available for the child to use to reach the face and operative area. A Papoose board and mummy restraint are whole body restraints and normally are not necessary for this type of surgery. A Posey belt or jacket allows movement of the arms and is usually used to keep the child in bed or in a wheelchair. (8:466–469)
Nursing Process—Planning
Client Need—Safe, effective care environment

94 4. Unless the physician orders otherwise, most restraints are removed and reapplied every 2 hours. (8:467)
Nursing Process—Planning
Client Need—Safe, effective care environment

95 2. Anorexia, nausea, vomiting, mental depression, hypotension, confusion, abdominal distention, decreased bowel sounds, paralytic ileus, muscle weakness, absent or diminished deep tendon reflexes, leg cramps, electrocardiogram changes, and weak irregular pulse are signs and symptoms of hypokalemia. (8:478; 15:118)
Nursing Process—Collecting data
Client Need—Physiological integrity

96 2. A Hickman catheter normally is inserted into the jugular vein with the tip in the right atrium. This type of catheter normally exits by way of a subcutaneous tunnel on the right thorax or the sternum. The exit tip of the catheter is used to give parenteral nutrition and medications and withdraw blood for laboratory analysis. (8:481–482)
Nursing Process—Implementation
Client Need—Physiological integrity

97 2. The lateral decubitus position with the knees drawn up normally is used for a lumbar puncture. This position widens the space between the vertebrae to aid in insertion of the needle. (8:663)
Nursing Process—Implementation
Client Need—Safe, effective care environment

98 1. Cerebral palsy is not a progressive neuromuscular disease and is caused by an injury to the motor coordinating areas of the brain. Surgery on the brain cannot help or cure those with this disorder. Physical therapy and other disciplines, such as occupational, speech, and recreational therapy often are of great benefit to those with cerebral palsy. (8:666–668)
Nursing Process—Implementation
Client Need—Health promotion/maintenance

99 4. Rickets is caused by a lack of sufficient vitamin D in the diet. The vitamin is essential for proper calcium and phosphorus use in the body's normal bone and teeth development. The abnormal process of development in a child lacking sufficient vitamin D is responsible for such signs of rickets as a delay in the closure of fontanelles, delayed tooth growth, dental caries, and deformities of long bones. (15:295)
Nursing Process—Collecting data
Client Need—Health promotion/maintenance

100 4. Pallor, listlessness, and irritability are observable signs of iron-deficiency anemia. A client history also may reveal anorexia, weight loss, and a decrease in the normal activity of a child. The other signs and symptoms given in this question usually are not related to iron-deficiency anemia. (8:726)
Nursing Process—Collecting data
Client Need—Health promotion/maintenance

101 2. Thrush is the more common term for oral moniliasis. Hirschsprung's disease is another term for a congenital megacolon. Colic is intermittent ab-

dominal pain or distress, usually seen in infants. Threadworm is a parasitic infestation. (8:743)
Nursing Process—Implementation
Client Need—Health promotion/maintenance

102 1. Children with pinworm must wash their hands thoroughly after defecating or urinating to prevent reinfection, which occurs when the contaminated fingers are placed in the mouth. If the child does not routinely wash the hands thoroughly after using the toilet, the parents must supervise this activity. There is no need to isolate the child. Asymptomatic family members should be examined because treatment may be necessary. Treatment consists of a single dose of the drug. (8:752; 15:182)
Nursing Process—Implementation
Client Need—Health promotion/maintenance

103 2. A sustained diastolic pressure over 90 mm Hg indicates hypertension. (8:775)
Nursing Process—Evaluation
Client Need—Physiological integrity

104 2. An ice bag can be used safely as long as it is removed every 30 to 45 minutes to check the skin and allow the area to return to normal. Continuous application of cold results in vasoconstriction, which, if allowed to continue, could result in a loss of blood supply to the part and gangrene. (8:587)
Nursing Process—Implementation
Client Need—Safe, effective care environment

105 3. Parents with children having the same disability often are able to provide emotional support. When these parents meet, they share a common bond and a common burden and learn from one another how obstacles can be overcome. Recommending that Kevin be placed in a long-term health care facility, referring the parents to a social welfare agency, or giving them literature to read probably will not help them cope with their problems. (19:588; 8:651)
Nursing Process—Implementation
Client Need—Health promotion/maintenance

106 1. When a child has a heart defect, such as an atrial septal defect or patent ductus arteriosis, one primary nursing goal is to reduce the workload of the heart. Additional important goals may include improving respiration, maintaining fluid and electrolyte balance, improving nutrition, re-

ducing anxiety, and providing emotional support for the child and the family. (19:623)
Nursing Process—Implementation
Client Need—Physiological integrity

107 2. Of these four children, Mark is the child most likely suffering from child abuse. Child abuse may be emotional, physical, mental, or sexual. Although the other three children in this question have injuries and also could be abused children, Mark shows fear and avoids his parents. Most children brought to the hospital reach out for their parents and cry when their parents leave; Mark avoids his parents, which may be an indication of child abuse. (8:407–408)
Nursing Process—Collecting data
Client Need—Safe, effective care environment

108 4. Of these four people, Carl is the one most likely to be abusing drugs. Any unusual behavior, changes in personality, or signs that appear to be abnormal may indicate drug abuse. Examples of abnormal signs include depression, excitability, profuse perspiration, dilated pupils, extreme apathy, and repeated absence from school. Clayton's grades have not had a significant drop; a 2-point change would not be abnormal. Tiffany's avoidance of some of her friends often is seen in adolescence, when some friendships may be brief and stormy. Barbara's arguments with her sister are not abnormal unless Barbara uses physical action against her sisters or if the arguments are frequent and severe. (8:406–407)
Nursing Process—Collecting data
Client Need—Psychosocial integrity

109 3. Toddlers often climb up or go down stairs as part of their search for something new in their environment. A toddler can be left unattended on a sofa; this caution applies to an infant. A toddler would not understand the importance of having fun without getting hurt or the importance of safe play. (8:403–404)
Nursing Process—Implementation
Client Need—Safe, effective care environment

110 4. A Wilms' tumor is a congenital, cancerous tumor of the kidney. Feeling, touching, or handling the client's abdomen may result in a rupture of the renal capsule and a spread of cancerous tumor cells, by way of the bloodstream, to other organs. Feeding the client, combing the client's hair, or giving the client a book to read would not exert pressure on the renal capsule. (8:774)
Nursing Process—Implementation
Client Need—Safe, effective care environment

111   2. Impetigo contagiosa is a contagious disorder caused by a streptococcal or staphylococcal infection of the skin. The child should be isolated from others until the lesions have cleared. In some camps the child may be sent home because isolation is nearly impossible. Usually, antibiotics are prescribed, and the condition clears in approximately 1 week. Continuous wet soaks are not indicated and may help spread the infection to other areas. The crusts can be removed with soap and water. (16:836)

   Nursing Process—Implementation
   Client Need—Safe, effective care environment

Classification of Test Items

Unit III Review Test 5

Directions: After each question the correct answer is given as well as a classification of each test question. Compare the correct answer with your answer. If a question has been answered *incorrectly*, draw a line to the end of the four columns. When finished, add up your correct scores and place the results at the bottom of each column.

Score Calculation:

To determine the percentage of the number of questions you answered correctly, divide the **Number Correct** by the **Number Possible**, as example 94 (the number of questions answered correctly) divided by 111 (the number of questions in the test) = .846 or 85%.

NURSING PROCESS

C = Collecting data
P = Planning
I = Implementation
E = Evaluation

CLIENT NEEDS

S = Safe, effective care environment
P = Physiological integrity
M = Psychosocial integrity
H = Health promotion/maintenance

Question #	Answer #	Nursing Process				Client Needs			
		C	P	I	E	S	P	M	H
1	3	C					P		
2	2			I		S			
3	4			I		S			
4	4			I			P		
5	2	C				S			
6	2	C				S			
7	1		P				P		
8	1			I		S			
9	3			I		S			
10	3			I		S			
11	4			I			P		
12	2			I			P		
13	2	C					P		
14	1			I			P		
15	3			I		S			
16	1			I					H
17	4			I					H
18	2		P				P		

NURSING PROCESS

C = Collecting data
P = Planning
I = Implementation
E = Evaluation

CLIENT NEEDS

S = Safe, effective care environment
P = Physiological integrity
M = Psychosocial integrity
H = Health promotion/maintenance

Question #	Answer #	Nursing Process				Client Needs			
		C	P	I	E	S	P	M	H
19	3			I					H
20	1			I			P		
21	2				E		P		
22	2		P			S			
23	2		P				P		
24	3			I			P		
25	1	C					P		
26	4				E		P		
27	4			I			P		
28	1	C					P		
29	1			I			P		
30	3		P			S			
31	1			I					H
32	2			I					H
33	4			I					H
34	3			I		S			
35	4			I		S			
36	3	C					P		
37	1			I			P		
38	2			I			P		
39	1		P			S			
40	2			I				M	
41	1			I		S			
42	2			I			P		
43	3			I				M	
44	2		P			S			
45	2		P				P		
46	4				E		P		
47	1		P				P		
48	3	C					P		

NURSING PROCESS

C = Collecting data
P = Planning
I = Implementation
E = Evaluation

CLIENT NEEDS

S = Safe, effective care environment
P = Physiological integrity
M = Psychosocial integrity
H = Health promotion/maintenance

Question #	Answer #	Nursing Process				Client Needs			
		C	P	I	E	S	P	M	H
49	1			I		S			
50	4			I					H
51	4			I					H
52	1			I			P		
53	4	C						M	
54	4			I		S			
55	1			I				M	
56	1	C							H
57	3			I				M	
58	3			I		S			
59	2			I		S			
60	4			I					H
61	3			I					H
62	3	C					P		
63	1			I					H
64	2			I					H
65	1			I					H
66	3			I					H
67	2			I					H
68	4			I					H
69	1			I		S			
70	1		P						H
71	4			I			P		
72	1			I		S			
73	2			I					H
74	4			I					H
75	2			I					H
76	3	C							H
77	4			I					H
78	3			I					H

NURSING PROCESS

C = Collecting data
P = Planning
I = Implementation
E = Evaluation

CLIENT NEEDS

S = Safe, effective care environment
P = Physiological integrity
M = Psychosocial integrity
H = Health promotion/maintenance

Question #	Answer #	Nursing Process				Client Needs			
		C	P	I	E	S	P	M	H
79	2			I					H
80	3			I					H
81	1			I					H
82	2			I					H
83	1	C							H
84	3		P					M	
85	4			I		S			
86	2			I					H
87	4			I					H
88	3			I					H
89	1			I					H
90	2			I		S			
91	1			I			P		
92	1			I					H
93	3		P			S			
94	4		P			S			
95	2	C					P		
96	2			I			P		
97	2			I		S			
98	1			I					H
99	4	C							H
100	4	C							H
101	2			I					H
102	1			I					H
103	2				E		P		
104	2			I		S			
105	3			I					H
106	1			I			P		
107	2	C				S			
108	4	C						M	

NURSING PROCESS

C = Collecting data
P = Planning
I = Implementation
E = Evaluation

CLIENT NEEDS

S = Safe, effective care environment
P = Physiological integrity
M = Psychosocial integrity
H = Health promotion/maintenance

Question #	Answer #	Nursing Process				Client Needs			
		C	P	I	E	S	P	M	H
109	3			I		S			
110	4			I		S			
111	2			I		S			
Number Correct									
Number Possible	111	18	14	75	4	31	33	7	40
Percentage Correct									

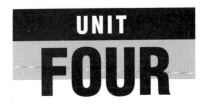

UNIT
FOUR

REVIEW TESTS 6 THROUGH 14

The Nursing Care of Adults with
Medical–Surgical Disorders

REVIEW TEST 6

The Nursing Care of Clients with Disorders of the Gastrointestinal System and Accessory Organs of Digestion

Nursing Care of Clients with Disorders of the Mouth
Nursing Care of Clients with Disorders of the Esophagus
Nursing Care of Clients with Disorders of the Stomach
Nursing Care of Clients with Disorders of the Small Intestine
Nursing Care of Clients with Disorders of the Large Intestine
Nursing Care of Clients with Disorders of the Rectum and Anus
Nursing Care of Clients with Disorders of the Gallbladder
Nursing Care of Clients with Disorders of the Liver
Nursing Care of Clients with Disorders of the Pancreas

Correct Answers and Rationale
Classification of Test Items

Directions: With a pencil, blacken the circle in front of the option you have chosen for your correct answer.

The Nursing Care of Clients with Disorders of the Gastrointestinal System and Accessory Organs of Digestion

NURSING CARE OF CLIENTS WITH DISORDERS OF THE MOUTH

Mr. Ron Stauffer, age 26, is admitted for diagnostic tests. He has been experiencing a cough, night sweats, and a low-grade fever. Mr. Stauffer has been taking a tetracycline antibiotic for the past 2 weeks.

1 While assessing Mr. Stauffer on admission, the nurse inspects his mouth. If the client has candidiasis, also known as moniliasis or thrush, which one of the following will the nurse observe?
   ○ 1. Clear, shiny, domed vesicles on the tongue
   ○ 2. Red, ulcerated patches at the gum margin
   ○ 3. White, curd-like patches throughout the mouth
   ○ 4. Dark, brown, flat lesions in the oropharynx

2 Mr. Stauffer asks the nurse how he may have acquired this oral infection. The most *accurate* explanation is that most individuals acquire candidiasis by
   ○ 1. being bitten by an insect like a fly or tick.
   ○ 2. having an unchecked growth of normal mouth organisms.
   ○ 3. inhaling moist droplets when someone sneezed.

   ○ 4. consuming contaminated water or tainted food.

3 The physician prescribes nystatin (Mycostatin) oral suspension. Which one of the following steps should the nurse plan to teach the client when administering this medication?
   ○ 1. Drink the medication through a straw.
   ○ 2. Dilute the medication with cold water.
   ○ 3. Retain the drug as long as possible in the mouth.
   ○ 4. Swish the drug in the mouth, but avoid swallowing it.

Mr. Frank Molzer, age 61, is being treated for cancer of the mouth. Evidence of his cancer was discovered during a routine dental examination.

4 As the nurse reads through Mr. Molzer's medical history, which one of the following factors is *most* associated with cancer of the mouth? The client
   ○ 1. has used smokeless tobacco most of his life.
   ○ 2. has worn dentures for 18 months.
   ○ 3. drinks decaffeinated coffee or tea daily.
   ○ 4. likes to chew sugarless gum occasionally.

5 The nurse prepares to provide oral hygiene for Mr. Molzer. Which one of the following techniques is *most* appropriate when caring for the client's dentures?

○ 1. Use hot water while brushing and rinsing his teeth.
○ 2. Hold the dentures over a basin of water or soft towel.
○ 3. Apply solvent to remove the oral adhesive from his teeth.
○ 4. Place the dentures in a clean, dry container when he's not using them.

6 To treat Mr. Molzer's oral cancer, the oncologist has implanted needles containing radioactive cesium inside his cheek. The sealed implant is attached to threads fastened externally to his face. Mr. Molzer has been feeling nauseated. Which one of the following additions to the care plan is essential if the client vomits?
○ 1. Inspect emesis for solid objects before disposing.
○ 2. Rinse emesis basin with diluted household bleach.
○ 3. Provide plastic emesis basin rather than metal.
○ 4. Cut threads fastened to cheek if vomiting occurs.

Faith O'Rourke has come to the gynecologist's office today to be fitted for a diaphragm. In the process of being prepared for her examination, she discusses with the nurse a fever blister she has on her mouth.

7 If Ms. O'Rourke makes all of the following statements about a herpes simplex type I infection, which one indicates that she is *misinformed*? She says that
○ 1. the lesion is a result of a viral infection.
○ 2. the infection is spread by direct contact.
○ 3. emotional stress can trigger a recurrence.
○ 4. the lesions only form on or within the mouth.

8 Ms. O'Rourke tells the nurse that she was given a prescription for acyclovir (Zovirax) by her family physician when the fever blister formed. Which one of the following statements indicates that she understands the use of the drug? Ms. O'Rourke says that this drug
○ 1. kills all of the virus causing the disease.
○ 2. shortens the episodes of the disease.
○ 3. prevents an outbreak from recurring.
○ 4. must be taken daily for her lifetime.

Sharon Fuller has just awakened following the delivery of a full-term infant during the night.

9 As the nurse provides the client with equipment for oral care, Sharon says to the nurse, "Some say that you should brush the teeth by making circles. Others say to move the toothbrush up and down. Just what is the best way to clean my teeth?" The best response from the nurse would be that the movement of the brush is not as important as
○ 1. stroking all the surfaces of the teeth.

○ 2. using a plaque-removing mouthwash afterwards.
○ 3. getting dental checkups every 6 months.
○ 4. replacing the toothbrush frequently.

NURSING CARE OF CLIENTS WITH DISORDERS OF THE ESOPHAGUS

Mr. Gordon Helman has been experiencing difficulty swallowing. Today the nurse is scheduling an appointment in the outpatient department for him. He will be having an esophagoscopy.

10 The nurse explains the procedure for esophagoscopy. Which one of the following indicates that Mr. Helman understands how he is to prepare himself for his diagnostic test? Mr. Helman says it is essential that he
○ 1. eat only a light breakfast before the examination.
○ 2. consume a low-residue diet until the test is done.
○ 3. avoid food and fluids after midnight before the test.
○ 4. drink a quart of liquid before arriving for the test.

The esophagoscopy reveals that Mr. Helman has a stricture near the end of his esophagus.

11 To help relieve Mr. Helman's discomfort, the best recommendation the nurse could make is to tell him to
○ 1. eat a variety of baby foods from now on.
○ 2. chew everything that is eaten very thoroughly.
○ 3. avoid drinking beverages while eating a meal.
○ 4. refrain from having milk and dairy products.

Mr. Robert Walters, age 38, is admitted with bleeding esophageal varices.

12 As the nurse reviews his medical record, which of the following factors is most likely related to his present condition? Mr. Walters
○ 1. works at an oil refinery.
○ 2. is a lacto-ovovegetarian.
○ 3. is extremely underweight.
○ 4. drinks alcohol heavily.

13 The team leader starts an infusion of whole blood. She asks the practical nurse to continue monitoring Mr. Walters during the blood transfusion. The nurse observes all of the following. Which one is the best indication that a *blood reaction* is occurring?
○ 1. The client's urine is very dark yellow.
○ 2. Mr. Walters becomes dyspneic suddenly.
○ 3. Mr. Walters' skin is pale and cool.
○ 4. Mr. Walters says he is extremely thirsty.

Ms. Victoria Hall has been diagnosed as having a hiatal hernia.

14 As the nurse gathers data from Ms. Hall, which one of the following is most likely to be this client's chief complaint?
- ○ 1. Vomiting
- ○ 2. Nausea
- ○ 3. Anorexia
- ○ 4. Heartburn

15 The nurse reviews a standardized care plan for the nursing diagnosis of *Altered Comfort related to esophageal reflux.* Which one of the following instructions should the nurse plan to include when teaching Ms. Hall how to manage her condition?
- ○ 1. Eat three well-balanced meals a day.
- ○ 2. Eat foods that are easy to swallow.
- ○ 3. Avoid lying down after eating food.
- ○ 4. Avoid skipping meals when hungry.

A barium swallow confirms that Anna Parker has esophageal diverticula.

16 Which one of the following findings is the nurse most likely to note during the physical assessment of Ms. Parker?
- ○ 1. External hemorrhoids
- ○ 2. Abdominal distention
- ○ 3. Foul-smelling breath
- ○ 4. Hypoactive bowel sounds

William Marvin has metastatic cancer of the esophagus. He ignored the difficulty he experienced with swallowing until he began to have pain. Surgery is no longer considered curative. He is undergoing palliative treatment with radiation.

17 The radiologist has used a red marking pencil identifying the radiation site. Which of the following actions is essential to Mr. Marvin's nursing care?
- ○ 1. Remove the marks by using ether or acetone.
- ○ 2. Do not rub or use lotion on that area of skin.
- ○ 3. Keep the irradiated skin exposed at all times.
- ○ 4. Use talcum powder to absorb skin perspiration.

Because of Mr. Marvin's inability to swallow food, his physician inserts a subclavian catheter for the purpose of providing the client with hyperalimentation, also known as total parenteral nutrition (TPN).

18 Which one of the following assessments is essential for the nurse to perform while Mr. Marvin receives TPN?
- ○ 1. Test the urine's specific gravity.
- ○ 2. Monitor the capillary blood glucose.
- ○ 3. Measure the arterial pulse pressure.
- ○ 4. Obtain an apical–radial pulse rate.

19 What is the best evidence the nurse could use to determine that Mr. Marvin is responding *favorably* to the administration of TPN?
- ○ 1. He remains alert.
- ○ 2. He gains weight.
- ○ 3. He feels hungry.
- ○ 4. He is pain free.

Anticipating that Mr. Marvin will be transferred to a nursing home or be discharged to home care, the physician inserts a gastrostomy tube for nourishment.

20 While administering liquid nourishment through the gastrostomy tube, Mr. Marvin says he feels full and nauseated. The best nursing measure at this time would be to
- ○ 1. measure the stomach residual.
- ○ 2. raise the height of the formula.
- ○ 3. stop the infusion temporarily.
- ○ 4. add water to dilute the formula.

21 Mr. Marvin looks away and does not speak while the nurse administers his tube feeding. Which one of the following statements would be best for encouraging him to express his feelings?
- ○ 1. "Are you feeling angry?"
- ○ 2. "It must be tough for you."
- ○ 3. "This may get better soon."
- ○ 4. "Lots of people eat this way."

NURSING CARE OF CLIENTS WITH DISORDERS OF THE STOMACH

Mr. Edward Knight is a 46-year-old plumber who is hospitalized to determine the cause of the gnawing epigastric pain he has been experiencing periodically.

22 When the admitting nurse obtains Mr. Knight's health history, if the pain is due to a peptic ulcer, he will most likely report that his discomfort goes away or is less intense when he
- ○ 1. skips a meal.
- ○ 2. goes to bed.
- ○ 3. eats food.
- ○ 4. bends over.

23 Which one of the following tests could the nurse perform to obtain additional supporting data that Mr. Knight's symptoms are due to a peptic ulcer? The nurse could check his
- ○ 1. urine for albumin.
- ○ 2. blood for glucose.
- ○ 3. stool for blood.
- ○ 4. emesis for pepsin.

24 Mr. Knight is scheduled for an x-ray of the upper gastrointestinal tract. After the nurse has explained the procedure, which one of the following statements indicates that Mr. Knight understands what this test involves?

○ 1. "A flexible tube will be inserted into my stomach."
○ 2. "Dye will be infused into my vein before the test."
○ 3. "My body will be placed within an imaging chamber."
○ 4. "I will have to swallow a large volume of barium."

Diagnostic tests reveal that Mr. Knight has a duodenal ulcer.

25 The physician writes an order for the nurse to give Mr. Knight 2 teaspoons of aluminum hydroxide gel (Amphojel) between meals and at bedtime. The nurse would be most correct in administering which one of the following equivalents?
○ 1. 30 mL
○ 2. 15 mL
○ 3. 10 mL
○ 4. 5 mL

26 Mr. Knight has been taking the aluminum hydroxide gel for 3 days. He tells the nurse all of the following information. Which one is most likely a *side effect* of the antacid he is taking?
○ 1. "I am constipated."
○ 2. "My skin itches."
○ 3. "My mouth is dry."
○ 4. "I feel tired."

The physician discontinues the administration of aluminum hydroxide gel. The physician then prescribes sucralfate (Carafate) for Mr. Knight.

27 When Mr. Knight asks the nurse to explain the action of the new medication, the most accurate response would be that sucralfate
○ 1. makes gastric secretions less acidic.
○ 2. covers the ulcer with a protective barrier.
○ 3. inhibits gastric acid production.
○ 4. blocks histamine receptors in the stomach.

28 The nurse caring for Mr. Knight works with the team leader in planning his discharge instructions. Their goal is to provide him with information that will help him prevent further gastric irritation. The plan should include the recommended use of which drug for occasional pain or discomfort?
○ 1. acetaminophen (Tylenol)
○ 2. aspirin (Anacin)
○ 3. ibuprofen (Advil)
○ 4. naproxen (Naprosyn)

The nurse is preparing Mr. Richard Eislen for abdominal surgery. Mr. Eislen has a history of chronic recurrent peptic ulcer disease.

29 As the nurse performs a head-to-toe physical assessment, which one of the following signs is *most in-*dicative that Mr. Eislen's ulcer has perforated? The client's
○ 1. skin appears ecchymotic.
○ 2. abdomen feels board-like.
○ 3. pupils are widely dilated.
○ 4. respirations are rapid.

30 The nurse helps the team leader insert a gastric sump tube. The nurse is asked to check its placement. An appropriate technique for determining that the distal end of the tube is in the stomach is to
○ 1. request a portable x-ray of the stomach.
○ 2. listen over the stomach as air is instilled.
○ 3. instill 100 mL of tap water into the tube.
○ 4. feel for air at the proximal end of the tube.

31 Mr. Eislen senses the critical nature of his condition. He says, "Nurse, am I going to make it?" The best response from the nurse would be:
○ 1. "We are doing everything we can to do just that."
○ 2. "That's something you'll have to ask your doctor."
○ 3. "Now what kind of a silly question is that?"
○ 4. "I've seen people in a whole lot worse shape."

A subtotal gastrectomy is performed on Mr. Eislen. Two thirds of his stomach, the pylorus, and a portion of the duodenum are removed. He is returned to his room after recovering from the anesthesia.

32 Mr. Eislen does not adequately cough and deep breathe because it increases the pain in his incision. Which one of the following nursing measures should the nurse plan to perform at this time?
○ 1. Explain that he is at high risk for developing pneumonia.
○ 2. Have him press a pillow against his incision when coughing.
○ 3. Ask the physician to order some form of oxygen for him.
○ 4. Keep the head of the bed elevated at all times of the day.

33 The nurse monitors the nasogastric tube and decompression. Which one of the following is essential to report to the nurse in charge?
○ 1. The client says his throat hurts.
○ 2. The client indicates he is thirsty.
○ 3. There is mucus accumulating in the nose.
○ 4. There is bright red bloody drainage.

34 Mr. Eislen's nasogastric tube is not draining. The nurse prepares to irrigate the tube. Which of the following actions is appropriate? The nurse
○ 1. instills 30 mL of sterile distilled water.
○ 2. administers oxygen before the irrigation.
○ 3. records the volume instilled and removed.
○ 4. asks the client to swallow frequently.

Discharge teaching is begun for Mr. Eislen. The charge nurse has written "Potential complication: Dumping syndrome" on Mr. Eislen's plan of care.

35 The nurse carries out the teaching plan developed by the charge nurse. Diet instructions are explained first. The best evidence that the client understands how altering his diet will prevent dumping syndrome is the statement:
- ○ 1. "I should drink a large volume of liquid at meals."
- ○ 2. "I should restrict eating sugary and starchy food."
- ○ 3. "It would be best to eat large meals during the day."
- ○ 4. "It would be best to reduce my intake of red meat."

36 Which one of the following activities should the nurse add to the teaching plan to help Mr. Eislen avoid experiencing dumping syndrome?
- ○ 1. Lie down for a short while after eating.
- ○ 2. Sleep with the head of the bed elevated.
- ○ 3. Walk several times a day between meals.
- ○ 4. Meditate or relax just prior to eating.

Mr. Fred Majors sought medical help for persistent indigestion, feeling of gastric fullness, and weight loss.

37 The nurse reviews the results of several diagnostic tests Mr. Majors has undergone. Which one of the following findings indicates a probability that Mr. Majors' symptoms are due to cancer of the stomach?
- ○ 1. Gastric analysis showed absence of hydrochloric acid.
- ○ 2. An elevated level of gastrin was found in the blood.
- ○ 3. Gastric irritation was noted during a gastroscopy.
- ○ 4. A urinalysis showed the presence of a few erythrocytes.

38 Mr. Majors' physician informed him that he will need lifelong vitamin therapy to prevent pernicious anemia following his total gastrectomy to treat stomach cancer. When questioned, the nurse would be most accurate in telling Mr. Majors that the name of the specific vitamin he will need is
- ○ 1. vitamin C.
- ○ 2. vitamin B_6.
- ○ 3. vitamin B_{12}.
- ○ 4. vitamin K.

NURSING CARE OF CLIENTS WITH DISORDERS OF THE SMALL INTESTINE

Ms. Connie Allen, age 19, has been having up to five loose stools per day. She is admitted for diagnostic testing and treatment.

39 The nurse collects a stool specimen that will be examined for ova and parasites. Which one of the following actions is appropriate? The nurse
- ○ 1. holds a specimen container under the client's rectum.
- ○ 2. places the collected specimen in a sterile container.
- ○ 3. refrigerates the covered container after collection.
- ○ 4. takes the specimen to the laboratory immediately.

40 The physician has prescribed diphenoxylate hydrochloride (Lomotil) 5 mg orally q.i.d. Which one of the following schedules shows that the team leader has scheduled the time for administering this drug correctly? The medication administration record indicates that this drug should be given at the following military times:
- ○ 1. 0730, 1130, 0430
- ○ 2. 0600, 1200, 1800, 0000
- ○ 3. 0900, 1300, 1700
- ○ 4. 0400, 0800, 1200, 1600, 2000

41 While Ms. Allen is having diarrhea, the physician restricts her intake to clear liquids. When Ms. Allen asks for some nourishment, which one of the following would be appropriate for the nurse to provide?
- ○ 1. Milk
- ○ 2. Pudding
- ○ 3. Gelatin
- ○ 4. Custard

42 Which one of the following findings would best indicate to the nurse that the client's fluid needs are being met?
- ○ 1. The blood pressure is normal.
- ○ 2. The client says she is thirsty.
- ○ 3. The lung sounds are clear.
- ○ 4. The urine appears dark yellow.

After a colonoscopy the physician tells Ms. Allen that she has Crohn's disease, which also is known as regional ileitis or regional enteritis.

43 Ms. Allen is eventually placed on a fiber-controlled diet. Ms. Allen is still confused after talking to the dietitian. She asks the nurse to re-explain what the term fiber means. The nurse would be most correct in telling her that fiber refers to
- ○ 1. foods that require chewing.
- ○ 2. the muscle found in red meat.
- ○ 3. the semisolid mass in the stomach.
- ○ 4. the indigestible part of plants.

Despite dietary and medication compliance, Ms. Allen eventually develops a draining fistula between a loop of the ileum and the skin.

44 The nurse accompanies the physician when he explains Ms. Allen's condition. Which one of the following statements indicates to the nurse that Ms. Allen understands the information provided by the physician? Ms. Allen describes a fistula as
  ○ 1. a communicating track between two structures.
  ○ 2. a mass protruding from the mucous membrane.
  ○ 3. hypertrophied scar tissue formed during healing.
  ○ 4. a local collection of pus in a body cavity.

45 The nursing team gathers to discuss Ms. Allen's plan for care. Based on the new complication, it would be essential to plan nursing measures for which one of the following problems?
  ○ 1. Incontinence
  ○ 2. Impaired skin
  ○ 3. Body image
  ○ 4. Depression

NURSING CARE OF CLIENTS WITH DISORDERS OF THE LARGE INTESTINE

Mr. Jerry Boland is admitted to the hospital for surgical repair of an inguinal hernia.

46 As the nurse obtains his history on admission, which one of the following facts is most likely associated with the acquisition of a hernia? The client
  ○ 1. experiences abdominal cramping when he drinks milk.
  ○ 2. does not get much physical exercise except at work.
  ○ 3. lifts heavy mail bags in his job as a postal worker.
  ○ 4. is approximately 10 pounds underweight.

47 Mr. Boland is not convinced that he needs surgery. He says it is possible for him to just push on the protrusion and it goes away from time to time. The nurse documents this information on the client's medical record. The most accurate term the nurse can use when charting what Mr. Boland described is that the hernia is
  ○ 1. idiopathic.
  ○ 2. strangulated.
  ○ 3. incarcerated.
  ○ 4. reducible.

48 Mr. Boland tells the nurse that he has been taking docusate calcium (Surfak) on a daily basis since his hernia was diagnosed. He asks the nurse why this medication was prescribed. The best response would be that docusate calcium
  ○ 1. strengthens the tone of the weakened abdominal muscle.
  ○ 2. softens the stool to avoid straining during defecation.

  ○ 3. prevents spasm of the tissue around the weak muscle.
  ○ 4. relieves the pain and discomfort from tissue swelling.

49 The nurse asks Mr. Boland to sign the operative consent stating that he is to have a right inguinal herniorrhaphy. What action would be most appropriate at this time if Mr. Boland says, "I hope I can get along without that section of my bowel"?
  ○ 1. Cancel the surgery.
  ○ 2. Notify the physician.
  ○ 3. Witness his signature.
  ○ 4. Administer an enema.

Mr. Boland returns from surgery.

50 Spinal anesthesia was used for Mr. Boland's surgery. Which one of the following postoperative orders should the nurse question before carrying it out?
  ○ 1. Diet as tolerated
  ○ 2. Fluids as desired
  ○ 3. Ambulate tomorrow
  ○ 4. Fowler's position

51 The nurse brings a suspensory, which is a sling-like support, to Mr. Boland's bedside. When asked why this is being applied, the best explanation from the nurse is that a suspensory is used to prevent
  ○ 1. sexual impotence.
  ○ 2. scrotal edema.
  ○ 3. strain on the incision.
  ○ 4. wound contamination.

52 Of the activities given below, the nurse should plan to teach Mr. Boland that postoperatively he should *avoid*
  ○ 1. forceful coughing.
  ○ 2. moving his legs.
  ○ 3. changing positions
  ○ 4. deep breathing.

Ms. Manuel, a 31-year-old woman, has a long history of ulcerative colitis. She is admitted to the hospital for an ileostomy.

53 In addition to having severe diarrhea, which other finding is the nurse likely to assess in clients with ulcerative colitis?
  ○ 1. Mucus and blood are present in the stool.
  ○ 2. The bowel sounds are hypoactive.
  ○ 3. The skin of the abdomen has striae.
  ○ 4. Shallow ulcerations are found in the mouth.

54 The team leader adds the nursing diagnosis of *Bowel Incontinence related to sudden urgency for defecation* on the care plan. Which one of the following should the nurse plan to *avoid* when carrying out the care of this client?
  ○ 1. Keeping the bedside commode nearby
  ○ 2. Answering her signal for help promptly
  ○ 3. Attaching a disposable diaper on her
  ○ 4. Helping her to the bathroom frequently

55 Ms. Manuel seems discouraged. She tells the nurse of the many hospitalizations she has had without much improvement in her condition. She says, "I am sure this surgery won't help either." In this situation it would be best for the nurse to say,
○ 1. "You are saying that you doubt that you will get better."
○ 2. "Do you want to talk to your doctor again before surgery?"
○ 3. "I'd recommend a more positive attitude this time around."
○ 4. "Of course it will. Others wish they'd had it done sooner."

56 After giving Ms. Manuel the preoperative medication consisting of 50 mg of meperidine hydrochloride (Demerol), 12.5 mg of hydroxyzine (Vistaril), and 0.3 mg of atropine sulfate, the most important nursing action would be to
○ 1. raise the side rails.
○ 2. help her to the toilet.
○ 3. provide oral hygiene.
○ 4. teach her leg exercises.

Ms. Manuel returns from the recovery room postoperatively.

57 Of the following vital signs, the one that should suggest to the nurse that Ms. Manuel is most probably going into shock is
○ 1. a bounding pulse.
○ 2. slowed respirations.
○ 3. low blood pressure.
○ 4. a high body temperature.

58 The time of day when it is best to plan stomal care and changing the appliance would be after Ms. Manuel
○ 1. awakens in the morning.
○ 2. has eaten breakfast.
○ 3. has been up and ambulated.
○ 4. finishes her last meal.

59 The nurse prepares to clean the skin around Ms. Manuel's stoma. The most appropriate technique would be to
○ 1. pat it with cotton balls.
○ 2. swab it with 70% alcohol.
○ 3. use water and mild soap.
○ 4. scrub it with peroxide.

60 When attaching the ileostomy appliance, the nurse should fit it so that
○ 1. the faceplate occludes the opening of the stoma.
○ 2. the appliance opening is ⅛ inches larger than the stoma.
○ 3. a ⅛-inch margin of the faceplate adheres to skin.
○ 4. the bag is directly at the waist or beltline.

61 Ms. Manuel tells the nurse she would like to do all of the following. Which one should the nurse tactfully inform her is *unrealistic*? Ms. Manuel wants to
○ 1. go swimming.
○ 2. play tennis.
○ 3. get pregnant again.
○ 4. control defecation.

Ms. Sherry Thompson is admitted with pain that is localized on the lower right side of the abdomen, halfway between the umbilicus and the crest of the ileum. Her physician suspects appendicitis.

62 Several laboratory tests were ordered on admission. Which one is *most* important for the nurse to monitor at this time?
○ 1. Bilirubin level
○ 2. Serum potassium
○ 3. Prothrombin time
○ 4. Leukocyte count

63 Which one of the following physical assessments would it be essential for the nurse to monitor frequently on a client with appendicitis?
○ 1. Body temperature
○ 2. Lung sounds
○ 3. Size of pupils
○ 4. Color of urine

Ms. Thompson's condition worsens. It is feared that her appendix has ruptured. She is prepared for emergency surgery.

64 Ms. Thompson discusses her self-care prior to admission with the nurse. Which one of Ms. Thompson's actions is most likely to have contributed to the rupturing of her appendix? Ms. Thompson says that she
○ 1. stopped eating and drinking.
○ 2. continued her usual activities.
○ 3. applied a hot water bottle to her lower abdomen.
○ 4. took acetaminophen (Tylenol) for her discomfort.

65 Ms. Thompson returns from surgery with an open drain extending from her incision. The drain, called a Penrose, is a flat, flexible, rubber tube. The drain is covered by a sterile dressing. Which one of the following body positions is best for the nurse to use for promoting drainage from the wound?
○ 1. Lithotomy
○ 2. Fowler's
○ 3. Recumbent
○ 4. Trendelenburg

66 Ms. Thompson is receiving a broad spectrum antibiotic, chloramphenicol (Chloromycetin) to treat the peritonitis, which is secondary to the ruptured appendix. Which one of the following should the nurse monitor to detect a life-threatening adverse reaction associated with this drug?

   ○ 1. Complete blood count
   ○ 2. Serum electrolytes
   ○ 3. Serum enzyme levels
   ○ 4. Routine urinalysis

Mr. Phillip Kauffman has noted blood in his stool for the past 6 months. He is seeing his physician because of this concern.

67 Besides rectal bleeding, which one of the following data in Mr. Kauffman's history indicates that he may have colon cancer?
   ○ 1. His bowel habits have changed.
   ○ 2. He has difficulty swallowing.
   ○ 3. He experiences chronic indigestion.
   ○ 4. Some foods give him intestinal gas.

68 The nurse prepares Mr. Kauffman for a sigmoidoscopy examination. Which one of the following indicates that the client needs more teaching? Mr. Kauffman says that
   ○ 1. he should sit on the toilet to give himself an enema.
   ○ 2. he can eat a light diet the evening before the examination.
   ○ 3. a flexible scope will be inserted into his rectum.
   ○ 4. this test is routinely performed on an outpatient basis.

69 The nurse who will be assisting with the sigmoidoscopy would be most correct in placing Mr. Kauffman in which position?
   ○ 1. Lithotomy
   ○ 2. Knee–chest
   ○ 3. Orthopneic
   ○ 4. Fowler's

Mr. Kauffman will undergo a bowel resection to remove the cancerous tumor.

70 A low-residue diet is prescribed for Mr. Kauffman during the preoperative period. Which of the following foods must the nurse indicate is *contraindicated* for him?
   ○ 1. Ground meat
   ○ 2. Bran cereal
   ○ 3. Orange juice
   ○ 4. Baked fish

71 Preoperatively Mr. Kauffman is to receive 1 g of neomycin sulfate (Mycifradin) orally every hour for four doses and then 1 g orally every 4 hours for the balance of the 24 hours. If the tablets come in a dosage strength of 500 mg per tablet, how many tablets should the nurse administer each time?
   ○ 1. ½ tablet
   ○ 2. 1 tablet
   ○ 3. 2 tablets
   ○ 4. 4 tablets

72 Mr. Kauffman asks the nurse why he must take the neomycin sulfate. The most accurate explanation in this situation is that it is given to
   ○ 1. treat any current infection he may have.
   ○ 2. suppress the growth of intestinal bacteria.
   ○ 3. prevent the onset of postoperative diarrhea.
   ○ 4. reduce the number of bacteria near the incision.

Ms. Frances Bucher has a distended abdomen. She is quite nauseated and has been experiencing persistent vomiting for the last 48 hours.

73 Which one of the following questions would be important for the nurse to ask to determine if Ms. Bucher has an intestinal obstruction?
   ○ 1. "When did you last eat a full meal?"
   ○ 2. "How much fluid are you vomiting?"
   ○ 3. "Does the emesis appear to contain feces?"
   ○ 4. "Has your appetite changed appreciably?"

The physician decides to insert a Miller-Abbott intestinal tube into Ms. Bucher.

74 Unlike a nasogastric tube, the main difference in the nursing care of the client with intestinal decompression is that immediately after the tube's insertion, the nurse would *not*
   ○ 1. stabilize the tube to the nose or face.
   ○ 2. connect the tube to mechanical suction.
   ○ 3. irrigate the tube to keep it patent.
   ○ 4. offer the client sips of water or ice.

The obstruction is not relieved. Ms. Bucher is scheduled for a laparotomy.

75 Ms. Bucher's preoperative orders include giving her meperidine hydrochloride (Demerol) 75 mg and atropine sulfate intramuscularly. The meperidine comes dispensed in a prefilled cartridge. It states that there is 100 mg/mL of meperidine in the cartridge. What volume of drug should the nurse give to administer 75 mg?
   ○ 1. 0.10 mL
   ○ 2. 0.25 mL
   ○ 3. 0.50 mL
   ○ 4. 0.75 mL

76 The written order for the atropine sulfate indicates that the nurse should administer 5 mg intramuscularly. The usual adult preoperative dose is 0.4 to 0.6 mg. Which nursing action is best at this time?
   ○ 1. Give a common preoperative dose of atropine.
   ○ 2. Administer just the meperidine at this time.
   ○ 3. Hold all the medication and notify the physician.
   ○ 4. Consult the pharmacist on the action to take.

77 The primary purpose for giving atropine sulfate to Ms. Bucher preoperatively is to

○ 1. dilate her pupils.
○ 2. relieve her anxiety.
○ 3. produce sleepiness.
○ 4. decrease secretions.

During surgery Ms. Bucher's bowel was found to be twisted. A portion of gangrenous bowel was removed and a colostomy was performed.

78 The nurse inspects Ms. Bucher's stoma postoperatively. Which one of the following findings indicates that the stoma's appearance is *normal*? The stoma appears
○ 1. pink and dry.
○ 2. red and moist.
○ 3. brown and wet.
○ 4. purple and sticky.

79 Ms. Bucher has a nasogastric tube in place. If all of the following nursing orders appear on her plan of care, which one should the nurse question because it is potentially unsafe?
○ 1. Encourage liberal fluid intake every hour.
○ 2. Offer throat lozenges every 4 hours as needed for discomfort.
○ 3. Irrigate nasogastric tube if drainage stops.
○ 4. Give oral hygiene every 4 hours during the day and as needed.

80 A few days after surgery, the physician orders the nurse to begin daily colostomy irrigations. Which position would be best for the client when carrying out this procedure?
○ 1. Lying on the left side
○ 2. Sitting on the toilet
○ 3. Standing at the sink
○ 4. Kneeling in the bathtub

81 During a conversation concerning her feelings about the colostomy, Ms. Bucher becomes silent. At this time it would be best for the nurse to
○ 1. change the subject to something more pleasant.
○ 2. refrain from interjecting comments or questions.
○ 3. provide information about care of the colostomy.
○ 4. offer a referral for psychologic counseling.

82 Ms. Bucher says to the nurse, "How will I ever adjust to this colostomy." In this case it would be best for the nurse to
○ 1. encourage the client to express her concerns.
○ 2. reassure her that adjustment will come with time.
○ 3. recommend she investigate care in a nursing home.
○ 4. say nothing, but quote her statement in the chart.

NURSING CARE OF CLIENTS WITH DISORDERS OF THE RECTUM AND ANUS

When a nurse visits a senior citizens' community meal site, several elderly individuals discreetly ask questions concerning constipation.

83 A person verbalizes her concerns about not having a daily bowel movement. The nurse would be most accurate in identifying that the *least* appropriate evidence of constipation is the
○ 1. frequency of defecation.
○ 2. consistency of the feces.
○ 3. effort in passing stool.
○ 4. volume of stool passed.

84 A gentleman tells the nurse that he cannot have a bowel movement without taking a daily laxative. What information is most essential for the nurse to explain?
○ 1. Chronic use of laxatives impairs natural bowel tone.
○ 2. Stool softeners are likely to be less harsh for him.
○ 3. Daily enemas would be more preferable than laxatives.
○ 4. Dilating the anal sphincter may aid bowel elimination.

85 Someone asks the nurse if there are any over-the-counter laxatives that should be avoided. It would be best for the nurse to explain that frequent use of which laxative can interfere with absorption of fat-soluble vitamins?
○ 1. Milk of magnesia
○ 2. Cascara sagrada
○ 3. Mineral oil
○ 4. Castor oil

A nurse who works at a nursing home cares for several individuals with bowel elimination problems.

86 Mr. John Carlson tells the nurse that he has a feeling of fullness in the rectum and is experiencing abdominal cramping. Which one of the following is an indication that the client may have a *fecal impaction*? Mr. Carlson
○ 1. passes small amounts of liquid stool.
○ 2. has extremely offending bad breath.
○ 3. requests medication for a headache.
○ 4. has not been eating well lately.

87 Which one of the following physical assessment techniques should the nurse plan to use to determine if a client has a fecal impaction?
○ 1. Auscultate the bowel sounds.
○ 2. Measure the abdominal girth.
○ 3. Insert a finger within the rectum.
○ 4. Inspect the appearance of the anus.

88 Ms. Edna Walker has a distended abdomen. She says she has "gas pains" but has not been able to pass

any flatus. Before inserting a rectal tube, which one of the following nursing measures would be most helpful for eliminating accumulating intestinal gas?
- ○ 1. Ambulate the client in the hall.
- ○ 2. Provide a carbonated beverage.
- ○ 3. Restrict the intake of solid food.
- ○ 4. Administer a narcotic analgesic.

89 If a rectal tube becomes necessary to relieve a client's distention and discomfort, what length of time should the nurse plan to leave the tube in place each time it is used?
- ○ 1. 5 minutes
- ○ 2. 20 minutes
- ○ 3. 45 minutes
- ○ 4. 1 hour

90 The nursing team gathers to discuss approaches for dealing with the bowel incontinence of a client. Which one of the following should be planned first before beginning bowel retraining?
- ○ 1. Limit the client's daytime physical activity.
- ○ 2. Record the time of day when incontinence occurs.
- ○ 3. Decrease the amount of food eaten at each meal.
- ○ 4. Empty the client's bowel with a soapsuds enema.

91 During the administration of a cleansing soapsuds enema, a client experiences cramping and has the urge to defecate. Which is the *best* nursing action at this time?
- ○ 1. Quickly finish instilling the remaining solution.
- ○ 2. Tell the client to hold his or her breath and bear down.
- ○ 3. Briefly stop the administration of the enema solution.
- ○ 4. Withdraw the tip of the enema tubing from the rectum.

92 The nurse prepares to insert a bisacodyl (Dulcolax) suppository to relieve a client's constipation. Which one of the following nursing actions is *inappropriate* when inserting the suppository? The nurse
- ○ 1. dons a clean glove on the dominant hand.
- ○ 2. positions the client on the left side.
- ○ 3. inserts the suppository approximately ½ in.
- ○ 4. tells the client to retain it briefly.

Mr. George Owens says his rectum is painful and itchy following a bowel movement. He also has observed that he has been passing blood with his stool. After an examination the physician tells him that the cause of his symptoms is hemorrhoids.

93 If Mr. Owens understands his physician's explanation of hemorrhoids, he will describe them as being
- ○ 1. swollen veins.
- ○ 2. tissue polyps.

- ○ 3. shallow ulcers.
- ○ 4. vascular tumors.

94 The nurse reviews Mr. Owens' health history. Which of the following most probably contributed to his developing hemorrhoids?
- ○ 1. He follows a low-sodium diet.
- ○ 2. He does not tolerate milk well.
- ○ 3. He is frequently constipated.
- ○ 4. He works as an accountant.

95 Besides increasing his consumption of bulk-forming foods, such as whole grains, fresh fruits, and vegetables, the best diet instruction the nurse can give Mr. Owens is to
- ○ 1. eat small meals frequently.
- ○ 2. drink eight glasses of fluid per day.
- ○ 3. avoid snacking between meals.
- ○ 4. reduce the intake of refined sugar.

Mr. Owens undergoes a hemorrhoidectomy.

96 The nurse gives Mr. Owens a sitz bath. Which one of the following is the best indication of its effectiveness?
- ○ 1. The client says his rectum is less painful.
- ○ 2. The client has no evidence of body odor.
- ○ 3. The client indicates that he feels refreshed.
- ○ 4. The client's body is pink, warm, and clean.

97 The physician prescribes docusate potassium (Dialose) for Mr. Owens. This drug promotes the retention of water in the stool. The nurse explains that the purpose for this medication is to
- ○ 1. ease bowel evacuation and its related discomfort.
- ○ 2. irritate the bowel and promote stool elimination.
- ○ 3. stimulate peristalsis to move wastes after digestion.
- ○ 4. reduce intestinal activity and decrease stool size.

Mr. Robert Park is admitted for the surgical treatment of a pilonidal cyst.

98 When the nurse performs the admission assessment, which of the following is a *common* finding among individuals with this diagnosis?
- ○ 1. There is a history of intermittent rectal bleeding.
- ○ 2. There is an open draining area near the coccyx.
- ○ 3. The client has experienced frequent bouts of diarrhea.
- ○ 4. The client has very little or baby fine anorectal hair.

Mr. Howard White is being treated for an anal fissure.

99 Which one of the following descriptions indicates that Mr. White correctly understands his condition? The client says that a fissure is a

 1. discolored skin area.
 2. flaking area of skin.
 3. fluid-filled pouch.
 4. narrow slit in tissue.

100 The physician recommends that Mr. White purchase and apply an over-the-counter anesthetic ointment called dibucaine (Nupercainal) to his anus to relieve the localized pain. Which one of the following drug application instructions would be essential for the nurse to provide?
 1. Use gloves when applying the ointment.
 2. Store the ointment in the refrigerator.
 3. Apply the ointment just before defecating.
 4. Clean the area before applying the drug.

NURSING CARE OF CLIENTS WITH DISORDERS OF THE GALLBLADDER

Ms. Beverly Fuller is being treated for cholecystitis, an inflamed gallbladder.

101 When Ms. Fuller describes her discomfort to the nurse, she is most likely to indicate that the pain she experiences becomes worse
 1. shortly after eating food.
 2. especially on an empty stomach.
 3. following periods of activity
 4. before arising in the morning.

102 Generally the pain from cholecystitis is localized in the right upper quadrant of the abdomen. However, if Ms. Fuller had referred pain, she would most likely describe to the nurse that it is felt
 1. in the right shoulder.
 2. in the midepigastrium.
 3. up the neck or jaw
 4. down the left arm.

103 The nurse reviews Ms. Fuller's medical record. If the cause of her inflamed gallbladder is due to cholelithiasis, which one of the following laboratory test results is a common finding? Ms. Fuller, like most individuals who develop stones in the gallbladder, will have a(n)
 1. low red blood cell count.
 2. low level of hemoglobin.
 3. elevated cholesterol level.
 4. elevated serum albumin.

104 A low-fat diet is prescribed for Ms. Fuller. After the dietitian explains the diet to Ms. Fuller, which one of the following statements indicates that Ms. Fuller needs *more* teaching. The client says she may eat
 1. broiled chicken.
 2. baked meatloaf.
 3. fried fish.
 4. roast turkey.

Ms. Edgerton, who was just admitted, will be having a battery of diagnostic x-rays. Tomorrow she is scheduled for a cholecystography, an x-ray of the gallbladder. The night before the test, the nurse is to administer several oral tablets that will facilitate a sharp x-ray image.

105 What information is essential for the nurse to know before administering the contrast substance to a client undergoing an x-ray of the gallbladder?
 1. Can the client tolerate holding still?
 2. How many x-rays has the client had?
 3. Is the client allergic to iodine?
 4. Does the client want any anesthesia?

The gallbladder is not visualized by cholecystography. An ultrasound of the gallbladder is scheduled for Ms. Edgerton.

106 Following the nurse's explanation of this test, which one of the following indicates that Ms. Fuller has an *accurate* understanding of the preparation for an ultrasound of the gallbladder? The client says that the preparation for this test involves
 1. withholding food for approximately 8 to 12 hours.
 2. drinking a container of barium just before the x-ray.
 3. eating a large test meal the night before the x-ray.
 4. inserting a large needle within one of the arm veins.

The ultrasound of Ms. Edgerton's gallbladder reveals that it is grossly enlarged and filled with many stones.

107 If gallstones obstruct the flow of bile, the nurse can expect that the client's stools will be
 1. black and tarry.
 2. light clay colored.
 3. very dark brown.
 4. greenish yellow.

The physician recommends that Ms. Edgerton have a cholecystectomy.

108 Ms. Edgerton's physician prescribes an intramuscular injection of menadiol sodium diphosphate (Synkayvite), a water-soluble derivative of vitamin K, on the day before surgery. When the client asks the nurse to explain the purpose for this drug, it would be most accurate to say it is used to promote
 1. wound healing.
 2. liver function.
 3. general health.
 4. blood clotting.

109 The prescribed dose of menadiol sodium diphosphate is 10 mg. The drug is supplied in a dosage strength of 5 mg/mL. The nurse prepares 2 mL of the drug. When selecting an intramuscular injection site, which one of the following should the nurse plan to *avoid* using?
 1. Dorsogluteal
 2. Ventrogluteal
 3. Vastus lateralis
 4. Deltoid

The surgeon performs a cholecystectomy on Ms. Edgerton. The client returns with a nasogastric tube, a T-tube for bile drainage, and a Jackson-Pratt tube for wound drainage.

110   When inspecting the tubes, which of the following would indicate to the nurse that the T-tube drainage is the color that should be expected? The color of the drainage is
   ○ 1. dark red or pale pink.
   ○ 2. clear or transparent.
   ○ 3. bright red or orange.
   ◉ 4. greenish yellow or brown.

111   The nurse prepares to change the abdominal dressing. Which of the following is the best technique for cleaning around the T-tube? Using an antiseptic,
   ○ 1. swab from the distal end of the tube toward the wound.
   ○ 2. wipe in a circular fashion toward the wound.
   ◉ 3. start at the wound and wipe in a circular fashion outward.
   ○ 4. rub back and forth where the tube exits from the skin.

112   The nurse empties the drainage in the Jackson-Pratt bulb reservoir before ambulating Ms. Edgerton. Which nursing action is essential for reestablishing the negative pressure within this drainage device? The nurse must
   ◉ 1. compress the bulb reservoir, and close the drainage valve.
   ○ 2. open the drainage valve allowing the bulb to fill with air.
   ○ 3. fill the bulb reservoir with sterile normal saline.
   ○ 4. secure the bulb reservoir to the skin near the wound.

NURSING CARE OF CLIENTS WITH DISORDERS OF THE LIVER

Ms. Sara Colbert, a 20-year-old college student, goes to the university health service because she has developed a sudden onset of flu-like symptoms, such as elevated temperature, chills, headache, anorexia, fatigue, nausea, and vomiting.

113   When monitoring the results of the laboratory tests performed on Ms. Colbert, which one is most indicative to the nurse that the client's symptoms are related to a liver disorder?
   ○ 1. Serum potassium
   ○ 2. Serum creatinine
   ○ 3. Blood urea nitrogen
   ○ 4. Amino transferase *Transaminase*

Hepatitis A is determined to be the cause of Ms. Colbert's symptoms.

114   Ms. Colbert asks the nurse how she acquired hepatitis A. The most likely route of hepatitis A transmission is from
   ○ 1. contaminated feces.
   ○ 2. insect carriers.
   ○ 3. infected blood.
   ○ 4. wound drainage.

115   The nursing team plans the infection control measures needed for the care of Ms. Colbert. Which one of the following would be essential to identify on the plan for care?
   ○ 1. Wear gloves whenever entering the client's room.
   ○ 2. Don a mask and gown when providing direct care.
   ○ 3. Maintain the client in a private room at all times.
   ◉ 4. Perform vigorous handwashing after leaving the room.

Several of Ms. Colbert's friends call the health service because they are concerned about their own risks for acquiring hepatitis A.

116   To prevent the spread of hepatitis A among Ms. Colbert's family and friends, the nurse could recommend that close contacts receive
   ○ 1. antibiotic therapy.
   ◉ 2. serum immunoglobulin.
   ○ 3. hepatitis vaccination.
   ○ 4. anti-inflammatory drugs.

Mr. Kent Fontaine is admitted to determine the cause of his jaundice.

117   When the nurse performs a physical assessment, the location where jaundice is first likely to be observed is in the
   ○ 1. stool.
   ○ 2. urine.
   ◉ 3. sclera.
   ○ 4. retina.

118   Rather than use the word jaundice in the assessment note, the nurse chooses to write an objective description of the client's skin color. The most accurate term the nurse can use to describe the color of jaundice is
   ○ 1. pink.
   ○ 2. blue.
   ○ 3. brown.
   ◉ 4. yellow.

119   Mr. Fontaine tells the nurse that his skin itches terribly. Which one of the following additions to the care plan would be appropriate for helping the client manage his discomfort?
   ○ 1. Discontinue all bathing temporarily.
   ◉ 2. Use only lanolin soap for bathing.
   ○ 3. Apply rubbing alcohol to skin.
   ○ 4. Provide a shower rather than a tub bath.

The cause of Mr. Fontaine's jaundice is hepatitis B infection.

120 Which one of the following facts in the client's social history would indicate to the nurse a possible source for acquiring hepatitis B infection? Mr. Fontaine
   ○ 1. lived in Alaska.
   ○ 2. is homosexual.
   ○ 3. abuses alcohol.
   ○ 4. is a carpenter.

121 Mr. Fontaine's appetite is very diminished. Besides asking that small, high-calorie foods be sent several times a day, which other approach may promote a higher intake of food?
   ○ 1. Request food the client particularly likes.
   ○ 2. Notify the dietitian to prepare only cold food.
   ○ 3. Ask that all desserts and sweets be eliminated.
   ○ 4. Restrict the amount of animal protein he eats.

122 Before discharging a client with hepatitis B, it is essential that the nurse inform him that for the remainder of his lifetime he must avoid
   ○ 1. sexual activity.
   ○ 2. donating blood.
   ○ 3. active exercise.
   ○ 4. foreign travel.

Mr. Nathan Gobel is seeking medical attention because he has been vomiting blood and passing bloody stools.

123 If Mr. Gobel has advanced cirrhosis of the liver, which one of the following signs will the nurse most likely find during the physical assessment?
   ○ 1. There will be excessive body hair.
   ○ 2. The abdomen will appear distended.
   ○ 3. The skin will look slightly cyanotic.
   ○ 4. Bowel sounds may be loud and hyperactive.

124 The nurse talks with Mr. Gobel's wife while he is changing into his hospital gown. If the client's wife mentions all of the following information, which one is most likely related to the development of cirrhosis?
   ○ 1. Mr. Gobel is a heavy user of alcohol.
   ○ 2. Mr. Gobel is a Viet Nam veteran.
   ○ 3. Mr. Gobel has osteoarthritis.
   ○ 4. Mr. Gobel has hypertension.

125 When the nurse inspects Mr. Gobel's skin, which of the following findings is *common* among individuals with cirrhosis?
   ○ 1. Spider-like blood vessels on the face
   ○ 2. Red butterfly pattern on the cheeks
   ○ 3. Patches of silvery scales on the elbows
   ○ 4. Multiple brown pigmented moles on the body

126 The nursing care plan indicates that the nurse should monitor Mr. Gobel's ascites each day. To carry out this nursing order, which one of the following nursing actions is appropriate?
   ○ 1. The apical and radial pulse rate should be counted.
   ○ 2. The lying and sitting blood pressure should be taken.
   ○ 3. The specific gravity of the urine should be checked.
   ○ 4. The circumference of the abdomen should be measured.

The physician tells Mr. Gobel that there is a danger in performing a liver biopsy. Instead, a magnetic resonance imaging (MRI) test will be performed.

127 The client asks the nurse what kind of danger the physician was referring to when he decided against doing a liver biopsy. The nurse would be accurate in identifying that the greatest risk associated with liver biopsy is
   ○ 1. hemorrhage.
   ○ 2. infection.
   ○ 3. blood clots.
   ○ 4. collapsed lung.

The MRI reveals hepatic cirrhosis and a large amount of fluid in the peritoneal cavity. A paracentesis is planned.

128 Which one of the following nursing actions is essential prior to assisting with the paracentesis? The nurse should
   ○ 1. ask the client to void.
   ○ 2. withhold food and water.
   ○ 3. insert a nasogastric tube.
   ○ 4. obtain a suction machine.

The physician prescribes the diuretic spironolactone (Aldactone) for Mr. Gobel.

129 The nurse would be most accurate in explaining to Mr. Gobel that the reason this particular type of diuretic is used is that it not only helps excrete water, it also
   ○ 1. limits the level of magnesium.
   ○ 2. conserves the supply of calcium.
   ○ 3. reduces the elimination of sodium.
   ○ 4. spares the excretion of potassium.

130 When administering an intramuscular injection to Mr. Gobel or any client with a liver disorder, which nursing action would be essential to perform?
   ○ 1. Cleanse the site with povidone-iodine (Betadine).
   ○ 2. Inject volumes of 1 mL or less in any one site.
   ○ 3. Use glass syringes rather than disposable plastic.
   ○ 4. Apply pressure longer than usual to the injection site.

Mr. John Foster is being treated for hepatic encephalopathy, which is secondary to cirrhosis.

131 Which laboratory test result would be most important for the nurse to monitor to assess the severity of Mr. Foster's condition?
○ 1. Serum creatinine
○ 2. Serum bilirubin
○ 3. Blood ammonia
○ 4. Blood urea nitrogen

132 Mr. Foster is on a low-protein diet to reduce the formation of the chemical that is toxic to his brain. If Ms. Foster asks the nurse if she can bring her husband some food from a fast food restaurant, which one of the following would be allowed?
○ 1. A milkshake
○ 2. A cheeseburger
○ 3. Chicken nuggets
○ 4. Onion rings

133 Which one of the following assessments would indicate to the nurse that Mr. Foster is bleeding from somewhere in his upper gastrointestinal tract?
○ 1. He has midepigastric pain.
○ 2. He feels very nauseated.
○ 3. His stools are black.
○ 4. His abdomen is distended.

134 A laxative and cleansing enema are ordered to remove blood that may be present in the intestine. When giving the enema to Mr. Foster, the nurse should insert the tip of the tubing a distance of approximately
○ 1. 1 to 2 in (2.5 to 5 cm).
○ 2. 3 to 4 in (7.5 to 10 cm).
○ 3. 6 to 8 in (15 to 20 cm).
○ 4. 9 to 10 in (22.5 to 25 cm).

135 Which one of the following assessment findings would most indicate that Mr. Foster's condition is worsening?
○ 1. He is difficult to arouse.
○ 2. His urine output is 100 mL/h.
○ 3. He snores when he is asleep.
○ 4. His blood pressure is 122/60

The seriousness of Mr. Foster's condition is explained to his wife. Ms. Foster is prepared for the possibility of her husband's death.

136 Ms. Foster cries as she recalls various significant events she and her husband shared together. Which action would be most therapeutic for the nurse at this time?
○ 1. Tell her to call a close family member.
○ 2. Listen to her express her thoughts.
○ 3. Suggest that she write in a diary.
○ 4. Ask about her future plans in life.

NURSING CARE OF THE CLIENT WITH DISORDERS OF THE PANCREAS

Mr. Raymond Stafford is brought to the emergency department because he has severe upper abdominal pain that came on suddenly a few hours ago. Nothing has relieved his pain. The nurse observes that the client is curled in a fetal position and is rocking back and forth.

137 Which one of the following nursing actions would help the nurse most to further assess Mr. Stafford's pain?
○ 1. Determine if the client can stop moving about.
○ 2. Ask the client to rate his pain from 1 to 10.
○ 3. Observe if the client is perspiring heavily.
○ 4. Give the client a prescribed pain-relieving drug.

138 Which one of the following laboratory tests, if elevated, is the best indication that Mr. Stafford's pain is caused by pancreatitis?
○ 1. Serum bilirubin
○ 2. Serum amylase
○ 3. Lactose tolerance
○ 4. Glucose tolerance

139 The charge nurse prepares to insert a gastric sump tube. So that the distal end will be located in the client's stomach, the nurse should place the tip of the tube at the client's nose and measure the distance from there to
○ 1. the jaw and then midway to the sternum.
○ 2. the mouth and then between the nipples.
○ 3. the midsternum and then to the umbilicus.
○ 4. the ear and then to the xiphoid process.

140 Before inserting the gastric sump tube, the assisting nurse watches the charge nurse inspect the nose to determine which nostril is larger and straighter. Which one of the following is *another* appropriate assessment technique used to select the nostril for inserting a nasogastric tube? The nurse occludes one nostril at a time and asks the client to
○ 1. sniff.
○ 2. exhale.
○ 3. smell a substance.
○ 4. blow air forcefully.

141 To aid in passing the gastric tube through the nose and pharynx the charge nurse lubricates the tip well. Which one of the following substances would be appropriate to use?
○ 1. An adhesive liquid, such as tincture of benzoin
○ 2. A water-soluble lubricant, such as K-Y jelly
○ 3. An oil-based lubricant, such as petroleum jelly
○ 4. An insoluble oil, such as mineral oil

142 Once the gastric sump tube is in the pharynx, which one of the following instructions from the nurse will help avoid placing the tube into the client's trachea? Tell the client to
○ 1. lower his chin to his chest.
○ 2. bend his head backward.
○ 3. turn his face to the side.
○ 4. keep his head perfectly straight.

143 Which one of the following actions would be most helpful for passing the gastric sump tube into the stomach. The nurse could ask the client to
○ 1. recite a nursery rhyme during insertion.
○ 2. swallow air or water through a straw.
○ 3. sing a favorite song as the tube is passed.
○ 4. chew a saltine cracker or dry piece of bread.

144 Which one of the following would indicate that the nasogastric tube has entered the respiratory tract rather than the stomach? The client turns blue, coughs, or
○ 1. cannot speak.
○ 2. cannot swallow.
○ 3. begins to sneeze.
○ 4. begins to vomit.

145 Mr. Stafford's fluid and nutritional needs are temporarily being met by administering intravenous fluid. While assessing the infusion, what finding should be reported to the charge nurse immediately?
○ 1. The tubing is coiled on the top of the mattress.
○ 2. The fluid is infusing in the client's dominant hand.
○ 3. The container has approximately 250 mL of fluid left.
○ 4. The intravenous site is pink, swollen, and tender.

146 After being kept NPO (nothing by mouth) for several days, Mr. Stafford is eventually placed on a bland, low-fat diet. If all of the following foods are on his breakfast tray, which one should the nurse *question*?
○ 1. Stewed prunes
○ 2. Skim milk
○ 3. Scrambled eggs
○ 4. Whole wheat toast

147 Before discharging Mr. Stafford, what information is essential for him to receive? The nurse must tell Mr. Stafford that for the rest of his life he must avoid
○ 1. donating blood.
○ 2. lifting heavy objects.

○ 3. drinking alcohol.
○ 4. taking laxatives.

Ms. Irene Blake is admitted with the diagnosis of cancer of the pancreas.

148 If Ms. Blake is typical of most others who develop cancer of the pancreas, the nurse can expect that one of the earliest problems for which the client sought treatment would be
○ 1. sharp pain.
○ 2. bleeding.
○ 3. jaundice.
○ 4. fainting.

Ms. Blake has constant pain in the upper abdomen and referred piercing pain in the back. The nurse notes that she regularly becomes uncomfortable 3 hours after receiving pain medication. Ms. Blake waits until her pain is almost unbearable before requesting an injection. Meperidine hydrochloride (Demerol), 50 mg, intramuscularly every 3 to 4 hours has been ordered for relief of pain.

149 Which of the following would be the best approach for the nurse to take to provide maximum comfort for Ms. Blake at this time?
○ 1. Give the medication immediately at her request.
○ 2. Offer the medication every 3 hours before she asks for it.
○ 3. Ask the physician to prescribe a higher dose.
○ 4. Administer the medication if the pain is severe.

Ms. Blake becomes thinner and weaker. She is no longer able to help with her hygiene.

150 During Ms. Blake's bath she says to the nurse, "Am I dying?" The best response from the nurse would be
○ 1. "Yes, I'm afraid that you are."
○ 2. "No, you are not going to die."
○ 3. "Do you think you are dying?"
○ 4. "Who would you like me to call?"

Correct Answers and Rationales

Two numbers appear in parentheses following each rationale. The first number identifies the textbook listed in the references, page 451, and the second number identifies the page(s) in that textbook on which the correct answer can be verified. Occasionally, two textbooks are given for verifying the correct answer.

Nursing Care of Clients with Disorders of the Gastrointestinal System and Accessory Organs of Digestion

NURSING CARE OF CLIENTS WITH DISORDERS OF THE MOUTH

1 3. Candidiasis causes small white patches on the mucous membrane of the mouth and tongue. Their appearance has been described as resembling milk curds. Red ulcerated patches near the margin of the teeth and gums are characteristic of gingivitis. Herpes simplex lesions are vesicles that become transformed to shallow ulcers. Herpes simplex is not restricted to the tongue. The last option does not describe any particular oral disease. (7:453)
Nursing Process—Collecting data
Client Need—Physiological integrity

2 2. An infection with the yeast organism, *Candida albicans*, is usually acquired from an overgrowth of normal flora found in and on the skin and mucous membranes of the gastrointestinal tract. Candidiasis is considered an opportunistic infection because the source of the infection is usually the client. Antibiotic therapy can upset the ecologic balance of organisms in the body, allowing some natural microbes to grow unchecked. Candidiasis is not transmitted from vectors, contaminated water, or food. Because the organisms are present in the mouth, it would be possible, but highly improbable, that the infection could be acquired by inhaling respiratory droplets from another individual. (7:453; 16:88)
Nursing Process—Implementation
Client Need—Health promotion/maintenance

3 3. Because nystatin is poorly absorbed from the gastrointestinal tract, holding the liquid suspension in the mouth as long as possible facilitates contact of the drug with the organism. The client is allowed to swallow the medication after swishing it around. There is no reason to use a straw or dilute the medication. (15:170)
Nursing Process—Planning
Client Need—Health promotion/maintenance

4 1. Factors that predispose to cancer of the mouth include any source of chronic irritation, such as holding a pipe in the mouth, holding chewing or smokeless tobacco in the mouth, consumption of alcohol, prolonged contact with rough dental appliances or jagged teeth. Wearing dentures for only 18 months is not generally long enough to cause cancerous changes. Certain processes for extracting caffeine have been linked with some forms of cancer but not cancer of the mouth. No hazards for cancer have been reported from chewing gum sweetened with aspartame (NutraSweet) at this time. (7:462; 16: 538)
Nursing Process—Collecting data
Client Need—Safe, effective care environment

5 2. Holding dentures over a basin of water or soft towel prevents breaking them if they slip from the hands. Hot water may warp the plastic from which some dentures are made. Oral adhesives do not require a special solvent for removal. Dentures should be kept moist to retain their fit and color. (18:101; 14:342)
Nursing Process—Implementation
Client Need—Physiological integrity

6 1. All emesis should be inspected to detect the presence of radioactive needles that may have been displaced. If one or more becomes dislodged, it should never be touched with the hands. It should be retrieved with long forceps and placed in a lead container. Bleach is not required for cleaning or disinfecting the emesis basin. There is no reason for using a plastic rather than metal emesis basin. The threads should never be cut; they should be counted each shift to make sure that the original number inserted are still present. (7:206; 14:709)
Nursing Process—Planning
Client Need—Safe, effective care environment

7 4. The lesions may also appear near the nose. It is possible to hand transfer the virus to the eyes and genital area. Handwashing and good personal hygiene must be used during the time the virus is replicating and being shed. All the other statements about herpes simplex I are true. (3:799; 7:730-731)

> Nursing Process—Evaluation
> Client Need—Health promotion/maintenance

8 2. Acyclovir does not cure the infection or prevent future outbreaks. It only shortens the time during which the virus is replicating and being shed. Some of the virus retreats within nerve fibers and escapes detection by the body's immune system where it remains dormant until stimulated. The drug is taken when the client first becomes aware of symptoms, such as an area of itching and tingling on the mucous membrane. Oral doses are generally taken for 10 days. (15:186-187; 7:731)

> Nursing Process—Evaluation
> Client Need—Health promotion/maintenance

9 1. The most important principle in cleaning the teeth and preventing decay is that all the surfaces of the teeth are brushed when performing oral hygiene. Though using a plaque-removing mouthwash is not inappropriate, it does not take precedence over brushing and flossing the teeth. The health of the teeth depends on a combination of conscientious daily care and regular dental checkups. A toothbrush should be replaced frequently, but replacing it is not the key to optimum oral care. (14:341; 18:102)

> Nursing Process—Implementation
> Client Need—Health promotion/maintenance

NURSING CARE OF CLIENTS WITH DISORDERS OF THE ESOPHAGUS

10 3. Food and fluid should be avoided to reduce the potential for aspiration. All other choices are incorrect because they involve eating or drinking. (7:199; 3:558)

> Nursing Process—Evaluation
> Client Need—Safe, effective care environment

11 2. Chewing food thoroughly will help the bolus slip through the narrowed stricture. Switching to baby food is too drastic at this time. Drinking liquids throughout a meal should be beneficial in thinning the bolus of food. Eliminating dairy products will not promote the ability to swallow food. (3:563; 14:862)

> Nursing Process—Implementation
> Client Need—Health promotion/maintenance

12 4. Chronic consumption of alcohol can damage the liver and interfere with blood flow from the esophagus and other abdominal organs. The hypertension created by the stagnation of blood causes esophageal veins to distend and bleed. None of the other facts in the client's social and medical history relate to his current condition. (3:565, 603; 16:598)

> Nursing Process—Collecting data
> Client Need—Safe, effective care environment

13 2. Dyspnea, hypotension, chest constriction, and back pain are some of the symptoms associated with an incompatibility reaction. An incompatibility reaction is life-threatening. The other assessments in this item are signs associated with hypovolemia. In this client's case the remaining signs and symptoms are probably due to blood loss. (18:675; 14:714)

> Nursing Process—Collecting data
> Client Need—Physiological integrity

14 4. A hiatal hernia results when a weakened area of the diaphragm allows a portion of the stomach to protrude into the esophagus. The acid contents of the stomach reflux into the esophagus causing irritation and inflammation, which the client describes as "heartburn." The remaining signs and symptoms are unrelated to the medical diagnosis. (14:862; 16:543)

> Nursing Process—Collecting data
> Client Need—Safe, effective care environment

15 3. An upright position for at least 2 hours after eating promotes the retention of swallowed food and gastric contents within the stomach by gravity. A person with a hiatal hernia is also encouraged to sleep with the head of his bed elevated. A client with this condition should eat small, frequent meals to avoid overdistending the stomach. Eating soft foods or eating when hungry has no effect on relieving the discomfort associated with this condition. (14:862; 16:545)

> Nursing Process—Planning
> Client Need—Health promotion/maintenance

16 3. The decomposition of swallowed food that becomes trapped in the blind pouches that form within the esophagus cause bad breath despite meticulous oral hygiene. The other assessments are unrelated to the data associated with esophageal diverticula. (16:542; 14:861)

> Nursing Process—Collecting data
> Client Need—Safe, effective care environment

17 2. Mechanical friction can further traumatize skin that has been affected by radiation. The skin can be cleaned with mild soap and tepid water and can be patted dry. The marks should never be removed because they are meant to remain on the skin throughout the interim of radiation therapy. The irradiated skin should be protected from direct sunlight. Clothing that covers the area of treatment should fit loosely. Powders containing metals should be avoided because they can absorb radiation and increase the potential for skin damage. (3:280; 14:708)

Nursing Process—Implementation
Client Need—Physiological integrity

18 2. It is essential to monitor the blood glucose levels frequently because TPN solutions contain high concentrations of glucose. Insulin coverage may be needed to maintain the blood sugar within an acceptable range. The specific gravity may become lower if the client begins to excrete higher volumes, but it is not generally monitored. Pulse pressure is the difference between the systolic and diastolic arterial pressure measurements. Pulse pressure usually is not affected by hyperalimentation. There would be no reason for taking the apical and radial pulses. (7:447; 3:567)

Nursing Process—Collecting data
Client Need—Safe, effective care environment

19 2. One of the best criteria that a client is responding favorably to TPN is a gradual and steady gain in weight. The client could remain alert despite improvement in his nutritional state. Hunger is both an emotional and physical phenomenon. Well-nourished, satiated people can feel hungry when they see, smell, or even think about food. The patient's tolerance of pain may increase with improved nutrition, but it would not be the best criterion for determining the effectiveness of TPN. (7:447; 18:153; 4:19)

Nursing Process—Evaluation
Client Need—Physiological integrity

20 3. It is important that the stomach not become overdistended. The stomach residual should be checked prior to administering an intermittent feeding. As a rule of thumb, the gastric residual should be no more than 100 to 150 mL of the previous intermittent feeding or, if continuous, no more than half of the previous hour's infusion volume. Raising the formula would cause the liquid nourishment to run in at a faster rate. Adding water to formula would add more volume. (18:150; 16:537)

Nursing Process—Implementation
Client Need—Physiological integrity

21 2. A nondirective approach is best for encouraging the client to discuss his feelings. Mr. Marvin is likely to deny feeling angry if asked a direct question. Telling him the situation may get better is false reassurance. The client knows the situation will not get better and will lose trust in the nurse's ability to be supportive. Just because "lots of people" are nourished by tube feedings doesn't necessarily make it easier for the client to cope. (17:67; 12:250)

Nursing Process—Implementation
Client Need—Psychosocial integrity

NURSING CARE OF CLIENTS WITH DISORDERS OF THE STOMACH

22 3. Individuals with peptic ulcers generally find that eating relieves their discomfort. The pain is caused by irritation of the eroded mucosa with hydrochloric acid and pepsin. Food tends to dilute the acid, thereby raising the *p*H of the secretions. This reduces irritation of the ulcerated tissue. Skipping a meal would increase the pain because the acid secretions would be very concentrated. Many ulcer clients report awakening at night with pain. Bending over would not cause or relieve the discomfort associated with an ulcer. (14:863; 7:467)

Nursing Process—Collecting data
Client Need—Physiologic integrity

23 3. A Hematest on stool can be performed by the nurse in the client's bathroom or dirty utility room. Blood in the stool is a significant finding. Its presence indicates that bleeding is occurring within the gastrointestinal tract. If the bleeding is occurring in the upper gastrointestinal tract, the stool will appear black. This finding is called *melana*. However, blood may be present without an obvious change in the normal color of stool. This finding is referred to as *occult blood*. Identifying blood in the stool is not proof that the client has an ulcer, but it aids the differential diagnosis. Albumin in the urine is a finding associated with kidney disease. Elevated glucose levels in the blood could be due to diabetes mellitus. Emesis is not tested for the presence of pepsin. (16:547; 14:863)

Nursing Process—Collecting data
Client Need—Physiological integrity

24 4. An upper gastrointestinal x-ray uses barium as a contrast medium. The client must drink the barium during the x-ray procedure. This opaque substance fills the hollow structures of the esophagus and stomach, improving their image. A gastroscopy involves inserting a flexible tube in the stomach. Intravenous dye may be used in some x-rays of the gallbladder. A client would be placed within a chamber when a computerized axial tomography scan is performed. (18:311; 14:848)

Nursing Process—Evaluation
Client Need—Safe, effective care environment

25 3. There is approximately 5 mL per teaspoon. The equivalent of 2 teaspoons is 10 mL. (15:9; 18:575)

Nursing Process—Implementation
Client Need—Physiological integrity

26 1. Constipation is a side effect of antacids containing aluminum and calcium. Antacids containing magnesium cause a laxative effect. None of the other symptoms the client described have been associated with antacid drug therapy. (15:275; 14:864)

Nursing Process—Collecting data
Client Need—Physiological integrity

27 2. Sucralfate forms a protective coating similar to mucus at the site of the ulcer. This layer then shields the irritated tissue from further irritation by hydrochloric acid and pepsin. Antacids neutralize gastric secretions, raising their pH. Histamine antagonists reduce gastric acid production by blocking H_2 receptors. (14:864; 15:271, 273)

Nursing Process—Implementation
Client Need—Health promotion/maintenance

28 1. Acetaminophen is the only safe analgesic in this list of drugs. Adverse reactions to acetaminophen include skin eruptions, hemolytic anemia, hypoglycemia, hepatotoxicity, and others. Acetaminophen is not associated with gastritis or ulcer formation. However, the link between salicylates, like aspirin, and the nonsteroidal anti-inflammatory drugs, like ibuprofen and naproxen, with ulcer formation and exacerbation is well documented. (14:863;3:574; 15:71-72)

Nursing Process—Planning
Client Need—Physiological integrity

29 2. When the stomach or other gastrointestinal structure perforates, the abdomen becomes very hard, rigid, and tender. The skin would become pale due to vasoconstriction associated with shock. Dilated pupils may be due to a variety of causes, such as mydriatic eye medication, eye surgery, cerebral anoxia, and so on. The respirations would be rapid, but this observation is not as significant as a tense abdomen. (14:864; 3:572)

Nursing Process—Collecting data
Client Need—Physiological integrity

30 2. Hearing a whooshing sound over the stomach as a bolus of air is instilled through the proximal end of the gastric tube is one method for determining placement. If the tube is in the esophagus, the client will belch. Another technique is to aspirate secretions from the tube and test the pH. If the secretions are coming from the stomach, the pH will be very acid. A portable x-ray would be an accurate method, but the cost and unnecessary radiation exposure make this method inappropriate. Liquids should never be instilled through a nasogastric tube until placement has been verified. If the tip was not in the stomach, aspiration could occur. Feeling for air is an unacceptable technique for determining placement. (18:139; 14:851)

Nursing Process—Collecting data
Client Need—Physiological integrity

31 1. The nurse offers the client a basis for hope by validating the conscientious efforts that are being made. The response is objective without giving false reassurance. The client may interpret the nurse's unwillingness to answer, in the second example, as an indication that his worst fear is confirmed. By implying that his serious question is frivolous, as in the third example, the client may be discouraged from attempting further communication about his fears and feelings. The last example shows a disregard for the client's unique perception and fears. (16:550; 14:470; 18:753)

Nursing Process—Implementation
Client Need—Psychosocial integrity

32 2. Splinting or supporting the incision promotes deeper inhalation and more forceful coughing. An explanation of his risks is not likely to encourage more active participation. Oxygen is not necessary unless respiratory complications occur, causing the client to become hypoxic. A high Fowler's position facilitates the potential for a larger volume of air, but unless the client actively uses his respiratory muscles, that will not happen. (14:448; 18:435)

Nursing Process—Planning
Client Need—Physiological integrity

33 4. This finding could be life-threatening. It would be important to use some comfort measure to relieve the sore throat, but the client's life is not endangered by the condition. The nurse could provide more frequent mouth care or offer the client sips of water or ice chips to relieve his thirst. The nurse could independently clean the nose with an applicator or moist face cloth. (7:471; 16:167)

Nursing Process—Implementation
Client Need—Safe, effective care environment

34 3. Any fluid instilled or removed should be recorded to maintain an accurate intake and output record. A nasogastric tube should be irrigated with normal saline, which does not have to be sterile. Oxygen should be administered prior to tracheobronchial suctioning. Swallowing will not affect a gastric tube irrigation. (18:152; 14:852)

Nursing Process—Implementation
Client Need—Physiological integrity

35 2. Consuming carbohydrates triggers the release of insulin, causing postparandial hypoglycemia. Therefore, to prevent this component of the dumping syndrome, postgastrectomy clients are taught to follow a low-carbohydrate diet. Fluids should not be consumed with meals because this increases the rapidity with which consumed food is dumped into the small intestine. Eating small meals is recommended for limiting the

bolus of food present in the stomach. Reducing the consumption of red meat is a healthy dietary change, but it will not prevent dumping syndrome. (16:553; 7:471)
　　Nursing Process—Evaluation
　　Client Need—Health promotion/maintenance

36 2. Lying down would delay the movement of food from the stomach into the small intestine. People with a hiatal hernia should sleep with the head of the bed elevated. Walking, meditation, and relaxation are healthy behaviors, but they are unrelated to preventing dumping syndrome. (16:553; 7:471)
　　Nursing Process—Planning
　　Client Need—Health promotion/maintenance

37 1. Absence of free hydrochloric acid in the stomach is associated with stomach cancer. This finding distinguishes the etiology of the symptoms from other causes, such as peptic ulcer, esophageal stricture, and so on. Gastrin is a hormone secreted by the mucosa of the pylorus and stomach. Gastrin causes hypersecretion of gastric acid. Gastritis is a common finding that can have multiple etiologies. The presence of a few red blood cells in the urine indicates blood loss within the urinary tract from conditions such as cystitis, glomerulonephritis, and others. (14:866; 16:549; 5:325)
　　Nursing Process—Collecting data
　　Client Need—Physiological integrity

38 3. Vitamin B_{12} cannot be absorbed in the absence of the stomach or absence of the intrinsic factor produced by the stomach. Regular injections of vitamin B_{12} are necessary following a total gastrectomy. Vitamins C and B_6 can be absorbed when nutrition is supplied orally or by other nutritional means, such as intestinal tube feeding or hyperalimentation. Vitamin K is synthesized by intestinal flora. It also is present in foods. Deficiency of vitamin K can occur when there is poor absorption of fats, as in gallbladder disease, celiac disease, ulcerative colitis, or when broad spectrum antibiotics such as neomycin sulfate and kanamycin (Kantrex) are administered. (7:464; 4:198)
　　Nursing Process—Implementation
　　Client Need—Health promotion/maintenance

NURSING CARE OF CLIENTS WITH DISORDERS OF THE SMALL INTESTINE

39 4. Stool specimens that may contain ova and parasites should be examined when the feces is fresh. Ova and parasites will not survive long below body temperature. Drying and cooling may destroy the organisms and result in invalid findings.

The client can use a bedpan or toilet for bowel elimination. The nurse can transfer a portion of stool to a waxed, covered container using a tongue blade. The specimen container need not be sterile. (14:371; 18:566; 5:228)
　　Nursing Process—Implementation
　　Client Need—Safe, effective care environment

40 2. The abbreviation *q.i.d.* means that the drug is to be administered four times a day. Scheduled hours may differ depending on the predetermined timetable set by the health agency. However, in following the order as it is written, administration can be no less or no more than four times during a 24-hour period. (18:577)
　　Nursing Process—Evaluation
　　Client Need—Safe, effective care environment

41 3. A clear liquid diet includes fat-free bouillon, tea or coffee, flavored gelatin, fruit ices, carbonated beverages like ginger ale, some clear fruit juices like apple and grape. Honey and sugar also may be used. No milk or milk products are permitted. (4:43; 14:245)
　　Nursing Process—Implementation
　　Client Need—Physiological integrity

42 1. A normal, stable blood pressure indicates that fluid volume is adequate in the extracellular and intracellular compartments. Blood is a component of body fluid. If fluid volumes are low within cells or in the interstitial spaces, intravascular fluid will move by osmosis to the areas of higher concentration. This depletion would cause the client to become hypotensive, feel light headed, and even faint during postural changes. Thirst is an indication that more fluid intake is needed. The lung sounds can remain clear despite dehydration. The urine in a well-hydrated person should be light yellow. (18:646-647; 16:112)
　　Nursing Process—Evaluation
　　Client Need—Physiological integrity

43 4. Fiber refers to the portion of fruits, vegetables, grains, and nuts that is not broken down and absorbed during the digestive process. Animal products are not a source of dietary fiber. Foods that require chewing is too limited a definition for fiber. The semisolid mass of food in the stomach is called chyme. (4:480-481; 14:221)
　　Nursing Process—Implementation
　　Client Need—Health promotion/maintenance

44 1. A fistula is an opening extending from one tissue surface to another. A polyp is a protruding mass. Hypertrophied scar tissue is referred to as a keloid. An abscess is a local collection of pus within injured or inflamed tissue. (14:286; 7:473)
　　Nursing Process—Evaluation
　　Client Need—Health promotion/maintenance

45 2. Ileal drainage contains enzymes and bile salts that are very damaging to the skin. There are not enough data indicating that the client is incontinent. Body image and depression are likely to occur whenever an individual develops a complication. However, standards for care would not be met if nursing measures for maintaining or restoring skin integrity were omitted from the nursing plan for care. (3:620; 16:581)
> Nursing Process—Planning
> Client Need—Physiological integrity

46 3. The most common cause of a hernia is performing an activity that increases intra-abdominal pressure, such as lifting heavy objects. When intra-abdominal pressure increases, it causes the intestine to protrude through areas in the abdominal musculature that are structurally weak. Discomfort related to ingesting milk products indicates lactose intolerance. Obesity accompanying inactivity does play a role in weakening abdominal muscles, but this person is reported to be thin. (3:579; 16:570)
> Nursing Process—Collecting data
> Client Need—Safe, effective care environment

47 4. A reducible hernia is one in which the protruding structures can be replaced in the abdominal cavity. Idiopathic is a term meaning without a known cause. A strangulated hernia is one that traps the intestine and cuts off its blood supply. An incarcerated hernia is another name for an irreducible hernia. This means that the protrusion is trapped and cannot be replaced. However, the blood supply is adequate. (16:570; 3:580)
> Nursing Process—Implementation
> Client Need—Safe, effective care environment

48 2. Docusate calcium is a stool softener that makes it easier to pass feces at the time of bowel elimination. Straining while having a bowel movement may make the abdominal defect larger or cause the intestine to become incarcerated or strangulated. This drug does not strengthen muscle tone, prevent spasm, or relieve pain. (3:579; 15:274)
> Nursing Process—Implementation
> Client Need—Health promotion/maintenance

49 2. The client's statement indicates that he has misunderstood his physician's explanation of the surgical procedure. For the consent to be valid, a person must understand that to which he is giving his consent. The physician is responsible for providing the explanation. The nurse is responsible for witnessing the client's signature and ensuring that the legal aspects of the contract are upheld. If the nurse determines that the client does not understand the information provided by the physician, the physician should be notified. If the client's misinformation is clarified, the surgery need not be canceled. The nurse should never allow a client to sign a contract he does not fully understand. An enema would only be given if the physician has written an order to do so. (18:76-77; 14:28; 7:102)
> Nursing Process—Implementation
> Client Need—Safe, effective care environment

50 4. To help prevent headaches after spinal anesthesia, it is customary to keep the client's head flat for 6 to 12 hours postoperatively. The remaining orders in this item are appropriate. (16:168; 7:114)
> Nursing Process—Implementation
> Client Need—Safe, effective care environment

51 2. A suspensory is used following a herniorrhaphy on a male patient to help prevent scrotal swelling. A suspensory does not prevent impotence, strain on the incision, or wound contamination. (16:571; 14:869)
> Nursing Process—Implementation
> Client Need—Health promotion/maintenance

52 1. To avoid undue strain and tension on the repaired muscle, the client should avoid any activity that increases intra-abdominal pressure. Coughing, heavy lifting, sneezing, and straining to have a bowel movement can lead to an incisional hernia until the repaired area has healed. (16:570; 14:869)
> Nursing Process—Planning
> Client Need—Health promotion/maintenance

53 1. The client with ulcerative colitis may have 12 or more diarrheal stools per day that contain blood and mucus along with fecal material. Bowel sounds are likely to be hyperactive. Striae are red or white streaks on the skin due to stretching. Because the client with ulcerative colitis suffers from weight loss and emaciation, this is not a common observation. Ulcers on the mucous membranes are confined to the colon. (16:560; 14:867)
> Nursing Process—Collecting data
> Client Need—Physiological integrity

54 3. Using a diaper on a person with fecal incontinence is usually emotionally distressing. It should be done only as a last resort, preferably with the client's permission. Keeping the bedside commode nearby, answering her signal promptly, and helping her to the bathroom frequently are acceptable methods for dealing with the urgency that results in incontinence. (18:552)
> Nursing Process—Planning
> Client Need—Psychosocial integrity

55 1. Reflecting is a response that lets the client know that both the content and the feelings are understood. The nurse avoids any emotional support or involvement by offering to arrange contact with the physician. Giving advice and disagreeing with a client are blocks to therapeutic communication. (9:139, 151)
Nursing Process—Implementation
Client Need—Psychosocial integrity

56 1. Once the preoperative medication is given, the side rails should be raised and the client instructed to remain in bed. Elimination and oral hygiene should be accomplished prior to giving the preanesthetic drugs. Meperidine and hydroxyzine would depress the central nervous system making it difficult for the client to remain alert during attempts at teaching leg exercises. (16:312; 18:443)
Nursing Process—Implementation
Client Need—Safe, effective care environment

57 3. A dropping blood pressure frequently suggests that the client is going into shock. A systolic pressure of 90 to 100 mm Hg indicates shock is approaching. Below 80 mm Hg, shock is present. Other signs of shock include a rapid, thready pulse; pale, cold, and clammy skin; rapid respirations; a falling body temperature; restlessness; and a decreased level of consciousness. (18:447; 16:167; 14:447)
Nursing Process—Evaluation
Client Need—Physiological integrity

58 1. The best time for changing an appliance and providing stomal care is when the bowel is somewhat inactive. This is usually in the morning before any food has been eaten. Exercise and eating tend to increase bowel activity, making it likely that intestinal contents will spill onto the skin if the procedure is done at that time. (16:580)
Nursing Process—Planning
Client Need—Physiological integrity

59 3. A mild soap and tepid water are most often recommended for cleaning the skin around the stoma. Patting the skin with cotton is ineffective for cleansing. Alcohol is drying and irritating to the skin. Scrubbing should be avoided because friction is likely to irritate the skin. (16:593; 18:560)
Nursing Process—Implementation
Client Need—Physiological integrity

60 2. The appliance opening should be large enough to avoid impairing circulation to the stoma, but small enough that ileal drainage will not damage the skin. There should be only a ¹⁄₁₆- to ¹⁄₈-in margin of skin exposed around the stoma. This allows room to attach the faceplate to the skin rather than to the stoma itself. However, it covers an adequate amount of skin to prevent excoriation due to contact with enzymes and bile salts in ileal drainage. The stomal opening should not be obstructed or stool will not be passed. The appliance would not remain adherent to the skin if only a ¹⁄₈-in margin was in contact with skin. The appliance must cover the stoma; the bag may or may not be directly at the waist or beltline. (18:560)
Nursing Process—Implementation
Client Need—Physiological integrity

61 4. Because the discharge from an ileostomy is high in water content, it is difficult for most to gain control of bowel elimination. It is realistic for people with an ileostomy to play tennis, swim, have sexual relations, get pregnant, and in general pursue careers and enjoy all manner of social activities. (3:623)
Nursing Process—Implementation
Client Need—Health promotion/maintenance

62 4. Appendicitis is an inflammation of the appendix. Infection often accompanies the inflammation. The white blood cells, also called leukocytes, increase when these conditions are present to wall off, destroy, or remove damaged tissue and pathogens. The bilirubin level is usually monitored on an adult with liver or gallbladder disease. The serum potassium would be important if the client had anorexia, vomiting, or diarrhea. The prothrombin time is generally monitored when the client is receiving the anticoagulant, warfarin sodium (Coumadin). (16:563; 14:869)
Nursing Process—Collecting data
Client Need—Physiological integrity

63 1. Fever accompanies the inflammation and infection of the appendix. The nurse should monitor the temperature at least every 4 hours and analyze its course. Following the trend of fever progression or regression helps to evaluate how the client is responding to treatment. Lung sounds ought to remain normal because uncomplicated appendicitis should not interfere with the exchange of air. The size of pupils would be assessed frequently on patients who have neurologic problems. The color of the urine should be observed and may change due to fluid volume deficit, but this assessment is not the most essential one to perform. (18:244; 14:374)
Nursing Process—Collecting data
Client Need—Physiological integrity

64 3. Applications of heat should be avoided whenever there is a possibility that abdominal discomfort is due to appendicitis. The heat will dilate blood vessels, increase swelling, and promote rupture of the veriform appendix. Withholding oral nourishment is advantageous if the symptoms are due to gastroenteritis or if emergency surgery is necessary. Pain generally limits activity. Because it did not in this case, the activity probably would not affect the course of the appendicitis. Acetaminophen is a nonsalicylate. It would lower a fever and relieve discomfort but would not predispose to rupturing the appendix. (14:870; 3:569)

Nursing Process—Evaluation
Client Need—Health promotion/maintenance

65 2. An open drain relies on gravity to remove secretions that are then deposited onto an absorbent dressing. Neither a lithotomy, recumbent, or Trendelenberg position would promote the collection of wound drainage near the drain. (18:480)

Nursing Process—Implementation
Client Need—Physiological integrity

66 1. Chloramphenicol is a potentially dangerous antibiotic. Its use is generally limited to severe infections in which less toxic drugs are ineffective or contraindicated. Serious and sometimes fatal blood dyscrasias have been documented as a result of its use. The nurse should observe for dropping erythrocyte, leukocyte, and thrombocyte cell counts. None of the other laboratory tests will reveal adverse reactions associated with the administration of chloramphenicol. (15:163)

Nursing Process—Collecting data
Client Need—Physiological integrity

67 1. A change in bowel habits is one of the seven danger signals for cancer identified by the American Cancer Society. Difficulty swallowing and indigestion also are warning signs of cancer. However, these symptoms are more likely associated with cancer of upper gastrointestinal structures, such as the esophagus and stomach. Most individuals experience an increased production of flatus from eating common gas-forming foods. (14:704)

Nursing Process—Collecting data
Client Need—Safe, effective care environment

68 1. An enema solution cannot be distributed very well in a sitting position. Overall there will be a less than desirable cleansing effect. Also, the person will usually experience a need to defecate sooner because of the pooling of solution within the rectum. (18:558; 5:747)

Nursing Process—Evaluation
Client Need—Safe, effective care environment

69 2. The knee–chest, also known as the genupectoral, position is appropriate for a sigmoidoscopic examination. In some cases a special bed or tilt table is used to help the client assume and maintain this position. A lithotomy position would be used for cystoscopy and vaginal examinations. An orthopneic position is helpful for promoting rest for dyspneic individuals. Fowler's position can be used for many reasons, one of which is improving ventilation. (18:307; 5:746)

Nursing Process—Implementation
Client Need—Safe, effective care environment

70 2. A low-residue diet contains no fruits, vegetables, or whole grain breads and cereals. Fruit and vegetable juices, with the exception of prune juice, are allowed in minimal amounts. Tender or ground meat can be eaten, as can refined carbohydrates, such as pasta. (4:480-481)

Nursing Process—Implementation
Client Need—Safe, effective care environment

71 3. There are 1000 mg in 1 g. To administer 1 g of neomycin the nurse should give the client two 500 mg tablets. A common formula to compute proper dosage is as follows (15:12; 18:574):

$$\frac{\text{dosage desired}}{\text{dosage on hand}} \times \text{quantity}$$

$$= \text{amount to administer}$$

$$\frac{1000 \text{ mg}}{500 \text{ mg}} \times 1 \text{ tablet} = \frac{1000}{500}$$

$$= 2 \text{ tablets to administer}$$

Nursing Process—Implementation
Client Need—Physiological integrity

72 2. During the operative procedure the bowel is opened, and the contents are likely to be transferred within the peritoneum. The neomycin destroys intestinal bacteria and reduces the risk of a postoperative infection. (15:163; 7:465)

Nursing Process—Implementation
Client Need—Health promotion/maintenance

73 3. When an obstruction interferes with the movement of intestinal contents toward the rectum for elimination, the client begins to experience distention and vomiting. At first the emesis contains gastric contents. As time passes the vomitus may contain fecal matter and have a foul odor. The other questions may be appropriate to ask, but they will not necessarily provide information associated with an intestinal obstruction. (7:461; 16:566)

Nursing Process—Collecting data
Client Need—Safe, effective care environment

74 1. While the intestinal tube is advancing further into the intestinal tract, the tube should not be taped to the client's face or pinned to the gown or bedding. There are multiple ports in intestinal tubes through which drainage and secretions

can be removed by suction. Intestinal tubes may need frequent irrigation to maintain their patency. Though the client is not allowed to drink or eat, small sips of water or ice chips may be offered to relieve a dry mouth. (15:535; 7:461)
Nursing Process—Implementation
Client Need—Safe, effective care environment

75 4. The nurse should use 0.75 mL to give the prescribed dose of 75 mg. A common formula to compute proper dosage is as follows (15:12; 18:580):

$$\frac{\text{dosage desired}}{\text{dosage on hand}} \times \text{quantity}$$

$$= \text{amount to administer}$$

$$\frac{75 \text{ mg}}{100 \text{ mg}} \times 1 \text{ mL} = \frac{75}{100}$$

$$= 0.75 \text{ mL to administer}$$

Nursing Process—Implementation
Client Need—Physiological integrity

76 3. Any written order that is unclear or unsafe must be questioned. This includes a drug dose that is higher or lower than the dosages given in approved references. The nurse should never administer a different dose until consulting with a physician. Written orders for combined preoperative medication indicate they should be given together. The pharmacist is a reliable source for obtaining drug information; however, the only person who can revise the order is the physician. (15:16; 18:582)
Nursing Process—Implementation
Client Need—Physiological integrity

77 4. The primary purpose for administering atropine sulfate preoperatively is to decrease oral and respiratory secretions. Atropine sulfate will dilate the pupils and produce drowsiness in some people, but this is not the primary reason for its preoperative use. (15:309-310)
Nursing Process—Implementation
Client Need—Safe, effective care environment

78 2. The stoma should appear pink or red. It should look shiny and feel moist because it is everted mucous membrane. A bluish or purple appearance indicates impairment of circulation to the stoma. This finding should be reported to the physician. The stoma should never appear brown or dry. (3:616; 16:578-580)
Nursing Process—Collecting data
Client Need—Physiological integrity

79 1. It is usual to restrict the intake of a client with a nasogastric tube to just a few ice chips or very small sips of water. A liberal fluid intake promotes the dilution and removal of a large quan-

tity of chemicals from the stomach. This predisposes the client to electrolyte and acid–base imbalances. Relieving throat discomfort and providing oral hygiene are appropriate nursing care. Irrigating a nasogastric tube is not unsafe. However, the nurse should follow the physician's written order or the agency's standards for care when carrying out this procedure. (18:140, 144, 679; 3:564)
Nursing Process—Implementation
Client Need—Physiological integrity

80 2. The best position for performing a colostomy irrigation is sitting on the toilet. This position and the environment simulate normal bowel elimination. The toilet also is convenient for hanging the distal end of the irrigating sleeve. The stool can be easily flushed away along with the drained irrigating solution. Because it may take some time for the bowel evacuation to be complete, clients often appreciate the privacy that the bathroom provides. If sitting on the toilet is not possible, provide privacy while the client sits on or in bed with the end of the sleeve placed within a bedpan. (18:562)
Nursing Process—Implementation
Client Need—Physiological integrity

81 2. Silence, when used appropriately, is a powerful means of communicating without verbalizing. Among other things, silence can convey acceptance, provide the client time to collect his thoughts, allow relief from emotionally charged content, and give the client the opportunity to proceed when ready. Changing the subject is nontherapeutic. It indicates that the nurse cannot handle the topic of conversation. Switching the discussion to physical care is a form of changing the subject. Active listening, rather than psychologic counseling, would be sufficient based on the data in the situation. (12:263)
Nursing Process—Implementation
Client Need—Psychosocial integrity

82 1. Encouraging the expression of concerns provides the client an opportunity to ventilate feelings without fear of retaliation. An open discussion can effectively lower a client's frustration level. Reassurance, in this case, is somewhat premature. The client needs to verbalize and clarify the specific problems she perceives. With the assistance of the nurse and other health care professionals, the client ought to achieve the ability to accomplish self-care. Maintaining the client's independence is more preferable than institutionalized care. Saying nothing may indicate to the client that the nurse prefers not to become involved with emotional problems. Quoting a client, however, is always appropriate when documenting information. (1:97; 17:67-68)

> Nursing Process—Implementation
> Client Need—Psychosocial integrity

NURSING CARE OF CLIENTS WITH DISORDERS OF THE RECTUM AND ANUS

83 4. Although a constipated stool is often small because it is lower in water content, the amount of stool is probably the most unreliable criterion. The volume of normal stool varies greatly with the amount and type of food a person eats. The consistency of the stool and the effort required for elimination are of more importance than the interval between defecations. (18:546)

> Nursing Process—Implementation
> Client Need—Health promotion/maintenance

84 1. Long-term use of laxatives causes the bowel to become sluggish because it is repeatedly subjected to artificial stimulation. Stool softeners are less harsh than laxatives. However, it would be best to determine the cause of the constipation and treat the etiology with life-style changes rather than continue to rely on pharmaceutical interventions. Daily enemas are just as habituating as laxative abuse. Dilating the anal sphincter is not usually a technique for promoting bowel elimination. (15:278; 18:547)

> Nursing Process—Implementation
> Client Need—Health promotion/maintenance

85 3. Mineral oil is a petroleum product that has lubricating properties. Humans lack the ability to digest and absorb mineral oil. It passes through the digestive system unchanged. Any fat-soluble vitamins present when food is consumed with mineral oil will not be absorbed. Occasional use of mineral oil, if taken at bedtime, may not be harmful, but frequent use should be avoided. None of the other laxatives interfere with the absorption of fat-soluble vitamins. (15:278; 4:518)

> Nursing Process—Implementation
> Client Need—Health promotion/maintenance

86 1. A client with a fecal impaction may expel liquid stool around the hardened mass. Bad breath is not usually a sign of constipation or fecal impaction. If halitosis is chronic, the nurse should suspect dental disease, ineffective oral hygiene, or esophageal diverticula. Headaches have been anecdotally associated with constipation, but a relationship has not been proven scientifically. Loss of appetite may be either the cause or the effect of impaired bowel elimination. Its presence is not necessarily an indication of a fecal impaction. (18:547; 3:189)

> Nursing Process—Collecting data
> Client Need—Physiological integrity

87 3. The only reliable method for confirming the presence of hard dry stool within the rectum is digital examination. The nurse should liberally lubricate a gloved finger and insert it within the client's rectum. If stool is present, the nurse may attempt to break up the mass of dry feces with a finger. This action may be preceded by the administration of an oil retention enema. Auscultating bowel sounds, measuring abdominal girth, and inspecting the anus are all appropriate physical assessment techniques, but they will not aid in determining if the client has a fecal impaction. (18:547; 7:291)

> Nursing Process—Planning
> Client Need—Physiological integrity

88 1. Activity promotes the movement of gas toward the anal sphincter where it can be released. Carbonated beverages can increase gas accumulation. Restricting food is inappropriate. It may prevent additional gas from forming, but it will not help eliminate what is already present. Narcotic analgesics tend to slow peristalsis and contribute to the retention of stool and intestinal gas. (18:550)

> Nursing Process—Implementation
> Client Need—Physiological integrity

89 2. A rectal tube should remain in place only approximately 20 to 30 minutes at one time when it is being used to help relieve distention from accumulating gas. Placement for only 5 minutes is not likely to achieve an optimal effect, yet longer than 30 minutes is unnecessary. The tube can be removed and replaced again in 1 to 2 hours if gas continues to accumulate. (18:551; 14:362)

> Nursing Process—Planning
> Client Need—Physiological integrity

90 2. Bowel elimination tends to occur in a cyclic pattern. Assessing the bowel elimination pattern should precede selecting interventions. Limiting activity would impair rather than promote bowel elimination. The diet should have adequate amounts of water and bulk-forming foods to help the client form soft, rather than constipated, stool. The regular administration of enemas may eventually help to regulate bowel elimination, but it would not be the first step in a bowel retraining program. (18:552; 14:768)

> Nursing Process—Planning
> Client Need—Physiological integrity

91 3. Interrupting the instillation of enema solution allows time for the bowel to adjust to the distention. Rapidly instilling the remaining solution may cause the client to lose control of his elimination. Taking deep breaths or panting rather than holding the breath will relieve some of the discomfort. To finish administering the remaining enema solution, the withdrawn tip will need to be reinserted. (18:555; 14:360)
Nursing Process—Implementation
Client Need—Physiological integrity

92 3. A rectal suppository should be inserted approximately 2 to 4 in. For the best effect, the suppository should be beyond the internal sphincter. A glove should be used to avoid contact with organisms in the rectum, stool, or blood. A left lateral position provides anatomic access to the rectal area. Retaining the suppository until feeling an urge to defecate will ensure its effectiveness. (18:553; 14:362)
Nursing Process—Implementation
Client Need—Physiological integrity

93 1. Hemorrhoids are dilated veins similar to varicose veins. A polyp is a mass of tissue protruding from mucous membrane. An ulcer is an area where the surface of the tissue is eroded. A tumor is an uncontrolled growth of tissue. (16:573; 7:473)
Nursing Process—Evaluation
Client Need—Health promotion/maintenance

94 3. Chronic constipation, hereditary factors, and conditions that increase venous pressure in the abdomen and pelvic area, such as pregnancy, ascites, and liver disease, foster the development of hemorrhoids. A low-sodium diet would tend to keep venous fluid volume within a low to normal level. Lactose intolerance is more likely to cause bloating, gaseousness, cramping, and diarrhea. An occupation that interferes with the use of the toilet when feeling the urge to defecate can predispose to constipation and the development of hemorrhoids. However, generally the work of an accountant would not fit that category. (16:573; 7:473)
Nursing Process—Collecting data
Client Need—Safe, effective care environment

95 2. The cellulose that remains after eating high-fiber foods absorbs water in the bowel. Lack of adequate fluid may make constipation more severe. None of the other recommendations will aid in preventing or eliminating constipation. (4:484; 18:546)
Nursing Process—Implementation
Client Need—Health promotion/maintenance

96 1. A sitz bath is primarily a comfort measure. The warmth of the water soothes the discomfort in the surgical area. Secondarily, a sitz bath keeps the incisional area clean and promotes healing. Because only the buttocks are submerged in water, evidence of personal hygiene is not an appropriate criterion for effectiveness. (3:582; 7:474)
Nursing Process—Evaluation
Client Need—Physiological integrity

97 1. Docusate potassium is a stool softener. Retaining water in the stool softens the mass and makes the stool easier and less painful to pass. Some categories of laxatives, like castor oil, stimulate bowel evacuation by irritating the intestinal mucosa. Bulk-forming laxatives, like psyllium (Metamucil), stimulate peristalsis by adding bulk and water to the stool. A drug that reduces intestinal activity would promote constipation rather than promote stool elimination. (15:274; 3:582)
Nursing Process—Implementation
Client Need—Health promotion/maintenance

98 2. A pilonidal cyst is actually a sinus with one or more openings onto the skin. Once the integrity of the skin is impaired, microorganisms enter and cause subsequent infection evidenced by purulent drainage. Neither rectal bleeding nor diarrhea are associated with a pilonidal cyst. The word pilonidal means a "nest of hair." The growth of stiff body hair in the anorectal area at puberty often precipitates irritation within the sinus tract. (3:582; 16:574)
Nursing Process—Collecting data
Client Need—Safe, effective care environment

99 4. A fissure is a cleft or crack in the skin or mucous membrane. A discolored skin area could fit the description of ecchymosis, nevi, freckles, and so on. Flaking skin is referred to as desquamation or scales. Among various possibilities, a fluid-filled pouch is a characteristic of a vesicle, abscess, and pustule. (14:720; 7:473)
Nursing Process—Evaluation
Client Need—Health promotion/maintenance

100 4. Cleaning the area where a topical medication will be applied ensures that it will be maximally absorbed. When the client will be applying a topical drug to himself, wearing gloves is not essential. Handwashing before and after the application, however, is important. For comfort an ointment that will be applied to a sensitive area should be kept at room temperature unless otherwise directed by the manufacturer. It is more appropriate to apply this type of medication immediately following a bowel movement, because pain would be greater at that time. In addition this drug can be routinely applied in the morning and evening. (18:588)

Nursing Process—Implementation
Client Need—Health promotion/maintenance

NURSING CARE OF CLIENTS WITH DISORDERS OF THE GALLBLADDER

101 1. The characteristic pain of cholecystitis comes on after eating. It is especially aggravated when the meal has a high fat content. Besides pain, the fat intolerance due to impaired flow of bile causes nausea, vomiting, distention, and flatulence. Ulcers are more likely to cause pain when the stomach is empty. Activity ought not to influence the discomfort of cholecystitis. The volume and type of food are more of a factor in the symptoms of gallbladder disease than the time of day. (7:485; 16:606)

Nursing Process—Collecting data
Client Need—Safe, effective care environment

102 1. The referred pain of cholecystitis is felt either in the right shoulder or some describe it as being in the back at the level of the shoulder blades. Ulcers and esophageal reflux cause pain felt in the midepigastric region. Angina pectoris may be experienced as pain in the neck, jaw, or down the left arm. (7:485; 3:595)

Nursing Process—Collecting data
Client Need—Physiological integrity

103 3. Evidence suggests that an elevated cholesterol level predisposes one to developing gallstones. The majority of gallstones are thought to form when bile in the gallbladder is thick, high in cholesterol, and low in bile acids. A low red cell count and hemoglobin are commonly found in people with bleeding, nutritional deficiency, or bone marrow disorders. Elevated serum albumin is not generally a common laboratory finding with any pathologic condition. (14:877; 7:485; 5:368)

Nursing Process—Collecting data
Client Need—Physiological integrity

104 3. Greasy fried foods and fatty meats are not allowed on a low-fat diet. Baked fish, poultry, and lean meat are allowed. Leaner cuts of beef, like round steak, could be ground and used in recipes that call for hamburger. Hard cheese, cream, gravies, salad oil, rich desserts, and nuts are restricted. Whole milk, butter or margarine, and sometimes eggs can be used in limited amounts. (4:486; 14:878)

Nursing Process—Evaluation
Client Need—Health promotion/maintenance

105 3. Radiography of the gallbladder involves the use of an oral iodine contrast medium. If a client is allergic to iodine, he is at risk for experiencing an allergic reaction to the radiopaque substance. Allergic reactions can be life-threatening. Most clients can cooperate by holding still for the brief amount of time required during the gallbladder x-ray. Determining the number of previous x-rays may be appropriate in terms of teaching and preparing a client. However, all individuals should receive an explanation before any procedure is performed. No anesthesia is given prior to or during an x-ray of the gallbladder. (5:655)

Nursing Process—Collecting data
Client Need—Safe, effective care environment

106 1. The person undergoing an ultrasound of the gallbladder should not eat food for approximately 8 to 12 hours before the test. Restricting food helps to eliminate the presence of gas. Intestinal gas can interfere with the transmission of sound waves toward the gallbladder and the scan of the structure's image. Water is permitted. Barium is used as a contrast medium for upper and lower gastrointestinal x-rays. During ultrasonography the gallbladder is imaged by applying a water-soluble lubricant to a hand-held transducer and passing it across the abdomen. (5:787; 7:443)

Nursing Process—Evaluation
Client Need—Safe, effective care environment

107 2. Bile pigments cause the normal brown appearance of stool. If bile is prevented from entering the small intestine, the stool that forms is likely to appear clay colored. Black, tarry stools indicate bleeding high in the gastrointestinal tract or the administration of oral iron therapy. Dark brown stool is normal; the shade may vary depending on the food that has been eaten. Greenish yellow stool is more often associated with diarrhea. (14:357; 5:233)

Nursing Process—Collecting data
Client Need—Physiological integrity

108 4. Biliary obstruction is often accompanied by hypoprothrombinemia. The preoperative administration of vitamin K will reduce the risk of hemorrhage. A single dose usually restores the normal prothrombin time within 8 to 24 hours. Vitamins A and C promote wound healing. Adequate intake of all water- and fat-soluble vitamins is necessary for general health. No specific vitamin will promote liver function. (15:296; 14:878; 3:596)

Nursing Process—Implementation
Client Need—Health promotion/maintenance

109 4. The deltoid muscle is not capable of absorbing large amounts of solution. Intramuscular injections into the deltoid muscle of an adult should be limited to 1 mL of solution. The deltoid should not be used as a site for injecting medication in an infant or child because it is not sufficiently developed to absorb medication adequately. The dorsogluteal, ventrogluteal, and vastus lateralis are large muscle sites that can absorb greater volumes of injected drugs. (18:611; 14:492)

  Nursing Process—Planning
  Client Need—Physiological integrity

110 4. The pigment found in bile is derived from hemoglobin. Depending on the concentration of pigment, the normal appearance of bile drainage can be described as being greenish yellow to orange brown. Bile is generally clear, but clear is not a color. Dark red drainage may indicate that venous blood is mixed with the biliary drainage. Bright red drainage is a sign of fresh or arterial bleeding. (3:596)

  Nursing Process—Collecting data
  Client Need—Physiological integrity

111 3. Wound cleansing should always be performed in a manner in which pathogens and debris are moved away from the impaired skin. A T-tube is inserted through a stab wound in the skin, so wiping outward in a circular fashion would be most correct. The other options describe techniques in which the components of more contaminated areas are brought toward the wound. (18:473; 3:240)

  Nursing Process—Implementation
  Client Need—Physiological integrity

112 1. To establish negative pressure, air and drainage must be emptied from the bulb reservoir and the opening capped before releasing the squeezed bulb. A Jackson-Pratt drain is an example of a closed drainage device. The Jackson-Pratt device could drain by gravity, not negative pressure, if the drainage valve was left open. The bulb reservoir is never filled with normal saline. The reservoir may be secured to the skin with tape. However, this is to prevent tension on the tubing and possibly pulling it from its insertion site. (3:240; 18:480-481)

  Nursing Process—Implementation
  Client Need—Safe, effective care environment

NURSING CARE OF CLIENTS WITH DISORDERS OF THE LIVER

113 4. Alanine and aspartate amino transferase, previously called transaminase, are blood tests performed to assess liver function. Liver and other organ disease and damage will result in elevated levels of these particular enzymes. The tests are repeated periodically to evaluate the client's response to treatment. Serum potassium is performed to monitor electrolyte balance when a client's nutritional or fluid balance may have been altered. Serum creatinine and blood urea nitrogen tests are performed to monitor kidney function. (3:599; 5:344; 7:476)

  Nursing Process—Collecting data
  Client Need—Physiological integrity

114 1. Infectious hepatitis A is generally spread by the oral–fecal route. In other words the stool contains the virus, and the pathogen is spread to the mouth of a susceptible individual. The transmission may be direct following contact with the excrement of an infected person or indirectly by ingesting fecally contaminated food or water or food handled by an individual with the virus. This virus also is present in the blood and saliva of infected individuals. However, transmission through these routes is more rare. (14:876; 16:600)

  Nursing Process—Implementation
  Client Need—Health promotion/maintenance

115 4. Conscientious handwashing is the best defense against the transmission of disease. Gloves need only be worn when nursing care involves direct contact with the client, his excrement, or other body fluids. Wearing gloves does not eliminate the need for handwashing. A gown may be used if soiling is possible, but a mask is not necessary. Only individuals who cannot be relied on to practice good handwashing are placed in a private room. (18:358-359; 3:598)

  Nursing Process—Planning
  Client Need—Safe, effective care environment

116 2. Immunoglobulin, formerly known as gamma globulin, is recommended for postexposure to an infected person with hepatitis A. It is most effective if administered within 48 hours to 2 weeks following exposure. Antibiotic therapy is ineffective in preventing or eliminating a viral infection. The current vaccine that is available is used to prevent hepatitis B infection. Anti-inflammatory drugs, such as salicylates, nonsalicylates, and steroids, are not effective therapy in preventing the spread of hepatitis A. (16:600-601; 3:600)

  Nursing Process—Implementation
  Client Need—Health promotion/maintenance

117 3. Jaundice is a yellow discoloration of tissue due to the accumulation of bilirubin in the blood. Jaundice is generally detected first in the sclera, or white area of the eyes. The stool of a jaundiced person is often gray due to lack of bile. The urine of a jaundiced person is dark brown due to the excretion of bilirubin. The appear-

ance of the retina does not change as a result of jaundice. (7:477; 14:875)
    Nursing Process—Collecting data
    Client Need—Safe, effective care environment

118 4. Jaundice is a term that refers to the yellow discoloration of tissue due to the excessive concentration of bilirubin in the blood. Pink is a normal color of white people. Cyanotic skin is a blue color. Other races, such as African Americans and Hispanics, normally have varying shades of brown skin tones. (14:874; 18:287)
    Nursing Process—Implementation
    Client Need—Safe, effective care environment

119 2. Lanolin is an emollient. It softens skin and prevents moisture loss. Dry skin can add to the itching sensation caused by the release of bile salts onto the skin. Bathing should not be discontinued altogether. Even in the worst situations, the skin can be bathed with tepid water. Alcohol is drying to the skin. Its use would contribute to itching. There would be no advantage to substituting a shower for a tub bath. (18:119; 16:838)
    Nursing Process—Planning
    Client Need—Physiological integrity

120 2. Homosexual men are at particularly high risk for acquiring blood-borne infections. The source of the hepatitis B virus is the blood of infected people or carriers. The virus can be present in semen, saliva, and blood. It can be transmitted by sexual contact, contaminated blood products, or accidental puncture with objects that contain traces of infected blood. There is no more connection between having lived in Alaska than any other state. Abusing alcohol compounds the liver damage concurrent with hepatitis, but it is not a cause of it. Being a carpenter is not a known risk factor in acquiring hepatitis B. (7:476; 3:598)
    Nursing Process—Collecting data
    Client Need—Safe, effective care environment

121 1. Food preferences are highly individualized. No one knows better the type of foods that are appealing than the client himself. Obtaining foods that the client particularly likes will often entice an individual with a poor appetite to eat considerably more. There is no advantage to serving all cold food. Food is more appetizing if there is a variety of colors, textures, and temperatures. Desserts need not be totally eliminated because a sufficient intake of carbohydrate spares the breakdown of body protein for energy. Complete protein is needed for the repair and growth of damaged liver cells. (14:241; 4:485)
    Nursing Process—Implementation
    Client Need—Physiological integrity

122 2. Donating blood is not recommended for people who have had hepatitis. The virus remains in the blood, even years after the person has had the acute illness, and can be passed on to others. Blood collection personnel are taught to screen and reject any potential donor who indicates that he has had jaundice in the past. Safe sex may be practiced, which would include using a latex condom. Convalescence may be prolonged following the acute phase of hepatitis, but eventually there should not to be any permanent physical restrictions. Individuals with hepatitis antibodies are not barred from foreign travel. (14:876)
    Nursing Process—Implementation
    Client Need—Safe, effective care environment

123 2. The abdomen of a person with cirrhosis is enlarged. This may be due to an increase in the liver size from repeated repair and regeneration of cells, an accumulation of fluid in the peritoneal cavity, or both. There is usually scant body hair on someone with cirrhosis. The skin will appear normal to jaundiced depending on the amount of liver damage. Bowel sounds are active but may be faint or distant because the sounds are muffled by fluid within the abdomen. (14:875; 16:597)
    Nursing Process—Collecting data
    Client Need—Safe, effective care environment

124 1. The etiology for Laënnec's portal cirrhosis, the most common form in the United States, is chronic malnutrition and alcoholism. Malnutrition is often a consequence of alcoholism. Viet Nam veterans were exposed to toxic chemicals during their military service, but their medical problems have not resulted in a predominant incidence of cirrhosis. If Mr. Gobel uses salicylates or nonsteroidal anti-inflammatory drugs, it may be a factor in his gastrointestinal bleeding but not the cirrhosis. The hypertension could be secondary to his alcohol abuse. (16:597; 3:602; 7:478)
    Nursing Process—Collecting data
    Client Need—Safe, effective care environment

125 1. The skin of a person with cirrhosis usually manifests multiple vascular lesions with a central red body with radiating branches. These are known as spider angiomas. They also may be referred to as telangiectasias, spider nevi, or vascular spiders. They may be found on the face, upper thorax, and shoulders. A butterfly pattern on the cheeks is a characteristic of lupus erythematosis. Silver scales are associated with psoriasis. Brown moles are common and are unrelated to cirrhosis. (16:597; 7:479)
    Nursing Process—Collecting data
    Client Need—Safe, effective care environment

126 4. Ascites is the collection of fluid within the peritoneal cavity. An appropriate technique for monitoring the increase or decrease in this condition is measuring the abdominal girth. Either the apical or radial pulse measurement would be appropriate for a general assessment. The position in which the blood pressure is measured should be consistent, but it may be taken either while the client is lying down or sitting. The specific gravity usually is monitored when there is a problem with intravascular fluid volume or renal disease. (7:480; 14:875)

   Nursing Process—Collecting data
   Client Need—Safe, effective care environment

127 1. After a liver biopsy the client must be monitored closely for signs of hemorrhage. The nurse should position the client so that body weight puts pressure on the needle site. A person with cirrhosis is at especially high risk for bleeding because liver disease results in diminished prothrombin. Prothrombinemia causes a prolonged delay in the time it takes for blood to clot. (7:442; 14:847)

   Nursing Process—Implementation
   Client Need—Health promotion/maintenance

128 1. The bladder should be emptied just prior to a paracentesis. A full bladder may be punctured as the needle is inserted through the abdominal wall. The client can eat and drink before the test. There is no need for a nasogastric tube or suction machine. (16:598; 18:317)

   Nursing Process—Implementation
   Client Need—Safe, effective care environment

129 4. Spironolactone is a diuretic that promotes sodium and water excretion while retaining potassium. In cirrhosis ascites is in part due to the overproduction of aldosterone. Aldosterone causes sodium and water retention and potassium excretion. Loss of potassium is dangerous. The advantage of this drug is its potassium-sparing quality. Spironolactone does not limit magnesium, conserve calcium, or reduce the elimination of sodium. (15:122)

   Nursing Process—Implementation
   Client Need—Health promotion/maintenance

130 4. Due to the tendency to bleed, the nurse should apply sustained pressure for a longer period to prevent hematoma formation and bruising. There is no scientific rationale for performing any of the other actions. (14:874; 16:604)

   Nursing Process—Implementation
   Client Need—Safe, effective care environment

131 3. Rising levels of ammonia in the blood are toxic to the central nervous system. Serum bilirubin would be monitored to assess the ability of the liver to form bile and send it to the gallbladder for concentration. Serum creatinine and blood urea nitrogen are tests used to monitor renal function. (3:603; 7:483)

   Nursing Process—Collecting data
   Client Need—Physiological integrity

132 4. Onions contain very little protein. The batter would add a certain amount of carbohydrate. The major nutrient in onion rings is the fat in which they were prepared. Besides protein, salt also may be a restricted item for the client with liver disease. Dairy products and meat are good sources of protein. Their consumption would be limited on a low-protein diet. The nurse could refer the client's wife to the dietitian so that other adjustments in his daily meal plan would allow him to eat these foods. (4:486, 626)

   Nursing Process—Implementation
   Client Need—Health promotion/maintenance

133 3. Stool that appears black or tarry is an indication that a significant amount of blood is being lost from the stomach or somewhere in the proximal end of the intestine. Gastric hemorrhage is not usually accompanied by pain, nausea, or abdominal distention. (14:357)

   Nursing Process—Collecting data
   Client Need—Safe, effective care environment

134 2. The tip of the enema tubing should be inserted approximately 3 to 4 in (7.5 to 10 cm) when giving a cleansing enema. This allows the tube to enter the anal canal and pass the internal sphincter, where the solution should be introduced into the rectum. Introducing the tube farther may injure mucous membranes. Introducing it a shorter distance places the solution in the rectum and causes the client to expel the enema before it has had a chance to be effective. (18:555; 14:359)

   Nursing Process—Implementation
   Client Need—Physiological integrity

135 1. Difficulty in arousing Mr. Foster indicates a significant neurologic change. It is a sign that the client may be progressing into hepatic coma. The client's physiologic and safety needs become even more important at this time. Convulsions may occur. The urine output and blood pressure are within normal limits. The fact that he snores is unrelated to his mental status. (7:483; 16:598)

   Nursing Process—Collecting data
   Client Need—Physiological integrity

136 2. Grief work involves dealing with the loss. Reviewing one's life is often a task that takes place in anticipatory grieving. This is therapeutic and should not be suppressed. Suggesting that a close family member be called is an example of changing the subject. Writing in a diary may be therapeutic. However, this action would be more appropriate at a later time. At the moment spontaneous verbalization is most therapeutic. It is unrealistic to expect that the client's wife is able to think about future plans before she has dealt with the reality of the loss. (9:316; 12:362)

> Nursing Process—Implementation
> Client Need—Psychosocial integrity

NURSING CARE OF CLIENTS WITH DISORDERS OF THE PANCREAS

137 2. Pain is a subjective experience. Asking the client to rate his pain numerically helps the nurse to assess its intensity. The rating scale can be used later to evaluate the effectiveness of pain relief techniques that may be used. Noting if a client can stop moving about is not a valid assessment technique. A cooperative client may make an effort to stop moving despite the continuation of severe pain. Perspiration is a physiologic sign that may accompany pain. However, because many factors can affect perspiration, its presence or absence is not the best assessment technique. Administering an analgesic is an intervention, not a form of assessment. (14:463; 7:133)

> Nursing Process—Collecting data
> Client Need—Physiological integrity

138 2. Elevated serum amylase is the most reliable evidence of pancreatitis. The bilirubin level may be elevated if the cause of the pancreatitis is due to an obstruction of the common bile duct or pancreatic duct. Glucose tolerance test abnormalities may indicate dysfunction of the endocrine functions of the pancreas, which may be secondary to pancreatitis. Elevated bilirubin and abnormal glucose tolerance tests, in and of themselves, are not the best indication of pancreatitis. Lactose tolerance test results have no relationship to pancreatitis. (3:604; 5:340)

> Nursing Process—Collecting data
> Client Need—Physiological integrity

139 4. The distance from the nose (N) to the earlobe (E) to the xiphoid (X) is called the NEX measurement. It is used to determine the approximate distance to the stomach. None of the other landmarks are correct for approximating the length that a nasogastric tube should be inserted. (18:137)

> Nursing Process—Collecting data
> Client Need—Physiological integrity

140 2. If the size and shape of each nostril appear equal, the nurse may ask the client to exhale while oc-

cluding one and then the other nostril. The nurse evaluates if air passes more freely through one or the other. If there is no difference, either nostril may be used. It is not necessary to blow forcefully to assess the ability to move air through each nostril. Sniffing and smelling are not appropriate assessment techniques. (18:138)

> Nursing Process—Collecting data
> Client Need—Physiological integrity

141 2. A water-soluble lubricant is the safest substance to use. It is preferred in case the tube is accidentally inserted into the airway. The solubility of the lubricant would prevent the client from possibly developing pneumonia. Remnants of an oil-based lubricant or insoluble oil in the airway can irritate the respiratory mucosa and cause pneumonia. Tincture of benzoin is a good substance to use externally on the skin to promote adhesion; it is inappropriate as a lubricant. (18:137; 16:534)

> Nursing Process—Implementation
> Client Need—Safe, effective care environment

142 1. Bringing the head forward helps close the trachea and open the esophagus. None of the other head positions will facilitate avoiding placement of the nasogastric tube within the airway. (18:138; 14:851)

> Nursing Process—Implementation
> Client Need—Safe, effective care environment

143 2. Swallowing will close the epiglottis, the cartilage that covers the larynx. The contraction of throat muscles during swallowing also helps direct the tube toward the stomach rather than the airway passages. Chewing may cause salivation but will not help the tube enter the stomach. Talking and singing are not appropriate during the passage of a gastric tube. (18:138; 14:851)

> Nursing Process—Implementation
> Client Need—Safe, effective care environment

144 1. The presence of the tube between the folds of the vocal cords interferes with vibration and the ability to speak. The tube should be withdrawn to the level of the oropharynx while the client reestablishes his ability to breathe. Swallowing would not be affected. Sneezing and vomiting are not appropriate signs to evaluate if a gastric tube is in the wrong location. (18:138)

> Nursing Process—Evaluation
> Client Need—Physiological integrity

145 4. Redness, swelling, and tenderness are signs of inflammation. The site needs to be changed as soon as possible. The infusion can flow by gravity with the tubing coiled on the bed. Though the nondominant hand is preferred for an intravenous infusion, its alternate placement is not an important finding to report. Most infusion rates are between 100 and 125 mL/h. There is ample time, with 250 mL left, to postpone reporting the information temporarily. (18:668-669;14:495)

> Nursing Process—Evaluation
> Client Need—Physiological integrity

146 3. The nurse should question if the client on a low-fat diet should have scrambled eggs. The intake of eggs should be limited on a low-fat diet. One scrambled egg made with milk and butter has approximately 8 g of fat. One cup of cooked unsweetened prunes has only a trace of fat. One cup of nonfat skim milk has a trace of fat. One slice of unbuttered whole wheat toast has 1 g of fat. (4:550, 556, 572, 578)

> Nursing Process—Evaluation
> Client Need—Physiological integrity

147 3. There is an established relationship between the chronic consumption of alcohol and the incidence of pancreatitis. Once an acute attack of pancreatitis has occurred, the client is at risk for chronic pancreatitis. Use of alcohol can lead to continued inflammation of this organ. It is essential to protect the pancreas from further irritation because complications include destruction of the organ itself, peritonitis, shock, and even death. Having had pancreatitis would not disqualify someone from donating blood, performing heavy lifting, or taking laxatives. (3:604; 16:613)

> Nursing Process—Implementation
> Client Need—Health promotion/maintenance

148 3. Pancreatic cancer, like most other forms of cancer, does not usually cause acute pain in the early stages. Jaundice is often the first noticeable symptom. Usually by the time the client seeks treatment, the tumor has spread. Severe anorexia and weight loss are signs and symptoms that also accompany cancer of the pancreas. Pain is a late sign; its severity increases as the tumor becomes larger. Bleeding is not usually a problem unless the cancer also has affected the liver. Fainting, unless from weight and fluid loss, is not a common sign of cancer of the pancreas. (14:878; 7:490)

> Nursing Process—Collecting data
> Client Need—Safe, effective care environment

149 2. It is better to control pain before it escalates. When pain is intense, relief is more difficult to achieve. Peaks and valleys of pain can be reduced by administering pain-relieving drugs on a routine schedule throughout the 24-hour period rather than just when it becomes absolutely necessary to do so. The goal is to keep the client free from pain yet not dull his consciousness or ability to communicate. Asking the physician to increase the current dose at this time may do just that. Tolerance is likely to develop later. It would be appropriate at that time for the nurse to consult the physician about changing the medication order. (18:762; 14:464)

> Nursing Process—Implementation
> Client Need—Physiological integrity

150 3. The most therapeutic response in this situation is to encourage the client to talk about his thoughts and feelings. People who are dying often know they are terminal without being told. It is important to support a client's hope than to bluntly confirm suspicions. It would be unethical to deny that the terminal client will improve. It would be appropriate to act as a liaison in contacting someone that will help the client take care of unfinished business. However, this would not be the first or best nursing response in this case. (9:312-313)

> Nursing Process—Implementation
> Client Need—Psychosocial integrity

Classification of Test Items

Unit IV Review Test 6

Directions: After each question the correct answer is given as well as a classification of each test question. Compare the correct answer with your answer. If a question has been answered *incorrectly*, draw a line to the end of the four columns. When finished, add up your correct scores and place the results at the bottom of each column.

Score Calculation:

To determine the percentage of the number of questions you answered correctly, divide the **Number Correct** by the **Number Possible**, as example 135 (the number of questions answered correctly) divided by 150 (the number of questions in the test) = .90 or 90%.

NURSING PROCESS

C = Collecting data
P = Planning
I = Implementation
E = Evaluation

CLIENT NEEDS

S = Safe, effective care environment
P = Physiological integrity
M = Psychosocial integrity
H = Health promotion/maintenance

Question #	Answer #	Nursing Process C	Nursing Process P	Nursing Process I	Nursing Process E	Client Needs S	Client Needs P	Client Needs M	Client Needs H
1	3	C					P		
2	2			I					H
3	3		P						H
4	1	C				S			
5	2			I			P		
6	1		P			S			
7	4				E				H
8	2				E				H
9	1			I					H
10	3				E	S			
11	2			I					H
12	4	C				S			
13	2	C					P		
14	4	C				S			
15	3		P						H
16	3	C				S			
17	2			I			P		
18	2	C				S			
19	2				E		P		

NURSING PROCESS

C = Collecting data
P = Planning
I = Implementation
E = Evaluation

CLIENT NEEDS

S = Safe, effective care environment
P = Physiological integrity
M = Psychosocial integrity
H = Health promotion/maintenance

Question #	Answer #	Nursing Process				Client Needs			
		C	P	I	E	S	P	M	H
20	3			I			P		
21	2			I				M	
22	3	C					P		
23	3	C					P		
24	4				E	S			
25	3			I			P		
26	1	C					P		
27	2			I					H
28	1		P				P		
29	2	C					P		
30	2	C					P		
31	1			I				M	
32	2		P				P		
33	4			I		S			
34	3			I			P		
35	2				E				H
36	2		P						H
37	1	C					P		
38	3			I					H
39	4			I		S			
40	2				E	S			
41	3			I			P		
42	1				E		P		
43	4			I					H
44	1				E				H
45	2		P				P		
46	3	C				S			
47	4			I		S			
48	2			I					H
49	2			I		S			

176

NURSING PROCESS

C = Collecting data
P = Planning
I = Implementation
E = Evaluation

CLIENT NEEDS

S = Safe, effective care environment
P = Physiological integrity
M = Psychosocial integrity
H = Health promotion/maintenance

Quetion #	Answer #	Nursing Process				Client Needs			
		C	P	I	E	S	P	M	H
50	4			I		S			
51	2			I					H
52	1		P						H
53	1	C					P		
54	3		P					M	
55	1			I				M	
56	1			I		S			
57	3				E		P		
58	1		P				P		
59	3			I			P		
60	2			I			P		
61	4			I					H
62	4	C					P		
63	1	C					P		
64	3				E				H
65	2			I			P		
66	1	C					P		
67	1	C				S			
68	1				E	S			
69	2			I		S			
70	2			I		S			
71	3			I			P		
72	2			I					H
73	3	C				S			
74	1			I		S			
75	4			I			P		
76	3			I			P		
77	4			I		S			
78	2	C					P		
79	1			I			P		

NURSING PROCESS

C = Collecting data
P = Planning
I = Implementation
E = Evaluation

CLIENT NEEDS

S = Safe, effective care environment
P = Physiological integrity
M = Psychosocial integrity
H = Health promotion/maintenance

Question #	Answer #	Nursing Process				Client Needs			
		C	P	I	E	S	P	M	H
80	2			I			P		
81	2			I				M	
82	1			I				M	
83	4			I					H
84	1			I					H
85	3			I					H
86	1	C					P		
87	3		P				P		
88	1			I			P		
89	2		P				P		
90	2		P				P		
91	3			I			P		
92	3			I			P		
93	1				E				H
94	3	C				S			
95	2			I					H
96	1				E		P		
97	1			I					H
98	2	C				S			
99	4				E				H
100	4			I					H
101	1	C				S			
102	1	C					P		
103	3	C					P		
104	3				E				H
105	3	C				S			
106	1				E	S			
107	2	C					P		
108	4			I					H
109	4		P				P		

NURSING PROCESS

C = Collecting data
P = Planning
I = Implementation
E = Evaluation

CLIENT NEEDS

S = Safe, effective care environment
P = Physiological integrity
M = Psychosocial integrity
H = Health promotion/maintenance

Question #	Answer #	Nursing Process				Client Needs			
		C	P	I	E	S	P	M	H
110	4	C					P		
111	3			I			P		
112	1			I		S			
113	4	C					P		
114	1			I					H
115	4		P			S			
116	2			I					H
117	3	C				S			
118	4			I		S			
119	2		P				P		
120	2	C				S			
121	1			I			P		
122	2			I		S			
123	2	C				S			
124	1	C				S			
125	1	C				S			
126	4	C				S			
127	1			I					H
128	1			I		S			
129	4			I					H
130	4			I		S			
131	3	C					P		
132	4			I					H
133	3	C				S			
134	2			I			P		
135	1	C					P		
136	2			I				M	
137	2	C					P		
138	2	C					P		
139	4	C					P		

NURSING PROCESS

C = Collecting data
P = Planning
I = Implementation
E = Evaluation

CLIENT NEEDS

S = Safe, effective care environment
P = Physiological integrity
M = Psychosocial integrity
H = Health promotion/maintenance

Question #	Answer #	Nursing Process				Client Needs			
		C	P	I	E	S	P	M	H
140	2	C					P		
141	2			I		S			
142	1			I		S			
143	2			I		S			
144	1				E		P		
145	4				E		P		
146	3				E		P		
147	3			I					H
148	3	C				S			
149	2			I			P		
150	3			I				M	
Number Correct									
Number Possible	150	45	16	69	20	45	62	8	35
Percentage Correct									

REVIEW TEST 7

The Nursing Care of Clients with Disorders of the Musculoskeletal System

The Nursing Care of Clients with Disorders of the Integumentary System

Correct Answers and Rationale
Classification of Test Items

Directions: with a pencil, blacken the circle in front of the option you have chosen for your correct answer.

The Nursing Care of Clients with Disorders of the Musculoskeletal System

NURSING CARE OF CLIENTS WITH STRAINS, SPRAINS, AND DISLOCATIONS

Mr. Brian MacKenzie is an enthusiastic golfer. He plays nine or 18 holes at least twice a week. Lately while playing golf, he has experienced pain when moving his right wrist. The physician has diagnosed his condition as tendinitis.

1 The physician tells Mr. MacKenzie that the cause of his problem is repetitive stress on his wrist. He is told to avoid overusing it. If Mr. MacKenzie made all of the following statements to the nurse, which one is the *best* action for him to take at this time? Mr. MacKenzie says that he should
   ○ 1. keep his hand as still as possible.
   ○ 2. stop playing golf for the time being.
   ○ 3. try playing miniature golf instead.
   ○ 4. wear a tight leather glove for golf.

Following an injury in which Ms. Leona Elkins slipped while climbing stairs, she experienced immediate swelling of her ankle and pain on movement. Her physician has sent her to the hospital for an x-ray.

2 The physician talks to the nurse in the emergency department on the phone. He describes his physical assessment of Ms. Elkins. He says that there is some edema and ecchymosis of the client's ankle. The nurse would understand that ecchymosis is a term meaning the skin appears
   ○ 1. freckled.
   ○ 2. mottled.
   ○ 3. bruised.
   ○ 4. blanched.

3 Which one of the following nursing measures would be most helpful for relieving the swelling

Timby B, Scherer JC: LIPPINCOTT'S REVIEW FOR NCLEX–PN. © 1994 J.B. Lippincott Company.

while preparing to obtain the x-ray of Ms. Elkins' lower leg?

○ 1. Dangle the foot.
○ 2. Elevate the foot.
○ 3. Exercise the foot.
○ 4. Immobilize the foot.

The x-ray reveals that the bones are intact. The physician tells Ms. Elkins that she has a severely sprained ankle.

4 The physician directs the nurse to wrap Ms. Elkins' foot with an elastic roller bandage referred to by some as an Ace bandage. Where should the nurse *begin* applying the bandage?

○ 1. Below the knee
○ 2. Above the ankle
○ 3. Across the phalanges
○ 4. At the metatarsals

The nurse anchors the roller bandage with a circular turn followed with several spiral turns.

5 Which turn would be most correct to use when wrapping the roller bandage around Ms. Elkins' ankle joint?

○ 1. Figure-of-eight turn
○ 2. Spiral reverse turn
○ 3. Recurrent turn
○ 4. Spica turn

Before Ms. Elkins leaves the emergency department, the nurse demonstrates how to apply the roller bandage. She is told to remove it for approximately 20 minutes and reapply it three times a day.

6 It is essential that the nurse tell Ms. Elkins to *loosen* the bandage if

○ 1. her toes feel fairly warm.
○ 2. her ankle feels painful.
○ 3. her toes appear swollen.
○ 4. she wears a cotton sock.

While falling from a short step ladder, Mr. Herbert West dislocates his shoulder.

7 The nurse examines Mr. West before he is seen by the physician. Which one of the following is more likely to be present with a dislocation than a sprain?

○ 1. Intense pain
○ 2. Severe swelling
○ 3. Impaired movement
○ 4. Obvious deformity

8 Mr. West asks the nurse what his physician meant when he said he would correct the dislocation by manipulation. The best explanation is that a manipulation involves

○ 1. making an incision to realign the bones.
○ 2. inserting a pin or wire into the joint.
○ 3. repositioning the bone ends manually.
○ 4. strengthening the joint with exercise.

Mr. West cannot afford the cost of a canvas sling. The nurse must teach him how to apply a triangular sling made from muslin.

9 If Mr. West makes all of the following statements, which one indicates that he needs more teaching? He says that

○ 1. his hand should be elevated higher than the elbow.
○ 2. the knot should be tied at the back of his neck.
○ 3. his elbow should be flexed when wearing the sling.
○ 4. the sling is used to elevate and support his arm.

NURSING CARE OF CLIENTS WITH ARTHRITIS

Ms. Rizak has acute rheumatoid arthritis. Her hands and spine are involved.

10 When the nurse admits Ms. Rizak, she is most likely to tell the nurse that the *first* symptom that caused her to seek health care was

○ 1. stiff, sore joints.
○ 2. generalized fatigue.
○ 3. stabbing hand pain.
○ 4. disuse of fingers.

11 Ms. Rizak takes a total of 5 g of acetylsalicylic acid (Bayer aspirin) per day. If each tablet contains 5 grains, how many tablets should the nurse make sure are stocked in the medicine cart for Ms. Rizak in each 24-hour period?

○ 1. 5 tablets
○ 2. 10 tablets
○ 3. 15 tablets
○ 4. 20 tablets

12 Ms. Rizak tells the nurse that she gets an upset stomach when she takes the aspirin. Which one of the following changes would be most appropriate to add to the client's plan of care to relieve the discomfort she experiences when taking the aspirin?

○ 1. Give aspirin before meals only.
○ 2. Give aspirin with cold water.
○ 3. Give aspirin with hot tea.
○ 4. Give aspirin with food or meals.

13 Ms. Rizak says she is surprised the physician prescribed such a common drug as aspirin. The nurse would be most correct in explaining that aspirin is one of the best drugs used in the treatment of arthritis because it relieves discomfort and

○ 1. stimulates the immune system.
○ 2. relaxes skeletal muscles.
○ 3. reduces joint inflammation.
○ 4. interrupts nerve synapses.

14 If Ms. Rizak shows signs and symptoms of aspirin toxicity, called salicylism, the nurse's *first* course of action should be to

○ 1. give buffered aspirin. It is less toxic than plain aspirin.

○ 2. continue giving the aspirin. The client requires the drug.

○ 3. omit a dose of the drug. This usually relieves toxic symptoms.

○ 4. notify the charge nurse. The medication order needs to be changed.

15 Ms. Rizak says that when she watches television her discomfort is decreased. Which of the following interpretations of Ms. Rizak's observation is most probably the correct one? The client is probably

○ 1. improving due to electronic signals.

○ 2. having less pain than she thinks.

○ 3. experiencing only a slight case of arthritis.

○ 4. being distracted from her pain.

Ms. Dorothy Kirby has been a long-term client at the arthritis clinic. Her hands and wrists are affected by rheumatoid arthritis.

16 When the nurse examines Ms. Kirby's hands, which finger joints are most often damaged by rheumatoid arthritis?

○ 1. Proximal finger joints

○ 2. Medial finger joints

○ 3. Distal finger joints

○ 4. Lateral finger joints

17 If Ms. Kirby is typical of most people with rheumatoid arthritis, the nurse would expect that she first developed symptoms

○ 1. in very early childhood.

○ 2. at the onset of puberty.

○ 3. during young adulthood.

○ 4. as she neared retirement.

18 If Ms. Kirby had all of the following laboratory tests when she first developed her joint symptoms, which one would be most diagnostic for rheumatoid arthritis?

○ 1. Erythrocyte sedimentation rate

○ 2. Partial thromboplastin time (PTT)

○ 3. Fasting blood sugar

○ 4. Blood urea nitrogen (BUN)

19 Which one of the following recommendations by the nurse would be most helpful in sustaining Ms. Kirby's ability to care for herself?

○ 1. Learn to play a musical instrument.

○ 2. Buy clothes that can be slipped on.

○ 3. Enroll in an aerobic exercise class.

○ 4. Eat food without chemical additives.

Ms. Muriel Wells has not responded to the usual drug therapy for arthritis. She now takes prednisone (Meticorten) daily.

20 While Ms. Wells takes prednisone, a corticosteroid, which one of the following assessments is most essential for the nurse to monitor?

○ 1. Daily weight

○ 2. Pulse rate

○ 3. Bowel sounds

○ 4. Skin integrity

21 If Ms. Wells makes all of the following statements about corticosteroid therapy, which one is *incorrect*? Ms. Wells says that

○ 1. she is very susceptible to getting infections.

○ 2. she should never stop taking her medication abruptly.

○ 3. she may develop low blood sugar and need glucose.

○ 4. she may become very depressed and perhaps suicidal.

22 The joints of Ms. Wells' hands are swollen, hot, and painful. The physician asks the nurse to apply a splint to each. The nurse would be most accurate in explaining to Ms. Wells that the primary purpose of the splints is to

○ 1. rest the affected joints.

○ 2. cure her joint disease.

○ 3. improve her hand strength.

○ 4. increase her range of motion.

A friend of Ms. Wells told her that her arthritis was cured by wearing copper bracelets. Ms. Wells is thinking of doing the same.

23 Which one of the following is the best information the nurse can provide the client with arthritis about wearing copper bracelets? The relief of arthritis symptoms while wearing a copper bracelet can be attributed to

○ 1. spontaneous remission.

○ 2. electrolyte balance.

○ 3. metallic attraction.

○ 4. chemical restoration.

24 The physician recommends that the nurse apply heat to Ms. Wells' hands to relieve some of her discomfort. If all of the following are available, which one will generally be most effective for the nurse to use?

○ 1. Hot water bottle

○ 2. Electric heating pad

○ 3. Warm moist compresses

○ 4. Infrared heat lamp

Mr. Lawrence Klein has a degenerative joint disease called osteoarthritis. For several years he has experienced pain and stiffness in his left hip joint. He is now seeing his physician because his range of motion is limited in this hip, and he can no longer walk with comfort.

25 The physician tells Mr. Klein that he could apply a heating pad to his hip periodically. It would be essential for the nurse to tell Mr. Klein that when he uses the heating pad,

○ 1. it should be kept on the low setting.
○ 2. he should secure it with safety pins.
○ 3. it should be covered with plastic.
○ 4. he should apply it for approximately 2 hours.

26 Mr. Klein asks the nurse if there are special foods that would help treat his arthritis. The most accurate information the nurse can provide is that there is no specific diet, but he can *minimize* the stress on his painful joint by
○ 1. maintaining normal weight.
○ 2. eating green leafy vegetables.
○ 3. increasing his intake of fruit.
○ 4. becoming more physically active.

27 Mr. Klein uses a cane when ambulating. The nurse observes Mr. Klein while he walks. Which one of the following observations indicates that the client needs more teaching about using a cane?
○ 1. The tip of the cane is covered with a rubber cap.
○ 2. The client wears athletic shoes with nonskid soles.
○ 3. The client uses the cane on his painful side.
○ 4. He holds his head up and looks ahead when walking.

28 Mr. Klein takes 600 mg of ibuprofen (Motrin) four times a day. Which one of the following questions would be important to ask a client who takes a non-steroidal anti-inflammatory drug (NSAID) to determine if a common side effect is occurring?
○ 1. Have you noticed any hand tremors?
○ 2. Do you take your medication with food?
○ 3. What is the color of your stools?
○ 4. Has your interest in sex changed?

Mr. Carl Eaton has been admitted to the hospital. He is to have a total hip replacement for osteoarthritis.

29 Mr. Eaton asks the nurse why the physician told him to stop taking his enteric coated aspirin (Ecotrin) 1 week ago. The most accurate rationale for the physician's instruction is that aspirin
○ 1. increases the risk of wound infection.
○ 2. impairs the ability to control bleeding.
○ 3. makes it difficult to assess his pain.
○ 4. interferes with the ability to heal.

30 The nurse teaches Mr. Eaton how to use an incentive spirometer. Which one of the following statements indicates that the client has a correct understanding of its use? He says that he should position the mouthpiece and
○ 1. inhale deeply.
○ 2. exhale forcefully.
○ 3. cough effectively.
○ 4. breathe naturally.

Mr. Eaton has been showering the last few days with an antibacterial soap. Just before surgery the nurse pre-

pares to shave a wide section of skin in the operative area.

31 Which of the following describes the best technique the nurse should use for shaving the hair from around the operative site?
○ 1. Avoid using soap to see the hair better.
○ 2. Press the razor deeply into the skin while shaving.
○ 3. Use long strokes in a medial to lateral direction.
○ 4. Pull the razor in the direction of hair growth.

Mr. Eaton returns to his hospital room after recovering from the operation in the postanesthesia reacting room.

32 It is essential for the nurse to maintain Mr. Eaton's operative hip in a position of
○ 1. adduction.
○ 2. abduction.
○ 3. flexion.
○ 4. rotation.

33 Which one of the following modifications to Mr. Eaton's bed should the nurse plan to make to facilitate his nursing care? The nurse should obtain
○ 1. a bed cradle.
○ 2. a bed board.
○ 3. an overhead trapeze.
○ 4. lower side rails.

34 Which of the following items would be best for the nurse to use to prevent external rotation of Mr. Eaton's operative leg?
○ 1. A foot board
○ 2. A trochanter roll
○ 3. A turning sheet
○ 4. A foam mattress

Mr. Ed Sperry is about to be discharged following his recovery from a total hip replacement. A list of discharge instructions is prepared by the team leader. The nurse caring for Mr. Sperry implements one portion of the discharge teaching by instructing him on positions he must avoid.

35 Which of the following statements indicates that the client has a correct understanding of the restrictions he must follow? Mr. Sperry says he should not
○ 1. cross his legs.
○ 2. point his toes.
○ 3. lie flat in bed.
○ 4. stand upright.

36 Before being discharged, it would be essential that the nurse tell Mr. Sperry to obtain which of the following items for his home care?
○ 1. A wheelchair
○ 2. A hospital bed
○ 3. A raised toilet seat
○ 4. A mechanical lift

37 Which one of the following areas of health teaching is essential for the nurse to include in the discharge instructions of a client who has undergone a total hip replacement?
○ 1. Obtaining assistance with dressing
○ 2. Using special equipment for eating
○ 3. Taking daily supplemental vitamins
○ 4. Avoiding bowel elimination problems

Mr. Arthur Clark has had a knee arthroplasty. An artificial joint has been used to replace his natural knee joint damaged by osteoarthritis. A continuous passive motion (CPM) machine will be used postoperatively.

38 It would be most correct for the nurse to explain to Mr. Clark that the primary purpose for using the CPM machine is to
○ 1. strengthen leg muscles.
○ 2. relieve foot swelling.
○ 3. reduce surgical pain.
○ 4. restore joint function.

39 To document the client's progress while using a CPM machine, it is essential that the charting indicate the degree of joint flexion, the number of cycles per minute, and the
○ 1. condition of the sutures around the incision.
○ 2. amount of time the client used the machine.
○ 3. characteristics of drainage from the wound.
○ 4. presence and quality of arterial pulses.

Mr. Joseph Carr is being treated for gout.

40 When the nurse examines Mr. Carr, which of the following structures is most likely to be affected by gout?
○ 1. Great toe
○ 2. Index finger
○ 3. Sacrococcygeal vertebrae
○ 4. Temporomandibular joint

41 If the physician orders all of the following laboratory tests, which one can the nurse expect to be elevated in a client who has gout?
○ 1. Creatinine clearance
○ 2. BUN
○ 3. Serum uric acid
○ 4. Serum calcium

42 While the client with gout is experiencing an acute attack, which one of the following items would be essential to use to promote his comfort?
○ 1. A bed cradle
○ 2. An electric fan
○ 3. A foam mattress
○ 4. A fracture bedpan

43 Mr. Carr is on a low-purine diet. Which one of the following foods should the nurse question if it was served on his dietary tray?
○ 1. Beets
○ 2. Milk
○ 3. Eggs
○ 4. Liver

During the acute attack of gout, the physician prescribes colchicine to be given every hour until the client's pain is relieved.

44 Which of the following, if it occurred, would also be an indication for the nurse to stop administering colchicine? The client develops
○ 1. vomiting.
○ 2. dizziness.
○ 3. drowsiness.
○ 4. a headache.

The nursing care plan indicates that Mr. Carr should have 3000 mL of fluid daily to prevent renal complications.

45 The time in the day when it is best to plan to offer proportionately greater amounts of fluid to Mr. Carr is
○ 1. before bedtime.
○ 2. early evening.
○ 3. in the morning.
○ 4. midafternoon.

46 The nurse advises Mr. Carr to continue consuming a high intake of fluid following discharge. Which one of the following should the nurse tell Mr. Carr to avoid, even in small amounts?
○ 1. Coffee
○ 2. Alcohol
○ 3. Cranberry juice
○ 4. Carbonated drinks

NURSING CARE OF CLIENTS WITH FRACTURES

While backpacking with a church group, Jerry Hendrick, age 16, steps into a hole. Because of the deformity in the appearance of the leg, a nurse with the group suspects that the fall caused a fracture of the tibia.

47 To immobilize the injured bone, it would be most correct to apply a splint from
○ 1. below the knee to above the hip.
○ 2. above the knee to below the hip.
○ 3. above the ankle to below the knee.
○ 4. below the ankle to above the knee.

The nurse accompanies Jerry to the nearest hospital. An x-ray reveals a comminuted fracture of the distal tibia.

48 The nurse would be most correct in explaining to Jerry that a comminuted fracture is one in which
○ 1. one bone end is driven into the other.
○ 2. the bone is splintered into pieces.
○ 3. there is no open break in the skin.
○ 4. a portion of the bone is split away.

Jerry needs surgery to realign the fractured bone.

49 From whom should consent be obtained to perform the surgical procedure?
   ○ 1. Jerry himself
   ○ 2. Jerry's physician
   ○ 3. Jerry's minister
   ○ 4. Jerry's parent

50 What should the hospital nurse do with the class ring that Jerry is wearing?
   ○ 1. Put it in the bedside stand.
   ○ 2. Leave it on the client's finger.
   ○ 3. Give it to a security guard.
   ○ 4. Lock it up with his valuables.

51 After scrubbing Jerry's skin prior to surgery, the hospital nurse prepares to cover the area with sterile gauze and sterile towels. Which *additional* item is essential?
   ○ 1. Sterile tape
   ○ 2. Sterile gloves
   ○ 3. Antiseptic swabs
   ○ 4. Elastic stocking

52 After surgery Jerry is observed closely for signs and symptoms of a fat embolism. One of the first signs of a fat embolism the nurse would observe is
   ○ 1. respiratory distress.
   ○ 2. abdominal distention.
   ○ 3. difficulty swallowing.
   ○ 4. absent bowel sounds.

Ms. Sylvia Major is rear-ended by another automobile while driving home from work. She has several fractured ribs as a result of being thrown against the steering wheel.

53 When the nurse examines Ms. Major, which system should be the major focus during assessment?
   ○ 1. Cardiovascular
   ○ 2. Respiratory
   ○ 3. Neurologic
   ○ 4. Gastrointestinal

Ms. Valerie Simmons has fractured her wrist trying to break a fall with an outstretched hand.

54 Which one of the following observations would indicate to the nurse that Ms. Simmons is developing compartment syndrome?
   ○ 1. The client experiences severe pain.
   ○ 2. The client's hand becomes reddened.
   ○ 3. The fingers develop muscle spasms.
   ○ 4. The radial pulse feels bounding.

Ms. Hunderford receives emergency care at the site of an automobile accident. A nurse who stopped to assist finds Ms. Hunderford lying on the pavement. It is assumed that she was not wearing a seat belt and was thrown from the car.

55 Of the following emergency measures, which one should the rescuer take first?
   ○ 1. Check the victim's breathing.
   ○ 2. Cover the victim with a blanket.
   ○ 3. Move the victim to the curb.
   ○ 4. Look for signs of injuries.

Ms. Hunderford complains of back and thigh pain. The nurse sees that the skin on the thigh is broken. A piece of broken bone protrudes. There is profuse bleeding from the wound.

56 The best technique the nurse could use in this situation to control the bleeding is to
   ○ 1. place a tourniquet around the leg.
   ○ 2. apply direct pressure at the wound.
   ○ 3. compress the femoral artery.
   ○ 4. elevate the injured extremity.

57 The nurse suspects that Ms. Hunderford may have a broken back. When the emergency personnel arrive, the nurse can expect that the preferred position in which the victim with a back injury will be transported to a health care agency is the
   ○ 1. side-lying position.
   ○ 2. face-lying position.
   ○ 3. back-lying position.
   ○ 4. semisitting position.

Ms. Rita Courtland is hospitalized with a fracture between the trochanters of her right femur.

58 During her admission assessment, the most typical sign of an intertrochanteric fracture of the hip the nurse will observe is
   ○ 1. paralysis of the affected leg.
   ○ 2. bruising of the affected leg.
   ○ 3. lengthening of the affected leg.
   ○ 4. external rotation of the leg.

59 If the nurse finds all of the following information in Ms. Courtland's medical record, which one places her at higher risk than others for sustaining a fracture? The client
   ○ 1. is postmenopausal.
   ○ 2. is somewhat obese.
   ○ 3. likes to do gardening.
   ○ 4. was born in England.

Ms. Courtland has surgery. An internal fixation device, known as a nail, is placed within the fractured area to stabilize the broken bone.

60 Because of her inactivity, the nurse teaches Ms. Courtland to perform an isometric exercise, known as quadriceps setting, with her unaffected leg. If Ms. Courtland does this exercise correctly, the nurse will observe her
   ○ 1. move her toes toward and away from her head.

○ 2. contract and relax the muscles of her thigh.
○ 3. lift her lower leg up and down from the bed.
○ 4. bend her knee and pull her lower leg upward.

61 Ms. Courtland wears knee-high antiembolism stockings. She asks the nurse how they prevent blood clots from forming. The nurse would be most accurate by explaining that the stockings
○ 1. prevent blood from pooling in the legs.
○ 2. reduce blood flowing to the extremities.
○ 3. keep the blood pressure lower in the legs.
○ 4. decrease the volume of red blood cells.

62 The nursing assistant helps with the care of Ms. Courtland. Which of the following indicates that the nursing assistant has applied the elastic stockings correctly? The nursing assistant applies the stockings to Ms. Courtland
○ 1. before getting her out of bed.
○ 2. just before doing leg exercises.
○ 3. when her legs are cool or swollen.
○ 4. at night prior to her bedtime.

Mr. Victor Marshall has had a fractured hip. The break occurred just below the head of his right femur. His intracapsular fracture has been repaired by removing the proximal end and inserting a metal device called an Austin-Moore prosthesis.

63 Before turning Mr. Marshall onto his unoperative side, the nurse should first
○ 1. place pillows between his legs.
○ 2. have him point his toes downward.
○ 3. flex his knee on the affected side.
○ 4. elevate the head of his hospital bed.

64 When Mr. Marshall is allowed to get up in a chair without bearing weight on his right foot, it would be best for the nurse to place the chair
○ 1. at the end of the bed.
○ 2. perpendicular to the bed.
○ 3. parallel with the bed.
○ 4. against a side wall.

65 Eventually Mr. Marshall is taught to use a three-point partial weightbearing gait when ambulating with a walker. Which of the following is evidence that he is performing this gait correctly? The nurse observes Mr. Marshall advance the walker and his operative leg while putting most of his weight on
○ 1. the hand grips of the walker.
○ 2. the back legs of the walker.
○ 3. the toes of his operative leg.
○ 4. the heel of his unoperative leg.

NURSING CARE OF CLIENTS WITH CASTS

Mr. Andrew Watson has an incomplete fracture of his radius. The physician plans to place his arm in a plaster cylinder cast.

66 When planning the preparation for the cast application, what information should the nurse tell the client before the cast is applied?
○ 1. The cast will feel very tight as it is applied.
○ 2. His arm will feel warm as the wet plaster sets.
○ 3. There will be a foul odor until the cast is dry.
○ 4. He may notice slight itching while the cast is wet.

67 While the physician wraps the arm with rolls of wet plaster, the nurse should support the wet cast
○ 1. on a soft mattress.
○ 2. on a firm surface.
○ 3. With the tips of the fingers.
○ 4. With the palms of the hand.

68 Mr. Watson asks the nurse to identify an advantage to having a cast of synthetic material rather than plaster of Paris. One advantage the nurse could mention is that a synthetic cast is
○ 1. less expensive.
○ 2. more lightweight.
○ 3. more flexible.
○ 4. less restrictive.

Ms. Juanita Kirk has a long leg plaster cast applied following an open reduction of a fractured femur.

69 When the client returns to her room after surgery, what should the nurse place under the cast?
○ 1. Synthetic sheepskin
○ 2. A vinyl sheet
○ 3. An absorbent pad
○ 4. Several pillows

70 Which of the following actions would be best for the nurse to use to dry the plaster cast?
○ 1. Leave the leg in the cast uncovered.
○ 2. Apply a heating blanket to the cast.
○ 3. Use a hair dryer to blow hot air.
○ 4. Place a heat lamp above the cast.

71 The nurse observes bloody drainage on the cast. What is the next action that the nurse should take?
○ 1. Document the finding in the medical record.
○ 2. Call the physician and report the finding.
○ 3. Circle it with ink and write down the time.
○ 4. Apply an ice bag over the spot of drainage.

72 Which of the following techniques is best for assessing the circulation in Ms. Kirk's extremity?
○ 1. Ask Ms. Kirk if the cast feels exceptionally heavy.
○ 2. Feel the cast to determine if it is unusually cold.
○ 3. Depress the nailbed and time the return of color.
○ 4. See if there is room to insert a finger in the cast.

While riding his motorcycle in a rain storm, Mr. Greg Haskins lost control and fractured the shaft of his femur. The fracture has been realigned. Mr. Haskins has a hip spica cast. It covers his trunk, one full leg, and the thigh of the other leg.

73 Mr. Haskins tells the nurse, "My father is furious about this accident. He says I should be in school instead of working." Of the following responses the nurse could make, it would be best to say
○ 1. "As they say, 'Father knows best.' "
○ 2. "All parents want their children to finish school."
○ 3. "It can be frustrating when a father and son disagree."
○ 4. "You are adult enough to make your own decisions now."

74 The nurse analyzes the communicated information with Mr. Haskins. It suggests that Mr. Haskins, like most young adults, is struggling with the developmental task that involves
○ 1. searching for his sexual identity.
○ 2. testing his physical abilities.
○ 3. acquiring his own independence.
○ 4. learning to control his emotions.

75 While giving care to Mr. Haskins, what equipment should the nurse plan to use to facilitate bowel elimination?
○ 1. A bedside commode
○ 2. A fracture bedpan
○ 3. A mechanical lift
○ 4. A raised toilet seat

76 Mr. Haskins asks the nurse to explain the purpose of the bar that runs from the plaster on one thigh to the other. The most accurate answer is that the bar is used for
○ 1. lifting and turning clients.
○ 2. performing physical exercise.
○ 3. strengthening the cast.
○ 4. hanging personal items.

77 Mr. Haskins tells the nurse that his skin itches terribly beneath the cast. What would be the best method the nurse could use to help relieve Mr. Haskins discomfort?
○ 1. Give him his prescribed analgesic medication frequently.
○ 2. Show him how to instill air inside his cast with a syringe.
○ 3. Bend a wire coat hanger so he can scratch inside the cast.
○ 4. Drop an ice cube down inside the cast and let it melt.

Mr. Henry Ward has had his hip spica cast for nearly 3 weeks.

78 The nurse detects a foul odor about Mr. Ward's cast. The nurse reports this finding promptly because an unpleasant smell is usually a sign that
○ 1. the plaster has dried improperly.
○ 2. there is bleeding under the cast.
○ 3. the cast is disintegrating.
○ 4. there is an infected wound.

79 The physician cuts a small window in the cast to inspect the underlying tissue. What should the nurse do with the piece of plaster cast that has been removed?
○ 1. Dispose of it in a plastic bag.
○ 2. Replace it in the hole with tape.
○ 3. Save it in the dirty utility room.
○ 4. Send it to the laboratory for a culture.

80 Mr. Ward's cast edges are beginning to crumble. The best technique the nurse can use for repairing it is to
○ 1. line the edge with strips of adhesive tape.
○ 2. apply a fresh strip of plaster to the edge.
○ 3. remove the crumbling edge with a cast cutter.
○ 4. cover the cast edge with a gauze dressing.

NURSING CARE OF CLIENTS WITH TRACTION

Before undergoing surgery for a fractured hip, Ms. Mabel Sullivan's leg is placed in Buck's traction.

81 When changing the linen on Ms. Sullivan's bed, it would be best for the nurse to
○ 1. roll her from one side of the bed to the other.
○ 2. apply the linen from the foot to top of the bed.
○ 3. leave the bottom sheets in place.
○ 4. raise her with a mechanical lift.

82 While providing nursing care for Ms. Sullivan, which one of the following indicates a need for action?
○ 1. The traction weights are hanging above the floor.
○ 2. The leg is in line with the pull of the traction.
○ 3. The client's foot is touching the end of the bed.
○ 4. The rope is in the groove of the traction pulley.

83 Which one of the following techniques would be best for assessing the circulation in the leg in traction?
○ 1. Observe if the client can wiggle or move her toes.
○ 2. Palpate for pulsation of the dorsalis pedis artery.
○ 3. Take the blood pressure on the leg with a thigh cuff.

○ 4. See if the client can feel sharp and dull sensations.

Mr. Thomas Skinner has been placed in Russell's traction while awaiting surgery to repair his fractured hip.

84 Where is it essential to inspect the skin while Mr. Skinner is in Russell's traction?
○ 1. Over the ischial spines
○ 2. In the popliteal space
○ 3. Near the iliac crests
○ 4. At the zygomatic arch

85 On the day of surgery Mr. Skinner is to be transported to the operating room in his bed. Which of the following techniques is correct? The nurse should
○ 1. leave the traction just as it is.
○ 2. remove the weights during his transport.
○ 3. rest the weights on the end of the bed.
○ 4. take his leg out of the traction.

Mr. Robert Evans' leg is in skeletal traction. There is a pin through the distal femur. The leg in traction is supported by balanced suspension.

86 Which finding would suggest to the nurse that Mr. Evans may have an infection at the pin site? The nurse observes that there is
○ 1. serous drainage.
○ 2. bloody drainage.
○ 3. mucoid drainage.
○ 4. purulent drainage.

87 The physician orders antibiotic therapy. If Mr. Evans is allergic to penicillin, an order for which one of the following types of antibiotics should be questioned?
○ 1. Aminoglycosides, like gentamicin sulfate (Garamycin)
○ 2. Cephalosporins, like cefaclor (Ceclor)
○ 3. Tetracyclines, like doxycycline (Vibramycin)
○ 4. Sulfonamides, like cotrimoxazole (Bactrim)

88 Mr. Evans feels the need to have a bowel movement. To place the bedpan the nurse should instruct him to
○ 1. roll to his side using the side rail.
○ 2. elevate his hips using his hands.
○ 3. move himself up using his legs.
○ 4. lift himself up using the trapeze.

Ms. Angela Freeman has acute low back pain. She has pelvic-belt traction, which she uses intermittently throughout the day.

89 When the nurse helps Ms. Freeman apply the pelvic traction, it would be best to place the *top* of the belt
○ 1. just below the rib cage.
○ 2. even with her waistline.

○ 3. level with the iliac crest.
○ 4. where it is most comfortable.

90 When it is time to take Ms. Freeman to physical therapy, what should the nurse do *first*?
○ 1. Unfasten the pelvic belt.
○ 2. Remove the traction weights.
○ 3. Hand her the overhead trapeze.
○ 4. Help her apply a back brace.

NURSING CARE OF CLIENTS HAVING AMPUTATIONS

During a farming accident Mr. Steve Rumsey's arm gets caught in a corn auger. His lower left arm and hand are crushed.

91 Which of the following assessments would the nurse typically find when the paramedics bring Mr. Rumsey to the hospital in shock? The client would have
○ 1. decreasing heart rate.
○ 2. decreasing blood pressure.
○ 3. increasing bowel sounds.
○ 4. increasing urine output.

92 In what position should the nurse place Mr. Rumsey while continuing with his assessment and care?
○ 1. Prone
○ 2. Supine
○ 3. On his back with his legs elevated
○ 4. On his side with his neck extended

Mr. Rumsey, who has not regained consciousness, is rushed to surgery where his arm is amputated above the elbow.

93 When Mr. Rumsey reacts from the anesthesia, he sees that his forearm is missing. He screams obscenities and sobs uncontrollably. Which of the following is the best action the nurse can take at this time?
○ 1. Leave the room until he has worked through his anger.
○ 2. Stay with him quietly in the room at his bedside.
○ 3. Tell him to get control of himself.
○ 4. Call the hospital chaplain for him.

94 Mr. Rumsey says, "I know my arm is not there, but I feel as though it is throbbing. It's driving me crazy." It would be helpful for the nurse to explain that he is experiencing
○ 1. referred pain.
○ 2. phantom pain.
○ 3. psychogenic pain.
○ 4. intractable pain.

The physician orders transcutaneous electric nerve stimulation (TENS) to relieve Mr. Rumsey's discomfort. The nurse applies the electrodes to the client's normal hand in the location where he describes the discomfort in his amputated hand.

95 When Mr. Rumsey asks how the TENS unit is supposed to help, the best explanation from the nurse would be that supposedly the sensation created by the TENS machine
○ 1. block's the brain's perception of pain impulses.
○ 2. travels to the nerve root of the amputated arm.
○ 3. destroys the brain's pain center.
○ 4. weakens the arm's sensory nerves.

Ms. Shirley Knight, a diabetic, is admitted with vascular problems. Some toes on her left foot are black. She is scheduled for a below-the-knee amputation.

96 When planning Ms. Knight's postoperative care, which position would it be most important for the nurse to *avoid*?
○ 1. Prone
○ 2. Supine
○ 3. Sitting
○ 4. Side-lying

Ms. Knight will use a three-point non–weight-bearing gait when she first begins ambulating.

97 The nursing team gathers to develop a plan to help strengthen Ms. Knight's muscles to prepare her for ambulation. If all of the following activities are suggested, which one should be started *immediately*?
○ 1. Stand at the side of the bed.
○ 2. Balance between parallel bars.
○ 3. Lift herself with the trapeze.
○ 4. Transfer from bed to chair.

98 When the nurse is changing the stump dressing, Ms. Knight says, "I just can't look at it!" Of the following comments the nurse could make, which one is best in this situation?
○ 1. "Look away until you feel ready."
○ 2. "Maybe you should get counseling."
○ 3. "I'd be curious to see how it looks."
○ 4. "Come on! It doesn't look that bad."

99 Ms. Knight asks the nurse why the stump is wrapped with elastic roller bandages several times a day. The best explanation for stump bandaging is that it is done to
○ 1. lengthen and tone muscles.
○ 2. shrink and shape the stump.
○ 3. maintain joint flexibility.
○ 4. absorb blood and drainage.

Just before his 18th birthday, Mr. Mike Collins was diagnosed as having a cancerous bone tumor in his femur. An above-the-knee amputation has been performed.

100 During Mike's immediate postoperative care, which one of the following assessments is essential for the nurse to perform? The nurse should
○ 1. look underneath the stump.
○ 2. dorsiflex the client's foot.
○ 3. take the client's temperature.
○ 4. inspect the skin on his back.

101 The nursing care plan says that the foot of Mike's bed is to be elevated. A nursing assistant asks why this measure is being taken. The best explanation from the nurse is that this position reduces stump swelling and
○ 1. decreases the risk for pneumonia.
○ 2. promotes drainage from the stump.
○ 3. prevents hip flexion contracture.
○ 4. stimulates intestinal peristalsis.

A rigid plaster shell surrounds the stump. A pylon, or temporary prosthesis, allows Mike to ambulate with crutches soon after surgery.

102 Which one of the following observations should indicate to the nurse that the crutches Mike is using need further adjustment?
○ 1. The client stands straight without bending forward.
○ 2. The top bars of the crutches fit snugly into the axilla.
○ 3. The elbows are slightly flexed when standing in place.
○ 4. The wrists are hyperextended when grasping the handgrips.

NURSING CARE OF CLIENTS WITH A HERNIATED INTERVERTEBRAL DISK

Mr. Barry Heywood, a construction worker, has been experiencing periodic bouts of low back pain. Now, in addition to the pain that radiates into his buttocks, he has some numbness and tingling in his leg. The physician suspects that Mr. Heywood has a herniated intervertebral disk in the lumbar spine.

103 While assessing the characteristics of Mr. Heywood's pain, it would be typical of a person with a herniated disk to indicate that the pain is *increased* when
○ 1. eating.
○ 2. sneezing.
○ 3. resting.
○ 4. urinating.

104 Mr. Heywood is receiving 10 mg of diazepam (Valium) orally t.i.d. Besides diminishing anxiety, the nurse explains that this medication also is used to
○ 1. reduce emotional depression.
○ 2. relax skeletal muscles.
○ 3. promote restful sleep.
○ 4. relieve inflammation.

Mr. Heywood is to remain in bed for the time being.

105 Which position would the nurse find gives Mr. Heywood the most comfort?
- ○ 1. On his back with the head and knees elevated
- ○ 2. On his side with hips and legs straight
- ○ 3. On his abdomen with his head to the side
- ○ 4. On his back with his head and knees straight

106 Which one of the following should the nurse use to provide support to Mr. Heywood's spine?
- ○ 1. A sheepskin pad
- ○ 2. An air mattress
- ○ 3. A bed board
- ○ 4. A foam square

107 Before turning Mr. Heywood to wash his back, which instruction should the nurse provide to minimize his discomfort?
- ○ 1. "Hold your breath as you are turning."
- ○ 2. "Move your upper body first then legs."
- ○ 3. "Curl up in a ball before you move."
- ○ 4. "Avoid twisting your body while moving."

108 Which one of the following observations would most indicate to the nurse that the skin over Mr. Heywood's coccyx is becoming impaired? The skin
- ○ 1. looks shiny over bony prominences.
- ○ 2. appears red when pressure is relieved.
- ○ 3. feels cool and clammy.
- ○ 4. is moist and warm.

109 The nurse applies a commercially made hot moist pack, called a hydrocollator pack, to the client's lower back. To reduce the potential for a thermal injury the nurse should plan to
- ○ 1. wrap the pack in several thick towels.
- ○ 2. rub skin lotion over the back area.
- ○ 3. place a pillow between him and the pack.
- ○ 4. position the client on a rubber ring.

Before being discharged, Mr. Heywood must be taught principles of good body mechanics.

110 The nurse would be correct in telling Mr. Heywood that when he picks something up, he should
- ○ 1. flex both his knees.
- ○ 2. keep his feet together.
- ○ 3. lift with arms extended.
- ○ 4. bend from the waist.

Conservative treatment no longer relieves Ms. Alma Reber's recurrent problems with a herniated disk. Surgery is recommended. Ms. Reber will have a laminectomy and spinal fusion in the lumbar area of the spine.

111 While practicing deep breathing exercises preoperatively with Ms. Reber, she tells the nurse that she is feeling dizzy and light-headed. The nurse explains that this is a common experience when breathing too

- ○ 1. slowly.
- ○ 2. deeply.
- ○ 3. rapidly.
- ○ 4. shallowly.

112 Postoperatively, it is essential that the nurse keep Ms. Reber's spine in a position of
- ○ 1. flexion.
- ○ 2. extension.
- ○ 3. hyperextension.
- ○ 4. circumduction.

113 The nurse administers 10 mg of intramuscular morphine sulfate to Ms. Reber for pain. Which one of the following observations indicates that she is experiencing an *adverse* reaction to the morphine? Ms. Reber's
- ○ 1. respirations are 8 breaths per minute.
- ○ 2. heart rate is 68 beats per minute.
- ○ 3. oral temperature is 97.8°F.
- ○ 4. systolic blood pressure is 138 mm Hg.

114 Which one of the following drugs should the nurse have on hand to counteract the adverse effects of the morphine sulfate?
- ○ 1. methadone hydrochloride (Dolophine)
- ○ 2. meperidine hydrochloride (Demerol)
- ○ 3. naloxone hydrochloride (Narcan)
- ○ 4. propoxyphene hydrochloride (Darvon)

115 The nurse helps the client take care of her hygiene needs. What hair care aid would be most helpful in grooming the hair of an African American client like Ms. Reber?
- ○ 1. A wire hairbrush
- ○ 2. A rat-tail comb
- ○ 3. A large-toothed pick
- ○ 4. A hot-air blow dryer

The Nursing Care of Clients with Disorders of the Integumentary System

NURSING CARE OF CLIENTS WITH HERPES ZOSTER (SHINGLES)

Mr. Stan Wagner, age 43, is complaining of redness on his lower chest and upper abdomen and is seen by a physician.

116 Which one of the following should the nurse include in an initial health history before Mr. Wagner sees his physician?
- ○ 1. The apparent cause of the reddened area
- ○ 2. Why the redness occurred in this particular area
- ○ 3. When and where the problem first appeared
- ○ 4. The relationship of the redness to his other medical problems

The physician determines that Mr. Wagner most probably has shingles (herpes zoster) and prescribes acyclovir (Zovirax).

117 Mr. Wagner asks the nurse what causes shingles. The most correct reply is based on the fact that shingles is caused by
  ○ 1. a reactivation of the varicella-zoster virus, which lies dormant in sensory ganglia.
  ○ 2. exposure to the mumps virus in the past month.
  ○ 3. a previous *Staphylococcus* infection.
  ○ 4. a drug allergy.

118 Mr. Wagner asks the nurse if the drug prescribed by the physician will cure his shingles. The most correct reply is based on the fact that this drug
  ○ 1. appears to prevent future attacks of shingles.
  ○ 2. may prevent the lesions from forming crusts.
  ○ 3. may reduce the severity of symptoms and prevent the development of further lesions.
  ○ 4. causes the lesions to disappear in approximately 48 hours.

NURSING CARE OF CLIENTS WITH PSORIASIS

Ms. Betty Lynch, age 29, notes that she has recently developed a skin problem and makes an appointment to be seen in a clinic specializing in the treatment of integumentary disorders. A diagnosis of psoriasis is made by the physician.

119 When examining Ms. Lynch's skin for areas of psoriasis, the nurse should look for
  ○ 1. weeping lesions on the trunk of the body.
  ○ 2. patches of redness covered with silvery scales.
  ○ 3. areas of redness surrounded by crusts.
  ○ 4. a rash characterized by raised, pus-filled lesions.

120 To reduce anxiety which one of the following is *most* important when the nurse examines Ms. Lynch's skin lesions?
  ○ 1. Being calm
  ○ 2. Not examining unaffected areas
  ○ 3. Being thorough
  ○ 4. Not showing repulsion

NURSING CARE OF CLIENTS WITH SKIN CANCER

Mr. Ed Hall, age 73, sees his physician because he has noticed a growth on his right temple. Biopsy reveals that the lesion is a basal cell carcinoma. The physician plans to remove the lesion with cryosurgery.

121 Mr. Hall asks the nurse what cryosurgery is. The most correct reply would describe this type of surgery as one that removes the lesion by means of
  ○ 1. the application of liquid nitrogen, which is a deep-freezing substance.
  ○ 2. cutting away the tumor with a laser beam.
  ○ 3. burning the tumor with an electric current.
  ○ 4. injecting the tumor area with a cancer-fighting drug.

122 Mr. Hall's lesion is removed by cryosurgery. Which one of the following should be included in teaching Mr. Hall about the care of the treatment site?
  ○ 1. Apply warm, wet soaks to the area until the scab falls off.
  ○ 2. The scab must be allowed to dry and fall off.
  ○ 3. Apply petroleum jelly to aid in removal of the scab.
  ○ 4. Use an ice pack for 24 hours to prevent the spread of cancer cells.

NURSING CARE OF CLIENTS WITH A STASIS ULCER

Mr. Tom Marshall, age 78, has a stasis ulcer due to arterial insufficiency. He is admitted to the hospital for more intensive treatment of the disorder.

123 Mr. Marshall asks the nurse if there is anything that can be done to lessen his pain. The most appropriate nursing action is to
  ○ 1. keep the affected area exposed to air.
  ○ 2. avoid chilling of the extremities.
  ○ 3. elevate the legs whenever the client is sitting.
  ○ 4. keep the client in bed until the ulcer has healed.

124 A topical enzyme preparation is to be applied to the stasis ulcer. Which one of the following techniques is *most* appropriate?
  ○ 1. Wash the area with alcohol before applying the topical enzyme.
  ○ 2. To reduce pain apply ice to the area before applying the topical enzyme.
  ○ 3. Cover the area with a restrictive dressing after applying the topical enzyme.
  ○ 4. Apply the topical enzyme with care because the area is painful.

NURSING CARE OF CLIENTS WITH A BURN INJURY

Ms. Shelley Ferris, age 29, was trapped in her home by a fire. The firemen arrive on the scene as the victim runs from the house. Her clothing and hair are on fire.

125 A nurse working as a volunteer fire fighter is first at the scene. The initial emergency treatment of this victim should include
  ○ 1. applying petroleum jelly to the burned areas.
  ○ 2. wrapping the affected areas in sterile gauze.
  ○ 3. pouring normal saline over the affected areas.
  ○ 4. smothering the flames by wrapping the victim in a blanket.

126 The next most important step in the emergency treatment of Ms. Ferris is
○ 1. obtaining her vital signs.
○ 2. establishing a patent airway.
○ 3. identifying the victim.
○ 4. determining the extent and type of burns.

Ms. Ferris is admitted to the hospital for treatment of her burns.

127 The nurse performing an initial assessment of Ms. Ferris should be aware that an early problem associated with extensive burns is
○ 1. shock.
○ 2. fever.
○ 3. thirst.
○ 4. diaphoresis.

128 The physician orders the insertion of a urethral catheter connected to a closed drainage system. The nurse should know that the primary purpose of an indwelling catheter for this client is to
○ 1. prevent decubiti.
○ 2. accurately measure urinary output.
○ 3. prevent damage to the bladder.
○ 4. determine the need for electrolyte replacement.

129 The physician states that Ms. Ferris should be observed for a fluid volume deficit, which may occur because of
○ 1. a decrease in urinary output.
○ 2. the movement of fluid from body cells to the plasma.
○ 3. a loss of skin integrity.
○ 4. an inability to administer fluids by the parenteral route.

Ms. Ferris has second- and third-degree burns over 35% of her body and is to be treated by the open method.

130 The nurse must be constantly aware of the major problem that may occur with this method of treatment, which is
○ 1. infection.
○ 2. abnormal eschar formation.
○ 3. itching.
○ 4. absence of eschar formation.

131 The nurse reviews the physician's orders and notes that a topical drug is to be applied to the burned areas. A topical drug is applied
○ 1. only when the eschar becomes soft.
○ 2. using clean technique.
○ 3. using aseptic technique.
○ 4. immediately before the client receives hydrotherapy.

132 The nursing care plan developed for Ms. Ferris includes proper positioning and the use of an alternating pressure mattress. When reviewing the plan of care, the nurse should understand that proper positioning
○ 1. decreases lung capacity.
○ 2. prevents contractures.
○ 3. decreases blood flow to the burned areas.
○ 4. prevents infection of noninjured areas.

133 The health care team is informed that skin grafting is planned for Ms. Ferris. Which one of the following should be considered when formulating a postoperative plan of care for the client having an autograft?
○ 1. A graft will be taken from a cadaver.
○ 2. There will be a donor site and a recipient site.
○ 3. Mesh will be used as a temporary graft.
○ 4. An animal skin will be used to provide a temporary graft.

134 Which one of the following is most appropriate for the postoperative plan of care when Ms. Ferris has skin grafts?
○ 1. Minimizing movement to prevent disruption of skin graft contact with underlying tissues
○ 2. Changing the dressing over the graft every 8 hours
○ 3. Reinforcing the dressing if drainage occurs
○ 4. Removing the dressing and applying wet soaks to the graft every 4 hours

NURSING CARE OF CLIENTS WITH A DECUBITUS ULCER

Mr. Richard Keller, age 74, is admitted to the hospital for treatment of medical problems including respiratory difficulty, diabetes, and fever. When the nurse performs an initial physical assessment, it is noted that Mr. Keller has decubitus ulcers on his left hip and sacrum.

135 To develop a care plan, the nurse should know that a decubitus ulcer usually results from
○ 1. an allergic reaction to drugs.
○ 2. a lack of blood supply to tissue.
○ 3. poor personal hygiene.
○ 4. a lack of dietary vitamin B.

136 The best method of preventing decubitus ulcer formation is
○ 1. the application of a skin-toughening agent to susceptible areas.
○ 2. keeping the head of the bed elevated 30 degrees during daytime hours.
○ 3. providing a low-protein diet.
○ 4. turning and repositioning the client every 2 hours.

137 The physician orders a pressure-reducing/relieving mattress for Mr. Keller. This device is placed
○ 1. under the client's hips.
○ 2. over the regular bed mattress.

○ 3. on top of the bed covers.
○ 4. under the regular bed mattress.

INDIVIDUAL TEST ITEMS

138 Ms. Link has dermatitis medicamentosa. Which one of the following would be *most* important when obtaining a health history?
○ 1. A family history of skin cancer
○ 2. A history of exposure to chickenpox or measles
○ 3. A history of kidney disease
○ 4. An allergy history

139 A client is seen in the emergency department for frostbite. Which one of the following measures should the nurse be prepared to use for treatment of this problem?
○ 1. A warm solution with a temperature of approximately 100°F
○ 2. Shaved ice enclosed in a plastic bag
○ 3. A heating pad
○ 4. A hot solution with a temperature of approximately 140°F

140 The nurse at a summer resort must be prepared to treat simple emergencies. Which one of the following maneuvers may be used to remove a tick from a client's skin?
○ 1. Crush the tick with a tweezers.
○ 2. Squeeze the tick between the fingers.
○ 3. Use a hot needle to make the tick release its hold.
○ 4. Wrap the tick in gauze and pull it quickly from the skin.

141 The nurse working at a summer resort also must be aware of problems such as athlete's foot (tinea pedis). Which of the following are the *common* symptoms of this disorder?
○ 1. Blisters forming on the top of the feet
○ 2. Red, scaly, sore cracks between the toes
○ 3. Wart-like growths found on the edges and soles of the feet
○ 4. Changes in the appearance of the toenails

142 A client has pruritus. Which one of the following measures could the nurse use to lessen this client's discomfort?
○ 1. Use hypoallergenic or glycerin soap for bathing.
○ 2. Add extra blankets to the bedding to decrease evaporation of moisture from the skin.
○ 3. Use cold water for bathing.
○ 4. Rub the skin dry after bathing.

143 Which one of the following should the nurse include in a teaching plan for a client with a herpes simplex virus type 1 infection?
○ 1. Apply petroleum jelly to the lesions to prevent spread to adjacent areas.
○ 2. Do not clean the affected areas.
○ 3. Use good personal hygiene to prevent spreading the virus to other body parts.
○ 4. Remove the scabs daily by soaking with hot compresses.

Correct Answers and Rationales

Two numbers appear in parentheses following each rationale. The first number identifies the textbook listed in the references, page 451, and the second number identifies the page(s) in that textbook on which the correct answer can be verified. Occasionally, two textbooks are given for verifying the correct answer.

The Nursing Care of Clients with Disorders of the Musculoskeletal System

NURSING CARE OF CLIENTS WITH STRAINS, SPRAINS, AND DISLOCATIONS

1 2. Temporarily eliminating the activity that has injured the tendons is the best action to take at this time. It is unnecessary to keep the hand and wrist immobile. Playing miniature golf would continue to pull or tear the tendons. Golfers wear gloves to prevent their skin from becoming blistered. Wearing a tight glove would not protect the joint from injury. (14:758; 3:656)
Nursing Process—Evaluation
Client Need—Physiological integrity

2 3. Ecchymosis refers to the black and blue skin discoloration caused by the rupture of small blood vessels with bleeding into the skin. Freckled skin would be scattered small brown pigmented spots on the skin. Mottled skin contains patchy areas that are light colored or blue. This observation is seen primarily in hypothermic infants and dying clients. Blanched skin appears pale. (7:777; 18:287)
Nursing Process—Collecting data
Client Need—Physiological integrity

3 2. Elevating a swollen extremity relieves swelling through the use of gravity. Dangling the foot would put the foot in a dependent position and increase the amount of swelling. Exercise would cause pain and further swelling in the early stage of the injury. Immobilization would be used to relieve pain and promote healing. (16:780; 14:749)
Nursing Process—Implementation
Client Need—Physiological integrity

4 4. The roller bandage should be started at the metatarsals. The metatarsal bones form the ball of the foot and instep. The toes, or phalanges, are left uncovered to assess circulation. To relieve swelling the injured area should be wrapped distally to proximally. If wrapped from below the knee toward the foot, swelling would not be relieved. (18:486; 14:394)
Nursing Process—Implementation
Client Need—Physiological integrity

5 1. The figure-of-eight turn is made by overlapping the roller bandage in an alternately ascending and descending oblique pattern around a joint. Each turn crosses the one preceding it so that it resembles the number eight. A spiral reverse turn is used to bandage a cone-shaped body part, such as the thigh or leg. The recurrent turn is used to cover the tip of a body part, such as the stump of an amputated limb. A spica turn is an adaptation of the figure-of-eight wrap. It is used when the wrap must go around an adjacent body part, such as the thumb and hand, thigh and hip, and so on. (18:486-487)
Nursing Process—Implementation
Client Need—Physiological integrity

6 3. Venous blood and lymph may be trapped in the toes and produce a swollen appearance if the roller bandage has been applied too tightly. Loosening the bandage and elevating the extremity should restore or improve circulation. Warm toes indicate that blood flow is adequate. The roller bandage will only lessen the pain. The injured area will not be pain free. Wearing a cotton sock would not be an indication for loosening the elastic bandage. (14:394)
Nursing Process—Implementation
Client Need—Health promotion/maintenance

7 4. A dislocation results in the temporary displacement of a bone from its normal position within a joint. This is caused by the tearing of the ligaments that connect two bone ends within a joint. Sprains do not interrupt the continuity of one bone with another; therefore, there is no obvious deformity. Both sprains and dislocations are accompanied by pain, swelling, and impaired movement. (16:779; 7:777)
Nursing Process—Collecting data
Client Need—Physiological integrity

8 3. To restore the normal function of the joint, the physician will reposition the two adjacent bones so that they are again in contact with one another. The repositioning is done manually with or without anesthesia. A surgical incision is necessary when doing a procedure called an open reduction. Inserting a pin or wire would be a type of internal fixation. Exercise would only be prescribed after a period of stabilization to allow time for healing. (16:779; 7:777)

Nursing Process—Implementation
Client Need—Health promotion/maintenance

9 2. The knot should be tied at the side of the neck to avoid pressure on the cervical vertebrae. All the other statements indicate correct information concerning the application and use of a sling. (14:419; 18:687)

Nursing Process—Evaluation
Client Need—Health promotion/maintenance

NURSING CARE OF CLIENTS WITH ARTHRITIS

10 1. The first symptom a person with rheumatoid arthritis is likely to report is joint stiffness when they awaken. It may be accompanied by swelling and discomfort in the affected joints. People with rheumatoid arthritis do tend to tire easily, but this is not usually the earliest symptom that causes concern. The pain is more of a continuous aching. Movement contributes to pain. Consequently, the person may avoid using the joints that are painful. However, it may be some time before the joints are destroyed and fixated. (16:800; 7:771)

Nursing Process—Collecting data
Client Need—Safe, effective care environment

11 3. A person who is to have 5 g of drug supplied in a dosage strength of 5 grains per tablet, will require 15 tablets in a 24-hour period.

1 g contains approximately 15 grains
5 g contains 75 grains (5 × 15 = 75)

To solve the problem using a ratio and proportion method, use the following steps (15:12; 18:574):

$$\frac{5 \text{ grains}}{1 \text{ tablet}} = \frac{75 \text{ grains}}{X \text{ tablets}}$$
$$5X = 75$$
$$X = 15 \text{ tablets}$$

Nursing Process—Implementation
Client Need—Physiological integrity

12 4. Taking irritating drugs with food or at mealtime helps decrease gastric distress. Aspirin, especially in large doses, tends to irritate the stomach mucosa. Giving aspirin on an empty stomach increases discomfort. Cold water or hot tea are not substances that will alter the acidity of the stomach or the aspirin. The caffeine in tea may

actually stimulate an increase in the production of stomach acid. (15:73)

Nursing Process—Planning
Client Need—Physiological integrity

13 3. Aspirin has the ability to produce analgesic, anti-inflammatory, and antipyretic effects. Its analgesic and anti-inflammatory effects are probably achieved by inhibiting chemicals called prostaglandins and not by interrupting nerve synapses. Prostaglandins increase sensitivity of peripheral pain receptors. Aspirin does not relax skeletal muscles or stimulate the immune system. (15:70)

Nursing Process—Implementation
Client Need—Health promotion/maintenance

14 4. It is best to notify the charge nurse promptly when signs or symptoms of aspirin toxicity appear. The physician needs to be consulted to change the dosage or to prescribe another type of drug. Buffering the aspirin only reduces the gastric irritation; it will not reduce its toxicity. It is not advisable to continue giving the aspirin if toxic symptoms have been noted. Withholding one dose will not effectively relieve toxic symptoms. (15:73; 18:575-576)

Nursing Process—Implementation
Client Need—Physiological integrity

15 4. Distraction is a legitimate and often very effective method for the relief of discomfort. Watching television is one method of distraction. There are no reports that electronic television signals are an effective treatment for arthritis. If the client had only a slight case of arthritis, she would be likely also to feel pain relief at times other than just watching television. (18:181; 3:216)

Nursing Process—Evaluation
Client Need—Physiological integrity

16 1. The proximal finger joints are affected the most in rheumatoid arthritis. There may be so much involvement that the fingers will actually turn laterally. In osteoarthritis the distal finger joints are more often deformed. Traumatic arthritis, which is associated with a specific injury, may affect any joint. (16:801, 803)

Nursing Process—Collecting data
Client Need—Physiological integrity

17 3. Though many people have juvenile arthritis, most individuals with rheumatoid arthritis experience the onset of the disease early in their adult life. The disease profoundly affects their ability to maintain employment during the productive years of life. (7:660; 16:800)

Nursing Process—Collecting data
Client Need—Safe, effective care environment

18 1. The erythrocyte sedimentation rate is a nonspecific test that indicates the presence and progress of an inflammatory disease. It may be elevated in a number of inflammatory conditions including rheumatoid arthritis. A PTT time is ordered to determine a person's ability to clot blood. It is commonly ordered when a person is on heparin therapy. A fasting blood sugar is performed to diagnose and evaluate the treatment of diabetes mellitus. The BUN is a common test for assessing renal function. (3:663; 7:772)

    Nursing Process—Collecting data
    Client Need—Physiological integrity

19 2. Hand deformity and muscle atrophy make it difficult to perform fine motor movement with the fingers. Purchasing clothes that can be pulled on or slipped on enables the client with rheumatoid arthritis to maintain a degree of independence. It is important for the person with arthritis to maintain joint mobility through exercise. However, it is unlikely that the client would be able to perform the finger coordination required to play a musical instrument. Aerobic exercise is unrealistic because it is likely to be too strenuous. Clients with rheumatoid arthritis are often anemic and tire easily. There is no known connection between chemical additives and the symptoms of arthritis. (14:755; 3:665)

    Nursing Process—Implementation
    Client Need—Health promotion/maintenance

20 1. Corticosteroid therapy can cause sodium and water retention. The consequence of hypernatremia is evidenced by weight gain. With an excess of fluid, blood pressure also may become elevated and should be closely monitored as well. The pulse rate is not likely to change appreciably. However, the pulse may feel bounding with an increase of fluid in the blood volume. Peristalsis is unaffected by corticosteroids. The skin of a person taking steroids may undergo various changes. However, the skin generally remains intact. The nurse may observe that the skin becomes thin and bruises easily. There may be increased hair growth, petechiae, redistribution of body fat, and striae. If the skin does become impaired as a result of injury or surgery, wound healing may be prolonged. (15:207; 3:662)

    Nursing Process—Collecting data
    Client Need—Physiological integrity

21 3. Individuals receiving corticosteroids tend to have elevated blood sugar. Diabetics may need to increase their dosage of insulin or oral hypoglycemic agents. Nondiabetics also should be monitored for hyperglycemia and glucosuria. Because steroids depress the inflammatory response, they place the client at high risk for acquiring infections. Steroids should be withdrawn gradually if therapy is to be discontinued to prevent acute adrenal insufficiency. Depression is common among individuals receiving corticosteroids. (15:207-208)

    Nursing Process—Evaluation
    Client Need—Health promotion/maintenance

22 1. During an acute attack, splints are used primarily to keep the inflamed joints somewhat inactive. Resting the part suppresses additional stress on the diseased joints caused by movement. The acute inflammation subsides with a combination of drug therapy and the body's natural healing processes. Secondarily, a certain amount of strength and joint flexibility will be preserved by limiting the damage during the acute attack. (3:662, 664; 7:772)

    Nursing Process—Implementation
    Client Need—Safe, effective care environment

23 1. The symptoms of rheumatoid arthritis can spontaneously go away. Many give credit for their remission to some unrelated activity or unorthodox treatment. The use of copper bracelets in the treatment of arthritis is a common folk medicine myth. Because people who suffer from chronic and incurable diseases, like arthritis, are desperate for something that will cure their illness, they are extremely vulnerable to fraudulent treatment. Through health teaching, the nurse helps individuals with incurable or terminal diseases avoid becoming victims of quackery. (3:662; 18:757-758)

    Nursing Process—Implementation
    Client Need—Health promotion/maintenance

24 3. Moist heat is more effective than forms of dry heat like a hot water bottle, electric heating pad, or infrared heat lamp. This phenomenon is attributed to the fact that water is a better conductor of heat than air. Whenever any form of heat is used, the nurse must take care that the client is not accidentally burned. (14:387; 3:666)

    Nursing Process—Implementation
    Client Need—Physiological integrity

25 1. To avoid burning the skin, a heating pad should be kept on a low setting. The client should be cautioned not to turn the heat setting higher when he becomes adapted to the sensation of warmth. It is hazardous to use safety pins. There is a potential for electric shock if metal pins puncture a heating wire. A heating pad should be covered with fabric, such as flannel. Heat should not be applied for longer than 20 to 30 minutes at a time. (3:666; 18:494-495)

    Nursing Process—Implementation
    Client Need—Safe, effective care environment

26 1. Obesity puts additional stress on a weight-bearing joint and contributes to discomfort. Eating green leafy vegetables and fruit are healthy behaviors, but they will not directly relieve the effects of the arthritis. Physical activity is likely to cause more discomfort because walking is painful for him. (3:665; 16:803)

Nursing Process—Implementation
Client Need—Health promotion/maintenance

27 3. A cane should be held on the uninvolved side. By doing so the client can transfer or redistribute his body weight from the painful joint to his hand when taking a step. Covering the tip with a rubber cap, wearing supportive shoes, and maintaining good posture are all appropriate techniques for using a cane. (18:419)

Nursing Process—Evaluation
Client Need—Health promotion/maintenance

28 3. A common side effect of NSAIDs is gastrointestinal symptoms. They include nausea, vomiting, diarrhea, constipation, epigastric pain, indigestion, and gastrointestinal bleeding, to name a few. This category of drugs should be used cautiously in individuals with a history of peptic ulcer disease. By asking the client to identify the color of his stools, the nurse would be assessing if the drug is causing gastrointestinal bleeding. NSAIDS are not known to cause changes in libido or hand tremors. Asking the client whether he takes his medication with food would be important once the nurse determines that the client is experiencing gastrointestinal side effects. (15:72-73)

Nursing Process—Collecting data
Client Need—Physiological integrity

29 2. Aspirin increases the possibility of postoperative bleeding. It interferes with the ability of platelets to clump together, one of the first mechanisms in clot formation. Aspirin does not increase the risk of wound infection or the ability to heal. Aspirin would not be discontinued to facilitate the assessment of the client's pain. (15:73; 16:810)

Nursing Process—Implementation
Client Need—Health promotion/maintenance

30 1. An incentive spirometer helps a client measure the effectiveness of deep inhalation. It is important postoperatively for the client to breathe deeply to open the airways and alveoli. This helps to improve the oxygenation of blood, eliminate carbon dioxide, and prevent atelectasis and pneumonia. None of the other three options indicates a correct use of an incentive spirometer. (18:434; 14:449)

Nursing Process—Evaluation
Client Need—Health promotion/maintenance

31 4. The strokes with the razor should be made with the grain of the hair shaft. This technique avoids nicking or scraping the skin. Impairing the integrity of the skin and bleeding increase the risk of postoperative wound infections. Soap is used to decrease the numbers of transient skin organisms. The razor should be held so that it glides across the surface of the skin. The direction of the razor strokes is determined by the direction of the hair growth. (7:105; 18:100, 436, 438)

Nursing Process—Implementation
Client Need—Safe, effective care environment

32 2. The hip of a client who has undergone an arthroplasty must be maintained in a position of abduction. If the client flexes his hip more than 90 degrees or adducts the hip, the prosthetic femoral head may become dislocated. A triangular foam wedge is generally kept between the client's legs while he is in bed. (16:811; 3:667)

Nursing Process—Implementation
Client Need—Physiological integrity

33 3. A trapeze is an item that allows the client to help move and lift himself. Encouraging the client to participate actively helps maintain his muscular strength and reduces the effort the nurse must provide when moving and positioning a client. A bed cradle is used to keep bed linen off of lower extremities. A bed board is used to support the client's spine. Lower side rails would be appropriate to maintain the safety of a confused client or one with a perceptual disorder. (16:812; 18:380)

Nursing Process—Planning
Client Need—Physiological integrity

34 2. A trochanter roll is used to maintain the hip in a position of extension. Placing this positioning device at the trochanter helps keep the hip from rotating outward. A foot board is used to prevent plantar flexion and foot drop deformity. A turning sheet is used to reposition a client. A foam mattress helps to relieve pressure from bony prominences. (18:379)

Nursing Process—Implementation
Client Need—Physiological integrity

35 1. A client with a total hip replacement must be told that he may not cross his legs. Crossing the legs places the hip in a position of adduction and flexion. These two positions can displace the prosthetic device. Pointing the toes as in plantar flexion or dorsiflexion will not impair the surgical procedure. Lying flat and standing upright will not be harmful. (16:812; 3:669)

Nursing Process—Evaluation
Client Need—Health promotion/maintenance

36 3. Postoperatively and for an extended time in his home care, the client will need to use a device that elevates his buttocks. This is necessary so that when he sits on the toilet or any other seat his hip is not flexed more than 90 degrees. The client will not need a wheelchair. He will ambulate using a walker. The client can continue to use his own bed at home. The client will be taught how to transfer himself from his bed to a chair. Therefore, a mechanical lift is unnecessary. (3:669; 16:812)

Nursing Process—Implementation
Client Need—Health promotion/maintenance

37 1. The client with a total hip replacement should avoid bending over to put on or take off socks, pants, and shoes. Someone should be available to help with these items of clothing. Another approach would be to modify the clothing so that the client can slip them on without flexing the hip more than 90 degrees. No special equipment is needed for eating. Taking supplemental vitamins is not necessary as long as the client consumes an adequate diet. It would be helpful to discuss how to avoid bowel elimination problems with any client that was prone to constipation or diarrhea. However, this would not be unique to the care of the client with a total hip replacement. (16:812; 3:669)

Nursing Process—Planning
Client Need—Health promotion/maintenance

38 4. A CPM machine is used primarily to restore full range of joint motion. Clients with knee joint replacement often are reluctant to exercise the operative knee actively because of pain. Exercise will tone and strengthen muscles. However, this is not the primary reason for using a passive motion machine. Exercise promotes venous circulation. Therefore, the machine would relieve dependent swelling. However, this is a secondary benefit from using a CPM machine. Use of the machine will be accompanied by discomfort. It would be appropriate for the nurse to administer a prescribed analgesic before using the CPM machine. (18:699; 7:774)

Nursing Process—Implementation
Client Need—Safe, effective care environment

39 2. How long the client used the CPM machine would be one indication of his response to treatment. Reviewing all the pertinent information in the documentation helps evaluate how the client is progressing in his recovery. Inspecting and documenting the appearance of the wound, the drainage on the dressing, and the presence and quality of arterial pulses are important data to record. However, this information would be documented with the physical assessment findings. (18:701)

Nursing Process—Implementation
Client Need—Safe, effective care environment

40 1. Gout can affect any joint, but approximately 80% of the people who have gout experience symptoms in their great toe. (3:665; 7:774; 14:756)

Nursing Process—Collecting data
Client Need—Physiological integrity

41 3. A serum uric acid level is used to diagnose gout. It may be elevated along with the creatinine clearance and BUN in renal failure. Serum calcium may be elevated in hyperparathyroidism; primary cancers, such as Hodgkin's disease or multiple myeloma; and metastasis to the bone. (16:803; 5:318)

Nursing Process—Collecting data
Client Need—Physiological integrity

42 1. A bed cradle is needed to prevent the affected joints from being touched or bumped. There is no relationship between gout and the need for an electric fan, foam mattress, or fracture bedpan. (14:756)

Nursing Process—Implementation
Client Need—Physiological integrity

43 4. Organ meats, such as liver, kidney, brain, and sweetbreads, are high in purines. Other high sources are fish roe, sardines, and anchovies. Foods that are moderately high in purines are meats, seafood, dried beans, lentils, spinach, and peas. (4:516; 14:756)

Nursing Process—Implementation
Client Need—Physiological integrity

44 1. The nurse should withhold the administration of colchicine when the client manifests gastrointestinal disturbances, such as nausea and vomiting, abdominal pain, or diarrhea. Dizziness, drowsiness, and headache are not signs of an adverse reaction to colchicine. (16:803; 15:319)

Nursing Process—Implementation
Client Need—Physiological integrity

45 3. Because the client usually has not had fluids during sleeping hours, it is best to serve the greater share of fluid in the morning. Serving a large volume of fluid after a meal may contribute to gastrointestinal fullness or upset. Consuming large amounts of fluid during evening hours or before bedtime usually interferes with sleep. The client is likely to be awakened with a full bladder and the need to urinate. (18:648)

Nursing Process—Planning
Client Need—Physiological integrity

46 2. There seems to be a relationship between the consumption of alcohol and the recurrence of gout symptoms. The client with gout should abstain from drinking alcohol. Coffee, cranberry juice, and carbonated beverages are safe to consume. (16:803; 3:665)

Nursing Process—Implementation
Client Need—Health promotion/maintenance

NURSING CARE OF CLIENTS WITH FRACTURES

47 4. To immobilize a broken bone, a splint must be applied so that it prevents movement of the joints above and below the injury. The tibia is between the knee and the ankle. Therefore, the splint should be applied from below the ankle to above the knee. (18:686)

Nursing Process—Implementation
Client Need—Physiological integrity

48 2. A comminuted fracture means that there are pieces or fragments of bone in the area where the bone was broken. An impacted fracture is one in which the bone ends are driven together. A simple, or closed, fracture is one in which there is no break in the skin. A greenstick fracture is the name given to a fracture in which the bone splits, but it does not break clear through. (16:780-781; 3:647)

Nursing Process—Implementation
Client Need—Health promotion/maintenance

49 4. The hospital must first attempt to obtain permission from a minor's parent or guardian. Minors cannot give permission under most circumstances. If permission is obtained over the telephone, at least two people must hear the verbal consent and cosign as witnesses to what they heard. (18:452; 3:228)

Nursing Process—Implementation
Client Need—Safe, effective care environment

50 4. Jewelry should be removed preoperatively, itemized, identified, and locked in a secure area. Another alternative is to give the client's valuables to a member of his family. The nurse has a responsibility to document in the client's record the items that were taken and how they are being kept secure. In some agencies the client is given a receipt for his property. If a client asks that a wedding ring be left on, the nurse can secure it to the finger or hand with tape or a strip of gauze. Class rings generally contain multiple grooves or crevices. These trap and hold microorganisms. It is best to reduce the number of pathogens as best possible before a client goes to surgery. The ring would be subject to theft if left in the bedside stand. Security guards usually

are not responsible for the safekeeping of personal valuables. (14:440; 18:442)

Nursing Process—Implementation
Client Need—Safe, effective care environment

51 2. The nurse will need to don sterile gloves once the packages of sterile gauze and sterile towels are opened. To maintain surgical asepsis only sterile items can come in contact with other sterile items. Regardless of how well handwashing is performed, the hands are never free of all organisms. Once the skin surface has been covered, the nurse can remove the gloves and secure the outside of the covering with clean tape. Antiseptic swabs are not needed; the skin was already scrubbed with an antimicrobial substance. An elastic stocking would not be applied over sterile gauze and towels. (18:440-441)

Nursing Process—Implementation
Client Need—Safe, effective care environment

52 1. Most fat emboli travel to the pulmonary circulation. Once the emboli partially or totally occlude blood flow through a pulmonary vessel, the client will experience dyspnea, rapid breathing and heart rate, cyanosis, chest pain, cough, blood-streaked sputum, and a feeling of doom. Emboli also may travel to the brain, causing confusion, agitation, and coma. (3:652; 7:781)

Nursing Process—Collecting data
Client Need—Physiological integrity

53 2. The ribs enclose the lungs. This makes injuries to the pulmonary system the prime complication associated with fractured ribs. The broken ribs may puncture the pleura and collapse a lung. As time passes, the client may develop pneumonia because of ineffective coughing and shallow breathing. The heart also is in the thorax but somewhat better protected in the center of the chest. It is not likely that a client whose injuries are limited to fractured ribs would have neurologic or gastrointestinal complications. (16:783)

Nursing Process—Collecting data
Client Need—Physiological integrity

54 1. Sharp pain is the first symptom of compartment syndrome. The pain is due to ischemia, the impairment of arterial blood flow, caused by swelling of the surrounding muscle within the inelastic fascia. Paralysis and sensory loss follow as nerves become damaged by compression and lack of blood supply. The hand would appear pale or white and cold from inadequate arterial blood. If the radial artery is assessed, the nurse would find that it is weak or absent. (7:782; 14:748)

Nursing Process—Collecting data
Client Need—Physiological integrity

55 1. All of the measures described in this item may become necessary in an emergency, but the first step a rescuer should take is to see that the victim is breathing. Maintaining ventilation is a priority to sustain life. (16:178; 18:734; 14:428)
Nursing Process—Implementation
Client Need—Physiological integrity

56 3. The best method for controlling bleeding in the case of a compound fracture is compressing the major artery above the site of the injury. Direct pressure on the wound itself may cause additional injuries to the soft tissue surrounding the fracture. A tourniquet should only be used if all other efforts to control bleeding are unsuccessful. If used, a tourniquet should be periodically released to allow oxygenated blood to the distal tissue. Elevation of the extremity may be helpful after applying pressure on the artery. (16:178)
Nursing Process—Implementation
Client Need—Physiological integrity

57 3. An accident victim with a suspected spinal injury should have his neck and back immobilized. A neck support should be applied. The victim should be flat on his back and secured to a rigid stretcher before being moved and transported. Rescuers need to keep the spine extended. Flexion may cause more injury to the vertebrae or the spinal cord. (16:455-456; 7:651)
Nursing Process—Implementation
Client Need—Physiological integrity

58 4. Typical signs of a fractured hip include external rotation and shortening of the affected leg. Bruising may or may not be present depending on the cause of the fracture. Sensation should be intact. Movement will result in increased pain. (16:786; 7:780)
Nursing Process—Collecting data
Client Need—Physiological integrity

59 1. Estrogen deficiency is linked to loss of calcium from the bones. Decreased bone mass weakens the skeletal system increasing a person's susceptibility for fractures. Being overweight would exert more stress on the skeletal system, but as long as the integrity of the bones is intact, the risk for fractures would be the same as for the general population. Doing gardening and being born in England would not potentiate the client's risk for a fracture. (3:665; 7:241)
Nursing Process—Collecting data
Client Need—Safe, effective care environment

60 2. Isometric exercises are performed by tensing and releasing muscles. They do not involve any appreciable movement of a joint. The quadriceps muscles are on the anterior of the thigh. All of the other options in this item describe iso-

tonic exercises that involve joint movement. (3:185; 18:416)
Nursing Process—Evaluation
Client Need—Physiological integrity

61 1. Elastic stockings, known as antiembolism or thomboembolic disease hose, support the valves within veins. As venous blood moves toward the heart, the supported valves prevent it from falling back into the lower legs and feet. When blood moves, rather than stands still, it is less likely to clot. Antiembolism stockings should not restrict arterial blood from flowing into the extremities. The arterial pressure should not be affected by wearing antiembolism stockings. Red blood cells, or erythrocytes, do not play a role in forming blood clots. Platelets, or thrombocytes, are the type of blood cells that clump together, especially when there has been an injury. (18:434, 436; 3:514)
Nursing Process—Implementation
Client Need—Safe, effective care environment

62 1. To prevent trapping venous blood in the lower extremities, elastic stockings should be applied while in a nondependent position. The best time to apply these stockings is in the morning before getting out of bed or after elevating the legs a short time. Elastic stockings should be worn almost continuously. They may be removed once per shift or once per day to assess the skin. (3:414; 18:438)
Nursing Process—Evaluation
Client Need—Safe, effective care environment

63 1. A client who has had a prosthesis inserted to repair a fractured hip should be turned using sufficient pillows so that his operative leg remains slightly abducted. This prevents displacement of the fixation device. Pointing the toes, flexing his knee, or elevating his head will not promote hip abduction. (7:781; 14:752)
Nursing Process—Implementation
Client Need—Physiological integrity

64 3. When helping a client transfer from the bed to a chair, it is best to place the chair parallel to and near the head of the bed. The nurse makes the distance as short as possible to promote safety when the client is weak or may lose his balance. Transferring to a chair at the end of the bed or against a side wall will require much more physical effort and involve safety hazards. Placing the chair perpendicularly would interfere with assisting the client. (18:399; 14:324)
Nursing Process—Implementation
Client Need—Safe, effective care environment

65 1. In a three-point partial weight-bearing gait, the weaker leg and walker are advanced together.

The majority of the weight is supported by the hands while the stronger leg is lifted and advanced. (18:421; 14:738)

    Nursing Process—Evaluation
    Client Need—Physiological integrity

NURSING CARE OF CLIENTS WITH CASTS

66 2. When plaster combines with water a chemical reaction takes place. Energy is given off in the form of heat. The client should be warned that his arm may feel quite warm temporarily. Steam or heat waves may even be seen rising from the surface of the wet cast. The cast supports the broken bone, but it should not constrict the underlying tissue. Wet plaster does not produce a disagreeable odor. Itching is not a common experience at the time a cast is applied. (18:688; 14:740)

    Nursing Process—Implementation
    Client Need—Safe, effective care environment

67 4. A wet cast should be held and supported with the palms of the hands. Using the fingers is likely to cause indentations in the cast. The inward dents then create pressure areas on the underlying tissue. After the cast has been applied, it should be allowed to dry on a soft surface. If the wet cast is on a hard surface is can become flattened. (18:689; 14:740)

    Nursing Process—Implementation
    Client Need—Safe, effective care environment

68 2. A cast made of synthetic materials has several advantages. It weighs much less than a plaster cast. A synthetic cast dries more quickly. It is more durable and not likely to soften if the cast becomes wet. It is no less flexible or less restrictive than plaster casts. The major disadvantage is that it is more expensive than traditional plaster casts. (14:740; 18:688)

    Nursing Process—Implementation
    Client Need—Health promotion/maintenance

69 4. A wet cast should be supported along its entire length with soft pillows as it dries. The soft support distributes the weight of the cast over a greater surface and prevents flattening of the underlying portion. Use of pillows also helps in elevating the extremity to relieve temporary swelling. A synthetic sheepskin or vinyl sheet would interfere with evaporation of water from the wet plaster. An absorbent pad would not cushion the weight of the cast sufficiently. (18:689; 14:740)

    Nursing Process—Implementation
    Client Need—Physiological integrity

70 1. Natural evaporation is the best way to dry a cast. This process may take 24 to 48 hours. It will in- volve turning the client at frequent intervals so that the entire cast circumference is exposed to the air. Intense heat such as with a heating blanket, hair drying, or heat lamp, should never be used to speed the drying process. Heat may burn the client or just dry the superficial surface of the cast. (16:788; 18:689)

    Nursing Process—Implementation
    Client Need—Physiological integrity

71 3. Circling the outer margin of the drainage on the cast helps the nurse evaluate the status of the bleeding. The nurse needs to return soon for another assessment. By comparing the subsequent size of the bloody spot, the nurse can evaluate how serious the situation is. It would be important to monitor the vital signs each time the drainage is assessed as well. All information should be documented. If the bleeding does not seem to be controlled, and the vital signs indicate that the client's condition is changing, the physician should be notified immediately. An ice bag is generally used to control swelling postoperatively. In some small way it also may decrease bleeding. (18:690; 16:790)

    Nursing Process—Implementation
    Client Need—Physiological integrity

72 3. The nurse assesses circulation in an extremity by performing the blanching test to determine capillary refill time. After releasing pressure on the nailbed, the color should return within 2 to 3 seconds. The assessment also should be performed on the opposite extremity. If the capillary refill time is similar in both extremities, the cast or tissue swelling is not a factor. Asking if the cast feels heavy or palpating it to feel the cast temperature are not appropriate techniques for assessing circulation. Determining that there is space between the cast and the skin is not a totally reliable assessment technique. If the circulation is impaired due to compartment syndrome, there may still be room to insert a finger at the margins of the cast. (18:692; 3:640)

    Nursing Process—Collecting data
    Client Need—Physiological integrity

73 3. When a client expresses a concern, it is best for the nurse to verbalize the feeling or message that the sender conveyed. This response shows understanding and a willingness to listen. Using clichés, agreeing with the client, or stereotyping the family interaction are all nontherapeutic. They will be of little help to a client who is struggling with a personal problem. (12:264)

    Nursing Process—Implementation
    Client Need—Psychosocial integrity

74 3. Most young adults seek to become independent of their parents. Developmental tasks concerned with self-identity, sexuality, testing the body's abilities, and learning to control emotional behavior occur more commonly before young adulthood. (16:24-25)

Nursing Process—Evaluation
Client Need—Health promotion/maintenance

75 2. The client with a hip spica cast is unable to flex his hips. A fracture bedpan elevates the buttocks just slightly enough to be used for bowel elimination. Because this client cannot sit, a bedside commode, mechanical lift, and raised toilet seat are inappropriate. (18:688)

Nursing Process—Planning
Client Need—Safe, effective care environment

76 3. One of the weakest areas of a hip spica cast is at the groin areas. This area tends to crack because it is stressed when turning and repositioning the client. The bar should never be used for lifting or turning, performing physical exercise, or hanging personal items. (18:688)

Nursing Process—Implementation
Client Need—Safe, effective care environment

77 2. Blowing air inside the cast can help relieve itching to a certain extent. The client must be cautioned about not scratching the skin. If the integrity of the skin is impaired, organisms may begin to grow in the warm, dark, moist environment. Administering an analgesic for itching is inappropriate. Moisture from melting ice cubes could eventually soften a plaster cast. (18:693-694; 3:640)

Nursing Process—Implementation
Client Need—Physiological integrity

78 4. The most frequent cause of an odor from a cast is an infected wound. Infected wounds produce purulent drainage. There is often an unpleasant odor as pus accumulates. To confirm the suspicion that an infection exists, the nurse should monitor the client for a cluster of additional signs and symptoms. Data that would support that a wound infection exists are an elevated temperature, tachycardia, anorexia, and malaise. (3:640; 18:692)

Nursing Process—Collect data
Client Need—Physiological integrity

79 2. The piece of plaster that was removed to make a window should not be thrown away. It should be replaced and secured with tape or a roller bandage. If the window remains open, tissue tends to bulge into the opening. The uneven pressure on the skin can cause it to break down. (18:690)

Nursing Process—Implementation
Client Need—Physiological Integrity

80 1. Rough or crumbling edges of a plaster cast can be repaired by making adhesive petals. Petals are rectangular or oval pieces of tape. The nurse inserts one end on the inside of the cast and folds down the other end on the outside edge of the cast. The strips are made to overlap, resembling the appearance of flower petals. The physician usually applies more plaster strips or uses a cast cutter if it is needed. Trimming a cast does not usually stop it from crumbling. Fragments of plaster are likely to continue breaking off if the nurse uses gauze to cover the cast edge. (7:757; 18:694)

Nursing Process—Implementation
Client Need—Physiological integrity

NURSING CARE OF CLIENTS WITH TRACTION

81 2. The leg of the client in Buck's traction should remain in alignment with the pull of the traction. This means that rather than making the bed as usual from side to side, the nurse removes and applies linen at the top or bottom of the bed and pulls it underneath the client. A person in Buck's traction should not be turned from side to side or raised with a mechanical lift. A client in traction, as any other hospitalized client, should have bed linen changed whenever it is soiled, wet, or needs replacement. (18:698; 7:764)

Nursing Process—Implementation
Client Need—Safe, effective care environment

82 3. To maintain countertraction, the client's foot should never press against the foot of the bed. If this is observed, the nurse should help pull the client back up toward the head of the bed. The weights should always hang free rather than rest on the floor or the bed. The body should be in alignment with the pull of the traction. The traction rope should move freely within the groove of the pulley. (18:697; 3:644)

Nursing Process—Evaluation
Client Need—Physiological integrity

83 2. The best technique for assessing circulation among the options provided is to palpate the distal peripheral pulse. The dorsalis pedis artery is on the top of the foot. Other pertinent circulatory assessments include observing the color and temperature of the skin, capillary refill time, and subjective complaints concerning pain. Checking movement and sensation are neurologic assessment techniques. Taking the blood pressure on the thigh rather than the arm is unnecessary. (16:794; 18:256)

Nursing Process—Collecting data
Client Need—Physiological integrity

84 2. The popliteal space behind the knee is especially prone to pressure and irritation when Russell's traction is used. This area is suspended in a sling,

which can become wrinkled. A piece of thick felt is sometimes used to line the sling to keep the surface smooth. The ischial spines are part of the inferior portion of the pelvic bones. The iliac crests are the upper flared portion of the bony pelvis. The zygomatic arches are in the cheek. (7:762; 18:698)
> Nursing Process—Collecting data
> Client Need—Physiological integrity

85 1. Preoperatively the traction should remain applied to the client. Its purpose is to relieve muscle spasm causing pain and immobilize the fractured bone. If the traction is removed or the weights released, muscle spasms will recur. Any realignment that may have been achieved with the use of traction may be jeopardized. (16:793; 14:745)
> Nursing Process—Implementation
> Client Need—Physiological integrity

86 4. Purulent drainage is sometimes referred to as pus. Purulent drainage is a collection of fluid containing white blood cells and pathogens. The presence of white blood cells indicates that the body is attempting to destroy and remove infecting organisms. Serous drainage is clear; it is made up of plasma or serum. Bloody drainage would indicate trauma. Mucoid drainage is sticky and transparent. It is released from mucous membranes. (18:460; 16:64)
> Nursing Process—Collecting data
> Client Need—Physiological integrity

87 2. There is a high probability that individuals who are allergic to penicillin also will exhibit a cross-sensitivity to cephalosporins. Both of these drugs are very similar in their structure. Though anyone with a drug sensitivity should be observed when a new medication, especially an antibiotic, is administered, individuals with a penicillin allergy seem to react more often to the cephalosporins than others. (15:156)
> Nursing Process—Implementation
> Client Need—Physiological integrity

88 4. The client should be told to raise his buttocks while pushing down with his unaffected foot and pulling himself up with the trapeze. The suspension will adjust with the movement and the line of traction remains unchanged. (7:762; 14:742)
> Nursing Process—Implementation
> Client Need—Safe, effective care environment

89 3. The uppermost edge of a pelvic belt should hug the client's hips. The pelvic belt helps to relieve spasms and pain in the muscles in the lumbar area. Placing the belt below the rib cage or at midabdomen would not promote the maximum effectiveness from its use. Though using pelvic belt traction will promote comfort, the location for its application is not arbitrarily determined on that basis. (14:742)
> Nursing Process—Implementation
> Client Need—Physiological integrity

90 2. The traction weights on both sides of the pelvic belt should be removed gradually and simultaneously. They should be reapplied in the same manner. Unfastening the belt first would cause the weights to drop to the floor. The trapeze would not be needed until the client is being helped from bed. If a back brace is used, it would be applied after removing the pelvic belt. (14:742)
> Nursing Process—Implementation
> Client Need—Physiological integrity

NURSING CARE OF CLIENTS HAVING AMPUTATIONS

91 2. In shock the blood pressure falls, and urine output decreases. The heart rate increases. As the bowel is deprived of an adequate blood supply, it may become less active causing bowel sounds to be diminished. (16:188-189; 14:414)
> Nursing Process—Collecting data
> Client Need—Physiological integrity

92 3. With very few exceptions, a person in shock should be kept flat with the lower extremities slightly elevated. Gravity helps to maintain blood in the area of the vital organs. Supine position is a back-lying position, but this would not provide the added benefit of elevating the legs. Prone is a face-lying position. Keeping the client on his side would interfere with the emergency assessment and care. (7:95; 16:192)
> Nursing Process—Implementation
> Client Need—Physiological integrity

93 2. Staying with a grief-stricken client indicates that the nurse is there for his emotional support. The client will be more likely to feel that he can depend on the nurse to be available and respond to his future needs. Leaving an uncomfortable situation is one method health professionals use to cope with their own feelings of inadequacy. The client will likely interpret the desertion as a sign that the nurse is not a caring individual. It is therapeutic for a person to release his rage as long as it does not endanger himself or others. Feeling angry is one of the early steps in the grieving process. The hospital chaplain may be helpful later, but the nurse should not leave the client alone for the time being. (14:753)
> Nursing Process—Implementation
> Client Need—Psychosocial integrity

94 2. Phantom pain or sensation is a phenomenon experienced by some people who have a limb am-

putated. The person feels a physical sensation in the missing limb. The feeling may range from a sense that the amputated part is still there or any number of sensations that cause discomfort, such as pain, cramping, burning, and itching. Referred pain is discomfort that is experienced in a location that is distant from the actual area of pathology. Psychogenic pain is discomfort that is emotional in origin. Intractable pain is severe and unrelenting. (18:176; 14:753)

Nursing Process—Implementation
Client Need—Health promotion/maintenance

95 1. Most believe that the nerve stimulation generates sensations that the brain perceives in place of the pain from the missing limb. This phenomenon is referred to as the *gate-control theory*. The process can be compared to a car waiting while a train crosses the highway. The impulses from the TENS unit are like the train. As long as the TENS impulses flood the brain, the pain impulses are blocked. (7:787; 18:186)

Nursing Process—Implementation
Client Need—Safe, effective care environment

96 3. Below-the-knee amputees are prone to developing knee flexion contractures. A contracture of this sort would interfere with wearing a prosthesis and being able to walk again. The stump should be kept in an extended or neutral position as much as possible. The prone and supine positions provide extension of the stump. It is possible for the stump to be extended or in a neutral position while lying on a side. (16:819; 7:785)

Nursing Process—Planning
Client Need—Physiological integrity

97 3. The muscles that will need strengthening most are those in the arms, neck, shoulders, chest, and back. Almost immediately after surgery, the nurse can encourage the client to lift up using the trapeze. The client also may squeeze rubber balls and perform arm push-ups. Doing arm push-ups involves placing the palms flat on the bed and raising the buttocks. Some provide the client with sawed-off crutches to use in bed to condition the same muscles that will be needed during ambulation. (7:279-280; 16:821; 18:420)

Nursing Process—Planning
Client Need—Physiological integrity

98 1. The nurse accepts the client's behavior and choice without judgment. This shows respect for the individual's unique effort to cope. The client's reaction is fairly normal. It is too early yet to determine that the client will need professional help to adjust. How the nurse would react is immaterial. Saying that the stump "doesn't look that bad" is an evaluative statement based on the nurse's standards and experiences. (12:235)

Nursing Process—Implementation
Client Need—Psychosocial integrity

99 2. Wrapping the stump decreases stump edema. A permanent prosthesis cannot be constructed until the stump is cone shaped and no longer undergoing changes in size. An equal amount of compression should be applied with each turn of the roller bandage. Isotonic and isometric exercises are used to tone muscles. Range of motion exercises maintain joint flexibility. Gauze dressings absorb blood and drainage. (16:818-819; 7:784)

Nursing Process—Implementation
Client Need—Safe, effective care environment

100 1. People undergoing amputations are at high risk for hemorrhage and shock. The dressing or compression cast should be examined, even underneath it, for signs of bleeding. Gravity may cause blood to accumulate underneath the stump. A tourniquet may be required for severe bleeding. Checking Homans' sign for thrombophlebitis, fever indicating infection, and skin impairment are all complications that may develop later in the postoperative period. (7:784; 16:818)

Nursing Process—Collecting data
Client Need—Physiological integrity

101 3. Elevating the entire foot of the bed, rather than just the stump, reduces stump swelling and prevents hip flexion contracture. Keeping the stump and uninvolved leg elevated would not reduce the risk for pneumonia, promote stump drainage, or stimulate peristalsis. (16:818; 7:785)

Nursing Process—Implementation
Client Need—Safe, effective care environment

102 2. There should be room for at least two fingers between the axilla and the axillary bar of the crutch. Prolonged pressure under the arm can affect circulation or impair nerve function resulting in permanent paralysis. All of the other observations are indications that the crutch length and the position of the handgrips are appropriate. (14:737; 18:420)

Nursing Process—Evaluation
Client Need—Physiological integrity

NURSING CARE OF CLIENTS WITH A HERNIATED INTERVERTEBRAL DISK

103 2. Any activity that increases intraspinal pressure, such as sneezing, causes the lower back pain to intensify. Other activities that make the pain more severe include coughing, lifting an object, and straining to have a bowel movement. Neither eating nor urinating should have an effect on the pain experience. Resting and inactivity should help to relieve the pain. (16:460; 3:348)

Nursing Process—Collecting data
Client Need—Physiological integrity

104 2. Diazepam relieves skeletal muscle spasm. By doing so, the client experiences a certain amount of relief from pain. Drugs in other chemical families would be used to reduce depression, promote sleep, and relieve inflammation. (15:253, 315; 16:460)

Nursing Process—Implementation
Client Need—Health promotion/maintenance

105 1. The position of comfort for most people who have a herniated disk is laying on the back with the head of the bed elevated and the knees flexed by gatching the bed. In the side-lying position, comfort is promoted by bending the hips and knees. These positions relieve tension on the lumbar and sacral nerves. (7:655)

Nursing Process—Implementation
Client Need—Physiological integrity

106 3. A wooden board placed beneath the mattress supports the skeletal system and keeps the vertebrae in good alignment. Soft, flexible, cushioning devices, such as a sheepskin pad, air mattress, and foam square, are better for relieving pressure on the skin. (16:460; 3:348)

Nursing Process—Implementation
Client Need—Physiological integrity

107 4. The client with a herniated disk should roll from side to side without twisting the spine. This type of movement prevents strain on the back during movement. Holding one's breath may increase discomfort if it is accompanied by bearing down. It would be difficult to turn a patient who is curled up in a ball. (16:461; 7:655)

Nursing Process—Implementation
Client Need—Safe, effective care environment

108 2. The chief sign of a pressure sore is redness. The skin does not return to normal color, even after pressure is relieved. Shiny skin may indicate local edema, which predisposes to the formation of a pressure sore. Normal skin is warm and dry. (18:462; 14:344)

Nursing Process—Collecting data
Client Need—Physiological integrity

109 1. A hot moist pack is generally hotter and applied longer than a soak. A hot moist pack should be enclosed at the core of thick layers of material like terry cloth towels, flannel, or a cotton bath blanket. The woven fabric absorbs the steam and conducts the warmth to the skin. The cover helps to retain the heat of the pack longer. A pil-

low would act as a barrier to the heat. Neither skin lotion nor using a rubber ring would prevent a burn. (18:496; 14:387; 3:349)

Nursing Process—Planning
Client Need—Safe, effective care environment

110 1. Bending both knees and keeping the back straight makes best use of the longest and strongest muscles in the body. The feet should be spread apart for a broad base of support. Extending the arms puts strain on weaker muscles by placing the weight of the lifted object outside the body's center of gravity. (18:160-161)

Nursing Process—Implementation
Client Need—Health promotion/maintenance

111 3. Feeling dizzy and light-headed is associated with breathing too rapidly. Hyperventilation does not allow enough time to exhale sufficient carbon dioxide. This can lead to dizziness, lightheadedness, weakness, tingling around the mouth and fingertips, and even fainting. The client should be instructed to slow down the rate of breathing, and exhale slowly for at least, or preferably more than, the amount of time it took to inhale. (18:432-433; 3:403)

Nursing Process—Implementation
Client Need—Safe, effective care environment

112 2. The major concern following a laminectomy and spinal fusion is keeping the back extended. The client must logroll from side to side or supine to prone position. A fracture bedpan should be used for elimination. There should always be sufficient help to avoid any twisting, flexion, or rotation at the operative area. (3:350; 16:462)

Nursing Process—Implementation
Client Need—Physiological integrity

113 1. Narcotic analgesics depress the respiratory center in the brain. If the respiratory rate is 10 or fewer breaths per minute, the physician should be notified immediately. All of the other vital sign measurements are generally considered normal for an adult. (15:65)

Nursing Process—Collecting data
Client Need—Physiological integrity

114 3. The administration of naloxone hydrochloride reverses the effects of opiates like morphine sulfate. Methadone, meperidine, and propoxyphene are all synthetic narcotics. If given, the latter would contribute to, rather than reverse, the adverse effects associated with morphine sulfate. (15:67)

Nursing Process—Implementation
Client Need—Physiological integrity

115 3. A large-toothed comb or pick is best for very thick or curly hair. A wire hairbrush or rat-tail comb, which has small, short, fine teeth, would

tend to break the shafts of hair from an African American client. African Americans benefit from using oil, rather than hot air, to moisturize their hair, which tends to be dry and coarse. (18:115)
> Nursing Process—Implementation
> Client Need—Physiological integrity

The Nursing Care of Clients with Disorders of the Integumentary System

NURSING CARE OF CLIENTS WITH HERPES ZOSTER (SHINGLES)

116 3. The length of time a skin disorder has been present and the area(s) where it first appeared may be significant in diagnosing and treating skin disorders. The client cannot be expected to know the cause of the disorder, why it occurred in a particular area, or the relationship of the symptoms to his other medical disorders. (16:829)
> Nursing Process—Collecting data
> Client Need—Physiological integrity

117 1. Shingles results from a reactivation of the varicella-zoster virus, which lies dormant in the sensory ganglia after a previous infection with chickenpox. The individual with shingles usually gives a history of chickenpox in childhood. Shingles also may occur in those who have not had chickenpox but come in contact with someone who has chickenpox or is immunocompromised (an immune system that is incapable of developing immunity to one or more specific antigens). Shingles is not caused by the mumps virus, a previous *Staphylococcus* infection, or a drug allergy. (16:414)
> Nursing Process—Implementation
> Client Need—Health promotion/maintenance

118 3. Acyclovir (Zovirax) is an antiviral drug used in the treatment of herpes simplex and shingles. This drug may reduce the severity of the symptoms (pain later followed by severe itching) and prevent the development of further lesions. Acyclovir does not prevent the lesions from forming crusts, prevent future attacks of shingles, or cause the lesions to disappear. Acyclovir must be taken within 48 hours of the first appearance of the symptoms to be effective. (16:414)
> Nursing Process—Implementation
> Client Need—Health promotion/maintenance

NURSING CARE OF CLIENTS WITH PSORIASIS

119 2. Psoriasis is characterized by areas of redness covered with silvery scales. Areas affected usually include the elbows, knees, and scalp, al-

though other areas also may be affected. (16:836; 7:724)
> Nursing Process—Collecting data
> Client Need—Physiological integrity

120 4. Clients with a skin disorder usually are very sensitive about their appearance and to reactions of those who see the skin lesions. The nurse must show acceptance of the skin disorder and not display any outward distaste or repulsion when examining the client. The nurse can show acceptance by touching the skin lesions, even though gloves are worn. A kind and sympathetic attitude often reduces anxiety and makes the client feel accepted, despite the appearance of the lesions. Being calm or thorough or not examining unaffected areas is not as important as showing acceptance and thus reducing anxiety. (7:726)
> Nursing Process—Collecting data
> Client Need—Psychosocial integrity

NURSING CARE OF CLIENTS WITH SKIN CANCER

121 1. Cryo means cold. Cryosurgery is the application of liquid nitrogen, which is extremely cold, to a lesion. The cold kills the cells, and a scab forms. The area usually scars. (16:840-841)
> Nursing Process—Implementing
> Client Need—Health promotion/maintenance

122 2. The client is warned not to pull or try to remove the scab because it must be allowed to dry and fall off. Applying wet soaks or petroleum jelly would remove the scab and possibly cause bleeding or an infection. Ice packs would not prevent the spread of cancer. (16:840-841)
> Nursing Process—Implementation
> Client Need—Health promotion/maintenance

NURSING CARE OF CLIENTS WITH A STASIS ULCER

123 2. Avoiding injury to and chilling of the affected area may relieve some pain. A blanket or lap robe should be provided when the client is allowed out of bed. If a bed cradle is prescribed, it may be covered with a blanket. Those with *arterial* insufficiency should not elevate their legs when sitting; this is appropriate when the client has venous insufficiency. Remaining in bed is not necessary unless the physician orders complete bed rest as part of the treatment regimen. Keeping the affected area exposed to air may increase rather than decrease pain. (16:841-843)
> Nursing Process—Implementation
> Client Need—Safe, effective care environment

124 4. The nurse must exercise care when applying a topical preparation to a stasis ulcer because these areas usually are painful. Washing the area with alcohol or applying ice are inappropriate measures because alcohol would cause severe burning, and ice would induce arterial spasm, which would increase pain. Applying a tight (restrictive) dressing would decrease circulation to the area and thus impede healing. (16:841-843)

Nursing Process—Implementing
Client Need—Physiological integrity

NURSING CARE OF CLIENTS WITH A BURN INJURY

125 4. The flames should be smothered by wrapping the victim in a blanket or rolling the victim on the ground. Ointments should not be applied to the skin until the victim is examined by a physician. Sterile gauze is not applied at the scene of the emergency unless the burned areas are small and only involve an extremity. When there are large burned areas the victim is wrapped in a sterile sheet before being transported to the hospital. Pouring normal saline over the burned areas is not appropriate at this time because the victim should be transported to a hospital as quickly as possible. (7:739)

Nursing Process—Implementation
Client Need—Physiological integrity

126 2. Once the flames are extinguished, establishing and maintaining a patent airway is of vital importance in the initial management of all burn victims. Many of these victims additionally inhale smoke, which irritates the air passages and results in increased respiratory secretions and edema of the air passages. Vital signs are important and should be obtained *after* a patent airway is established. Identifying the victim and determining the extent and type of burns are less important than making sure the victim is able to breathe. (16:851-852)

Nursing Process—Implementation
Client Need—Physiological integrity

127 1. Shock is a serious problem for the burned victim, especially those with extensive burns. Shock can be seen in those with what appears to be a minor burn injury that only involves a small area. Shock, when it occurs, usually is seen shortly after the initial injury and must be treated immediately. Fever also may occur, but this is usually seen later and may be the result of infection in the burned areas. Thirst and diaphoresis on unburned areas could occur immediately or later but is not a major problem at this time and is less important than identifying and treating shock. (7:739, 741)

Nursing Process—Collecting data
Client Need—Physiological integrity

128 2. The urinary output and the fluid intake must be *accurately* measured on all victims of a burn injury. The determination of intravenous fluid replacement is partially based on urinary output and other measurements, such as central venous pressure readings. While an indwelling catheter may prevent decubiti in any client, the primary purpose here is to measure urinary output. An indwelling catheter does not prevent damage to the bladder or help in determining the need for electrolyte replacement. (16:852)

Nursing Process—Implementation
Client Need—Physiological integrity

129 3. Burned areas lose body fluids because the integrity of the skin is lost. Fluids can be administered by vein if one is available. If a vein is not available, a surgical incision over the vein (cutdown) may be necessary. Total parenteral nutrition also may be used to supply fluids and electrolytes by means of a catheter inserted into the superior vena cava. Initially, body fluid moves from the plasma to the interstitial (between cells) compartment. Later, the fluid moves in the opposite direction. A decrease in urinary output does not cause a fluid volume deficit. (7:742-743)

Nursing Process—Collecting data
Client Need—Physiological integrity

130 1. Infection is a major problem associated with the open method of burn treatment because the affected areas are exposed to the microorganisms present in the air. (3:809)

Nursing Process—Implementation
Client Need—Safe, effective care environment

131 3. Unless the physician orders otherwise, aseptic technique is used when a topical drug is applied to a burned area. Wound infection is a major problem associated with burn injuries because the damaged skin provides an entrance for microorganisms. Topical drugs usually are applied after hydrotherapy. Application of a topical drug does not depend on the condition of the eschar. (3:810)

Nursing Process—Implementation
Client Need—Physiological integrity

132 2. Proper positioning is important in the prevention of contractures, decubitus ulcer formation, foot drop, and impaired pulmonary function. (7:746)

Nursing Process—Implementation
Client Need—Physiological integrity

133 2. An autograft uses the client's own skin and is taken from an uninjured area. The care plan must consider the care of two sites, namely the donor site or the area from which the graft is taken and the recipient site, where the graft is placed.

When an animal skin is used this is called a heterograft or xenograft. Using skin from another individual (usually a cadaver) is called an allograft or homograft. (16:846-847)
Nursing Process—Planning
Client Need—Physiological integrity

134 1. The physician usually desires minimal movement of the grafted area for approximately 48 hours after the procedure to prevent disturbing the contact between the skin graft and underlying tissues. Disturbance of the graft may result in problems, such as failure to adhere to underlying tissues, infection, and tissue necrosis. The graft dressing is only changed or reinforced by the physician. Wet soaks would not be applied to the graft because this may disturb the contact between the graft and underlying tissues. (7:745)
Nursing Process—Implementation
Client Need—Physiological integrity

NURSING CARE OF CLIENTS WITH A DECUBITUS ULCER

135 2. Decubitus ulcers, also called pressure ulcers, most always result from a lack of blood supply to tissue. Prolonged pressure on an area, usually a bony prominence such as the heels, sacrum, and hips, results in a loss of blood supply to the area. As the superficial tissues die and slough, underlying skin structures and bone may be exposed. Decubitus ulcers are not *directly* caused by drugs, poor personal hygiene, or a lack of vitamin B. (7:712)
Nursing Process—Planning
Client Need—Physiological integrity

136 4. Repositioning the client every 2 hours is the best method of preventing decubitus ulcers. Application of a skin-toughening agent and a diet high in protein are of value in maintaining skin integrity, but neither are effective if the client's position is not changed at frequent intervals. Keeping the head of the bed elevated is of no value in preventing this problem. (7:712)
Nursing Process—Implementation
Client Need—Safe, effective care environment

137 2. A pressure reducing/relieving device, such as an alternating pressure mattress, is placed over the regular bed mattress and under the full length of the client's body. (7:717)
Nursing Process—Implementation
Client Need—Safe, effective care environment

INDIVIDUAL TEST ITEMS

138 4. A history of allergies, especially to drugs, would be important information. Dermatitis medica-

mentosa is an allergic skin response to one or more drugs. (7:722)
Nursing Process—Collecting data
Client Need—Safe, effective care environment

139 1. A bath with a warm solution is recommended for the treatment of frostbite. Ice or snow is never rubbed onto the affected area because this produces additional frostbite. A heating pad should not be used because it may cause further tissue damage. (16:184)
Nursing Process—Planning
Client Need—Physiological integrity

140 3. Using a hot needle or a few drops of turpentine makes the tick release its hold on the skin surface. Tweezers may then be used to gently remove the tick. Crushing the tick with a tweezers, pulling it quickly from the skin, or squeezing the tick between the fingers could induce pathogenic microorganisms, such as those causing Lyme disease, into underlying tissues. (7:181)
Nursing Process—Implementation
Client Need—Physiological integrity

141 2. Red, scaly cracks between the toes are the more common symptoms of athlete's foot (tinea pedis). Burning also may be noted. (7:836)
Nursing Process—Collecting data
Client Need—Safe, effective care environment

142 1. Hypoallergenic or glycerin soap decreases skin irritation and therefore may lessen itching. Regular soap may contain a substance that adds to or causes itching. Light cotton bedding and clothing are recommended to allow normal evaporation of moisture from the skin. Tepid water, rather than hot or cold water, is recommended for bathing. Patting the skin dry rather than rubbing may reduce skin irritation and itching. (7:838)
Nursing Process—Implementation
Client Need—Safe, effective care environment

143 3. Herpes simplex virus type 1 also is commonly known as "cold sores" or "fever blisters." Clients with this type of infection are cautioned to use good personal hygiene to prevent the spread of the infection to other areas, such as the eyes and genitals. The application of petroleum jelly will not prevent the spread of the infection. Scabs, should they form, should be allowed to dry and fall off. When cleaning the affected areas, care is taken to use tissues or gauze to gently clean and remove any fluid that has formed on the lesions. The tissues or gauze are used only once and then discarded. (3:799)
Nursing Process—Implementation
Client Need—Health promotion/maintenance

Classification of Test Items

Unit IV Review Test 7

Directions: After each question the correct answer is given as well as a classification of each test question. Compare the correct answer with your answer. If a question has been answered *incorrectly*, draw a line to the end of the four columns. When finished, add up your correct scores and place the results at the bottom of each column.
Score Calculation:

   To determine the percentage of the number of questions you answered correctly, divide the **Number Correct** by the **Number Possible**, as example 125 (the number of questions answered correctly) divided by 143 (the number of questions in the test) = .874 or 87%.

NURSING PROCESS

C = Collecting data
P = Planning
I = Implementation
E = Evaluation

CLIENT NEEDS

S = Safe, effective care environment
P = Physiological integrity
M = Psychosocial integrity
H = Health promotion/maintenance

Question #	Answer #	Nursing Process				Client Needs			
		C	P	I	E	S	P	M	H
1	2				E		P		
2	3	C					P		
3	2			I			P		
4	4			I			P		
5	1			I			P		
6	3			I					H
7	4	C					P		
8	3			I					H
9	2				E				H
10	1	C				S			
11	3			I			P		
12	4		P				P		
13	3			I					H
14	4			I			P		
15	4				E		P		
16	1	C					P		
17	3	C				S			
18	1	C					P		
19	2			I					H
20	1	C					P		

NURSING PROCESS

C = Collecting data
P = Planning
I = Implementation
E = Evaluation

CLIENT NEEDS

S = Safe, effective care environment
P = Physiological integrity
M = Psychosocial integrity
H = Health promotion/maintenance

Question #	Answer #	Nursing Process				Client Needs			
		C	P	I	E	S	P	M	H
21	3				E				H
22	1			I		S			
23	1			I					H
24	3			I			P		
25	1			I		S			
26	1			I					H
27	3				E				H
28	3	C					P		
29	2			I					H
30	1				E				H
31	4			I		S			
32	2			I			P		
33	3		P				P		
34	2			I			P		
35	1				E				H
36	3			I					H
37	1		P						H
38	4			I		S			
39	2			I		S			
40	1	C					P		
41	3	C					P		
42	1			I			P		
43	4			I			P		
44	1			I			P		
45	3		P				P		
46	2			I					H
47	4			I			P		
48	2			I					H
49	4			I		S			
50	4			I		S			
51	2			I		S			
52	1	C					P		

NURSING PROCESS

C = Collecting data
P = Planning
I = Implementation
E = Evaluation

CLIENT NEEDS

S = Safe, effective care environment
P = Physiological integrity
M = Psychosocial integrity
H = Health promotion/maintenance

Question #	Answer #	Nursing Process				Client Needs			
		C	P	I	E	S	P	M	H
53	2	C					P		
54	1	C					P		
55	1			I			P		
56	3			I			P		
57	3			I			P		
58	4	C					P		
59	1	C				S			
60	2				E		P		
61	1			I		S			
62	1				E	S			
63	1			I			P		
64	3			I		S			
65	1				E		P		
66	2			I		S			
67	4			I		S			
68	2			I					H
69	4			I			P		
70	1			I			P		
71	3			I			P		
72	3	C					P		
73	3			I				M	
74	3				E				H
75	2		P			S			
76	3			I		S			
77	2			I			P		
78	4	C					P		
79	2			I			P		
80	1			I			P		
81	2			I		S			
82	3				E		P		
83	2	C					P		
84	2	C					P		

NURSING PROCESS

C = Collecting data
P = Planning
I = Implementation
E = Evaluation

CLIENT NEEDS

S = Safe, effective care environment
P = Physiological integrity
M = Psychosocial integrity
H = Health promotion/maintenance

Question #	Answer #	Nursing Process				Client Needs			
		C	P	I	E	S	P	M	H
85	1			I			P		
86	4	C					P		
87	2			I			P		
88	4			I		S			
89	3			I			P		
90	2			I			P		
91	2	C					P		
92	3			I			P		
93	2			I				M	
94	2			I					H
95	1			I		S			
96	3		P				P		
97	3		P				P		
98	1			I				M	
99	2			I		S			
100	1	C					P		
101	3			I		S			
102	2				E		P		
103	2	C					P		
104	2			I					H
105	1			I			P		
106	3			I			P		
107	4			I		S			
108	2	C					P		
109	1		P			S			
110	1			I					H
111	3			I		S			
112	2			I			P		
113	1	C					P		
114	3			I			P		
115	3			I			P		
116	3	C					P		

NURSING PROCESS

C = Collecting data
P = Planning
I = Implementation
E = Evaluation

CLIENT NEEDS

S = Safe, effective care environment
P = Physiological integrity
M = Psychosocial integrity
H = Health promotion/maintenance

Question #	Answer #	Nursing Process				Client Needs			
		C	P	I	E	S	P	M	H
117	1			I					H
118	3			I					H
119	2	C					P		
120	4	C						M	
121	1			I					H
122	2			I					H
123	2			I		S			
124	4			I			P		
125	4			I			P		
126	2			I			P		
127	1	C					P		
128	2			I			P		
129	3	C					P		
130	1			I		S			
131	3			I			P		
132	2			I			P		
133	2		P				P		
134	1			I			P		
135	2		P				P		
136	4			I		S			
137	2			I		S			
138	4	C				S			
139	1		P				P		
140	3			I			P		
141	2	C				S			
142	1			I		S			
143	3			I					H
Number Correct									
Number Possible	143	32	11	87	13	34	79	4	26
Percentage Correct									

REVIEW TEST 8

The Nursing Care of Clients with Vascular Disorders and Disorders of the Blood and Lymphatic Systems

Correct Answers and Rationales
Classification of Test Items

Directions: With a pencil, blacken the circle in front of the option you have chosen for your correct answer.

The Nursing Care of Clients with Vascular Disorders and Disorders of the Blood and Lymphatic Systems

NURSING CARE OF CLIENTS WITH AN AORTIC ANEURYSM

While undergoing a computed tomography (CT) scan, the radiologist detects that Mr. Charles Lewis has an abdominal aortic aneurysm.

1 If Mr. Lewis has a correct understanding of the physician's explanation of his condition, he will tell the nurse that an aneurysm is
- ○ 1. a weakened valve in a major blood vessel.
- ○ 2. a stationary blood clot in a large vein.
- ○ 3. a fatty deposit in the wall of an artery.
- ○ 4. an outpouching in the wall of an artery.

For the time being, Mr. Lewis's physician prescribes 250 mg of methyldopa (Aldomet) orally t.i.d.

2 When Mr. Lewis asks why he must take methyldopa, the best explanation the nurse can provide is that this drug
- ○ 1. lowers the pressure within the artery.
- ○ 2. alters the clotting mechanisms in blood.
- ○ 3. slows the formation of cholesterol.
- ○ 4. improves the circulation of venous blood.

3 Of the following side effects, which one would the nurse be correct in associating with the administration of methyldopa?
- ○ 1. Drowsiness
- ○ 2. Constipation
- ○ 3. Nervousness
- ○ 4. Perspiration

4 The nurse would be most correct in administering a medication ordered t.i.d.
- ○ 1. once a day.
- ○ 2. twice a day.
- ○ 3. three times a day.
- ○ 4. four times a day.

After monitoring Mr. Lewis's response to the medication, the physician increases his dosage of methyldopa to 1 g orally b.i.d.

5 Each tablet of methyldopa (Aldomet) contains 250 mg. How many tablets should the nurse give Mr. Lewis to administer 1 g of this medication?

○ 1. 2 tablets
○ 2. 4 tablets
○ 3. 6 tablets
○ 4. 8 tablets

6 If Mr. Lewis asks the nurse what benefit there is in taking methyldopa (Aldomet), the best answer would be that this drug will
○ 1. reduce his risk for hemorrhage.
○ 2. keep other aneurysms from forming.
○ 3. allow him to remain active.
○ 4. slow his disease process.

Mr. Phillip Borden has been admitted for the regulation of diabetes mellitus.

7 Which one of the following physical assessments should lead the nurse to think that Mr. Borden may have an abdominal aortic aneurysm?
○ 1. The nurse palpates a pulsating mass in his abdomen.
○ 2. The nurse hears an extra heart sound during auscultation.
○ 3. During inspection, the nurse sees uneven chest movements.
○ 4. While percussing the abdomen, a hollow sound is heard.

Ms. Stella Graber resides in a long-term care facility. She has advanced atherosclerotic heart disease. The physician has documented that she has an abdominal aortic aneurysm. Ms. Graber has refused surgical treatment.

8 Which one of the following symptoms is Ms. Graber likely to manifest if the aneurysm becomes *larger* or begins to *dissect*?
○ 1. Hematuria
○ 2. Indigestion
○ 3. Rectal bleeding
○ 4. Low back pain

Several years ago Ms. Graber told her physician that she did not want heroic measures performed to maintain her life. The physician wrote a "do not resuscitate" order on her medical record.

9 If Ms. Graber loses consciousness and remains unresponsive, the nurse should
○ 1. have her transferred to the hospital.
○ 2. call the local ambulance service.
○ 3. notify her attending physician.
○ 4. perform cardiopulmonary resuscitation.

NURSING CARE OF CLIENTS WITH THROMBOPHLEBITIS

Following a total abdominal hysterectomy, Ms. Sara Fleming develops a slightly elevated temperature and swelling in the right calf of her leg.

10 When the nurse dorsiflexes Ms. Fleming's right foot, she says she experiences pain in her calf. The nurse would be most accurate in reporting to the team leader that Ms. Fleming has a positive
○ 1. Babinski's sign
○ 2. Homans' sign
○ 3. Chadwick's sign
○ 4. Romberg's sign

11 Based on the fact that the nurse's assessments indicate that Ms. Fleming has a possible thrombophlebitis, which one of the following changes should be noted on the nursing care plan?
○ 1. Ambulate twice each shift.
○ 2. Refrain from massaging legs.
○ 3. Caution to avoid leg elevation.
○ 4. Encourage active leg exercises.

The physician prescribes warm moist compresses for the client's affected leg.

12 Which of the following nursing actions is *correct* when applying the warm moist compress? The nurse
○ 1. heats the water to 120°F.
○ 2. uses sterile technique.
○ 3. inspects the skin every 4 hours.
○ 4. covers the wet gauze with a towel.

13 Which one of the following would indicate to the nurse that the stationary thrombus in Ms. Fleming's leg has become a moving embolus? Ms. Fleming suddenly develops
○ 1. chest pain.
○ 2. leg cramps.
○ 3. numbness in the foot.
○ 4. swelling of the knee.

Mr. Dennis Sommerlott has developed a thrombophlebitis in a leg vein following weeks of bed rest. His physician has ordered a one-time administration of heparin calcium (Calciparine) 7500 U subcutaneously.

14 When Mr. Sommerlott asks why he is receiving this injection of medication, the best explanation the nurse can give is that heparin acts on a blood clot by helping to
○ 1. shrink it.
○ 2. dissolve it.
○ 3. prevent it from becoming larger.
○ 4. prevent it from becoming dislodged.

15 The heparin calcium comes supplied in a dosage strength of 5000 U/mL. To administer 7500 U of heparin, the nurse must fill the syringe with
○ 1. 0.7 mL
○ 2. 0.15 mL
○ 3. 1.2 mL
○ 4. 1.5 mL

16 When the nurse withdraws the medication from the vial, which of the following is *correct*? The nurse

○ 1. removes the rubber stopper in the top of the vial.

○ 2. instills the same volume of air as liquid that will be removed.

○ 3. mixes the drug by rolling it in the palms of the hands.

○ 4. shakes the drug vigorously to distribute the drug evenly.

17 When the nurse administers the heparin, which of the following actions is *correct*? The nurse

○ 1. selects the dorsogluteal site.

○ 2. uses a 1½-inch 22-gauge needle.

○ 3. inserts the needle at a 45-degree angle.

○ 4. massages the site afterward.

The physician rewrites the order for heparin each day for the next 3 days.

18 When Mr. Sommerlott asks why he can't have the heparin orally rather than the injection, the most accurate information the nurse can provide is that

○ 1. the oral form of heparin has a bitter taste.

○ 2. heparin is inactivated by stomach secretions.

○ 3. heparin taken orally causes stomach upset.

○ 4. the injectable form of heparin works better.

19 The nurse gathers all of the following data on Mr. Sommerlott, which one should be reported *immediately*?

○ 1. Mr. Sommerlott says bathing makes him very tired.

○ 2. Mr. Sommerlott never eats all the food on his tray.

○ 3. Mr. Sommerlott's gums bleed after brushing his teeth.

○ 4. Mr. Sommerlott says he has a hard time falling asleep.

20 When Mr. Sommerlott improves, he talks about taking a trip by automobile across the United States. Based on his history of thrombophlebitis, which of the following suggestions would be most important for the nurse to offer?

○ 1. Eat meals regularly during the trip.

○ 2. Don't drive after it becomes dark.

○ 3. Get out and walk about every hour.

○ 4. Use major highways and expressways.

Mr. Joseph Cooper, who is recovering from open heart surgery, has been receiving heparin postoperatively on a daily basis to prevent forming a thrombus.

21 If the physician orders all of the following for the care of Mr. Cooper, which one should the nurse *question*?

○ 1. Performing active leg exercises

○ 2. Giving penicillin intramuscularly

○ 3. Applying antiembolism stockings

○ 4. Ambulating three times a day

22 Which laboratory test should the nurse monitor and report when a client is receiving anticoagulant therapy using heparin?

○ 1. Partial thromboplastin time (PTT)

○ 2. Protein electrophoresis (PEP)

○ 3. Packed cell volume (PCV)

○ 4. Prothrombin time (PT)

23 The drug the nurse should plan to have available in case it becomes necessary to overcome the effects of the heparin that Mr. Cooper is receiving is

○ 1. calcium lactate.

○ 2. sodium benzoate.

○ 3. protamine sulfate.

○ 4. aluminum phosphate.

Eventually Mr. Cooper's physician discontinues the administration of heparin. He orders warfarin sodium (Coumadin) in its place.

24 Which one of the following laboratory test results must the nurse report before the physician will prescribe the daily dosage of warfarin sodium?

○ 1. PTT

○ 2. Total iron binding capacity

○ 3. Red blood cell count

○ 4. PT

25 While Mr. Cooper is taking warfarin sodium, the drug the nurse would expect the physician to prescribe if Mr. Cooper was in danger of hemorrhaging is

○ 1. protamine sulfate.

○ 2. sodium citrate.

○ 3. vitamin K.

○ 4. vitamin E.

NURSING CARE OF CLIENTS WITH VARICOSE VEINS

Ms. JoAnne Penrod, who works as a cashier in a grocery store, makes an appointment with a physician for her yearly pelvic examination and Pap test.

26 Which one of the following observations made by the nurse while helping Ms. Penrod into stirrups would most likely indicate that she has varicose veins?

○ 1. Ms. Penrod's feet look swollen.

○ 2. Ms. Penrod's feet look purple.

○ 3. The veins in Ms. Penrod's legs protrude from the skin.

○ 4. The veins in Ms. Penrod's legs are difficult to see.

27 Which one of the following statements made by Ms. Penrod to the nurse would most correlate with having varicose veins?

○ 1. "My legs feel heavy and tired by evening."
○ 2. "My feet perspire heavily during the day."
○ 3. "I wake up at night with leg cramps."
○ 4. "I have pain in my shins when I jog."

28 Which one of the following suggestions would be most beneficial in helping to relieve Ms. Penrod's symptoms caused by varicose veins?
○ 1. Elevate your legs frequently during the day.
○ 2. Wear two pair of thick cotton socks.
○ 3. Walk about when experiencing leg cramps.
○ 4. Take up a less active sport, such as fishing.

29 Which one of the following should the nurse tell Ms. Penrod to wear while working?
○ 1. A full support bra
○ 2. Support pantyhose
○ 3. Soft leather shoes
○ 4. Cotton underwear

Mr. Joseph Giddings, a truck driver, is scheduled for a vein stripping procedure as treatment for his varicose veins.

30 If the nurse reads all of the following information in Mr. Giddings' health history, which one is most related to his development of varicose veins?
○ 1. Mr. Giddings' mother also has varicose veins.
○ 2. Mr. Giddings has smoked cigarettes for 20 years.
○ 3. Mr. Giddings was a track athlete in high school.
○ 4. Mr. Giddings tries to follow a vegetarian diet.

31 After the physician explains the operation to Mr. Giddings, he asks the nurse how his blood will circulate in his legs after surgery. The best explanation the nurse can provide is that
○ 1. some of the arteries begin to function as veins.
○ 2. new veins grow to replace those removed.
○ 3. other veins take over the work of those removed.
○ 4. the ends of the removed veins are reconnected to others.

32 All of the following nursing actions are important. Which one is of highest priority when planning the postoperative care of a client following a vein stripping?
○ 1. Providing the client with nutritious food
○ 2. Orienting the client to his surroundings
○ 3. Ambulating the client frequently
○ 4. Offering regular oral hygiene

Mr. Giddings asks the nurse for medication for his pain. The physician has ordered propoxyphene hydrochloride (Darvon), 65 mg, orally every 4 hours as needed for pain.

33 Mr. Giddings says to the nurse when offered the propoxyphene, "If that's Darvon, I don't want it. It makes me sick to my stomach." The best action the nurse can take at this time is to
○ 1. tell the client that the drug is propoxyphene.
○ 2. explain that this is what the physician ordered.
○ 3. advise him to take the drug with lots of water.
○ 4. report the information to the nurse in charge.

34 Which of the following information would be essential when the nursing team plans the discharge instructions for Mr. Giddings?
○ 1. "Do not cross your legs when sitting."
○ 2. "Try to get 8 hours of sleep at night."
○ 3. "Think about finding a new occupation."
○ 4. "Drink two or more cups of milk daily."

NURSING CARE OF CLIENTS WITH PERIPHERAL VASCULAR DISORDERS

Ms. Virginia Drake, a nursing home resident, has poor circulation in her extremities.

35 Which of the following physical assessments is common among individuals with peripheral vascular disease?
○ 1. The toenails are thick and hard.
○ 2. Hair growth on the legs is extensive.
○ 3. Knee jerk reflexes are hyperactive.
○ 4. Peripheral pulses are bounding.

36 If Ms. Drake tells the nurse her feet are cold, which of the following nursing actions would be best?
○ 1. Apply a hot water bottle.
○ 2. Use an electric heating pad.
○ 3. Wrap them in a warm blanket.
○ 4. Elevate her feet on a stool.

The hospital has acquired a Doppler ultrasound device. At a special staff inservice meeting, a nurse demonstrates how to use this new equipment. A staff volunteer is requested to act as a client.

37 The nurse prepares to show how to use the Doppler ultrasound device to assess blood flow through the dorsalis pedis artery. Which of the following actions is *correct*? The nurse
○ 1. places the probe beside the ankle.
○ 2. applies acoustic jelly to the skin.
○ 3. records the time of capillary refill.
○ 4. measures the temperature of the skin.

A client is admitted with a stasis ulcer on the lower leg.

38 When the nurse assesses this type of lesion, the most characteristic finding is that the impaired skin appears
○ 1. to contain purulent drainage.
○ 2. blanched around the open area.
○ 3. dark brown, dry, and crusty.
○ 4. as a fluid-filled blister.

The physician writes an order directing the nurse to apply continuous wet-to-dry dressings to the stasis ulcer.

39 When the client asks why this type of dressing is being applied, the best explanation the nurse can provide is that wet-to-dry dressings are generally used to
○ 1. pull away dead tissue.
○ 2. absorb liquid drainage.
○ 3. prevent skin infection.
○ 4. keep the wound clean.

Eventually the wet-to-dry dressings are discontinued. The physician tells the nurse to cover the client's ulcer with DuoDERM, a type of air occlusive dressing.

40 The nurse would be most correct in telling the client that the main advantage in using this type of dressing is that it
○ 1. reduces the formation of scar tissue.
○ 2. relieves pain from skin irritation.
○ 3. is less expensive than gauze dressings.
○ 4. speeds healing by keeping the wound moist.

41 Which of the following signs indicates that the client's stasis ulcer is *healing*?
○ 1. A margin of pinkish-red tissue lines the wound.
○ 2. The ulcer turns dark brownish-black.
○ 3. A shallow layer of pale tissue forms in the center.
○ 4. The drainage becomes milky white in appearance.

Ms. Adler has had Raynaud's disease for several years.

42 In which part of the body would the nurse expect Ms. Adler's symptoms to be localized?
○ 1. In her legs
○ 2. In her hands
○ 3. In her chest
○ 4. In her neck

43 Which one of the following would Ms. Adler most likely correlate with the onset of her discomfort?
○ 1. Exposure to heat
○ 2. Exposure to cold
○ 3. Exposure to sun
○ 4. Exposure to wind

44 The teaching plan for people like Ms. Adler with Raynaud's disease should include explaining that it is important to *avoid*
○ 1. wearing gloves.
○ 2. emotional stress.
○ 3. drinking alcoholic beverages.
○ 4. bathing with perfumed soap.

Mr. Carl Bennett, age 32, has been diagnosed as having thromboangiitis obliterans, also known as Buerger's disease.

45 When Mr. Bennett describes his earliest symptoms, he is most likely to tell the nurse that he experienced
○ 1. a heavy feeling in his lower extremities.
○ 2. frequent problems with ingrown toenails.
○ 3. leg pain accompanying walking or exercise.
○ 4. swollen feet at the end of the day.

46 When the nurse palpates the peripheral pulses in Mr. Bennett's lower extremities, the most common finding is that they will feel
○ 1. strong.
○ 2. normal.
○ 3. full.
○ 4. weak.

47 If Mr. Bennett understands the potential complications from his disease process, he will tell the nurse that it is *most* important for him to regularly see a(n)
○ 1. podiatrist for foot care.
○ 2. dietitian for weight control.
○ 3. ophthalmologist for eye care.
○ 4. counselor for emotional therapy.

The physician discusses the possibility of treating Mr. Bennett's disease by performing a sympathectomy.

48 The best evidence that Mr. Bennett understood the physician's explanation of this surgical procedure is when he says that a sympathectomy will
○ 1. promote vasodilation.
○ 2. aid muscle relaxation.
○ 3. relieve mental stress.
○ 4. slow his heart rate.

Mr. Bennett is taught to perform Buerger-Allen exercises.

49 When Mr. Bennett returns the nurse's demonstration, he is performing these exercises *correctly* if he lies flat with his legs elevated for several minutes and then
○ 1. sits on the edge of the bed.
○ 2. stands and touches his toes.
○ 3. jogs in place at the bedside
○ 4. pretends to climb stairs.

50 When preparing Mr. Bennett to manage his disease, it is essential that the nurse plan to inform Mr. Bennett and other people with Buerger's disease that
○ 1. heavy lifting is contraindicated.
○ 2. use of tobacco must be avoided.
○ 3. airplane travel is restricted.
○ 4. sexual activity is prohibited.

NURSING CARE OF CLIENTS WITH VARIOUS TYPES OF ANEMIA

Ms. Heather Warren, who has been attending college for several months, goes to the university's medical service.

She has been feeling extremely tired and is concerned that this symptom may be due to a health problem.

51 Which one of the following laboratory tests could the nurse expect to be abnormal if the cause of Heather's fatigue is due to nutritional anemia?
- ○ 1. Prothrombin time
- ○ 2. Bleeding time
- ○ 3. Fibrinogen level
- ○ 4. Hemoglobin level

52 A complete blood count is performed. The report indicates that the red blood cells are hypochromic. This means that
- ○ 1. there is a low number of cells.
- ○ 2. there is a small volume of blood.
- ○ 3. the cells lack normal color.
- ○ 4. the cells are small in size.

53 Heather provides the health service nurse with all of the following information, which one is related to her anemia?
- ○ 1. She has chronic constipation.
- ○ 2. She experiences menstrual cramps.
- ○ 3. She feels chilled most of the time.
- ○ 4. She had rheumatic fever as a child.

The nurse takes a diet history from Heather.

54 If Heather says she *does not* consume any of the following foods, which one is most likely to be associated with her nutritional anemia?
- ○ 1. Milk
- ○ 2. Meat
- ○ 3. Oranges
- ○ 4. Candy

The physician prescribes ferrous sulfate (Feosol) 1 tablet orally t.i.d. for Heather.

55 The nurse explains the directions to Heather for taking the ferrous sulfate. For the best absorption of oral iron preparations it would be best for the nurse to tell Heather to take the drug
- ○ 1. between meals.
- ○ 2. with each meal.
- ○ 3. just before eating.
- ○ 4. just before bedtime.

56 If Heather understands the nurse's explanation concerning the effects from taking iron, she will say that this drug will cause her stools to become
- ○ 1. medium brown.
- ○ 2. quite black.
- ○ 3. clay colored.
- ○ 4. light green.

57 Rather than taking the ferrous sulfate with water, to enhance the absorption of the iron supplement, the nurse may advise Heather to take the tablet with
- ○ 1. milk.
- ○ 2. tea.
- ○ 3. a soft drink.
- ○ 4. orange juice.

Ms. Evelyn Ware, who resides in a nursing home, has difficulty swallowing the capsule of iron that the physician has prescribed. The physician changes the medical order to a liquid preparation.

58 When the nurse plans the administration of the liquid iron preparation, it is essential that it be given
- ○ 1. through a straw.
- ○ 2. in a paper cup.
- ○ 3. with a metal spoon.
- ○ 4. without any water.

Ms. Carol Weiss develops anemia due to heavy menstrual blood loss.

59 When the office nurse interviews Ms. Weiss, which of the following information is most likely related to her anemia?
- ○ 1. She fainted last week at work.
- ○ 2. She has occasional insomnia.
- ○ 3. Her gall bladder has been removed.
- ○ 4. Her abdomen is somewhat tender.

60 During the physical assessment of Ms. Weiss, the nurse is most likely to observe that her skin appears
- ○ 1. mottled.
- ○ 2. flushed.
- ○ 3. pale.
- ○ 4. blue.

The physician instructs his office nurse to administer iron dextran (Imferon) intramuscularly. The nurse plans to administer the injection by Z-track (zig-zag) technique.

61 Which one of the following muscles would be best for the nurse to plan on using when giving the injection by Z-track technique?
- ○ 1. Deltoid
- ○ 2. Trapezius
- ○ 3. Gluteus medius
- ○ 4. Latissimus dorsi

62 The best reason the nurse can give Ms. Weiss for administering the injection by Z-track technique is that iron dextran is irritating to subcutaneous tissue; therefore, it must be
- ○ 1. absorbed slowly.
- ○ 2. deposited deeply.
- ○ 3. instilled quickly.
- ○ 4. massaged vigorously.

63 Just before inserting the needle into the muscle, the nurse would be correct to pull the tissue at the site
- ○ 1. laterally.
- ○ 2. diagonally.
- ○ 3. downward.
- ○ 4. upward.

Ms. Orr, a 50-year-old woman, is suspected of having pernicious anemia. She is hospitalized for diagnostic purposes.

64 If the nurse writes all of the following information on a traditional, source-oriented record using narrative charting, which one contains *inappropriate* information in the nurses' notes?
  ○ 1. States, "I get nauseated when I eat."
  ○ 2. Has Medicare insurance for health care.
  ○ 3. Skin over back and buttocks is flushed.
  ○ 4. Has asked to see a Presbyterian minister.

65 When the nurse inspects Ms. Orr's mouth, a common finding among individuals with pernicious anemia is
  ○ 1. a red beefy tongue.
  ○ 2. many dental cavities.
  ○ 3. large pallatine tonsils.
  ○ 4. dry mucous membranes.

66 If Ms. Orr has developed neurologic symptoms associated with pernicious anemia, she is most likely to describe to the nurse that she has
  ○ 1. numbness and tingling in the extremities.
  ○ 2. morning headaches and sudden dizziness.
  ○ 3. restlessness and sleep pattern disturbances.
  ○ 4. periods of temporary amnesia and fainting.

The physician orders a Schilling test.

67 The nurse should tell Ms. Orr and the nursing assistant assigned to her care that this test will involve collecting
  ○ 1. urine.
  ○ 2. blood.
  ○ 3. stool.
  ○ 4. sputum.

The Schilling test confirms that Ms. Orr has pernicious anemia.

68 If Ms. Orr understands the physician's explanation of pernicious anemia, she will tell the nurse that her condition has developed due to a deficiency of
  ○ 1. intrinsic factor.
  ○ 2. bile salts.
  ○ 3. lipase.
  ○ 4. pepsinogen.

69 The nurse should expect that to treat Ms. Orr's pernicious anemia the physician will prescribe
  ○ 1. blood transfusions.
  ○ 2. iron medication.
  ○ 3. vitamin B_{12} injections.
  ○ 4. vitamin K injections.

Ms. Angela Rogers is hospitalized because her red blood cell count is low, and the physician is unsure of what is causing it. The physician intends to aspirate bone marrow for more diagnostic information. The nurse in-

forms Ms. Rogers that the sample of bone marrow will be taken from the iliac crest.

70 If the nurse has explained the anatomic location in terms that the client can understand, where will Ms. Rogers point when asked to identify the site for the bone marrow aspiration?
  ○ 1. The posterior hip
  ○ 2. The center chest
  ○ 3. The upper arm
  ○ 4. The groin area

71 One of the major responsibilities of the nurse during a bone marrow aspiration is helping to
  ○ 1. minimize discomfort.
  ○ 2. hold instruments.
  ○ 3. regulate suction.
  ○ 4. administer oxygen.

72 After a bone marrow aspiration has been completed, it is essential for the nurse to monitor
  ○ 1. trends in the blood pressure.
  ○ 2. bleeding from the puncture site.
  ○ 3. changes in the client's pulse.
  ○ 4. the client's level of consciousness.

The bone marrow aspiration reveals that Ms. Orr has low levels of erythrocytes, leukocytes, and platelets. The physician concludes that she has aplastic anemia.

73 When Ms. Orr is bathing, which one of the following observations is the best indication that she is having difficulty tolerating the current level of activity?
  ○ 1. She becomes short of breath.
  ○ 2. She feels extremely nauseated.
  ○ 3. Her pulse rate drops below 60.
  ○ 4. Her skin becomes moist and cool.

74 Which one of the following physical assessment findings is due to a low number of platelets?
  ○ 1. Multiple bruises
  ○ 2. Coarse body hair
  ○ 3. Thick toenails
  ○ 4. Cool extremities

75 Because Ms. Orr has a reduced leukocyte count, it is most important for all caregivers to
  ○ 1. perform conscientious handwashing.
  ○ 2. relieve pressure over bony prominences.
  ○ 3. provide daily high protein nourishment.
  ○ 4. monitor heart rate and rhythm each shift.

The physician tells Ms. Orr that she will be receiving 2 U of packed blood cells.

76 Ms. Orr asks how packed cells are different from the usual blood transfusion. The nurse is most correct in explaining that packed cells
  ○ 1. contain the same blood cells in less fluid volume.

○ 2. contain more blood cells in the same fluid volume.

○ 3. are less likely to cause an allergic reaction.

○ 4. will stimulate her own bone marrow to function.

Ms. Orr is typed and crossmatched for the 2 U of packed cells. Ms. Orr's blood type is A, Rh positive.

77 The nurse goes to the blood bank to obtain the first unit of packed cells. Which one of the following blood types of donated blood would be *incompatible* if transfused into Ms. Orr?

○ 1. A, Rh negative

○ 2. O, Rh positive

○ 3. O, Rh negative

○ 4. AB, Rh positive

Ms. LuEllen Majors also has aplastic anemia. She tells the nurse that she has been receiving corticosteroid treatment for more than 1 year in an effort to treat her disease.

78 While the nurse examines Ms. Majors, which one of the following is most likely due to the administration of corticosteroids. The client's

○ 1. voice is quite husky.

○ 2. face is moon-shaped.

○ 3. muscles are large.

○ 4. skin looks tanned.

79 Which one of the following statements may indicate that Ms. Majors has a complication from the use of corticosteroid administration? Ms. Majors says

○ 1. "I've been experiencing such heartburn lately."

○ 2. "I've been taking long naps during the day."

○ 3. "I seem to have lost my appetite."

○ 4. "Bright lights cause me discomfort."

Because corticosteroid therapy has not been effective, Ms. Majors has consented to have a bone marrow transplant to cure her aplastic anemia. She undergoes total body irradiation.

80 Just prior to and for several weeks following the bone marrow transplant, the *highest* priority when planning the nursing care of Ms. Majors will be

○ 1. relieving depression.

○ 2. promoting nutrition.

○ 3. preventing infection.

○ 4. monitoring hydration.

Mr. Bruno Argos has had a splenectomy. The surgical procedure was performed to treat a rare type of anemia called thalassemia. While assessing him postoperatively, the nurse notes that Mr. Argos has a subcostal incision.

81 Due to the location of the operative incision, Mr. Argos is at especially high risk for developing one of the following complications. It is essential that the nursing care plan identify measures that will prevent

○ 1. vomiting.

○ 2. dehydration.

○ 3. distention.

○ 4. pneumonia.

82 Before being discharged, the nurse should plan to inform the client who has had a splenectomy that he should consult with his physician as soon as possible if he

○ 1. acquires an infection.

○ 2. feels unusually fatigued.

○ 3. plans any foreign travel.

○ 4. develops gastric upset.

The nursing unit is informed to expect a new male admission. The client is experiencing a sickle cell crisis.

83 If this new admission fits the profile of individuals in the United States with sickle cell anemia, the nurse can expect that his cultural background is

○ 1. Mexican American

○ 2. Asian American

○ 3. Native American

○ 4. African American

84 During the admission assessment, which one of the following should the nurse attribute to the client's blood disease?

○ 1. His tongue is white.

○ 2. His urine is cloudy.

○ 3. He is jaundiced.

○ 4. He is nauseated.

85 The nurse observes that the client's knee is swollen and painful. Consequently, which one of the following nursing measures should be carried out?

○ 1. Perform passive range of motion during each shift.

○ 2. Help to change positions to achieve comfort.

○ 3. Ambulate with him at frequent intervals.

○ 4. Encourage quadriceps setting exercises.

86 Which one of the following nursing interventions is the best approach for maintaining tissue perfusion during a sickle cell crisis?

○ 1. Provide a large intake of fluids.

○ 2. Apply thigh-high elastic stockings.

○ 3. Elevate the lower extremities.

○ 4. Dangle on the side of the bed.

87 The client tells the nurse that he intends to marry a woman who has sickle cell trait. Which one of the following would be the best recommendation at this time? He should be advised to

○ 1. obtain genetic counseling.

○ 2. adopt all his children.

○ 3. undergo a vasectomy.

○ 4. have only two children.

NURSING CARE OF CLIENTS WITH ACQUIRED IMMUNODEFICIENCY SYNDROME

Mr. Peter Gates makes an appointment with his physician because he has been losing weight and has noted swollen lymph nodes in his armpits and groins.

88 If Mr. Gates tells the nurse all of the following, which one places him at high risk for acquired immunodeficiency syndrome (AIDS)?
○ 1. He had surgery 6 months ago.
○ 2. He went to Mexico on his vacation.
○ 3. He breeds and sells poodles.
○ 4. He is an intravenous drug user.

89 The physician orders several laboratory tests. Which one would the nurse expect to be performed to identify antibodies to the human immunodeficiency virus (HIV)?
○ 1. Schick test
○ 2. Dick test
○ 3. Enzyme-linked immunosorbent assay test (ELISA)
○ 4. Veneral disease research laboratory (VDRL) test

90 The nurse reviews the results of Mr. Gates' complete blood count. If Mr. Gates has AIDS, which blood cell count will be especially low?
○ 1. Erythrocytes
○ 2. Thrombocytes
○ 3. Lymphocytes
○ 4. Reticulocytes

91 Which one of the following infection control policies should be implemented for a person who is diagnosed as HIV positive?
○ 1. Drainage and secretion precautions
○ 2. Blood and body fluid precautions
○ 3. Strict isolation
○ 4. Respiratory isolation

A client with AIDS is admitted with an opportunistic respiratory infection. He makes statements to the nurse that imply a sense of hopelessness.

92 Which one of the following nursing approaches would be most therapeutic to plan at this time?
○ 1. Encouraging him to set small, daily goals
○ 2. Making a referral to the hospital chaplain
○ 3. Planning periodic distractions, such as television
○ 4. Recommending that he contact a lawyer

93 During which of the following nursing interventions performed for a client with AIDS would it be most important for the nurse to wear gloves?
○ 1. Giving a bed bath
○ 2. Providing oral care
○ 3. Changing a dressing
○ 4. Feeding the client

NURSING CARE OF CLIENTS WITH THROMBOCYTOPENIA

The nurse reads the physician's report of the history and physical performed on a new male client. Based on the findings, the physician has made a tentative medical diagnosis of idiopathic thrombocytopenia purpura.

94 While giving a report to the nursing team on the next shift, a nursing assistant asks the nurse to explain what the term *idiopathic* means. The best explanation of this word is that the cause of the disease is
○ 1. abnormal cell growth.
○ 2. exposure to a toxin.
○ 3. probably an allergy.
○ 4. basically unexplainable.

95 The physician has indicated that the client has purpura. When conducting the physical assessment the nurse would look for
○ 1. small skin hemorrhages.
○ 2. dark areas of cyanosis.
○ 3. flushed red skin.
○ 4. protruding veins.

96 When the nursing team plans the care of the client with thrombocytopenia, one of the priorities must include
○ 1. preventing injury.
○ 2. promoting activity.
○ 3. restricting visitors.
○ 4. encouraging fluids.

NURSING CARE OF CLIENTS WITH POLYCYTHEMIA

97 A client with polycythemia has an enlarged spleen. The position that will provide the most comfort for this person is
○ 1. sitting upright.
○ 2. lying on the back.
○ 3. lying on the side.
○ 4. elevating the legs.

98 To prevent the formation of blood clots when a person has polycythemia, the best nursing action would be to
○ 1. provide protein foods.
○ 2. increase fluid intake.
○ 3. restrict dietary sodium.
○ 4. encourage weight loss.

The physician tells the patient with polycythemia that a phlebotomy will be performed.

99 The client understands the procedure if he tells the nurse that
○ 1. blood will be removed from his vein.
○ 2. tourniquets will be applied to his arms.
○ 3. some veins will be surgically occluded.
○ 4. he will receive a blood transfusion.

NURSING CARE OF CLIENTS WITH HEMOPHILIA

Ms. Anne Hershey has a 4-year-old child who has inherited classic hemophilia A. Ms. Hershey is now pregnant and has undergone an amniocentesis. The fetus has been determined to be female.

100 Which one of the following statements by Ms. Hershey can the nurse confirm is true?
- ○ 1. "This baby will manifest the symptoms of hemophilia."
- ○ 2. "This baby will have a much milder form of hemophilia."
- ○ 3. "This baby will carry the genetic trait for hemophilia."
- ○ 4. "This baby will not inherit any genes for hemophilia."

An adult man with hemophilia hits his head when involved in a minor automobile accident. Before discharging the client from the emergency department, the nurse reviews the signs and symptoms that would indicate bleeding.

101 The best evidence that the client has understood his discharge instructions would be if he identified which one of the following as an *early* indication of intracranial bleeding?
- ○ 1. Convulsions
- ○ 2. Drowsiness
- ○ 3. Ringing in the ears
- ○ 4. Diminished appetite

102 A client with hemophilia is concerned about becoming HIV positive from receiving donated blood. Which of the following would be the most accurate information from the nurse?
- ○ 1. Blood donors are tested before their blood is accepted.
- ○ 2. Donated blood is tested for AIDS antibodies once collected.
- ○ 3. No donated blood contains the virus causing AIDS anymore.
- ○ 4. There is no way to identify the AIDS virus in blood yet.

NURSING CARE OF CLIENTS WITH LEUKEMIA

103 The nurse collects the following data on a client who has chronic myelogenous leukemia. All of the information should be reported. Which one most indicates a possible infection?
- ○ 1. Blood in the stool
- ○ 2. Prolonged vomiting
- ○ 3. Cloudy urine
- ○ 4. Extreme fatigue

104 The nurse notes that the leukemia client's mouth bleeds after he brushes his teeth. Which of the following would be the best alternative for mouth care at this time?

- ○ 1. Use foam mouth swabs.
- ○ 2. Use only dental floss.
- ○ 3. Discontinue oral hygiene.
- ○ 4. Eliminate the use of toothpaste.

105 When the nurse helps the leukemia patient who has an ulcerated mouth select foods from his menu, which one of the following foods would be best?
- ○ 1. Spaghetti with meat balls
- ○ 2. Grilled cheese sandwich
- ○ 3. Salad with French dressing
- ○ 4. Creamed potato soup

106 A person with leukemia is receiving antineoplastic drugs to treat his disease. The nurse should plan to prepare the client for which one of the following common side effects?
- ○ 1. Hair loss
- ○ 2. Body rash
- ○ 3. Constipation
- ○ 4. Headaches

The physician tells a client who has been receiving drug therapy for his leukemia that his condition is in remission.

107 The client has understood what this term means if he tells the nurse that
- ○ 1. he will never need treatment again.
- ○ 2. he will need drugs again in a few months.
- ○ 3. his symptoms are gone.
- ○ 4. his disease is cured.

A client with terminal leukemia is no longer experiencing acute problems; he will be discharged in a few days. Though he is stable now, the physician has discussed with the client and his family that he will probably not survive more than 6 more months.

108 Which one of the following organizations would be the best place for referring this client and his family?
- ○ 1. Public Health Department
- ○ 2. Centers for Disease Control and Prevention
- ○ 3. National Hospice Organization
- ○ 4. The local Community Chest

NURSING CARE OF CLIENTS WITH INFECTIOUS MONONUCLEOSIS

109 A young college woman with infectious mononucleosis asks the health service nurse how she acquired this condition. The best answer would be that the virus causing this disease is transmitted by
- ○ 1. contact with blood or body fluids.
- ○ 2. direct contact with an infected person.
- ○ 3. consuming contaminated food or water.
- ○ 4. the bite of an insect, such as a mosquito.

110 Which one of the following is likely to have been one of the first symptoms experienced by a client with infectious mononucleosis?

○ 1. Increased thirst
○ 2. Frequent voiding
○ 3. Sore throat
○ 4. Intestinal upset

111 Which one of the following is essential for the nurse to stress when discussing this client's self-care?
○ 1. Complying with antibiotic therapy
○ 2. Restricting physical activity
○ 3. Taking supplemental vitamins
○ 4. Returning for blood transfusions

NURSING CARE OF CLIENTS WITH LYMPHOMA

Mr. Martin Swift, a person with Hodgkin's disease, is being admitted to the hospital

112 If Mr. Swift is typical of most people who develop Hodgkin's disease, his age is most probably
○ 1. under 20 years.
○ 2. between 20 and 35 years.
○ 3. between 35 to 45 years.
○ 4. over 65 years.

113 When inspecting and palpating the lymph nodes of a person with Hodgkin's disease, which one of the following findings is the nurse most likely to assess? The lymph nodes will be
○ 1. enlarged and painless.
○ 2. small and firm.
○ 3. swollen and tender.
○ 4. fixed and hard.

Mr. Swift will undergo treatment of his Hodgkin's disease with external radiation therapy. The cervical and axillary lymph nodes are the areas that will be irradiated. The nurse consults with the team leader and radiology department concerning how to prepare the client for his treatment.

114 Which of the following instructions should the teaching plan include when preparing a client for radiation therapy?
○ 1. "Don't get the skin in your armpits and neck wet."
○ 2. "Don't use any deodorants with aluminum hydroxide."
○ 3. "Shave the hair from your neck and axilla daily."
○ 4. "After each treatment apply zinc oxide ointment."

115 What is the best response from the nurse when Mr. Swift becomes concerned that his skin is reddened?
○ 1. Explain that this is a normal reaction with radiation.
○ 2. Tell him that the heat from radiation causes vasodilation.
○ 3. Inform him that the redness indicates superficial bleeding.

○ 4. Reassure him that the redness is hardly noticeable.

Mr. Swift will continue his radiation treatment as an outpatient following his hospital discharge.

116 Before Mr. Swift leaves the nursing unit, the most important information to include in his discharge instructions is that when he goes outside, he should
○ 1. wear several layers of warm clothing.
○ 2. avoid becoming chilled or too warm.
○ 3. wear a mask to filter dust and pollen.
○ 4. protect his irradiated skin from sunlight.

Mr. Gregory Swisher has advanced non-Hodgkin's lymphoma. Antineoplastic drugs are being given to control his condition.

117 Which one of the following should be reported immediately because it indicates that a client receiving cancer chemotherapy needs to be placed in reverse (protective) isolation?
○ 1. The client has anorexia and loses weight.
○ 2. The client experiences frequent diarrhea.
○ 3. The client's white blood cell count drops.
○ 4. The client becomes disoriented and confused.

Mr. Swisher is not responding to medical treatment. The physician asks the nurse to accompany him when he tells the client that his condition is terminal.

118 Which one of the following nursing actions would help Mr. Swisher most come to grips with his impending death?
○ 1. Provide literature on death and dying.
○ 2. Allow him privacy to think by himself.
○ 3. Let him talk about how he is feeling.
○ 4. Encourage him to get a second opinion.

NURSING CARE OF A CLIENT WITH LYMPHEDEMA

Ms. Margaret Ross is admitted to a nursing home. Before performing the initial assessment, the nurse reads in the medical record that Ms. Ross has lymphedema of the right arm.

119 Which one of the following is most likely to have contributed to the development of the lymphedema? The client
○ 1. has a healed fracture of the humerus.
○ 2. had a radical mastectomy years ago.
○ 3. is being treated for pernicious anemia.
○ 4. was immunized for smallpox as a child.

120 Because Ms. Ross has lymphedema, which one of the following is essential when planning her care?
○ 1. Avoid turning the client on her right side.
○ 2. Avoid giving injections in her right arm.
○ 3. Avoid active exercise of her right arm.
○ 4. Avoid use of nail polish on her right hand.

Correct Answers and Rationales

Two numbers appear in parentheses following each rationale. The first number identifies the textbook listed in the references, page 451, and the second number identifies the page(s) in that textbook on which the correct answer can be verified. Occasionally, two textbooks are given for verifying the correct answer.

1 4. An aneurysm is a balloon-like outpouching in the wall of an artery. Aneurysms commonly occur in the thoracic or abdominal aorta and in cerebral arteries. Weakened valves in veins cause blood vessels in the legs to appear distended and twisted. A stationary blood clot is referred to as a thrombus. A fatty deposit in the wall of an artery is called a plaque. (16:320; 3:513)

   Nursing Process—Collecting data
   Client Need—Health promotion/maintenance

2 1. Methyldopa (Aldomet) is a centrally acting antiadrenergic agent that is given to control hypertension. Though an aneurysm will not improve with drug therapy, rupture of the aneurysm and subsequent hemorrhage can be prevented by lowering the pressure within the artery. Methyldopa does not alter clotting mechanisms, slow the formation of cholesterol, or improve venous circulation. (15:43; 7:385)

   Nursing Process—Implementation
   Client Need—Health promotion/maintenance

3 1. Drowsiness is a side effect associated with centrally acting antiadrenergic drugs. This reaction may occur because drugs in this category decrease the activity of the sympathetic nervous system. Other side effects of methyldopa (Aldomet) include bradycardia, nausea, vomiting, rash, and headache. Constipation, nervousness, and perspiration are not side effects of methyldopa. (15:43, 129)

   Nursing Process—Collecting data
   Client Need—Physiological integrity

4 3. The abbreviation *t.i.d.* means three times a day. The abbreviation for administering a drug once a day is *q.d.* Twice a day administration is indicated by the abbreviation *b.i.d.* Giving a medication four times a day is indicated by the abbreviation *q.i.d.* (18:576; 14:486)

   Nursing Process—Implementation
   Client Need—Physiological integrity

5 2. The correct number of tablets necessary to administer 1 g or 1000 mg of methyldopa when the dosage strength is 250-mg per tablet is four

tablets. A common formula used to compute proper dosage is as follows (15:12; 18:574):

$$\frac{\text{Dosage desired}}{\text{Dosage on hand}} \times \text{quantity} = \text{Amount to administer}$$

$$\frac{1000 \text{ mg}}{250 \text{ mg}} \times 1 \text{ tablet} = \frac{1000}{250} = 4 \text{ tablets}$$

   Nursing Process—Implementation
   Client Need—Physiological integrity

6 1. Antihypertensives are given to individuals with aneurysms to reduce the risk for rupture of the weakened arterial wall with subsequent hemorrhage. Antihypertensives will not keep other arterial defects from forming, alter his level of activity, or slow the atherosclerotic disease process. (16:321; 7:385)

   Nursing Process—Implementation
   Client Need—Health promotion/maintenance

7 1. When the portion of the descending aorta containing the aneurysm becomes larger and larger, an examiner may be able to feel a pulsating mass. Extra heart sounds are associated with disorders of the conduction system or congestive heart failure. Uneven chest movements are more often a sign of a pneumothorax or flail chest. It would be normal to hear a hollow sound when percussing most areas of the abdomen. A dull sound would indicate the presence of a solid organ, such as the liver, or tissue mass, such as a tumor. (16:321; 7:385)

   Nursing Process—Collecting data
   Client Need—Physiological integrity

8 4. Pressure from an enlarging or dissecting abdominal aortic aneurysm is most likely to be manifested as low back pain. The client may indicate that no position or nursing measure relieves the pain. Because the blood loss from a dissecting aneurysm is internal, the cause of rectal bleeding or blood in the urine would be from some other cause. The client may complain of cramping abdominal pain but not indigestion if the intestine's blood supply is inadequate. (3:513; 16:321)

   Nursing Process—Collecting data
   Client Need—Physiological integrity

9 3. The nurse should inform the physician of the change in the client's condition. Pertinent assessments, such as vital signs and skin color, should be reported at the same time. If the client were not breathing and pulseless, it would be unethical to violate her wishes by performing cardiopulmonary resuscitation. The nurse would not be following the physician's written order if resuscitation efforts were initiated. The physician would be the one to decide about transferring the client using the local ambulance service based on the information the nurse communicates. (18:752; 14:468)
Nursing Process—Implementation
Client Need—Safe, effective care environment

NURSING CARE OF CLIENTS WITH THROMBOPHLEBITIS

10 2. Pain in the calf when the foot is dorsiflexed is referred to as a positive Homans' sign. This phenomenon was named after a surgeon, Dr. John Homans, who noted the finding in individuals who developed thrombi in the deep veins of the calf. An abnormal Babinski's reflex is present if the great toe of an adult extends and the other toes fan out when the bottom of the foot is stroked. A client would manifest a positive Romberg's sign if balance could not be maintained with the eyes closed and feet together. Chadwick's sign is the term used when the mucous membrane of the vagina takes on a bluish color at approximately the fourth week of pregnancy. (16:316; 14:563)
Nursing Process—Implementation
Client Need—Safe, effective care environment

11 2. Whenever a thrombophlebitis is suspected, the legs should not be massaged. Activity is generally restricted. Ambulation, exercise, or massage may cause a blood clot, if present, to break away from the vessel wall and circulate in the bloodstream. Though there is some controversy, elevating the legs is recommended by some to relieve local swelling. At no time, however, should pillows be placed under the knees or the bed gatched at the knees. (14:807; 3:511; 7:387)
Nursing Process—Implementation
Client Need—Safe, effective care environment

12 4. A dry towel and a waterproof cover act as insulators and prevent rapid heat and moisture loss from the compress. To avoid burning the skin, the temperature of the compress solution should be between 98°F and 105°F. The skin should be inspected at least every 30 minutes to monitor for thermal injury. Sterile technique is not nec-

essary as long as the skin is intact. (18:493; 14:388)
Nursing Process—Implementation
Client Need—Physiological integrity

13 1. An embolism, or moving blood clot, can be carried in the circulation to other vital organs. If the embolus becomes wedged in the blood vessels supplying the lungs, the client is likely to complain of sudden, sharp chest pain and breathing difficulty and will exhibit a cough and bloody sputum. An embolus also could cause confusion and paralysis if it travels to cerebral vessels in the brain. If lodged in the coronary blood vessels, the client suffers a heart attack. Leg cramps, local swelling, and numbness are not signs or symptoms associated with a pulmonary, cerebral, or coronary embolism. (14:807; 7:332)
Nursing Process—Collecting data
Client Need—Physiological integrity

14 3. Heparin prevents future clots from forming. Heparin is an anticoagulant that inhibits the conversion of fibrinogen to fibrin. Only thrombolytic agents, such as streptokinase, will shrink and dissolve clots that have already formed. The use of thrombolytic agents is extremely hazardous. The risks usually outweigh the benefits in the case of thrombophlebitis. Drug therapy will not prevent a thrombus from becoming dislodged. (15:101; 3:511)
Nursing Process—Implementation
Client Need—Health promotion/maintenance

15 4. The nurse must administer a volume of 1.5 mL to give the client 7500 U of heparin that comes in a dosage strength of 5000 U/mL. A common formula used to compute proper dosage is as follows: (15:12; 18:574)

$$\frac{\text{dosage desired}}{\text{dosage on hand}} \times \text{quantity} = \text{amount}$$
$$\text{to administer}$$

$$\frac{7500 \text{ U}}{5000 \text{ U}} \times 1 \text{ mL} = \frac{7500}{5000} = 1.5 \text{ mL}$$

Nursing Process—Implementation
Client Need—Physiological integrity

16 2. When a drug is withdrawn from a vial, the nurse should instill a volume of air that will equal the amount of fluid that will be withdrawn. Adding air to the contents of a vial facilitates withdrawing the drug. If air is not instilled, a partial vacuum is created making it difficult to remove solution. If too much air is instilled, solution will surge into the syringe and in some cases force the plunger from the barrel of the syringe. If the rubber stopper is removed, the drug will not remain sterile. Modified insulins, not heparin,

should be rotated gently prior to withdrawal to mix the additive and insulin together. Heparin does not need to be shaken vigorously before withdrawing it from the vial. (18:606; 14:489)
    Nursing Process—Implementation
    Client Need—Physiological integrity

17 3. When the adult client is of average or thin size, it is acceptable practice to insert a needle intended for subcutaneous administration at a 45-degree angle to the skin. For obese adults it is recommended that the nurse use a 90-degree angle to insert the needle. The dorsogluteal site is used for intramuscular injections. The needle size for a subcutaneous injection should be between ½ and ⅝ inches and 23 to 26 gauge. The injection site following the administration of heparin should not be massaged because this can increase the tendency for local bleeding. (18:624)
    Nursing Process—Implementation
    Client Need—Physiological integrity

18 2. Heparin can only be injected because it is inactivated by the gastric acid in the stomach. Because of its rapid anticoagulant effect, heparin is used first to alter the clotting mechanism, and then an oral anticoagulant, such as warfarin sodium, is used for maintenance therapy. (15:101)
    Nursing Process—Implementation
    Client Need—Health promotion/maintenance

19 3. When a client receiving anticoagulant therapy manifests any sign of bleeding, it should be reported. Feeling tired, leaving food on the tray, and sleep pattern disturbance require further nursing assessment and care planning, but they are not as potentially dangerous as bleeding. (15:103)
    Nursing Process—Implementation
    Client Need—Physiological integrity

20 3. Individuals with a history of forming clots should take measures to prevent pooling of venous blood. Walking helps to move venous blood from the distal areas of the legs back to the right side of the heart. If walking is not possible, then isometric leg exercises should be performed. Maintaining adequate hydration also is helpful in preventing the recurrence of thrombophlebitis. (3:509, 511; 7:387)
    Nursing Process—Implementation
    Client Need—Health promotion/maintenance

21 2. Injections should be avoided, if possible, when a client is receiving anticoagulant therapy. If questioned, the penicillin could be prescribed by an alternate route, such as orally or intravenously. There is a tendency for a client with altered clotting mechanisms to have prolonged bleeding

from an injection site and to form painful hematomas. The nurse needs to apply firm pressure following any unavoidable injection. Performing leg exercises, applying antiembolism stockings, and ambulation would all be appropriate nursing measures to prevent the formation of a thrombus in the lower legs. (5:121; 15:102-103)
    Nursing Process—Implementation
    Client Need—Physiological integrity

22 1. The PTT is used to monitor the client's response to heparin therapy. The therapeutic range is 1.5 to 2.5 times the control time. PEP is a blood test used to diagnose multiple sclerosis. PCV is the same as a hematocrit. It measures the percentage of cells in a volume of blood. The PT, or pro-time as it is sometimes called, is a test that is used to monitor the response of a client who is receiving an oral anticoagulant, such as warfarin sodium. (15:101; 5:119)
    Nursing Process—Collecting data
    Client Need—Physiological integrity

23 3. Protamine sulfate is the antagonist for heparin. It would be given to counteract the anticoagulant effects of heparin and restore more normal clotting mechanisms. Calcium lactate is a mineral supplement. Sodium benzoate is used as a food preservative. Aluminum phosphate is an ingredient in some antacid products. (15:102)
    Nursing Process—Planning
    Client Need—Safe, effective care environment

24 4. The prothrombin time is measured daily on clients receiving an oral anticoagulant like warfarin sodium. The physician uses the results of this laboratory test to decide if the dosage of warfarin sodium should be increased, decreased, maintained, or omitted for that day. A partial thromboplastin time is used to monitor and prescribe heparin dosages. Total iron binding capacity is a blood test used to diagnose various anemias and blood diseases. A red blood cell count indicates the total number and types of erythrocytes in a sample of blood. (15:99; 5:120)
    Nursing Process—Implementation
    Client Need—Safe, effective care environment

25 3. Vitamin K would be given to increase the amount of a client's prothrombin that was dangerously reduced by the administration of warfarin sodium. During the clotting process, prothrombin is converted to thrombin. Production of prothrombin depends on sufficient vitamin K. Protamine sulfate is the antidote for heparin therapy. Sodium citrate is added to donated blood to prevent coagulation during storage. Vitamin E helps in red blood cell formation, protects essential fatty acids, and is thought to be

important for normal reproduction in animals. (15:99; 5:121)

    Nursing Process—Planning
    Client Need—Physiological integrity

NURSING CARE OF CLIENTS WITH VARICOSE VEINS

26 3. Most individuals with superficial varicose veins in the legs have large veins that stand out from the skin. They appear twisted and deep blue. Due to the venous congestion, the client's feet may eventually become swollen and may look cyanotic. However, swollen and cyanotic feet are not the classic signs associated with varicose veins. Dependent edema and cyanosis of the feet can be caused by any number of systemic diseases. Superficial varicose veins are not difficult to see. (14:808; 16:319)

    Nursing Process—Collecting data
    Client Need—Physiological integrity

27 1. Most people with varicose veins describe that their legs ache and feel heavy and tired. At night, symptoms should be relieved because the impaired circulation is most prominent when the person sits or stands for a long period of time. Leg pain during activity is more likely to be caused by inadequate arterial blood flow or a sport-related injury. (3:514; 7:388)

    Nursing Process—Collecting Data
    Client Need—Safe, effective care environment

28 1. Symptoms associated with varicose veins are relieved by elevating the legs periodically during the day. Other techniques that improve venous circulation, such as isometric or isotonic exercise, may also be helpful. Wearing cotton socks would not provide symptomatic relief from varicose veins; wearing elastic support hose, however, would be beneficial. Walking would help improve venous circulation, but this should be done frequently throughout the day. Fishing would not promote venous circulation because it generally involves sitting or standing for long periods of time. (7:388; 14:808)

    Nursing Process—Implementation
    Client Need—Health promotion/maintenance

29 2. Support hose or elastic stockings improve the function of incompetent valves within the leg veins. Wearing a full support bra may improve posture and relieve low back pain. Soft leather shoes provide comfort and help foot perspiration to evaporate. Wearing cotton underwear is recommended to prevent vaginal yeast infections. Girdles and clothing that would constrict blood flow in the lower body should be avoided. (14:808; 7:388)

    Nursing Process—Implementation
    Client Need—Health promotion/maintenance

30 1. Heredity is a predisposing factor in developing varicose veins. Other contributing factors include occupations that require prolonged standing or sitting, obesity, and the pressure on veins from an enlarging uterus during the later months of pregnancy. Though smoking is definitely unhealthy, nicotine has a major vasoconstricting effect on arterioles rather than veins. An active life-style or athletic exercise is more likely beneficial for the cardiovascular system. Eating a vegetarian diet, as long as it contains all the essential amino acids, generally promotes health rather than endangers it. (14:808; 16:319)

    Nursing Process—Collecting data
    Client Need—Safe, effective care environment

31 3. Following a vein-stripping procedure, blood returns to the right side of the heart through other veins that are deeper in the leg. Arteries cannot transport both oxygenated and unoxygenated blood. New veins are not formed as replacements. The ends of the removed veins are sutured closed. They are not reconnected to other blood vessels. (14:808; 16:319)

    Nursing Process—Implementation
    Client Need—Health promotion/maintenance

32 3. Early and frequent ambulation is essential following vein stripping and vein ligation surgery. During the immediate postoperative period, walking may be ordered hourly while the client is awake. Even during the night, the client is aroused and assisted to walk several times. Walking helps to promote venous circulation that has been temporarily compromised by the removal of some leg veins. Most individuals having surgery can reduce their intake of food for a short period of time without severe consequences. Orienting a confused person is important, but disorientation is not usually a problem among most surgical clients. Oral hygiene is a basic component of good nursing care. However, if ambulation is not performed, the client is at risk for developing postoperative complications. (14:808; 16:319)

    Nursing Process—Planning
    Client Need—Physiological integrity

33 4. When a person states that an unfavorable reaction is experienced when taking a particular medication, the drug should be withheld and the information reported to the nurse in charge or the physician. It is unethical to try to deceive a client by giving the generic name for a drug. A medical order can be changed by consulting with the physician. Taking propoxyphene with a lot of water is not likely to reduce or prevent gastrointestinal upset. (18:583; 14:486)

    Nursing Process—Implementation
    Client Need—Physiological integrity

34 1. It is essential that a client who has had a vein stripping be informed about ways to prevent congestion of blood in the lower extremities. Crossing the legs should be avoided. It puts pressure on blood vessels and interferes with circulation. Getting adequate sleep and consuming recommended amounts of milk are healthy suggestions, but promoting circulation is more important. This client's occupation probably contributes to problems with circulation. However, the surgical procedure and pertinent teaching about ways to promote circulation should help relieve his condition. (7:388; 14:808)

Nursing Process—Planning
Client Need—Health promotion/maintenance

NURSING CARE OF CLIENTS WITH PERIPHERAL VASCULAR DISORDERS

35 1. Individuals with peripheral vascular disease develop *trophic changes*, like thick, hard nails. Other signs include thin, shiny skin with little hair growth. Trophic changes are the result of chronic impaired blood flow to the epidermal tissues. The peripheral pulses are often weak and difficult to detect in a client with peripheral vascular disease. Hyperactive knee jerk reflexes are not a characteristic of peripheral vascular disease. (3:506; 14:806)

Nursing Process—Collecting data
Client Need—Physiological integrity

36 3. Extra clothing or blankets, rather than external heat sources, should be used whenever possible for individuals with peripheral vascular disease. Because of their disease process, they are often insensitive to warm temperatures and are at high risk for being burned. Layers of loosely woven fibers, especially of natural material like cotton or wool, help hold pockets of warm air close to the body surface. This promotes a feeling of warmth. Elevating the feet would relieve edema but would not necessarily make the feet feel warmer. (14:806; 18:490; 3:514)

Nursing Process—Implementation
Client Need—Physiological integrity

37 2. The nurse must apply acoustic jelly to the skin when using a Doppler ultrasound device. The gel helps beam the ultrasound toward the blood vessel being assessed. Movement of red blood cells through an artery produces an intermittent, pulsating sound. Movement of blood through a vein makes a continuous sound like whistling wind. The dorsalis pedis artery is on the top of the foot. The posterior tibialis artery is beside the ankle. When assessing capillary refill the nurse releases a compressed nailbed and counts the number of seconds it takes for blood to return. A Doppler ultrasound device will not measure skin temperature. (18:291)

Nursing Process—Implementation
Client Need—Safe, effective care environment

38 3. Stasis ulcers appear darkly pigmented, dry, and scaly. Venous congestion causes edema. The localized swelling interferes with adequate arterial blood flow causing poor oxygenation and nourishment of skin tissue. This combined with the retention of metabolic wastes leads to inflammation of the skin, sometimes referred to as cellulitis. The inflamed tissue chronically breaks open, forming craters that are difficult to heal. (3:506, 514)

Nursing Process—Collecting data
Client Need—Physiological integrity

39 1. Wet-to-dry dressings are used as a technique for débriding a wound. The moisture softens dried secretions and dead tissue. As the gauze dressing dries, the wound debris becomes trapped in the fibers of the dressing. When the dried dressing is removed, the wound is cleaned of substances that interfere with healing. Dry gauze dressings, rather than wet, have a greater capacity for absorbing liquid drainage, preventing skin infection, and keeping a wound clean. (7:710; 18:482)

Nursing Process—Implementation
Client Need—Health promotion/maintenance

40 4. A moist wound undergoes accelerated healing. An air occlusive dressing prevents evaporation of wound moisture. The moist environment allows healing by second intention to occur at a more rapid rate. Some feel that the reason healing is faster using an air occlusive dressing is that by preventing oxygen from reaching the wound externally, capillary growth to the wound is stimulated. This type of dressing can remain in place for up to 7 days unless it comes loose or there are signs of an infection. Air occlusive dressings, like DuoDERM, are initially more expensive than traditional gauze dressings. The need for less frequent changing tends to reduce the initial cost for some individuals. (18:467; 7:716)

Nursing Process—Implementation
Client Need—Health promotion/maintenance

41 1. *Granulation tissue* appears pinkish-red. This is a sign that new projections of capillaries are supplying regenerating cells in the area. An open wound, like an ulcer, heals from the outer margins inward. The presence of dark brownish-black tissue indicates unhealthy or necrotic tissue. Blanched pale tissue usually indicates inadequate arterial blood supply. Milky white, or pu-

rulent, drainage indicates that an infection is present. (18:458; 14:285; 16:154)
   Nursing Process—Evaluation
   Client Need—Physiological integrity

42 2. The symptoms of arterial vasospasm associated with Raynaud's disease are generally confined to an individual's hands or feet. The nose, ears, and chin are less commonly involved. The client experiences periodic episodes during which the affected areas feel cold, painful, numb, and prickly due to poor circulation. As blood flow resumes, the deprived areas become flushed and warm. A throbbing sensation is then experienced. (16:315; 14:809)
   Nursing Process—Collecting data
   Client Need—Safe, effective care environment

43 2. Conditions that lead to vasoconstriction, such as exposure to cold or emotional upsets, aggravate or exacerbate the symptoms experienced by individuals with Raynaud's disease. The effect of wind would depend on the temperature of the air. (3:513; 16:315)
   Nursing Process—Collecting data
   Client Need—Physiologic integrity

44 2. Stress stimulates the sympathetic nervous system, causing vasoconstriction. When the arterioles narrow, blood flow is impaired, and the client may experience an episodic attack of pain, numbness, pallor, and so on. Wearing warm gloves while out of doors in cold weather would be beneficial. Drinking alcoholic beverages and bathing with perfumed soap are not necessarily contraindicated for a person with Raynaud's disease. (14:809; 3:513)
   Nursing Process—Implementation
   Client Need—Health promotion or maintenance

45 3. Individuals with Buerger's disease report that they experience leg pain or muscle cramps during periods of active movement. This symptom is referred to as *intermittent claudication*. The discomfort is relieved by rest at first; eventually the pain may occur even while inactive. People with varicose veins report feeling a sense of heaviness in their legs. If a client with thromboangiitis obliterans has ingrown toenails, it is a coincidental finding and not related to the disease process. There seems to be a hereditary link to ingrown toenails. They also may be caused by poor fitting shoes and improper nail cutting. Edema may occur when the disease is far advanced. (16:297; 7:387)
   Nursing Process—Collecting data
   Client Need—Safe, effective care environment

46 4. Thromboangiitis obliterans is an acute inflammation of the arteries and veins in the lower extremities. This disease results in decreased blood flow in the legs and feet. The distal peripheral pulses are frequently found to be diminished or absent. A normal peripheral pulse feels strong or full. It is easily felt with only moderate pressure. (7:387)
   Nursing Process—Collecting data
   Client Need—Physiological integrity

47 1. Because of impaired arterial and venous circulation, a person with thromboangiitis obliterans can easily develop gangrene if the toes or feet are injured. A podiatrist is a professional who cares for feet. The services of a podiatrist should be used for nail care, corn treatment, callouses, and so on. Some individuals with this condition undergo amputation when foot ulcers or injuries become infected or do not heal. Weight control, visual examination, and seeking counseling for emotional problems are all positive health habits, but they are not directly related to the complications of Buerger's disease. (7:387; 14:809)
   Nursing Process—Collecting Data
   Client Need—Health promotion/maintenance

48 1. A sympathectomy is a procedure that promotes vasodilation of peripheral arterioles. It involves cutting sympathetic nerve fibers from the autonomic nervous system. Severing these particular nerve fibers will not produce skeletal muscle relaxation, relieve mental stress, or slow the heart rate. (3:508; 14:809)
   Nursing Process—Evaluation
   Client Need—Health promotion/maintenance

49 1. When Buerger-Allen exercises are performed, the legs are alternately elevated while lying down and then lowered to a dependent position by sitting on the edge of the bed or couch. When the legs flush, the client returns to lying flat in bed again. (3:508; 16:297)
   Nursing Process—Collecting data
   Client Need—Health promotion/maintenance

50 2. Because nicotine causes vasoconstriction, cigarette smoking should be avoided by a person with Buerger's disease. There are no contraindications for heavy lifting, traveling by air, or engaging in sexual activity based on the pathology involved in Buerger's disease. (7:387; 14:809)
   Nursing Process—Planning
   Client Need—Health promotion/maintenance

NURSING CARE OF CLIENTS WITH VARIOUS TYPES OF ANEMIA

51 4. One of the simplest ways to diagnose anemia is to measure the hemoglobin. If the hemoglobin level is below 12 g/dL in an adult female or 14 g/dL in a male, the person is considered anemic.

Other diagnostic tests would be required to determine the cause of the anemia. Prothrombin time, bleeding time, and fibrinogen level are all tests that might be performed if a person had a clotting problem or was at high risk for bleeding. (14:714; 16:373)

Nursing Process—Collecting data
Client Need—Physiological integrity

52 3. Hypochromic is a term meaning of paler color in comparison to normal. When this finding is a characteristic of the red blood cells, it generally means that there is insufficient hemoglobin. This is common when a person has iron-deficiency anemia, which is also known as nutritional anemia. (3:444; 7:416-417)

Nursing Process—Collecting data
Client Need—Physiological integrity

53 3. An anemic person is likely to feel colder than usual most of the time. This symptom is most likely due to impaired cellular oxygenation from reduced levels of hemoglobin. Without oxygen, the body's ability to produce calories of heat during metabolism is affected. Constipation, dysmenorrhea, and a history of rheumatic fever are not related to nutritional anemia. (14:714)

Nursing Process—Collecting data
Client Need—Safe, effective care environment

54 2. Omitting meat from the diet can cause iron-deficiency anemia. Good food sources of iron include meat, fish, certain beans, iron-enriched cereals, whole grain products, and green leafy vegetables. Iron is more poorly absorbed from plant sources. Milk, citrus fruits, and candy are not good sources of iron. Milk is a good source of calcium and protein. Citrus fruits are a good source of potassium and vitamin C. Candy is a source of empty calories. That is, it is high in calories without any appreciable contribution to nutrition. The health of a person who does not consume candy would not be harmed. (4:211, 289; 7:418)

Nursing Process—Collecting data
Client Need—Physiological integrity

55 1. Iron is absorbed very poorly from the gastrointestinal tract. Absorption occurs best when the drug is taken on an empty stomach with water. Taking the drug between meals, or at least 1 hour before meals, would be the best routine for maximum benefit. Taking the drug just before eating or with the meal would cause the drug to be present in the stomach with food. When food and some other drugs, like antacids, are taken at the same time as iron, its absorption is decreased. However, if a client experiences gastrointestinal upset while taking iron, rather than

discontinuing the medication, the client may reduce the discomfort by taking the ferrous sulfate with food or milk. If the client only took the ferrous sulfate before bedtime, she would not be following the prescribed daily schedule for taking this drug three times a day. (15:300; 14:715; 7:416)

Nursing Process—Implementation
Client Need—Health promotion/maintenance

56 2. Most individuals who take iron observe that their stools become jet black or dark green. Stool is normally a medium brown color. Clay colored stools are associated with liver or biliary disease. The stool may become light green with diarrhea, or it may assume this color from eating certain foods. (16:376; 14:715)

Nursing Process—Evaluation
Client Need—Health promotion/maintenance

57 4. The presence of vitamin C, found in orange or other citrus juices, improves the absorption of iron. For this reason some pharmaceutical companies combine iron and vitamin C in the same capsule or tablet. Iron taken with milk would interfere with its absorption. Taking iron with tea or a soft drink is not likely to be any more beneficial than taking it with water. (4:71; 7:416)

Nursing Process—Implementation
Client Need—Health promotion/maintenance

58 1. Liquid iron preparations stain the teeth. Drinking the medication through a straw minimizes contact of the drug with the teeth. Using a paper cup or metal spoon will not protect the teeth from unsightly staining. Diluting the liquid iron with at least 2 to 4 oz of water also will reduce the potential for staining teeth. (15:299; 14:715)

Nursing Process—Planning
Client Need—Physiological integrity

59 1. Individuals who are anemic from blood loss often experience dizziness and fainting. This is probably due to low blood volume or an inability to maintain adequate oxygenation to the brain. Anemia is more likely to cause an individual to feel tired and require more sleep. Having had the gall bladder removed and having a tender abdomen are unrelated to anemia from blood loss. (3:444; 7:415)

Nursing Process—Collecting data
Client Need—Safe, effective care environment

60 3. The skin of an anemic individual is most likely to appear pale. This is generally due to the fact that tissue oxygenation, which causes the skin and mucous membranes to appear pink, is impaired due to decreased amounts of hemoglobin or red blood cells. Cyanosis is more likely caused by the buildup of carbon dioxide in the blood. Flushed appearance is due to factors such as vasodilation, increased blood volume, and thermal injury. Mottled skin is a condition characterized by generalized purplish, spotted areas. It is often seen in newborns who are chilled or inactive. (3:444; 7:415)

    Nursing Process—Collecting data
    Client Need—Physiological integrity

61 3. The ventrogluteal site, which includes the gluteus medius and gluteus minimus muscles, is the preferred site for administering an injection by Z-track technique. Z-track injections should be given deeply into a large muscle. The deltoid muscle is used for intramuscular injections; however, it is a smaller muscle in comparison to other intramuscular injection sites. Neither the trapezius muscle, located in the back and shoulder, nor the latissimus dorsi, the widest muscle in the back, are used for injections. (18:620; 14:492)

    Nursing Process—Planning
    Client Need—Physiological integrity

62 2. Using a Z-track technique helps to deposit irritating substances deeply within the muscle so that it will not leak into subcutaneous tissues. Absorption would occur at the same rate as any other intramuscular injection. Z-track administration involves injecting the drug with slow, even pressure. The nurse should wait to remove the needle for approximately 10 seconds after all the drug has been instilled. Injections given by Z-track technique are not massaged afterwards. (18:611; 14:492)

    Nursing Process—Implementation
    Client Need—Health promotion/maintenance

63 1. When administering an injection using the Z-track technique, the tissue is pulled laterally until it is taut. It is held in that position during the injection as well. The position of the tissue is not released until after the needle has been withdrawn. (18:620; 14:493)

    Nursing Process—Implementation
    Client Need—Physiological integrity

64 2. The company and type of health insurance an individual has would be information gathered by personnel in the admissions or business office. The nurse should document subjective and objective assessment data, nursing care, treatment interventions, and the client's responses. (14:278, 18:59)

    Nursing Process—Evaluation
    Client Need—Safe, effective care environment

65 1. The tongue of a person with pernicious anemia is generally red, smooth, and sore. Dental cavi-

ties, large tonsils, and dry mucous membranes are not common characteristics of most individuals with pernicious anemia. (16:375; 7:418; 14:714)

    Nursing Process—Collecting data
    Client Need—Physiological integrity

66 1. Pernicious anemia may impair peripheral and spinal cord nerve fibers, causing symptoms such as tingling and numbness in the extremities, loss of position sense, a staggering gait, and partial or total paralysis. Headaches are not a classic complaint among individuals with pernicious anemia nor is restlessness or sleep disturbances. Some experience confusion, depression, personality changes, and memory loss but not to the point of amnesia. (7:418; 16:375)

    Nursing Process—Collecting data
    Client Need—Physiological integrity

67 1. All urine is collected for 24 to 48 hours after the client receives oral and injected doses of vitamin B_{12} when a Schilling test is performed. Subnormal levels of vitamin B_{12} in the urine suggest pernicious anemia. (16:370; 3:441)

    Nursing Process—Planning
    Client Need—Safe, effective care environment

68 1. Pernicious anemia results when the gastric mucosa fails to produce an adequate amount of *intrinsic factor*. Without the intrinsic factor, secreted by the parietal cells in the stomach, vitamin B_{12} cannot be absorbed from the small intestine. Vitamin B_{12} is necessary for normal blood cell formation. Reduced production of intrinsic factor is found as an inherited trait; it also may develop following a total or partial gastrectomy or removal of the ileum. Strict vegetarians may develop pernicious anemia because they do not consume animal protein foods that contain Vitamin B_{12}. Insufficient bile salts would occur with gall bladder disease. Lipase is an enzyme secreted by the pancreas. Pepsinogen is converted into pepsin, a component of gastric secretions, in the presence of gastric acid. (7:418; 16:375)

    Nursing Process—Evaluation
    Client Need—Health promotion/maintenance

69 3. Pernicious anemia is not curable, but the manifestations of the disease can be treated by life-long injections of vitamin B_{12}. Blood transfusions would be administered to someone who had hemolytic anemia or severe loss of red blood cells and hemoglobin. Iron preparations are given for nutritional anemia and when blood cells or hemoglobin are low, but the condition is not life-threatening. Vitamin K is administered for clotting disorders in which the client's prothrombin level is low. (3:444; 7:418)

    Nursing Process—Collecting data
    Client Need—Physiological integrity

70 1. The iliac crest is the curved rim along the upper border of the ilium. It can be felt in the hip area near the level of the waist. The sternum, or breastbone, located in the center of the chest is an alternate site for aspirating a sample of bone marrow. The iliac crest is generally the first choice as a site for this procedure because it contains more bone marrow than the sternum. The humerus, or upper arm, and the groin area are not sites from which bone marrow is aspirated. (11:92; 14:712)

    Nursing Process—Evaluation
    Client Need—Safe, effective care environment

71 1. This procedure is performed at the bedside. The client undergoing a bone marrow aspiration will likely need the help of the nurse in minimizing pain. Despite the use of local anesthesia, a person usually feels pressure as the needle is driven within the bone. Brief, but sharp pain is experienced as the needle finally enters the bone and marrow is withdrawn. Premedication may be helpful, as well as using distractive techniques and supportive encouragement. The physician generally needs no assistance with instruments during the procedure. A suction machine is not used. Oxygen ought not to be needed under most conditions. (3:441; 14:712)

    Nursing Process—Implementation
    Client Need—Physiological integrity

72 2. Bleeding from the puncture site is one of the most common problems following a bone marrow aspiration. If bleeding is not controlled, a painful hematoma may form. Firm pressure or an ice pack may be used to limit bleeding. Under usual circumstances, a bone marrow aspiration is not likely to cause shock. Though the blood pressure and pulse may fluctuate somewhat, it is usually due to anxiety and fear rather than from loss of blood volume. The client ought to remain awake and alert throughout and following the procedure. (3:441; 7:412)

    Nursing Process—Collecting data
    Client Need—Safe, effective care environment

73 1. Rapid or labored breathing indicates that an adequate amount of oxygen is not available for a client's metabolic needs. It would be important for the nurse at this time to provide the dyspneic client with a period of rest. Feeling nauseated is not generally associated with hypoxemia. The pulse rate should be expected to increase with activity, accompanied by decreased oxygena-

tion. Cool, moist skin accompanies a drop in blood pressure or other physical problems. It is not usually a classic sign of fatigue or intolerance of activity. (14:715; 16:376)

    Nursing Process—Collecting data
    Client Need—Physiological integrity

74 1. A low number of platelets, also known as thrombocytes, increases the risk for bleeding. Bruises indicate that there has been bleeding into the skin. Coarse body hair, thick toenails, and cool extremities are not associated with thrombocytopenia, or low level of platelets. (7:420; 3:438)

    Nursing Process—Collecting data
    Client Need—Physiological integrity

75 1. Thorough and conscientious handwashing is a priority responsibility when caring for any individual with a low white blood cell count. The white blood cells, or leukocytes, help reduce and remove disease-causing pathogens. A client with leukopenia is at high risk for infection. Handwashing is the best technique for reducing the spread of microorganisms. Maintaining skin integrity, adequate nourishment, and assessing vital signs are all components of good nursing care. However, these actions are not directly related to the depressed white blood cell count. (16:449; 7:421)

    Nursing Process—Implementation
    Client Need—Physiological integrity

76 1. Packed cells contain similar numbers of blood cells. A unit of packed blood cells is prepared by removing approximately two thirds of the plasma from a unit of whole blood. The administration of packed cells is preferred for clients who need a blood transfusion but for whom additional water within the circulatory system would be hazardous. Typically the candidate for packed cells is someone who is prone to congestive heart failure or who has poor kidney function. Packed cells pose the same risk for an allergic reaction as whole blood. Packed cells will not stimulate the bone marrow to produce blood cells. (16:129; 14:503)

    Nursing Process—Implementation
    Client Need—Safe, effective care environment

77 4. A person with blood type A, Rh positive would have a reaction if transfused with AB, Rh positive blood. It is always best to administer the same blood type. However, O type blood is referred to as the universal donor. In an emergency anyone may receive type O blood. People who are Rh positive may receive compatible blood types that are either Rh positive or Rh negative. The reverse is not true; in other words a person who

is Rh negative should never be given Rh positive blood. (7:412-413; 18:673)
Nursing Process—Collecting data
Client Need—Physiological integrity

78 2. Long-term administration of endogenous corticosteroids cause body changes like a "moon" face and "buffalo" hump on the back of the neck, which resemble signs of Cushing's syndrome caused by a hyperfunctioning adrenal cortex. The voice is not affected. There is apt to be muscle wasting with long-term corticosteroid use. Anabolic steroids cause muscle enlargement. Steroid administration causes the skin to appear thin and transparent. Purple striae may be found on the abdomen and hips. Bronzed skin is found in individuals who have Addison's disease due to an inadequately functioning adrenal cortex. (15:205; 14:664)
Nursing Process—Collecting data
Client Need—Physiological integrity

79 1. Steroids are known to cause peptic ulcer formation. For this reason the physician also may prescribe drugs to protect the gastric mucosa from erosion. Drowsiness, anorexia, and photophobia are not common problems experienced by individuals who take corticosteroids. (15:208; 14:664)
Nursing Process—Collecting data
Client Need—Physiological integrity

80 3. Total body irradiation destroys the client's bone marrow and places the individual at high risk for infection. People undergoing bone marrow transplant are placed in protective isolation, prophylactic antibiotics and antifungal medications are administered, and visitors may be restricted to prevent the client from acquiring an infection from which he may not recover. The nurse should never neglect to promote optimum nutrition and hydration and to help the client cope with fear and depression. However, if these problems occur, they are more easily treated than an infection. (7:421; 16:379)
Nursing Process—Planning
Client Need—Physiological integrity

81 4. A client with a subcostal incision, located below the ribs, often resists coughing and deep breathing postoperatively because these activities cause pain. Inadequate ventilation and stasis of secretions place the client at high risk for pneumonia. Any postoperative client can develop vomiting, dehydration, and abdominal distention, but these are not directly related to the fact that the incision is close to the diaphragm. (16:172-173; 3:242)
Nursing Process—Planning
Client Need—Physiological integrity

82 1. The spleen contains phagocytes, which engulf bacteria. Without the spleen, a person is at high risk for developing an infection, especially respiratory infections caused by the pneumococci organism. Individuals who undergo a splenectomy should receive immunizations against pneumococcal pneumonia. Antibiotics may be prescribed prophylactically when even a mild respiratory infection occurs. Feeling fatigued or developing gastric upset are annoying problems and should be reported if they persist or recur. Immunizations are mandated by law depending on the country in which foreign travel will take place. (3:454; 14:714)
Nursing Process—Planning
Client Need—Health promotion/maintenance

83 4. The gene for sickling in hemoglobin is found in 1 out of every 10 African Americans. In Africa the sickling effect developed as a genetic adaptation protecting Africans from malaria. When African Americans were forced into slavery in America and other western countries, the genetic characteristic continued to be passed on generation after generation. Because malaria in the United States is minimal, the genetic phenomenon is detrimental rather than protective. This disease also occurs in smaller numbers among people from Mediterranean and Middle Eastern countries. (14:715; 16:373)
Nursing Process—Collecting data
Client Need—Safe, effective care environment

84 3. Jaundice is commonly present in individuals with sickle cell anemia. It is due to the fact that sickled red blood cells are destroyed more rapidly than normal red blood cells. A white, coated tongue may indicate a fungal infection or mouth breathing. Cloudy urine is a sign associated with a urinary tract infection. Nausea has multiple causes, but it is not particularly a common symptom among people with sickle cell anemia. (7:420; 16:373)
Nursing Process—Collecting data
Client Need—Safe, effective care environment

85 2. It is important to change positions to avoid complications of immobility, but activity should be limited during a sickle cell crisis. No specific position is ideal; the goal is to relieve pressure and promote comfort. Exercise and ambulation would be contraindicated because they would increase the client's need for tissue oxygenation at a time when the oxygen-carrying capacity of red blood cells is very limited. (3:448; 7:420)
Nursing Process—Implementation
Client Need—Physiological integrity

86 1. Increasing and maintaining a high volume of fluid intake by oral or intravenous routes will promote the circulation of sickled blood cells through blood vessels. Elastic stockings promote venous return of blood; however, the arterial blood contains the oxygen needed by cells and tissue. Elevating the legs will relieve swelling associated with thrombus formation. However, in sickle cell crisis there are likely to be many microemboli. Neither elevating the legs nor dangling them will help move red blood cells that accumulate and form thrombi. (3:447-448; 7:420)
   Nursing Process—Implementation
   Client Need—Physiological integrity

87 1. The client with sickle cell anemia and his fiancée should be advised to obtain genetic counseling. The nurse has a duty to provide access to all the information on which they can make the best possible decision for the situation as it affects them. It would be unethical for a health care worker to recommend any specific family planning option in particular. Only the client and his future wife have the right to decide whether to have their own natural children, to adopt children, or to prevent conception by permanent sterilization. (3:447; 18:17, 76-77)
   Nursing Process—Planning
   Client Need—Safe, effective care environment

NURSING CARE OF CLIENTS WITH ACQUIRED IMMUNODEFICIENCY SYNDROME

88 4. Intravenous drug users who share needles, male homosexuals, bisexuals, women who have intercourse with these males, and infants of infected mothers are at greatest risk for developing AIDS. Haitians and Africans also have a high incidence of this disease among their native populations. Vacationing in Mexico, breeding dogs, and having had surgery in and of itself should not place the client at any greater risk for AIDS than other individuals. (14:699; 3:786)
   Nursing Process—Collecting data
   Client Need—Safe, effective care environment

89 3. The ELISA test detects the presence of antibodies to viral antigens. A reactive ELISA test is generally repeated. If it continues to be reactive, more specific tests for the HIV antibodies, such as the Western blot test or indirect fluorescent antibody test are performed before making a definitive diagnosis of AIDS. A VDRL test is used as a screening test for syphilis. The Schick test is used to determine if a person has antibodies to the bacterial toxins of the organism causing diphtheria. The Dick test is used to assess the immunologic status of a person to the toxins associated with an infection of scarlet fever. (7:807; 16:87)
   Nursing Process—Collecting data
   Client Need—Physiological integrity

90 3. The virus causing AIDS decreases the number and functioning of T4 lymphocytes, also known as helper lymphocytes. When the virus invades the lymphocyte, it uses components of the cell's DNA to complete the virus' genetic code. This allows the virus to continue reproducing itself. Once infected, the lymphocyte can no longer continue its role in promoting antibody production. Without adequate numbers of normal functioning lymphocytes, the person with AIDS is extremely susceptible to infection and tumor formation. Mature red blood cells, called erythrocytes; immature red blood cells, called reticulocytes; and thrombocytes, also known as platelets, are unaffected by HIV. (7:810; 16:86)
   Nursing Process—Collecting data
   Client Need—Physiological integrity

91 2. Following blood and body fluid precautions is the recommended infection control policy when caring for a person who is HIV positive or has other blood-borne diseases like hepatitis B. Universal blood and body substance precautions are used when caring for all clients. Drainage and secretion precautions are used when an individual has a condition in which there is infective purulent material, such as a wound abscess. Strict isolation is used when a person has a highly communicable disease, like chickenpox, which can be spread by contact and airborne routes. Respiratory isolation is recommended when microorganisms can be transmitted on droplets that can be coughed, sneezed, or breathed into the environment. (18:360; 3:109)
   Nursing Process—Implementation
   Client Need—Safe, effective care environment

92 1. Setting and reaching realistic daily goals can help the client experience a sense of hope. Hope is a powerful influence on a dying person's will to live and can do much to lift a depressed person's spirits. A referral to the chaplain is appropriate if the client requests contact with a clergyman. Distraction will not help a client deal with his feelings or promote a sense of hope. Contacting a lawyer may help an individual take care of unfinished business, but it too should only be arranged if the client indicates that he would like the nurse's assistance in this matter. (3:302)
   Nursing Process—Planning
   Client Need—Psychosocial integrity

93 3. The nurse would be at highest risk for transferring the virus present in blood when changing a dressing. Gloves should be worn as a barrier against contact with the reservoir of infection, in this case blood. For utmost safety gloves should be worn whenever there is a possibility that body substances may contain blood. However, though some body fluids have been found to contain the HIV virus, the Centers for Disease Control and Prevention indicates that stool, nasal secretions, sputum, saliva, urine, perspiration, tears, and vomitus are not considered vehicles of HIV transmission unless they contain visible blood. (18:357; 16:87)

> Nursing Process—Implementation
> Client Need—Safe, effective care environment

NURSING CARE OF CLIENTS WITH THROMBOCYTOPENIA

94 4. The term *idiopathic* is used to indicate that a disease exists, but whatever has caused the condition is unknown. For example individuals who have elevated blood pressure, the etiology of which cannot be explained, are said to have idiopathic hypertension. Idiopathic epilepsy would indicate a seizure disorder that has no known cause. (3:445; 14:774)

> Nursing Process—Implementation
> Client Need—Safe, effective care environment

95 1. Small hemorrhages in the skin, mucous membranes, or subcutaneous tissues are referred to as purpura. Bleeding also may occur internally when a person has thrombocytopenia. There is no other additional term for dark areas of cyanosis. The term for flushed red skin is *erythema*. Protruding veins are referred to as distended or as being *varicosities*. (16:386; 3:445)

> Nursing Process—Collecting data
> Client Need—Physiological integrity

96 1. Preventing injury must be a priority concern when caring for people with thrombocytopenia because they are prone to bleeding. The care plan may specify careful handling of the client, padding the side rails with soft material, avoiding injections, using a soft toothbrush for mouth care, using extended pressure when discontinuing intravenous infusions, and so on. Activity may be restricted to reduce the potential for injury. Generally, individuals with thrombocytopenia are not at high risk for infection; therefore, visitors are not restricted. A normal intake of oral fluid is appropriate unless a client experiences a large loss of blood volume. (14:639; 16:387)

> Nursing Process—Implementation
> Client Need—Safe, effective care environment

NURSING CARE OF CLIENTS WITH POLYCYTHEMIA

97 1. Sitting upright will allow abdominal organs, like the spleen, liver, and intestines, to fall away from the diaphragm. By reducing crowding of the diaphragm, dyspnea is more likely to be reduced, and the client will feel more comfortable. (18:384, 395)

> Nursing Process—Implementation
> Client Need—Physiological integrity

98 2. Keeping a person with polycythemia well hydrated will reduce the viscosity or thickness of the blood. Thrombi are less likely to form if the excessive numbers of blood cells are kept diluted within the plasma. In that way they can move more easily throughout the circulatory system, reducing the possibility of clumping together within a small blood vessel. Providing protein foods, restricting dietary sodium, and encouraging weight loss are healthful interventions, but they will not have a therapeutic effect on preventing the formation of blood clots. (3:445; 16:378)

> Nursing Process—Implementation
> Client Need—Physiological integrity

99 1. A phlebotomy involves removing blood from the circulatory system. In the case of polycythemia, sometimes as much as 500 mL of blood may be removed at one time in an effort to reduce the large number of cells in the circulation. The procedure is similar to when an individual donates blood to a blood bank. Applying tourniquets, surgically occluding blood vessels, and administering blood would all be contraindicated because they would increase the congestion of blood in an already overloaded circulatory system. (3:445; 7:422)

> Nursing Process—Evaluation
> Client Need—Safe, effective care environment

NURSING CARE OF CLIENTS WITH HEMOPHILIA

100 3. Females inherit the trait for classic hemophilia A and can pass that trait on to their own sons. Males who inherit the gene manifest the disease. Females who carry the trait do not manifest any symptoms. There are other types of hemophilia, but not classic hemophilia A, that can affect both women and men. (3:451; 14:718)

> Nursing Process—Evaluation
> Client Need—Health promotion/maintenance

101 2. Drowsiness, or a change in the level of consciousness, is one of the earliest signs of increased pressure from intracranial bleeding. Other signs may include headache, visual problems, vomiting, motor weakness or paralysis, and personality changes. Convulsions would occur later as the bleeding progressed. Tinnitus, or ringing in the ears, is not commonly associated with active intracranial bleeding. The individual may not lose his appetite but may vomit with or without nausea. (16:449; 14:772)

    Nursing Process—Evaluation
    Client Need—Health promotion/maintenance

102   2. Once collected, all donated blood is tested for HIV antibodies. Donated blood is the safest it has ever been since early 1985. However, it is still not 100% safe because some blood donors who have the virus in their blood may not have produced sufficient antibodies to cause a positive reaction when the blood is tested. All potential blood donors are asked questions about life-style behaviors that would indicate they are at risk for HIV infection, but some may not answer the questions honestly. Blood donors are encouraged to call the blood collection agency later and report an identifying number, but not their name, if they feel someone would be at risk if they received a unit of their donated blood. (14:699; 3:135-136; 18:673)

    Nursing Process—Implementation
    Client Need—Health promotion/maintenance

103   3. Cloudy urine is a common sign associated with a urinary tract infection. Other findings that suggest an infection may be occurring include fever, cough, increased respirations and heart rate, and ulcerated oral mucous membranes. Blood in the stool would be associated with altered clotting mechanisms. Prolonged vomiting may be a side effect of chemotherapy. Extreme fatigue would accompany reduced numbers of red blood cells, causing anemia. (16:382; 3:527)

    Nursing Process—Collecting data
    Client Need—Physiological integrity

104   1. Foam mouth swabs are less likely to traumatize the gums and oral mucous membranes. They may be substituted for the toothbrush temporarily. Oral hygiene should not be discontinued because the mouth contains organisms that can be the source of an opportunistic infection. The potential for injury would continue to exist if the nurse eliminated toothpaste but not the use of the toothbrush. (16:212; 18:104; 14:342)

    Nursing Process—Implementation
    Client Need—Physiological integrity

105   4. Soft, bland foods, such as creamed soups, cottage cheese, baked fish, macaroni and cheese, custard, and pudding, would help to maintain nutrition but relieve oral discomfort from coarse or irritating foods. Spicy foods should be avoided. (14:717; 16:212, 382)

    Nursing Process—Implementation
    Client Need—Physiological integrity

106   1. The client who receives antineoplastic drugs is likely to experience hair loss. The hair loss is not permanent; the hair will return when the drug therapy is discontinued. In the meantime the nurse should let the client discuss how he or she feels about the potential hair loss. If the client is troubled by this effect, the nurse can offer suggestions for disguising the fact that hair loss is occurring. Some possible alternatives include wearing a turban, baseball cap, scarf, or wig. (16:382; 3:287)

    Nursing Process—Planning
    Client Need—Safe, effective care environment

107   3. The term remission means that presently the person does not show signs of his original disease. However, this does not mean the condition is cured. Though this is a good sign, the client's prognosis continues to be guarded becuase it is difficult to predict how long the remission will last. If the disease is manifested again, treatment will be reinstituted at that time. For this reason it is very important to stress that the person maintain regular checkups with his physician. In the meantime they should be encouraged to live as fully and normally as possible. (14:1098; 7:845)

    Nursing Process—Evaluation
    Client Need—Health promotion/maintenance

108   3. The National Hospice Organization offers assistance to dying individuals with less than 6 months to live. They provide services to assist the family in caring for the terminally ill individual's physical and emotional needs. They continue working with the family, even after the client's death, in helping them resolve their grief. The public health department provides preventive services in the area of immunizations, care of well babies, diagnosing sexually transmitted and other communicable diseases, inspecting sanitary conditions of buildings and food establishments, and so on. The Centers for Disease Control and Prevention studies the incidence of communicable diseases and recommends practices for controlling their spread. The local Community Chest is a philanthropic organization that collects and distributes funds to many social welfare organizations in the community. (3:312; 7:225)

    Nursing Process—Implementation
    Client Need—Health promotion/maintenance

NURSING CARE OF CLIENTS WITH INFECTIOUS MONONUCLEOSIS

109   2. Mononucleosis is transmitted by direct contact with the droplets or oral secretions of another infected person. This disease has been referred

to as the "kissing disease" because the virus may be passed from one individual to another by the oral route. Sharing eating utensils and cigarettes also would be ways of transmitting this disease as well. (7:157; 14:672)

Nursing Process—Implementation
Client Need—Health promotion/maintenance

110 3. One of the first signs of infectious mononucleosis is a sore throat. This may be accompanied by a fever and headache. In severe cases the lymph nodes, including the spleen, become enlarged. Jaundice may occur in some individuals. Increased thirst and frequent urination are common in uncontrolled diabetes mellitus and diabetes insipidus, as well as other disease syndromes. Intestinal upset is not a common symptom in people with infectious mononucleosis. (7:157)

Nursing Process—Collecting data
Client Need—Safe, effective care environment

111 2. Rest is essential for the recovery from infectious mononucleosis. Physical activity, if not limited, is likely to intensify symptoms, prolong recovery, or contribute to complications involving the liver, spleen, heart, and nervous system. Treatment is usually symptomatic involving oral fluids, analgesics, and antipyretics. (14:672; 16:393)

Nursing Process—Implementation
Client Need—Health promotion/maintenance

112 2. Hodgkin's disease most often strikes males in young adulthood between the ages of 20 and 35 years. Though the cause of the disease remains unknown, there are some who believe that the abnormal lymph cells develop because of exposure to environmental toxins, such as pesticides or other harmful chemicals. (3:453; 7:422)

Nursing Process—Collecting data
Client Need—Physiological integrity

113 1. Hodgkin's disease is characterized by lymph nodes that are enlarged yet painless. The physical change in cervical lymph nodes is generally one of the first abnormal signs of this disease. Later the axillary and inguinal lymph nodes also may become involved. Regardless of the location in the body, cancerous growths are hardly ever painful in the early stages of the disease. This often explains why early warning signs of cancer tend to be ignored. (14:717; 16:394)

Nursing Process—Collecting data
Client Need—Safe, effective care environment

114 2. Deodorants or other skin preparations that contain metals must be avoided. They absorb the x-rays and increase skin irritation. The skin can be washed with tepid water, mild soap, and a soft wash cloth. The hair in the area need not be shaved. In fact, shaving may further impair the integrity of the skin, which will be somewhat damaged temporarily by the radiation. Zinc oxide also contains a metal and should not be applied to the skin. If the skin does become dry, blistered, or peeled, the physician may prescribe a topical application, such as vitamin A and D ointment, lanolin, pure aloe vera gel, or cortisone ointment. (3:280; 14:708)

Nursing Process—Planning
Client Need—Safe, effective care environment

115 1. Reddening or bronzing of the skin can be expected in the area that is being irradiated. It would be best if the client were informed about possible skin changes before therapy began. It should be stressed that the discoloration is only temporary. Though ionizing radiation used in cancer therapy is a form of energy, it does not produce heat or bleeding under the skin. The client's concern is not likely about the cosmetic change, but rather about his fear that an adverse reaction is occurring. Therefore, reassuring him that the redness is hardly noticeable is inappropriate. (3:280; 16:212)

Nursing Process—Implementation
Client Need—Safe, effective care environment

116 4. The most important information to give the client with irradiated skin is that it should be protected from direct sunlight. Advising the client to wear several layers of warm clothing would be appropriate if there was an accompanying problem with poor circulation. For comfort any individual should avoid becoming chilled or too warm. Wearing a face mask would only be warranted if the client had allergies to inhaled substances, had cardiovascular disease in which vasoconstriction could cause ischemia, or needed a barrier to infectious microorganisms or environmental pollutants. (16:212; 7:204)

Nursing Process—Planning
Client Need—Health promotion/maintenance

117 3. If the white blood cell count drops to dangerously low levels, the client becomes susceptible to infection. Chemotherapy drugs can depress bone marrow function. Periodic blood cell counts are monitored to assess for this potential side effect. Anorexia, nausea, vomiting, weight loss, and diarrhea also are side effects of cancer treatment, but they are not indications that the client should be placed in protective isolation. Confusion and disorientation suggest that the client is experiencing some neurologic problems. The client should be observed closely to protect his safety, but the symptoms would not justify implementing protective isolation. (16:210; 7:205)

Nursing Process—Collecting Data
Client Need—Safe, effective care environment

118 3. It is generally agreed that grieving is facilitated by discussing feelings with another person. The client should not be left alone immediately after hearing this information. It would be important for the nurse to stay with the client as he processed the information he was just given. The client also would benefit from talking with other supportive individuals, such as a spouse, family member, friend, or clergyman. Reading literature on the subject and thinking in private may help some people but are not believed to be as effective for most as verbalizing thoughts. If the client requested a second opinion, the request should not be denied. However, it would be inappropriate for the nurse to initiate the suggestion. It would be considered a form of false reassurance and could prolong denial. (18:755; 3:299)

    Nursing Process—Implementation
    Client Need—Psychosocial integrity

119 2. When the axillary lymph nodes are removed during a radical mastectomy, lymph circulation is impaired. The lymph collects and pools within the arm on the side of the mastectomy. The condition is generally permanent once it develops. Elevation of the affected arm and hand, applying an inflatable pressure sleeve or elasticized bandage, squeezing a rubber ball, and active exercise are immediate postoperative interventions designed to prevent, reduce, or eliminate the development of lymphedema. (3:453; 7:564)

    Nursing Process—Collecting data
    Client Need—Physiological integrity

120 2. Because circulation in the arm with lymphedema is impaired, certain nursing interventions, such as administering injections, taking a blood pressure, obtaining blood, or starting an intravenous infusion, should be avoided. Prolonged pressure during positioning should always be avoided, but there is no contraindication at this late date to lying on the affected side for brief periods. Active exercise should be encouraged. Though nail polish would interfere with assessing capillary refill, it is not necessary to totally discourage its use. (14:912; 16:704)

    Nursing Process—Planning
    Client Need—Physiological integrity

Classification of Test Items

Unit IV Review Test 8

Directions: After each question the correct answer is given as well as a classification of each test question. Compare the correct answer with your answer. If a question has been answered *incorrectly*, draw a line to the end of the four columns. When finished, add up your correct scores and place the results at the bottom of each column.

Score Calculation:
   To determine the percentage of the number of questions you answered correctly, divide the **Number Correct** by the **Number Possible**, as example 108 (the number of questions answered correctly) divided by 120 (the number of questions in the test) = .90 or 90%.

NURSING PROCESS

C = Collecting data
P = Planning
I = Implementation
E = Evaluation

CLIENT NEEDS

S = Safe, effective care environment
P = Physiological integrity
M = Psychosocial integrity
H = Health promotion/maintenance

Question #	Answer #	Nursing Process				Client Needs			
		C	P	I	E	S	P	M	H
1	4	C							H
2	1			I					H
3	1	C					P		
4	3			I			P		
5	2			I			P		
6	1			I					H
7	1	C					P		
8	4	C					P		
9	3			I		S			
10	2			I		S			
11	3			I		S			
12	4			I			P		
13	1	C					P		
14	3			I					H
15	4			I			P		
16	2			I			P		
17	3			I			P		
18	2			I					H
19	3			I			P		

NURSING PROCESS

C = Collecting data
P = Planning
I = Implementation
E = Evaluation

CLIENT NEEDS

S = Safe, effective care environment
P = Physiological integrity
M = Psychosocial integrity
H = Health promotion/maintenance

Question #	Answer #	Nursing Process				Client Needs			
		C	P	I	E	S	P	M	H
20	3			I					H
21	2			I			P		
22	1	C					P		
23	3		P			S			
24	4			I		S			
25	3		P				P		
26	3	C					P		
27	1	C				S			
28	1			I					H
29	2			I					H
30	1	C				S			
31	3			I					H
32	3		P				P		
33	4			I			P		
34	1		P						H
35	1	C					P		
36	3			I			P		
37	2			I		S			
38	3	C					P		
39	1			I					H
40	4			I					H
41	1				E		P		
42	2	C				S			
43	2	C					P		
44	2			I					H
45	3	C				S			
46	4	C					P		
47	1	C							H
48	1				E				H
49	1	C							H

NURSING PROCESS

C = Collecting data
P = Planning
I = Implementation
E = Evaluation

CLIENT NEEDS

S = Safe, effective care environment
P = Physiological integrity
M = Psychosocial integrity
H = Health promotion/maintenance

Question #	Answer #	Nursing Process				Client Needs			
		C	P	I	E	S	P	M	H
50	2		P						H
51	4	C					P		
52	3	C					P		
53	3	C				S			
54	2	C					P		
55	1			I					H
56	2				E				H
57	4			I					H
58	1		P				P		
59	1	C				S			
60	3	C					P		
61	3		P				P		
62	2			I					H
63	1			I			P		
64	2				E	S			
65	1	C					P		
66	1	C					P		
67	1		P			S			
68	1				E				H
69	3	C					P		
70	1				E	S			
71	1			I			P		
72	2	C				S			
73	1	C					P		
74	1	C					P		
75	1			I			P		
76	1			I		S			
77	4	C					P		
78	2	C					P		
79	1	C					P		

NURSING PROCESS

C = Collecting data
P = Planning
I = Implementation
E = Evaluation

CLIENT NEEDS

S = Safe, effective care environment
P = Physiological integrity
M = Psychosocial integrity
H = Health promotion/maintenance

Question #	Answer #	Nursing Process				Client Needs			
		C	P	I	E	S	P	M	H
80	3		P				P		
81	4		P				P		
82	1		P						H
83	4	C				S			
84	3	C				S			
85	2			I			P		
86	1			I			P		
87	1		P			S			
88	4	C				S			
89	3	C					P		
90	3	C					P		
91	2			I		S			
92	1		P					M	
93	3			I		S			
94	4			I		S			
95	1	C					P		
96	1			I		S			
97	1			I			P		
98	2			I			P		
99	1				E	S			
100	3				E				H
101	2				E				H
102	2			I					H
103	3	C					P		
104	1			I			P		
105	4			I			P		
106	1		P			S			
107	3				E				H
108	3			I					H
109	2			I					H
110	3	C				S			

NURSING PROCESS

C = Collecting data
P = Planning
I = Implementation
E = Evaluation

CLIENT NEEDS

S = Safe, effective care environment
P = Physiological integrity
M = Psychosocial integrity
H = Health promotion/maintenance

Question #	Answer #	Nursing Process				Client Needs			
		C	P	I	E	S	P	M	H
111	2			I					H
112	2	C					P		
113	1	C				S			
114	2		P			S			
115	1			I		S			
116	4		P						H
117	3	C				S			
118	3			I				M	
119	2	C					P		
120	2		P				P		
Number Correct									
Number Possible	120	44	17	49	10	31	56	2	31
Percentage Correct									

REVIEW TEST 9

The Nursing Care of Clients with Disorders of the Respiratory System

Nursing Care of Clients with a Common Cold
Nursing Care of Clients with Allergic Rhinitis
Nursing Care of Clients with Anaphylaxis
Nursing Care of Clients with Pneumonia
Nursing Care of Clients with Influenza
Nursing Care of Clients with Bronchitis
Nursing Care of Clients with Asthma
Nursing Care of Clients with Emphysema
Nursing Care of Clients with Tuberculosis
Nursing Care of Clients with Cancer of the Lung
Nursing Care of Clients with Chest Injuries
Nursing Care of Clients with Pulmonary Embolism
Nursing Care of Clients with a Tracheostomy
Individual Test Items

Correct Answers and Rationales
Classification of Test Items

Directions: With a pencil, blacken the circle in front of the option you have chosen for your correct answer.

The Nursing Care of Clients with Disorders of the Respiratory System

NURSING CARE OF CLIENTS WITH A COMMON COLD

1 Which symptom, if reported by a person with an upper respiratory infection, is the best indication that *complications* are developing? The client reports having
○ 1. nasal stuffiness.
○ 2. a dry cough.
○ 3. a high fever.
○ 4. scratchy throat.

2 Before recommending that a person with a cold use a nonprescription decongestant, the nurse should determine if the individual has
○ 1. arthritis.
○ 2. asthma
○ 3. hypertension.
○ 4. diabetes.

3 During a visit to the physician's office, a client complains to the nurse that the physician would not prescribe an antibiotic for a head cold. The best explanation the nurse could provide is that
○ 1. antibiotics are ineffective in treating viral infections.
○ 2. once cold symptoms develop, antibiotics are ineffective.
○ 3. antibiotics only prevent the spread of colds to others.
○ 4. they should only be used for immunosuppressed individuals.

4 A neighbor asks a nurse to recommend something to relieve the scratchy sore throat that accompanies her cold. A common comfort measure would be to recommend gargling with
○ 1. household bleach.
○ 2. vanilla extract.
○ 3. bourbon whiskey.
○ 4. salt water.

5 If the nurse observes all of the following after giving the person a lozenge, which one will do most to

Timby B, Scherer JC: LIPPINCOTT'S REVIEW FOR NCLEX–PN. © 1994 J.B. Lippincott Company.

decrease the effectiveness of the drug therapy? While the lozenge is in the client's mouth, he or she

- ○ 1. swallows saliva frequently.
- ○ 2. sucks on it for a long time.
- ○ 3. bites it into small pieces.
- ○ 4. talks while it is in his mouth.

6 A client receives a prescription for elixir of terpin hydrate with codeine to relieve a persistent cough. Which one of the following instructions should the nurse plan to provide?

- ○ 1. "Don't take the drug more frequently than prescribed."
- ○ 2. "Avoid taking the medication before going to sleep."
- ○ 3. "Drink extra fluids throughout your waking hours."
- ○ 4. "Warm the syrup to make the taste more acceptable."

7 The prescribed dose of a liquid cough syrup is 5 mL. Which household measurement would be the equivalent to recommend when teaching a client how to self-administer the medication

- ○ 1. 1 ounce
- ○ 2. 1 tablespoon
- ○ 3. 1 teaspoon
- ○ 4. 1 cup

NURSING CARE OF CLIENTS WITH ALLERGIC RHINITIS

Ms. Angela Dobson has noted that every fall her nasal passages become swollen, she sneezes endlessly, and her eyes become red, itchy, and watery. She makes an appointment with an allergist.

8 For symptomatic relief the physician prescribes terfenadine (Seldane), an antihistamine. The nurse should inform Ms. Dobson that while taking this drug, she is likely to experience

- ○ 1. weight loss.
- ○ 2. constipation.
- ○ 3. drowsiness.
- ○ 4. depression.

Ms. Dobson thinks her allergy is to ragweed pollen. The physician recommends that Ms. Dobson undergo skin testing.

9 When Ms. Dobson asks the nurse why skin testing would be beneficial because everyone else in her family is allergic to ragweed, the best explanation is that

- ○ 1. her symptoms may be due to more than one substance.
- ○ 2. skin testing helps to build up blocking antibodies.
- ○ 3. testing is an example of high quality medical care.

- ○ 4. insurance generally covers diagnostic skin testing.

Ms. Dobson is scheduled for scratch skin testing. The forearms are used.

10 Which of the following signs would indicate to the nurse that the area scratched has reacted to a substance? The skin at the test site will

- ○ 1. look red.
- ○ 2. look pale.
- ○ 3. feel painful
- ○ 4. feel numb.

Based on the outcome of the skin tests, Ms. Dobson has agreed to desensitization treatment. She will come back every week for allergy injections.

11 After receiving her injection, it would be most important for the nurse to inform Ms. Dobson to

- ○ 1. take a couple of aspirin before leaving.
- ○ 2. wait at least 20 minutes before going home.
- ○ 3. make sure someone else drives the car.
- ○ 4. call the office as soon as she arrives home.

NURSING CARE OF CLIENTS WITH ANAPHYLAXIS

12 Which one of the following is an early indication that a client is developing anaphylaxis? The client

- ○ 1. has difficulty breathing.
- ○ 2. complains of a headache.
- ○ 3. develops a sore throat.
- ○ 4. loses bladder control.

13 Which one of the following drugs should the nurse plan to have available whenever there is a possibility that a person may develop anaphylaxis?

- ○ 1. codeine sulfate
- ○ 2. morphine sulfate
- ○ 3. dopamine (Intropin)
- ○ 4. epinephrine (Adrenalin)

14 To monitor the effectiveness of the drug therapy administered to a client in anaphylaxis, it would be best for the nurse to frequently assess

- ○ 1. urine output.
- ○ 2. skin color.
- ○ 3. blood pressure.
- ○ 4. pupil response.

15 If a person experiencing anaphylaxis becomes unresponsive, which of the following actions should the nurse take first?

- ○ 1. Elevate the feet higher than the head.
- ○ 2. Loosen all constricting clothing.
- ○ 3. Lift the chin and tilt the head back.
- ○ 4. Cover the individual with a blanket.

NURSING CARE OF CLIENTS WITH PNEUMONIA

Mr. Paul Baker has an admitting diagnosis of pneumonia. When he arrives, the nurse observes that he has shaking chills and a fever of 104.2°F. A chest x-ray and sputum specimens for culture and sensitivity have been ordered.

16 Which of the following nursing actions would be essential before the chest x-ray is done?
  ○ 1. Make sure the client does not eat food.
  ○ 2. Remove the metal necklace he is wearing.
  ○ 3. Have the client swallow x-ray dye.
  ○ 4. Administer a parenteral analgesic.

17 The client's respiratory secretions are difficult to raise. If all of the measures below are possible, which one will help most when planning to obtain the sputum specimen?
  ○ 1. Providing the client with a generous fluid intake
  ○ 2. Encouraging the client to change positions regularly
  ○ 3. Asking the dietitian to send him food high in fiber
  ○ 4. Seeing to it that the client has frequent rest periods

18 At what time of the day would it be easiest to obtain a sputum specimen?
  ○ 1. Before bedtime
  ○ 2. After a meal
  ○ 3. Between meals
  ○ 4. Upon awakening

19 The client understands the nurse's instruction on handling the sputum specimen container if he says
  ○ 1. he should don gloves before opening the container.
  ○ 2. he should wipe the container with an alcohol swab.
  ○ 3. he cannot touch the outside of the container.
  ○ 4. he must not touch the inside of the container.

20 The nurse notes that the client's sputum is rust colored. The nurse would be accurate in assuming that the sputum contained
  ○ 1. food.
  ○ 2. blood.
  ○ 3. bile.
  ○ 4. saliva.

21 After collecting the sputum specimen, which one of the following nursing actions would be most appropriate?
  ○ 1. Administer oxygen.
  ○ 2. Provide mouth care.
  ○ 3. Offer nourishment.
  ○ 4. Encourage ambulation.

A client has been diagnosed with pneumococcal pneumonia. He is receiving penicillin by intramuscular injection.

22 The client asks the nurse why the physician chose to use penicillin to treat the pneumonia. The best response is that
  ○ 1. the sensitivity report showed the organism was easily killed by penicillin.
  ○ 2. most viral infections respond well when treated with penicillin drugs.
  ○ 3. penicillin is one of the safest yet most effective antibiotics.
  ○ 4. all antibiotics are similar; the choice of drug is not that important.

23 The nurse chooses to inject the penicillin using the dorsogluteal site. If the nurse selects the site appropriately, the injection will be administered into the
  ○ 1. hip.
  ○ 2. arm.
  ○ 3. thigh.
  ○ 4. buttock.

24 The recommended technique to help reduce discomfort when giving an intramuscular injection into the dorsogluteal site is to have the client
  ○ 1. point his toes inward.
  ○ 2. tighten his muscles.
  ○ 3. cross his legs.
  ○ 4. flex his knees.

25 If the client has an allergic reaction to penicillin, the nurse will most likely observe that the individual
  ○ 1. has a slow pulse.
  ○ 2. develops hives.
  ○ 3. feels sleepy.
  ○ 4. looks jaundiced.

NURSING CARE OF CLIENTS WITH INFLUENZA

The nurse working in a nursing home calls the physician because an elderly resident has a fever of 104.6°F, headache, dry cough, and sore muscles. The physician suspects the person has influenza because there have been multiple cases at this time in the community.

26 The nurse shares with the nursing assistant that the client needs to consume extra fluid. What would be an appropriate goal for oral intake in the next 24-hour period?
  ○ 1. 500 mL
  ○ 2. 1000 mL
  ○ 3. 1500 mL
  ○ 4. 3000 mL

The physician orders the nurse to give 10 grains of aspirin orally to the client every 4 hours as necessary for a fever over 102°F and to administer a tepid alcohol sponge bath at this time.

27 Alcohol is added to the water used for the sponge bath because it
○ 1. promotes skin integrity.
○ 2. destroys microorganisms.
○ 3 speeds liquid evaporation.
○ 4. feels soothing to the skin.

28 The nursing assistant helping with the sponge bath asks the nurse to explain what the word *tepid* means. The best explanation is that it means
○ 1. hot.
○ 2. cold.
○ 3. warm.
○ 4. icy.

29 If the client develops all of the following, which one is an indication that the sponge bath should be *discontinued*?
○ 1. Nausea
○ 2. Chills
○ 3. Flushing
○ 4. Confusion

30 Which of the following is the best indication that the tepid sponge bath is having a therapeutic effect?
○ 1. The client says she feels more comfortable.
○ 2. The client says she would like to eat lunch.
○ 3. The client's rectal temperature is 102.4°F.
○ 4. The client's headache is somewhat relieved.

31 Other than obtaining a vaccination against influenza, what is the best advice the nurse can give for preventing this type of infection?
○ 1. Consume adequate vitamin C.
○ 2. Avoid going to crowded places.
○ 3. Dress warmly in cold weather.
○ 4. Reduce daily stress and anxiety.

NURSING CARE OF CLIENTS WITH BRONCHITIS

32 A client with acute bronchitis is receiving aerosol therapy. The client understands the purpose of this treatment if he states that its use is intended to
○ 1. relieve tissue irritation.
○ 2. kill infectious organisms.
○ 3. dry respiratory passages.
○ 4. slow the respiratory rate.

33 A client with bronchitis asks the nurse why he is receiving guaifenesin (Robitussin A-C), an antitussive that contains codeine. The best explanation is that it
○ 1. liquefies thick mucus.
○ 2. dilates the bronchi.
○ 3. suppresses coughing.
○ 4. reduces inflammation.

34 If the client who receives an antitussive containing codeine experiences all of the following, which one is most likely an adverse effect to the codeine?

○ 1. Nausea
○ 2. Dyspnea
○ 3. Diarrhea
○ 4. Headaches

NURSING CARE OF CLIENTS WITH ASTHMA

Mr. Larry Carter has had asthma ever since early childhood. As he has aged, the attacks have become less frequent. He has come to the emergency department at this time because he is experiencing respiratory distress.

35 The nurse prepares to auscultate Mr. Carter's chest with a stethoscope. The position of choice for assessing lung sounds in this client is to have him
○ 1. sit up.
○ 2. stand.
○ 3. lie on his back.
○ 4. lie on his side.

36 When the nurse listens to Mr. Carter breathe, the most characteristic sound that is likely to be heard during the onset of an asthma attack is
○ 1. wet bubbling.
○ 2. dry crackling.
○ 3. soft blowing.
○ 4. noisy wheezing.

Pulse oximetry is used to monitor Mr. Carter's oxygenation status

37 The nurse would be most correct in applying the sensor of the pulse oximeter to Mr. Carter's
○ 1. arm.
○ 2. lip.
○ 3. ear.
○ 4. leg.

38 A blood sample is taken from the client's artery to measure blood gases. Immediately after the specimen has been drawn, the most essential nursing action would be to
○ 1. apply direct pressure to the site for 5 minutes.
○ 2. warm the blood in the specimen tube 5 minutes.
○ 3. assess the client's blood pressure in 5 minutes.
○ 4. elevate the client's arm for at least 5 minutes.

The physician orders 60% oxygen administration with a partial rebreathing mask and bag reservoir.

39 Which of the following observations when administering oxygen in this manner should be reported to the respiratory therapy department?
○ 1. Moisture accumulates inside the mask.
○ 2. The bag collapses during inspiration.
○ 3. The mask covers the mouth and nose.
○ 4. The strap about the head is snug.

The physician orders the nurse to administer 0.1 mg of epinephrine to the patient subcutaneously. The label indicates that the epinephrine is a 1:1000 dilution, which means that 1 g of epinephrine has been mixed with 1000 mL of liquid.

40 The correct volume needed to administer the prescribed dose of 0.1 mg of epinephrine is
- ○ 1. 0.1 mL.
- ○ 2. 1.0 mL.
- ○ 3. 10 mL.
- ○ 4. 0.001 mL.

41 Which one of the following nursing measures will help most to reduce the anxiety the client is experiencing during an asthma attack?
- ○ 1. Close the door to the examination room.
- ○ 2. Remain within the client's view.
- ○ 3. Pull the bedside privacy curtain.
- ○ 4. Cover the client with a light sheet.

NURSING CARE OF CLIENTS WITH EMPHYSEMA

Mr. Gary Dixon has emphysema. His condition has been complicated at this time due to a respiratory infection.

42 While assisting Mr. Dixon into a hospital gown, the nurse is most likely to find that his chest appears
- ○ 1. funnel shaped.
- ○ 2. barrel shaped.
- ○ 3. mottled.
- ○ 4. muscular.

The nurse prepares to administer oxygen to Mr. Dixon with a nasal cannula.

43 Which one of the following oxygen flow rates is most appropriate for a client with emphysema?
- ○ 1. 2 L/min
- ○ 2. 5 L/min
- ○ 3. 8 L/min
- ○ 4. 10 L/min

Mr. Dixon is receiving intravenous fluid that contains aminophylline.

44 The nurse explains to Mr. Dixon that the primary purpose for using this drug is to
- ○ 1. relieve persistent coughing.
- ○ 2. lessen sputum production.
- ○ 3. reduce respiratory distress.
- ○ 4. dilute thick secretions.

45 Which one of the following side effects should the nurse expect when a person receives aminophylline?
- ○ 1. Bronchospasm
- ○ 2. Hypotension
- ○ 3. Drowsiness
- ○ 4. Tachycardia

A nurse has been providing home care for Mr. Robert Turner who has emphysema.

46 When assisting the client with postural drainage, which one of the following nursing actions will help most to loosen secretions?
- ○ 1. Tell the client to take deep breaths.
- ○ 2. Strike the back with a cupped hand.
- ○ 3. Apply pressure below the diaphragm.
- ○ 4. Place the client in a sitting position.

47 Which of the following nursing observations is the best evidence that postural drainage has been effective?
- ○ 1. The client's respiratory rate is increased.
- ○ 2. The client's appetite is much improved.
- ○ 3. The client's sputum culture is negative.
- ○ 4. The client expectorates a large volume of sputum.

48 Before leaving Mr. Turner's home, he says to the nurse, "This disease has made me a prisoner in my own home." The best response from the nurse would be
- ○ 1. "Tell me more about how you're feeling."
- ○ 2. "There are lots of things you can still do."
- ○ 3. "You're just having a bad day today."
- ○ 4. "You'll probably feel better tomorrow."

NURSING CARE OF CLIENTS WITH TUBERCULOSIS

The nurse in a nursing home is required by the state's law to test all newly admitted clients for tuberculosis. The agency's policy is to administer a Mantoux intradermal skin test.

49 The nurse's technique is correct if the needle is inserted at a
- ○ 1. 10-degree angle.
- ○ 2. 45-degree angle.
- ○ 3. 90-degree angle.
- ○ 4. 180-degree angle.

50 When it has been determined that a tuberculin skin test is positive, the most accurate explanation to the client is that
- ○ 1. there is an active infection present.
- ○ 2. antibodies are present in his blood.
- ○ 3. he is immune to this type of disease.
- ○ 4. he needs to be in strict isolation.

51 Which one of the following is the nurse likely to find among individuals who have acquired tuberculosis?
- ○ 1. Foul breath
- ○ 2. Weight gain
- ○ 3. Night sweats
- ○ 4. High fever

52 For a client who is suspected of having tuberculosis, it would be essential for the nurse to plan on taking the temperature
○ 1. at predawn hours.
○ 2. in the afternoon.
○ 3. early evening.
○ 4. late at night.

Efforts at obtaining a sputum specimen from a client who is suspected of having tuberculosis have been unsuccessful. The physician intends to perform a gastric lavage.

53 The best explanation from the nurse as to the reason for performing this procedure is that the organism
○ 1. may be found in swallowed sputum.
○ 2. also infects gastric tissue.
○ 3. migrates from the lungs to the stomach.
○ 4. can be destroyed by instilling fluid.

The nurse follows up on the dietitian's instructions with a client with tuberculosis. This individual has a very low income.

54 If the client identified that his lunches often included the following menus, which meal would be the most *nutritious*?
○ 1. Tossed salad, vinegarette dressing, iced tea.
○ 2. Jelly sandwich on whole wheat bread, coffee.
○ 3. Meatless chili with beans, cornbread, milk.
○ 4. Chicken boullion, jello, sweetened lemonade.

The physician prescribes a combination of para-aminosalicylate sodium (PAS) and isoniazid, under the brand name Laniazid, to treat a client with tuberculosis.

55 When the client asks the nurse why he is taking two drugs, the best explanation is that when these drugs are combined
○ 1. one diminishes the side effects of the other.
○ 2. one kills the live organism, the other its spores.
○ 3. their toxic effects are reduced.
○ 4. bacterial resistance is slowed.

56 To avoid the gastrointestinal side effects associated with PAS, the best action the nurse could plan to take is to
○ 1. administer the drug on an empty stomach.
○ 2. give the drug with food or at mealtimes.
○ 3. encourage the client to drink lots of water.
○ 4. provide the client with a carbonated beverage.

A nurse from the public health department visits a newly diagnosed tuberculosis client at his home to evaluate his understanding and compliance with drug therapy.

57 The client asks the nurse how he can protect his family from acquiring this disease. The most practical recommendation would be to
○ 1. have them live with other relatives temporarily.
○ 2. cover his mouth and nose when coughing or sneezing.
○ 3. wear a paper face mask at all times.
○ 4. clean the house with disinfectant.

NURSING CARE OF CLIENTS WITH CANCER OF THE LUNG

Mr. Joseph Walton is undergoing diagnostic tests to determine if he has cancer of the lung.

58 If Mr. Walton is typical of most with this disease, which one of the following early warning signs did he most likely ignore?
○ 1. Difficulty swallowing
○ 2. Gradual weight loss
○ 3. Persistent cough
○ 4. Unusual bleeding

The physician requests that a sputum specimen be obtained and sent to the laboratory to see if it contains tumor cells.

59 Which one of the following nursing actions will ensure that an appropriate specimen is collected?
○ 1. Have the client gargle and expectorate the liquid.
○ 2. Tell the client to provide a large volume of saliva.
○ 3. Explain that he should attempt a deep, forceful cough.
○ 4. Swab the back of his throat to stimulate gagging.

A bronchoscopy has been scheduled.

60 Which one of the following would be most important for the nurse to plan prior to the bronchoscopy?
○ 1. Keep the client from eating and drinking.
○ 2. Have the client empty his bowel and bladder.
○ 3. Ensure that the client gets adequate sleep.
○ 4. Scrub the upper chest with an antiseptic.

61 Which one of the following assessments is most important for the nurse to make following a bronchoscopy?
○ 1. Level of consciousness
○ 2. Condition of mouth
○ 3. Respiratory effort
○ 4. Ability to speak

The nurse observes blood when suctioning the secretions that accumulate in Mr. Walton's mouth after bronchoscopy.

62 Which other assessment would be most important for the nurse to make at this time to evaluate the significance of the bleeding?
    ○ 1. Count the pulse rate.
    ○ 2. Listen to heart sounds.
    ○ 3. Check the pupil response.
    ○ 4. Measure chest expansion.

63 When the nurse empties the secretions from the suction container, which one of the following infection control measures is most important to perform?
    ○ 1. Wear a mask.
    ○ 2. Wear a gown.
    ○ 3. Wear goggles.
    ○ 4. Wear gloves.

Mr. Bailey, a client with lung cancer, is scheduled for a pneumonectomy.

64 If Mr. Bailey has an accurate understanding of the explanation the surgeon has provided, he will tell the nurse that during surgery
    ○ 1. one of his lungs will be removed.
    ○ 2. one lobe of his lung will be removed.
    ○ 3. a sample of tissue from his lung will be biopsied.
    ○ 4. a lung will be opened and examined during surgery.

65 While helping the team to develop the postoperative plan of care for Mr. Bailey, it would be essential to stress that this client should lie with his
    ○ 1. healthy lung uppermost.
    ○ 2. head lower than his heart.
    ○ 3. legs gatched at the knees.
    ○ 4. arms elevated on pillows.

NURSING CARE OF CLIENTS WITH CHEST INJURIES

66 Before treating and releasing a client with fractured ribs from the emergency department, which one of the following instructions should the nurse provide?
    ○ 1. Breathe deeply several times every hour.
    ○ 2. Breathe shallowly to avoid discomfort.
    ○ 3. Breathe rapidly to promote ventilation.
    ○ 4. Breathe into a paper bag every hour.

67 When assessing the victim of a motorcycle accident, which finding suggests that the individual has a flail chest?
    ○ 1. Sucking air can be heard by the chest.
    ○ 2. The trachea deviates from midline.
    ○ 3. A portion of chest moves inward during inspiration.

    ○ 4. The victim has severe chest pain during expiration.

During a mugging, a victim is stabbed in the chest, causing his lung to collapse. Two chest tubes are inserted.

68 Where is it most likely that the nurse will see bloody drainage?
    ○ 1. From the victim's nose
    ○ 2. From the victim's mouth
    ○ 3. From the tube in the upper chest
    ○ 4. From the tube in the lower chest

69 The chest tubes have been inserted into a commercial waterseal system. When the nurse monitors the waterseal chamber just after the chest tube insertion, which of the following findings suggests that it is functioning *appropriately*?
    ○ 1. The fluid rises and falls with respirations.
    ○ 2. The fluid level is lower than when first filled.
    ○ 3. The fluid bubbles continuously.
    ○ 4. The fluid looks frothy white.

70 When caring for the client, it is essential that the chest tubes
    ○ 1. hang below the opening in the drainage collector.
    ○ 2. hang straight from the bed into the container.
    ○ 3. be wrapped so as to encircle the client's chest.
    ○ 4. be tucked securely under the bed's mattress.

71 Which one of the following indicates that air is leaking into the tissue around the chest tube insertion site?
    ○ 1. The tissue has the appearance of a balloon.
    ○ 2. There is a hissing sound like a leaking tire.
    ○ 3. The skin crackles when touched.
    ○ 4. Air can be felt as it escapes.

72 A client with waterseal drainage must be transported for a chest x-ray. Which of the following nursing actions is appropriate?
    ○ 1. Clamp the chest tubes before leaving the room.
    ○ 2. Keep the drainage system below the insertion site.
    ○ 3. Attach a portable suction machine to the chest tubes.
    ○ 4. Provide mechanical ventilation during transport.

73 At the end of the shift what is the best way for determining the amount of drainage from the chest tube in a closed waterseal system?
    ○ 1. Empty the collection chamber and measure the volume.
    ○ 2. Subtract the client's fluid intake from his output.

○ 3. Instill sterile irrigation solution and measure the drainage.

○ 4. Subtract the previously marked volume from the current amount.

NURSING CARE OF CLIENTS WITH PULMONARY EMBOLISM

Following an abdominal hysterectomy, Ms. May Morton suddenly experiences severe chest pain and dyspnea. A pulmonary embolism is suspected.

74 Ms. Morton says, "Nurse, I'm dying." What would be the best response from the nurse?
   ○ 1. "You'll be just fine in a few minutes."
   ○ 2. "I'll stay with you while we wait for the doctor."
   ○ 3. "Why would you even think something like that?"
   ○ 4. "Let's talk about something more pleasant."

75 Which one of the following would be the most helpful nursing action to take at this time?
   ○ 1. Turn on the television for distraction.
   ○ 2. Administer oxygen by face mask.
   ○ 3. Offer the client a sip of water.
   ○ 4. Wipe her face with a cool cloth.

Ms. Morton becomes unresponsive and pulseless. The nurse initiates cardiopulmonary resuscitation.

76 How many breaths per minute should an adult receive during cardiopulmonary resuscitation?
   ○ 1. 8 per minute
   ○ 2. 12 per minute
   ○ 3. 15 per minute
   ○ 4. 20 per minute

To treat the hypotension Ms. Morton develops, dopamine is administered by intravenous infusion.

77 What is the most important action the nurse can take when it is observed that the fluid containing the dopamine has infiltrated and is leaking into subcutaneous tissue? The nurse should discontinue the infusion and
   ○ 1. notify the physician immediately.
   ○ 2. elevate the client's arm on pillows.
   ○ 3. apply an ice bag to the swollen area.
   ○ 4. check the client's respiratory rate.

Once Ms. Morton's condition is stabilized, a lung scan is ordered.

78 Which of the following questions must be asked before the client undergoes the lung scan?
   ○ 1. "Do you have a living will?"
   ○ 2. "Have you ever had radiation?"
   ○ 3. "Are you allergic to iodine?"
   ○ 4. "When did you urinate last?"

NURSING CARE OF CLIENTS WITH TRACHEOSTOMY

Mr. Rick Stone is recovering from multiple trauma after being involved in an automobile accident. A tracheostomy has been performed. He is receiving oxygen through a T-piece.

79 Which of the following nursing actions is essential when caring for a client receiving oxygen in this manner?
   ○ 1. Drain the condensed moisture in the tubing.
   ○ 2. Put his neck through range of motion hourly.
   ○ 3. Encourage him to breathe through his nose.
   ○ 4. Apply petroleum jelly to his stoma frequently.

80 Which of the following assessments indicates a need for the nurse to suction a client with a tracheostomy?
   ○ 1. Respirations are deep.
   ○ 2. Wet lung sounds are heard.
   ○ 3. The pulse rate is slow.
   ○ 4. Blood pressure is low.

81 Which nursing action is essential before performing tracheal suctioning?
   ○ 1. Provide mouth care.
   ○ 2. Grease the catheter.
   ○ 3. Clean around the stoma.
   ○ 4. Administer oxygen.

82 When should the nurse occlude the vent on the suction catheter when suctioning a client?
   ○ 1. Before inserting the catheter
   ○ 2. When inside the inner cannula
   ○ 3. While withdrawing the catheter
   ○ 4. When the client begins coughing

83 When in the airway, the nurse should apply suction for no longer than
   ○ 1. 5 to 7 seconds.
   ○ 2. 10 to 15 seconds.
   ○ 3. 15 to 20 seconds.
   ○ 4. 20 to 30 seconds.

84 While withdrawing the suction catheter, which one of the following nursing techniques is most *correct*?
   ○ 1. Remove the catheter slowly.
   ○ 2. Pinch and pull the catheter.
   ○ 3. Plunge the catheter up and down.
   ○ 4. Twist and rotate the catheter.

85 Which one of the following nursing actions is essential *after* suctioning a client?
   ○ 1. Administer oxygen.
   ○ 2. Give mouth care.
   ○ 3. Offer oral liquids.
   ○ 4. Assess blood pressure.

86 Which one of the following solutions would be best for the nurse to use when cleaning the inner cannula of a tracheostomy tube?

○ 1. Isopropyl alcohol
○ 2. Sodium hypochlorite
○ 3. Hydrogen peroxide
○ 4. Povidone-iodine

A nurse has been asked to be a peer evaluator when other nurses practice the procedure for tracheostomy care during an inservice program.

87 When performing the tracheostomy care demonstration, it would be correct for each nurse to
○ 1. cut a gauze square to fit around the stoma.
○ 2. secure the ties at the back of the neck.
○ 3. attach new ties before removing the old.
○ 4. replace the inner cannula after changing the ties.

INDIVIDUAL TEST ITEMS

88 Which position would be most correct for the nurse to place a client undergoing a thoracentesis?
○ 1. Lithotomy
○ 2. Sitting
○ 3. Prone
○ 4. Supine

89 The best evidence that an individual has understood the activity involved in a pulmonary function test is that the client states this test involves
○ 1. having an x-ray.
○ 2. drawing blood.
○ 3. breathing into a mouthpiece.
○ 4. examining expectorated sputum.

90 While the nurse conducts a physical assessment, which one of the following findings most indicates that the person has pleurisy?

○ 1. The client has a productive cough.
○ 2. The client has pain when breathing.
○ 3. The client's nailbeds are cyanotic.
○ 4. The client's heart rate is rapid.

91 Which one of the following blood *p*H measurements reported on an arterial blood gas test is considered *normal?*
○ 1. 7.20
○ 2. 7.30
○ 3. 7.40
○ 4. 7.50

92 Which one of the following explanations by the nurse to the nursing assistant is the most accurate reason for using a cuffed tracheostomy tube?
○ 1. The cuff prevents skin breakdown.
○ 2. The cuff prevents aspiration.
○ 3. The cuff provides more comfort.
○ 4. The cuff reduces infection.

93 Which one of the following nursing measures will help most to reverse respiratory alkalosis caused by hyperventilation? The nurse should have the client breathe
○ 1. through his nose.
○ 2. humidified oxygen.
○ 3. into a paper sack.
○ 4. from his diaphragm.

94 A nurse reports that a client is having Cheyne-Stokes respirations. The best description of this type of breathing is that it is one in which the respirations cycle through shallow breathing to deep breathing followed again by shallow breathing and
○ 1. pursed-lip breathing.
○ 2. abdominal grunting.
○ 3. loud, noisy snoring.
○ 4. a period of apnea.

Correct Answers and Rationales

Two numbers appear in parentheses following each rationale. The first number identifies the textbook listed in the references, page 451, and the second number identifies the page(s) in that textbook on which the correct answer can be verified. Occasionally, two textbooks are given for verifying the correct answer.

The Nursing Care of Clients with Disorders of the Respiratory System

NURSING CARE OF CLIENTS WITH A COMMON COLD

1 3. A high fever suggests that the client with a common cold has now acquired a secondary bacterial infection, such as bronchitis or pneumonia. Viral infections like the common cold are generally associated with a low-grade fever. Symptoms of the common cold are generally confined to the head and throat. They include nasal congestion and discharge, discomfort in the nose and throat, sneezing, and watery eyes. The person also may have a headache, feel chilled, and experience fatigue and loss of appetite. A dry cough may be due to nasal drainage passing into the pharynx causing irritation. A productive cough would indicate more that the infection also involves the lower respiratory tract. (3:396; 16:230)
    Nursing Process—Collecting data
    Client Need—Physiological integrity

2 3. Nonprescription decongestants should not be used by individuals with hypertension and heart disease. Most contain adrenergic drugs like ephedrine sulfate, which stimulate the sympathetic nervous system. They can cause tachycardia and increase blood pressure, even in normal individuals. Adrenergic drugs would not be contraindicated in individuals with arthritis, asthma, or diabetes unless they had accompanying cardiovascular disease. (15:263)
    Nursing Process—Collecting data
    Client Need—Physiological integrity

3 1. The common cold is a viral infection of the nasal passages and throat. Antibiotics are only useful in treating bacterial infections. No drug cures the common cold. An infection without additional secondary complications is self-limiting. (16:229; 3:378)
    Nursing Process—Implementation
    Client Need—Health promotion/maintenance

4 4. Gargling with a dilute mixture of salt dissolved in warm water is a common comfort measure for a sore throat. Household bleach is an excellent disinfectant, but it should not be used internally. Vanilla extract and whiskey contain alcohol, but they are not recommended for a topical medicinal effect. (16:230)
    Nursing Process—Implementation
    Client Need—Health promotion/maintenance

5 3. Biting a lozenge into small pieces would decrease the amount of time the ingredients in the solid disk would be distributed to irritated pharyngeal tissue. Swallowing the solid disk whole also would be inappropriate. The effectiveness of a lozenge is promoted by holding it in the mouth and swallowing the dissolved ingredients. As long as the lozenge remains in the mouth, talking will not affect its effectiveness. The client must stop talking periodically to swallow the dissolved medication as it becomes mixed with saliva. (18:594)
    Nursing Process—Evaluation
    Client Need—Physiological integrity

6 1. A patient taking a narcotic should be warned not to exceed the recommended dose. Extra self-administration can lead to sedation and habituation. Because narcotic antitussives would not interfere with sleep, their administration would not be contraindicated before retiring. Expectorants, not sedative antitussives, should be taken with extra fluids to thin mucoid secretions facilitating their expectoration. Chilling substances, rather than warming them, is more likely to disguise an unpleasant taste. (15:268)
    Nursing Process—Planning
    Client Need—Health promotion/maintenance

7 3. One teaspoon is the approximate household equivalent of 5 mL. Some manufacturers of nonprescription cough medications include a dosing cup marked with various household equivalents. To ensure safety, however, the nurse should include an explanation of the equivalent during discharge instructions. (18:575; 14:479)
    Nursing Process—Implementation
    Client Need—Health promotion/maintenance

NURSING CARE OF CLIENTS WITH ALLERGIC RHINITIS

8 3. Antihistamines commonly cause people to feel drowsy and fall asleep easily. They should be warned to use caution if driving or operating machinery while taking a drug in this category. Because activity is slowed, weight gain is common. Gastrointestinal side effects include increased appetite, nausea, and diarrhea but not constipation. (15:262; 14:511)

Nursing Process—Implementation
Client Need—Health promotion/maintenance

9 1. Many hypersensitive people are allergic to more than one substance. Testing does not promote the production of blocking antibodies. Even though skin testing is considered a standard of practice among allergy specialists and insurance companies may partially or completely pay for this service, most clients generally want to know how the proposed medical care will benefit them personally. (14:836, 993; 3:141)

Nursing Process—Implementation
Client Need—Safe, effective care environment

10 1. An area of local *erythema*, or redness, indicates a positive reaction to the antigen applied to the scratched skin. Swelling, known as *induration*, also may accompany a reaction. A positive reaction would not appear pale or feel especially painful or numb. (7:400; 16:95)

Nursing Process—Collect data
Client Need—Safe, effective care environment

11 2. The client undergoing desensitization should stay in the physician's office at least 20 minutes following the injection for observation. Occasionally a person has a severe allergic reaction to even the small amount of antigen used in the desensitization injection. The client's safety would be endangered if a severe reaction occurred and medical assistance was not immediately available. Antihistamines may reduce allergic symptoms, but aspirin would have no direct effect. If a client has waited 20 minutes, driving would not be contraindicated. The client need not call the office when arriving home. (17:802)

Nursing Process—Implementation
Client Need—Physiological integrity

NURSING CARE OF CLIENTS WITH ANAPHYLAXIS

12 1. Signs of anaphylaxis include difficult breathing, hives, and loss of consciousness as blood pressure falls. Headache, sore throat, and urinary incontinence are not associated with an anaphylactic reaction. (3:143; 14:985; 16:97)

Nursing Process—Collecting data
Client Need—Physiological integrity

13 4. Epinephrine is the drug of choice when a client experiences anaphylactic shock. This drug helps raise the blood pressure by constricting blood vessels and dilates the bronchi, thereby facilitating breathing. Without emergency treatment, victims of anaphylaxis can die in 5 to 10 minutes. Codeine and morphine are central nervous system depressants. They would potentiate hypotension. Dopamine is an adrenergic drug in the same family as epinephrine, but it is not the drug of choice during anaphylaxis. It is more often given to maintain the blood pressure of individuals who have experienced a myocardial infarction. (3:143; 16:97)

Nursing Process—Planning
Client Need—Physiological integrity

14 3. Because shock is one of the major problems during anaphylaxis, monitoring blood pressure would be the most appropriate technique for evaluating the effectiveness of treatment. The nurse would expect that the blood pressure would rise, breathing would become less labored, and the person would become alert. Maintaining adequate urine output would indicate that a person's circulatory volume was sufficient, but this assessment would be difficult unless a urinary catheter is in place. Skin color is not as valid an assessment, but it should go from pale to appropriate ethnic color once blood flow is restored to the periphery. As long as the brain is receiving adequate oxygen, the pupils should continue to respond by constricting when stimulated with direct light. (15:38; 17:803)

Nursing Process—Evaluation
Client Need—Physiological integrity

15 3. The nurse should maintain an open airway by lifting the chin and tilting the head. Placing the person in Trendelenburg position, loosening clothing, and covering the individual may be appropriate, but keeping the airway open is the first priority. (14:428; 17:393)

Nursing Process—Implementation
Client Need—Physiological integrity

NURSING CARE OF CLIENTS WITH PNEUMONIA

16 2. Any article containing metal must be removed before a chest x-ray is performed. The image of a metal object that remains in place during an x-ray may be misinterpreted as diseased tissue. Fasting is not required before a chest x-ray. No radiopaque dye is given for a chest x-ray. Analgesia is not necessary because there is no accompanying discomfort. (17:316; 18:311)

Nursing Process—Planning
Client Need—Safe, effective care environment

17 1. Respiratory secretions that are difficult to raise can be thinned when fluid intake is increased. Increasing moisture in inspired air through humidification also will help. Changing positions improves circulation and prevents pooling of respiratory secretions. High-fiber foods help to reduce or prevent constipation. Frequent rest relieves fatigue and activity intolerance. (18:709)
Nursing Process—Planning
Client Need—Physiological integrity

18 4. It is easiest to obtain a sputum specimen when awakening in the morning. Secretions tend to accumulate in the respiratory tract during the night. Pooled secretions are more easily raised, especially if the individual is not fatigued from activity. Forced coughing after a meal can lead to vomiting. (3:391; 18:709)
Nursing Process—Planning
Client Need—Safe, effective care environment

19 4. The client must not touch the inside of the sputum specimen container or the inside of its lid. The inside of the container must be kept sterile so that no other sources of microorganisms, other than what is present in the sputum, are collected. The hands contain abundant pathogens and nonpathogens. It would not be necessary to don gloves because the outside of the container can be touched. Wiping the outside of the container is not necessary because it is considered unclean anyway. (14:813; 18:709)
Nursing Process—Evaluation
Client Need—Safe, effective care environment

20 2. Sputum that appears rusty is likely to contain blood. Food or bile should not be present in sputum because sputum is produced within the respiratory tract. Saliva is clear. (14:811)
Nursing Process—Collecting data
Client Need—Physiological integrity

21 2. Mouth care is an appropriate hygiene measure after obtaining a sputum specimen. Expectorating sputum often causes a residual foul taste in the mouth or an unpleasant odor to the breath. Oxygen would be appropriate if the client were short of breath. Eating should be delayed until the client is rested and unlikely to become nauseous. Walking may cause further fatigue after the effort of coughing. (3:397; 18:709)
Nursing Process—Implementation
Client Need—Physiological integrity

22 1. Antibiotics are selected on the basis of their effect on the infectious organism. This information is obtained by performing a culture and sensitivity. The organism is first encouraged to grow in the laboratory medium. Then small disks of various drugs are placed in the growing colonies. If

growth is inhibited around a certain disk, it is a good drug to use. Antibiotics are ineffective in treating viral infections. Though widely used, penicillin, like any other drug, has dangerous side effects. Such things as drug effectiveness, cost, route of administration, the client's history of drug allergy, and other factors affect the physician's choice. (15:154; 14:499)
Nursing Process—Implementation
Client Need—Health promotion/maintenance

23 4. The dorsogluteal site is located in the buttock. The hip is the location of the ventrogluteal site. The deltoid site is located in the arm. The vastus lateralis and rectus femoris are injection sites located in the thigh. (14:492; 18:610-611)
Nursing Process—Implementation
Client Need—Physiological integrity

24 1. Pointing the toes inward reduces the discomfort when giving an injection into the dorsogluteal site. Tightening muscles increases discomfort. Crossing the legs and flexing the knees would place the client in an awkward position and would not help to relieve discomfort. (14:491; 18:610)
Nursing Process—Implementation
Client Need—Physiological integrity

25 2. A skin rash and hives, sometimes accompanied by itching, are common signs of an allergic reaction. Severe allergic reactions may include difficulty breathing and dramatic drop in blood pressure with loss of consciousness, pallor, diaphoresis, and tachycardia. Other signs and symptoms of an allergy include gastrointestinal symptoms like nausea, vomiting, and diarrhea. (14:984; 15:155)
Nursing Process—Collecting data
Client Need—Physiological integrity

NURSING CARE OF CLIENTS WITH INFLUENZA

26 4. An intake of 3000 mL would be safe in the absence of any preexisting cardiovascular or renal problems. The additional fluid will help to keep the client hydrated and aid in temperature regulation. Less than 3000 mL would not be adequate because the metabolic rate is increased as a result of the elevated body temperature. (3:397; 18:642)
Nursing Process—Planning
Client Need—Physiological integrity

27 3. Alcohol enhances rapid evaporation of the liquid from the skin's surface. Alcohol does inhibit the growth of microorganisms and causes drying of the skin; for some the application of alcohol may feel soothing. However, these are not reasons for

adding it to water used for a temperature-reducing bath. (14:391; 18:95)
Nursing Process—Implementation
Client Need—Physiological integrity

28 3. Tepid means a temperature that is lukewarm or slightly cool. Most authorities recommend that a tepid temperature is in the range of 80°F to 93°F. It would not be appropriate to use bath water that is hot when trying to reduce a fever. Cold or icy water should only be used if the client has severe hyperthermia, for example, from heat stroke. (18:491)
Nursing Process—Implementation
Client Need—Safe, effective care environment

29 2. Chilling is an indication that the body temperature is falling too rapidly. The muscle contraction that accompanies chilling will produce heat and interfere with reducing body temperature. It would be best to temporarily discontinue the sponge bath, dry the skin, and protect the client from any drafts. Nausea is not an adverse effect associated with sponge bathing. A feverish individual is likely to appear flushed and may become disoriented. These signs would indicate that nursing measures, such as the sponge bath, need to proceed to relieve the fever. (14:391; 18:96)
Nursing Process—Collecting data
Client Need—Safe, effective care environment

30 3. A decrease in the client's temperature is the best evidence that the tepid sponge bath is having a therapeutic effect. Feeling more comfortable and hungry, along with relief of the headache, are subjective responses that correlate with fever reduction. However, objective data tend to be considered more reliable. (14:392; 18:96)
Nursing Process—Evaluation
Client Need—Physiological integrity

31 2. All of the options provided can help reduce the potential for infection. However, because respiratory infections are primarily spread by direct contact with another sick individual, avoiding crowds would be the best advice. The U.S. Public Health Service Advisory Committee on Immunization recommends annual vaccination against influenza for people over the age of 65 and those with other chronic health problems. (3:388; 14:839)
Nursing Process—Implementation
Client Need—Health promotion/maintenance

NURSING CARE OF CLIENTS WITH BRONCHITIS

32 1. Aerosol therapy involves depositing small droplets of moisture onto respiratory tissue. The warmed moist air soothes the respiratory passages and liquefies secretions produced as a result of the inflammation. Other benefits can be obtained by adding medications to the vaporized water. Individuals with acute bronchitis are generally bothered initially by a nonproductive cough that is aggravated by dry air. Oral or parenteral antibiotic therapy would be used to kill infectious organisms. Respiratory mucosa should be moist. The respiratory rate may be lowered as ventilation is improved. However, this is a secondary benefit of aerosol therapy and not its primary purpose. (3:420; 17:320-321)
Nursing Process—Collect data
Client Need—Health promotion/maintenance

33 3. Codeine depresses the cough center in the brain. Antitussives that contain codeine or a similar synthetic chemical, dextromethorphan, are called sedative antitussives. They are indicated when a person's lungs are clear, but persistent coughing continues that serves no good purpose or could adversely affect recovery from other conditions. Expectorants liquefy secretions. Bronchodilators open respiratory passages. Salicylates and steroids are types of drugs that reduce inflammation. (15:267; 14:510-511)
Nursing Process—Implementation
Client Need—Health promotion/maintenance

34 1. Common adverse effects of codeine include nausea, vomiting, constipation, and excitement. Dyspnea, diarrhea, and headaches are not associated with the use of codeine. (15:267)
Nursing Process—Collecting data
Client Need—Physiological integrity

NURSING CARE OF CLIENTS WITH ASTHMA

35 1. A sitting position is preferred when auscultating the chest. This allows the nurse access to the anterior, lateral, and posterior areas of the chest. Changing positions during auscultation would further tax an already dyspneic client. A client in respiratory distress will generally not tolerate lying flat or on his side. Standing would be unsafe for a client who is having extreme difficulty breathing. (3:395; 18:288)
Nursing Process—Planning
Client Need—Safe, effective care environment

36 4. As air passages become narrowed, as in the onset of an asthmatic attack, the nurse is most likely to hear wheezing. This generally is noted during expiration. Wet bubbling sounds indicate accumulated secretions. This would more likely be heard during recovery from the asthmatic attack when thick secretions are able to move. Dry crackling sounds indicate that air is moving into and opening small airways, such as the terminal bronchioles and alveoli. Soft blowing sounds are normal in open, distal small airways of the lungs. (16:257; 14:836; 17:314)

    Nursing Process—Collecting data
    Client Need—Physiological integrity

37 3. The sensor of a pulse oximeter can be applied to the ear lobe, finger, thumb, toe, or bridge of the nose. The arm or leg would be too dense to allow light to transilluminate from tissue to the sensor. Applying the sensor to the lip may cause discomfort or be dislodged easily. (3:391)

    Nursing Process—Implementation
    Client Need—Safe, effective care environment

38 1. To avoid excessive blood loss and a painful hematoma from a punctured arterial site, it is essential to apply direct pressure for a minimum of 5 minutes. The specimen is cooled in ice once it is collected. The blood pressure is not likely to be affected by the loss of 5 to 10 mL of blood. Elevating the arm is one way to control bleeding from a vein, but it is not likely to be effective in the case of bleeding from an artery. (3:391; 17:315)

    Nursing Process—Implementation
    Client Need—Physiological integrity

39 2. The reservoir bag of a nonrebreathing mask should remain partially filled during inspiration. If the bag collapses completely, the equipment may be faulty. This information should be reported to the respiratory therapy department. The mask has been applied properly if it covers the mouth and nose and the strap fits the head snugly. Moisture is likely to accumulate because the oxygen is being humidified. This would not be significant information to report. The nurse can temporarily wipe the moisture away and reapply the mask. (18:730; 3:423)

    Nursing Process—Implementation
    Client Need—Safe, effective care environment

40 1. The volume of epinephrine 1:1000 that should be injected to administer 0.1 mg is 0.1 mL. To solve the problem using a ratio and proportion method, use the following steps (15:8-10; 18:580-581):

$$\frac{1000 \text{ mg } (1 \text{ g})}{1000 \text{ mL}} = \frac{0.1 \text{ mg}}{\text{X mL}}$$
$$1000\text{X} = 100$$
$$\text{X} = 0.1 \text{ mL}$$

    Nursing Process—Implementation
    Client Need—Physiological integrity

41 2. Remaining with the client provides reassurance that if he needs immediate help, someone is available. Anxiety is best reduced by being with another supportive individual. Closing the door, pulling the privacy curtain, and covering the client are confining actions. They are apt to increase the feeling of being suffocated. (16:261; 12:200)

    Nursing Process—Implementation
    Client Need—Physiological integrity

NURSING CARE OF CLIENTS WITH EMPHYSEMA

42 2. Individuals with long-standing emphysema develop a barrel shaped appearance to their chest. The physical change is probably due to chronic overdistention of the lungs due to impaired ability to exhale air. A person with emphysema would not usually have a funnel shaped, mottled, or muscular chest. (3:400; 14:838)

    Nursing Process—Collecting data
    Client Need—Physiological integrity

43 1. Giving oxygen at greater than 3 L would interfere with the brain's response to the hypoxic drive. The stimulus to breathe in a person with chronic obstructive lung disease comes from low levels of oxygen rather than higher than normal levels of carbon dioxide. Administering high concentrations of oxygen would depress the respiratory center. (17:330; 18:726)

    Nursing Process—Implementation
    Client Need—Physiological integrity

44 3. The therapeutic action of aminophylline is the reduction of respiratory distress. Aminophylline is classified as a bronchodilator. Aminophylline would not be expected to relieve coughing, decrease sputum production, or thin secretions. (15:264)

    Nursing Process—Implementation
    Client Need—Health promotion/maintenance

45 4. Aminophylline is likely to cause tachycardia because it affects the sympathetic nervous system. Other side effects include hypertension, insomnia, and restlessness. The therapeutic action of aminophylline is bronchodilation, not bronchospasm. (15:264)

    Nursing Process—Collecting data
    Client Need—Physiological integrity

46 2. Administering rhythmic gentle blows with a cupped hand, known as percussion, is used to cause thick secretions to break loose from within the airways. This technique also may be combined with vibration. Vibration involves producing wave-like tremors to the chest by making firm, circular movements with open hands. For draining all but the upper lobes of the lung, the client should be positioned so that the lower chest is elevated higher than the head. Deep breathing improves ventilation, but it does not necessarily move secretions. Applying pressure below the diaphragm is an emergency measure for relieving an obstructed airway. (18:706; 14:816-817)

> Nursing Process—Implementation
> Client Need—Physiological integrity

47 4. Expectorating a large volume of sputum is the best evidence that postural drainage has been effective. The respiratory rate should be lowered if hypoxia has been relieved. Though the return of an appetite is a good sign, it is not the best evidence that postural drainage has been effective. A negative sputum culture only indicates that an infectious process is not present. (17:420; 16:247)

> Nursing Process—Evaluation
> Client Need—Physiological integrity

48 1. It is therapeutic to encourage a person to express his or her feelings. It shows that the nurse is empathetic to the person's emotional condition and is willing to listen. Disagreeing with the client, belittling feelings, and using a reassuring cliché block the therapeutic effectiveness of communication. (9:138-139)

> Nursing Process—Implementation
> Client Need—Psychosocial integrity

NURSING CARE OF CLIENTS WITH TUBERCULOSIS

49 1. When administering an intradermal injection, the needle is inserted between the layers of skin at approximately a 10- to 15-degree angle. Subcutaneous injections are given at either a 45- or 90-degree angle depending on the size of the client. Intramuscular injections are given at a 90-degree angle. It would be incorrect to give any injection by inserting the needle at a 180-degree angle. (18:625; 14:493)

> Nursing Process—Implementation
> Client Need—Physiologic integrity

50 2. A positive tuberculin skin test indicates that at some time, the person's immune system developed antibodies against the tuberculin bacillus. It does not necessarily mean that there is a currently active infectious process taking place, nor does it mean that there is not an active infection. Anyone with a positive tuberculin skin test without any known history of having had the disease, should have a chest x-ray and sputum examinations. Drugs may be administered prophylactically to individuals who suddenly test positive after having a history of being negative. A positive skin test would not indicate protective immunity. This infectious disease is transmitted by direct contact. In the hospital strict isolation is not necessary. The Centers for Disease Control and Prevention recommends following Acid Fast Bacillus isolation precautions. Most newly diagnosed tuberculosis cases are treated as outpatients rather than being hospitalized. (16:251; 14:815, 842)

> Nursing Process—Implementation
> Client Need—Health promotion/maintenance

51 3. Common signs and symptoms among individuals with tuberculosis include night sweats, mild fever, gradual weight loss, cough, and the raising of bloody sputum. There could be many explanations for foul breath. It is not unique to people with tuberculosis. (17:151; 16:251)

> Nursing Process—Collecting data
> Client Need—Safe, effective care environment

52 2. Individuals with tuberculosis are more likely to have a temperature elevation during the afternoon. If the temperature is not taken during this time, its omission may delay diagnosis. The temperature may be within normal ranges during other times of the day. (14:842; 3:407)

> Nursing Process—Planning
> Client Need—Physiological integrity

53 1. Gastric lavage may be used to obtain a specimen from a person who swallows respiratory secretions rather than expectorating them. Tuberculosis can be spread to other tissues besides the lungs. However, the spread is generally by means of the bloodstream. The gastric secretions tend to destroy organisms. The instilled fluid provides sufficient liquid volume in the stomach to aid in removing the desired specimen. (16:251; 3:405, 407)

> Nursing Process—Implementation
> Client Need—Safe, effective care environment

54 3. Combining beans and a grain is an economic means of consuming all essential amino acids found in an animal source. Drinking milk also improves the nutrition of this meal choice. The alternative meals are economic. However, because they do not provide adequate sources of protein, they would not be considered nutritious choices. (18:126, 130; 4:250)

> Nursing Process—Implementation
> Client Need—Health promotion/maintenance

55 4. Bacterial resistance occurs more slowly when antitubercular drugs are used in combination rather than singly. Side effects are not reduced; they do not act at different periods during the organism's life cycle; and their toxic effects are not reduced when given in combination. (15:173; 14:842)

> Nursing Process—Implementation
> Client Need—Health promotion/maintenance

56 2. Giving medication with food protects the stomach from becoming upset. The potential for gastric upset is increased if irritating medications are administered on an empty stomach. Drinking water will not necessarily reduce gastrointestinal side effects. Though a carbonated beverage may relieve stomach distention, it is not the best approach for reducing the irritation caused by many drugs, including para-aminosalicylate sodium. (15:174; 3:408)

> Nursing Process—Planning
> Client Need—Physiological integrity

57 2. Covering the mouth and nose when coughing or sneezing limits the scattering of moist droplets that contain the infectious organism. Sunlight easily destroys tuberculosis organisms. Family members of an actively diseased person usually are prescribed antitubercular drugs prophylactically. Drug therapy is often effective in destroying the presence of the infectious organisms in the sputum within a few days. It would be unnecessary to separate family members, wear a paper mask continuously, or clean the house with a disinfectant. (3:409; 17:152)

> Nursing Process—Implementation
> Client Need—Safe, effective care environment

NURSING CARE OF CLIENTS WITH CANCER OF THE LUNG

58 3. A cough and dyspnea are generally the earliest signs of lung cancer. Most tend to ignore these signs rationalizing that they are a consequence of chronic smoking. Therefore, diagnosis and treatment often are delayed. Later signs of lung cancer include unexplained weight loss, blood-tinged sputum, fatigue, and respiratory distress. (3:843; 17:344)

> Nursing Process—Collecting data
> Client Need—Physiological integrity

59 3. Coughing is the best method for raising sputum. Saliva is not sputum. Gargled solution is not likely to contain adequate secretions or cells from the bronchial or deeper pulmonary structures. Stimulating a gag reflex is more likely to cause the client to vomit. (14:813; 16:224)

> Nursing Process—Implementation
> Client Need—Safe, effective care environment

60 1. Preparation for a bronchoscopy should include keeping the client from eating or drinking for at least 6 to 8 hours prior to the procedure. This reduces the risk of aspiration. Though emptying the bowel and bladder promotes comfort, the accidental loss of urine or stool would not be as life-threatening as aspiration. Adequate rest is desirable but not essential. The instrument used for bronchoscopy is introduced through the mouth. Therefore, scrubbing the upper chest is unnecessary. (3:390; 14:814)

> Nursing Process—Planning
> Client Need—Safe, effective care environment

61 3. Respiratory effort is the most critical assessment to make following a bronchoscopy. It would be one of the first responses to change if the client experienced edema and trauma in the airway. All the other assessment alternatives are appropriate but not as likely to indicate life-threatening consequences. (3:390-391; 14:814)

> Nursing Process—Collecting data
> Client Need—Physiological integrity

62 1. The pulse rate would be the best indication at this time as to whether the nurse should be concerned about the presence of blood in the secretions. Slight bleeding can be expected following bronchoscopy due to trauma. If hemorrhage or impaired ventilation is occurring, the pulse rate will be rapid. Pupillary changes are an indication of brain function. Heart sounds indicate how effectively blood is circulating through the chambers of the heart. Chest expansion is more likely to change if one lung is not filling adequately with air. (3:391; 17:125)

> Nursing Process—Collecting data
> Client Need—Physiological integrity

63 4. Gloves are the most important barrier garment in this situation. Gloves should be worn whenever there is a possibility for contact with body fluids containing blood. Because the nurse would be involved in holding the container, the hands should be protected. In addition to the gloves, it would be acceptable to don any or all of the other items. The choice of additional items is based on the nurse's judgment as to the potential for contact with blood by some other means such as splashing into the eyes, nose, or mouth or onto the uniform. (3:102; 18:361)

> Nursing Process—Implementation
> Client Need—Safe, effective care environment

64 1. The prefix "pneumo" refers to lung; the suffix "ectomy" means removal. The name of the procedure in which only a lobe of the lung is removed is "lobectomy." The other two choices are not as accurate an explanation. They do not include the main purpose for performing the surgical procedure. (17:344)

> Nursing Process—Evaluation
> Client Need—Safe, effective care environment

65 1. The client with a pneumonectomy should lie with his unoperative lung uppermost. Maintaining the collection of postoperative drainage within the empty cavity where the lung was removed promotes consolidation. Also by avoiding compression of the remaining healthy lung between the mattress and body weight, ventilation is facilitated. Lying with the head lowered may interfere with breathing because abdominal contents would press against the diaphragm. Gatching the knees would be a comfort measure but is not necessarily essential to this client's care. Elevating the arms on pillows would be an optional position to use if and when the client's breathing became labored. However, it would not be specified in the routine postoperative plan for care. (17:345; 3:413)

    Nursing Process—Implementation
    Client Need—Physiological integrity

NURSING CARE OF CLIENTS WITH CHEST INJURIES

66 1. To prevent the widespread collapse of alveoli, known as *atelectasis*, the client should be instructed to breathe deeply several times every hour. People with fractured ribs have a natural tendency to breathe shallowly to avoid discomfort. Shallow breathing promotes atelectasis. Breathing rapidly can lead to respiratory alkalosis. Breathing into a paper bag promotes an increased level of carbon dioxide in the blood. This is appropriate for individuals who are hyperventilating and becoming lightheaded. (17:333; 16:257)

    Nursing Process—Implementation
    Client Need—Health promotion/maintenance

67 3. Flail chest is a condition in which three or more ribs are broken in two or more places making the chest wall unstable. This condition is characterized by a paradoxic movement of the unstable section during inspiration and expiration. In other words when the client takes a breath, an area of the chest wall moves inward; when the client exhales, the area moves outward. A sucking chest wound and tracheal deviation are associated with chest trauma causing a pneumothorax. Chest pain only during expiration is not a common finding. (3:411)

    Nursing Process—Collecting data
    Client Need—Physiological integrity

68 4. Blood will collect and drain by gravity through the tube in the lower chest. Air in the chest rises and will exit through the tube in the upper chest. It is unlikely that any blood will be noted from the victim's nose or mouth if the injury is limited to a hemothorax or pneumothorax. (3:413; 14:826)

    Nursing Process—Collecting data
    Client Need—Physiological integrity

69 1. The fluid in the waterseal chamber should rise and fall in synchrony with respirations or bubble intermittently when it has just be inserted. Once the lung has expanded or if the tubing is kinked or plugged, these findings will not be seen. If the fluid level falls below the filling line of 2 cm, more fluid should be added. Continuous bub-

bling indicates that there is a leak in the system. The fluid should look clear and transparent. (16:273; 18:733)

    Nursing Process—Collecting data
    Client Need—Safe, effective care environment

70 2. To facilitate gravity drainage the chest tubes should hang straight from the bed into the drainage collector. If the tubes hang below the collector, drainage will be slowed or stopped. Wrapping the chest tube around the client's chest or tucking it under the bed's mattress will compress the lumen of the tubes and impair drainage. (18:733; 14:828)

    Nursing Process—Implementation
    Client Need—Safe, effective care environment

71 3. Air that is leaking and becoming trapped within the local tissue at the insertion site crackles when touched. The crackling sound, called *crepitus* or *subcutaneous emphysema*, resembles that of crisp rice cereal when mixed with milk. Puffs of air cannot be felt. There is no hissing sound because the air does not escape into the atmosphere. The air tends to diffuse into the tissue and rise to the upper part of the body. Eventually the face and neck may appear swollen, but the local tissue at the site would not look like a balloon. (16:273; 18:733)

    Nursing Process—Collecting data
    Client Need—Physiological integrity

72 2. The drainage collector should be kept below the tubes' insertion sites. As long as the waterseal is maintained, the lungs will be unaffected. Clamping the chest tubes for an appreciable amount of time can lead to a tension pneumothorax. Suction would not be applied directly to the chest tubes. Suction may be added to the waterseal system, but the waterseal system would be disconnected from the suction before leaving the room. Mechanical ventilation is only necessary if a client cannot maintain adequate oxygenation even with supplemental oxygen. (3:413; 18:733)

    Nursing Process—Implementation
    Client Need—Safe, effective care environment

73 4. Each nurse marks the level of drainage on the calibrated collection chamber at the end of the shift. The volume of drainage is calculated by subtracting the marked volume identified by the previous shift with the current volume. A closed waterseal system should never be opened to measure the drainage volume. Chest tubes are not irrigated. Subtracting fluid intake from output would only help in evaluating the status of the client's fluid balance. (3:413; 18:733)

    Nursing Process—Implementation
    Client Need—Safe, effective care environment

NURSING CARE OF CLIENTS WITH PULMONARY EMBOLISM

74 2. Staying with a frightened client is one of the best methods for relieving or reducing anxiety. Telling her she will be fine is a nontherapeutic communication technique called offering false reassurance. Asking a "why" question is a nontherapeutic technique because rather than accept the client's feeling, it demands that the client provide an explanation. Changing the subject also is an example of nontherapeutic communication. (12:356)
Nursing Process—Implementation
Client Need—Psychosocial integrity

75 2. Oxygen would relieve the dyspnea and chest pain. In this anxious state the client will not be easily distracted. Oral fluids should be avoided in case cardiopulmonary resuscitation may be needed. Recently ingested fluids or food could be aspirated. Wiping her face may show concern, but it is not likely to alter her symptoms or perception of the seriousness of the situation. (3:412; 16:256)
Nursing Process—Implementation
Client Need—Physiological integrity

76 2. Anyone over the age of 8 should be given rescue breaths at a rate of at least 12 per minute or once every 5 seconds. Children between the ages of 1 and 8 years should be given 15 breaths per minute. Children up to the age of 1 year should be given 20 breaths per minute. (14:430; 18:741)
Nursing Process—Implementation
Client Need—Physiological integrity

77 1. The information regarding infiltrated dopamine should be reported to the physician immediately. This drug can cause tissue to slough unless another drug, phentolamine (Regitine) is injected into the tissue. Elevating the client's arm and applying ice will reduce swelling, but it will not restore circulation. Checking the client's respiratory rate is an appropriate nursing measure, but it is not the most important action the nurse should take in this situation. (15:40)
Nursing Process—Implementation
Client Need—Physiological integrity

78 3. It is essential that the nurse assess for an allergy to iodine because the dye used for the scan may be iodine based. Alternative substances are available if the client is sensitive to iodine. Asking the client about a living will is likely to potentiate her anxiety. Having been exposed to radiation or knowing the approximate time of the last urination have no bearing on the performance of a lung scan. (3:390)
Nursing Process—Collecting data
Client Need—Safe, effective care environment

NURSING CARE OF CLIENTS WITH A TRACHEOSTOMY

79 1. Moisture that condenses within the tubing of the T-piece should be drained often. Collected moisture can drain into the tracheostomy and lead to aspiration. A wet tracheostomy dressing also can support the growth of pathogens. Range of motion need not be performed hourly. It is anatomically impossible for a person with a tracheostomy to breathe through the nose. Petroleum-based products should not be used around oxygen because of the potential for fire. (18:731)
Nursing Process—Implementation
Client Need—Safe, effective care environment

80 2. Wet lung sounds indicate that secretions are accumulating within the airway. Because a client with a tracheostomy lacks the ability to cough effectively, the nurse must protect and maintain an open airway for him. Deep respirations are not undesirable. A rapid pulse rate is more likely to indicate impaired ventilation, rather than slow. A low blood pressure is unrelated to the need for oxygenation. (17:318; 18:718)
Nursing Process—Collecting data
Client Need—Physiological integrity

81 4. To prevent hypoxia, oxygen should be administered before performing tracheal suctioning. Suctioning removes oxygen and tracheal secretions from the lungs. Clients with artificial airways should have frequent mouth care, but it is not essential before performing tracheal suctioning. The catheter is inserted into sterile normal saline to test the function of the suction machine and reduce the surface tension of the plastic catheter, but no lubricant is used. The stoma must be cleaned from time to time, but this does not have to be done before suctioning the airway. (17:318; 18:718)
Nursing Process—Implementation
Client Need—Physiological integrity

82 3. The vent should not be occluded until after the catheter has been fully inserted and is being withdrawn. This reduces the potential for causing hypoxia. Closing the vent before insertion or when just inside the inner cannula prolongs the time during which oxygen is removed from the airway. Coughing may or may not coincide with the proper time to occlude the vent. Therefore, it should not be used as a criterion for this action. (17:319; 18:718-719)
Nursing Process—Implementation
Client Need—Physiological integrity

83 2. Suctioning should not extend beyond 10 to 15 seconds. Some suggest that one's own breath be held during suctioning to be more aware of the air hunger the client is experiencing. Suctioning

for too little time may not effectively clear the airway. Suctioning beyond 10 to 15 seconds can cause hypoxia. (3:427-428; 18:719)
Nursing Process—Implementation
Client Need—Physiological integrity

84   4. Twisting and rotating the catheter during its withdrawal helps remove secretions that are located in all directions within the airway. Withdrawing the catheter slowly may cause the nurse to exceed the recommended time for suctioning beyond 10 to 15 seconds. Neither pinching and pulling nor plunging the catheter up and down are acceptable techniques during suctioning. (14:826; 16:240)
Nursing Process—Implementation
Client Need—Physiological integrity

85   1. Oxygen should be readministered to replace the deficit created during the suctioning process. Providing mouth care and assessing the blood pressure are appropriate nursing measures to perform, but they are not necessarily essential after suctioning a client. A person with a fresh tracheostomy is not usually allowed to eat or drink; even if the client has mastered swallowing and has a tracheostomy, offering oral liquids is not essential after suctioning. (3:428; 18:719)
Nursing Process—Implementation
Client Need—Physiological integrity

86   3. Hydrogen peroxide is the best solution to use when cleaning the inner cannula. It mechanically loosens and facilitates the removal of protein debris from the surface of the equipment. Isopropyl alcohol, sodium hypochlorite, and povidone iodine are good antiseptics, but they are best used for inhibiting and destroying microorganisms by topical application. (18:720; 14:826)
Nursing Process—Implementation
Client Need—Safe, effective care environment

87   3. To prevent the possibility that the client may cough the tracheostomy tube out of his airway, the old ties should not be removed until the replacement ties are secured. Gauze squares should not be cut to fashion a stomal dressing. The cut threads may enter the airway and irritate the tissue. Special drain gauze or tracheostomy dressing material should be used, or gauze can be folded rather than cut to fit around the stoma. The inner cannula should be replaced as soon as it has been cleaned, rinsed, and dried, or within at least 5 minutes. If there is a delay in replacing the inner cannla, mucous secretions may accumulate and dry in the outer cannula. This may alter the size of the opening and interfere with replacement. (18:720-721)
Nursing Process—Implementation
Client Need—Physiological integrity

88   2. It is best to place a client undergoing a thoracentesis in a sitting position so that the physician has access to the eighth or ninth rib space. Once sitting, it would be helpful for the client to rest his head and elevate his arms on the overbed table. If this position is impossible, the nurse may alternatively place the client on his unaffected side. Lithotomy position is used for procedures in which the caregiver needs access to structures in the area of the vaginal or urinary meatus and for some rectal procedures. It would be incorrect to place the client in a prone or supine position for a thoracentesis. (17:317; 18:317)
Nursing Process—Implementation
Client Need—Safe, effective care environment

89   3. A pulmonary function test is performed by having the client breathe in and out through a mouthpiece. A tube connects the mouthpiece to an air-filled drum. The drum rises and falls with ventilation. A graphic recording of the volume of air exchanged during breathing is obtained. (17:315-316; 16:224)
Nursing Process—Evaluation
Client Need—Safe, effective care environment

90   2. The most classic symptom associated with pleurisy is feeling a sharp, stabbing pain when taking a deep breath. Pleurisy is an inflammation of the pleural membranes surrounding the lungs. If a cough is present, it would be due to some other pulmonary problem. Cyanotic nailbeds and tachycardia can be caused by any number of cardiopulmonary diseases that interfere with tissue oxygenation. (3:398-399; 16:249)
Nursing Process—Collecting data
Client Need—Physiological integrity

91   3. The normal pH range for blood is between 7.35 and 7.45. If the arterial blood pH is below 7.35, the client is in a state of acidosis. If the pH is above 7.45, the client is in a state of alkalosis. (17:315; 16:223)
Nursing Process—Collecting data
Client Need—Physiological integrity

92   2. A cuff on a tracheostomy tube forms a tight seal preventing liquid nasopharyngeal secretions, stomach contents, or tube feeding formula from entering the lower respiratory passages. If the person also is receiving mechanical ventilation, the cuff ensures that the oxygenated air does not escape before it is delivered to the lower areas of the lungs. An inflated cuff may lead to tissue breakdown because the pressure occludes capillary blood flow. Using a cuffed tracheostomy tube does not provide more comfort or reduce infection any better than an uncuffed tracheostomy tube. (3:427; 16:239)
Nursing Process—Implementation
Client Need—Safe, effective care environment

93 3. Rebreathing exhaled carbon dioxide from a paper bag will increase the blood levels of P_{CO_2} restoring arterial blood gas ranges to normal. None of the other options would result in conserving and raising the level of carbon dioxide being lost by rapid breathing. (3:171; 14:697)

Nursing Process—Implementation

Client Need—Physiological integrity

94 4. Cheyne-Stokes breathing is a pattern in which the client cycles through shallow then rapid breathing, followed again by shallow breathing and ending in a period of apnea. Pursed-lip breathing is a therapeutic breathing technique performed by individuals with chronic obstructive pulmonary disease. Grunting respirations are common in children with congestive heart failure. Snoring may occur as a result of a deviated septum or may accompany periods of sleep apnea. (3:394; 17:313)

Nursing Process—Collecting Data

Client Need—Safe, effective care environment

Classification of Test Items

Unit IV Review Test 9

Directions: After each question the correct answer is given as well as a classification of each test question. Compare the correct answer with your answer. If a question has been answered *incorrectly*, draw a line to the end of the four columns. When finished, add up your correct scores and place the results at the bottom of each column.

Score Calculation:

To determine the percentage of the number of questions you answered correctly, divide the **Number Correct** by the **Number Possible**, as example 78 (the number of questions answered correctly) divided by 94 (the number of questions in the test) = .83 or 83%.

NURSING PROCESS

C = Collecting data
P = Planning
I = Implementation
E = Evaluation

CLIENT NEEDS

S = Safe, effective care environment
P = Physiological integrity
M = Psychosocial integrity
H = Health promotion/maintenance

Question #	Answer #	Nursing Process				Client Needs			
		C	P	I	E	S	P	M	H
1	3	C					P		
2	3	C					P		
3	1			I					H
4	4			I					H
5	3				E		P		
6	1		P						H
7	3			I					H
8	3			I					H
9	1			I		S			
10	1	C				S			
11	2			I			P		
12	1	C					P		
13	3		P				P		
14	3				E		P		
15	3			I			P		
16	2		P			S			
17	1		P				P		
18	4		P			S			
19	4				E	S			

NURSING PROCESS

C = Collecting data
P = Planning
I = Implementation
E = Evaluation

CLIENT NEEDS

S = Safe, effective care environment
P = Physiological integrity
M = Psychosocial integrity
H = Health promotion/maintenance

Question #	Answer #	Nursing Process				Client Needs			
		C	P	I	E	S	P	M	H
20	2	C					P		
21	2			I			P		
22	1			I					H
23	4			I			P		
24	1			I			P		
25	2	C					P		
26	4		P				P		
27	3			I			P		
28	3			I		S			
29	2	C				S			
30	3				E		P		
31	2			I					H
32	1	C							H
33	3			I					H
34	1	C					P		
35	1		P			S			
36	4	C					P		
37	3			I		S			
38	1			I			P		
39	2			I		S			
40	1			I			P		
41	2			I			P		
42	2	C					P		
43	1			I			P		
44	3			I					H
45	4	C					P		
46	2			I			P		
47	4				E		P		
48	1			I				M	
49	1			I			P		

NURSING PROCESS

C = Collecting data
P = Planning
I = Implementation
E = Evaluation

CLIENT NEEDS

S = Safe, effective care environment
P = Physiological integrity
M = Psychosocial integrity
H = Health promotion/maintenance

Question #	Answer #	Nursing Process				Client Needs			
		C	P	I	E	S	P	M	H
50	2			I					H
51	3	C				S			
52	2		P				P		
53	1			I		S			
54	3			I					H
55	4			I					H
56	2		P				P		
57	2			I		S			
58	3	C					P		
59	3			I		S			
60	1		P			S			
61	3	C					P		
62	1	C					P		
63	4			I		S			
64	1				E	S			
65	1			I			P		
66	1			I					H
67	3	C					P		
68	4	C					P		
69	1	C				S			
70	2			I		S			
71	3	C					P		
72	2			I		S			
73	4			I		S			
74	2			I				M	
75	2			I			P		
76	2			I			P		
77	1			I			P		
78	3	C				S			
79	1			I		S			
80	2	C					P		

NURSING PROCESS

C = Collecting data
P = Planning
I = Implementation
E = Evaluation

CLIENT NEEDS

S = Safe, effective care environment
P = Physiological integrity
M = Psychosocial integrity
H = Health promotion/maintenance

Question #	Answer #	Nursing Process				Client Needs			
		C	P	I	E	S	P	M	H
81	4			I			P		
82	3			I			P		
83	2			I			P		
84	4			I			P		
85	1			I			P		
86	3			I		S			
87	3			I			P		
88	2			I		S			
89	3				E	S			
90	2	C					P		
91	3	C					P		
92	2			I		S			
93	3			I			P		
94	4	C				S			
Number Correct									
Number Possible	94	25	10	52	7	28	50	2	14
Percentage Correct									

REVIEW TEST 10

The Nursing Care of Clients with Disorders of the Reproductive System

Nursing Care of Clients with Breast Cancer
Nursing Care of Clients Having a Hysterectomy
Nursing Care of Clients with Benign Prostatic Hypertrophy
Nursing Care of Clients with Cancer of the Prostate Gland
Nursing Care of Clients with a Sexually Transmitted Disease
Individual Test Items

The Nursing Care of Clients with Disorders of the Neurologic System

Nursing Care of Clients with a Seizure Disorder
Nursing Care of Clients with Parkinson's Disease
Nursing Care of Clients with Alzheimer's Disease
Nursing Care of Clients with a Cerebral Aneurysm
Nursing Care of Clients with a Brain Tumor
Nursing Care of Clients with a Cerebrovascular Accident
Nursing Care of Clients with a Spinal Cord Injury
Nursing Care of Clients with Multiple Sclerosis
Individual Test Items

Correct Answers and Rationale
Classification of Test Items

Directions: With a pencil, blacken the circle in front of the option you have chosen for your correct answer.

The Nursing Care of Clients with Disorders of the Reproductive System

NURSING CARE OF CLIENTS WITH BREAST CANCER

Ms. Ann Gibson, age 32, discovers a lump in her left breast and sees her physician, who recommends an immediate biopsy of the lesion.

1 Ms. Gibson is to have an aspiration biopsy, and the physician asks the nurse to explain the procedure to Ms. Gibson. The nurse can describe an aspiration biopsy as under
   ○ 1. local anesthesia a needle and syringe are used to remove a sample of tissue.
   ○ 2. general anesthesia a small knife is used to remove a sample of tissue.
   ○ 3. local anesthesia a suction machine is used to remove the entire lesion.

   ○ 4. general anesthesia liquid nitrogen is used to destroy the tumor.

Ms. Gibson has a malignant tumor of her left breast and is scheduled for a modified radical mastectomy.

2 The nurse helping to develop a postoperative care plan should know that this type of mastectomy involves removal of the
   ○ 1. tumor and a small amount of breast tissue.
   ○ 2. breast, axillary lymph nodes, and pectoral muscles.
   ○ 3. breast leaving the skin and nipple intact.
   ○ 4. breast and axillary lymph nodes.

3 Which one of the following should the nurse recognize as a postoperative *complication* of a modified radical mastectomy?
   ○ 1. Edema of the lower extremities
   ○ 2. Edema of the arm on the operative side

○ 3. Inability to move the arm for 1 to 2 days after surgery

○ 4. Lymph node enlargement

4 Which one of the following nursing tasks performed on Ms. Gibson is *incorrect*?

○ 1. Taking her pulse on the right arm

○ 2. Using her left arm to monitor the blood pressure

○ 3. Preparing material for an intravenous infusion to be started on her right arm

○ 4. Comparing the size of her left arm with her right arm

5 The nurse plans to encourage coughing and deep breathing. This nursing task is important for this client because the

○ 1. pectoral muscles have been removed.

○ 2. surgical dressing tends to restrict chest movement.

○ 3. urinary output tends to be low.

○ 4. accessory muscles of respiration have been removed.

6 During the immediate postoperative period, the nurse supports Ms. Gibson's left arm on a pillow raised above the level of her breast to prevent

○ 1. hemorrhage.

○ 2. edema.

○ 3. contractures.

○ 4. lymph node enlargement.

Ms. Gibson is scheduled for discharge from the hospital.

7 When instructing Ms. Gibson prior to her discharge from the hospital, the nurse should stress that

○ 1. a prosthesis should be worn immediately after going home.

○ 2. a foam rubber prosthesis provides a more comfortable fit.

○ 3. postmastectomy exercises must be practiced regularly.

○ 4. water should be taken sparingly to prevent swelling of the arm on the operative side.

8 Which one of the following should the nurse include in teaching Ms. Gibson skin care of the operative area?

○ 1. Apply a cream or ointment to soften the surgical scar.

○ 2. Wear sterile gloves when washing the operative area.

○ 3. Avoid washing the operative site for 3 to 4 weeks.

○ 4. Wash the area gently with soap and a soft washcloth.

9 The nurse plans to teach Ms. Gibson the technique of examining her remaining breast. This examination should be performed

○ 1. weekly.

○ 2. every 2 weeks.

○ 3. every month on the first day of the month.

○ 4. every month, 1 week after menstruation.

10 Which one of the following is part of a breast self-examination (BSE) and should be included in instructions given to Ms. Gibson?

○ 1. The entire examination is performed while lying on the back with the arm down at the side.

○ 2. Stand in front of a mirror to detect any changes in the breast.

○ 3. Lie on the abdomen to detect any breast pain or tenderness.

○ 4. Lie prone or sit when examining the breast.

The nurse shows Ms. Gibson how to examine her breast.

11 Which part of the hand is Ms. Gibson instructed to use when examining her breast?

○ 1. The heel of the hand

○ 2. The index finger and thumb

○ 3. The index finger

○ 4. The pads of the four fingertips

NURSING CARE OF CLIENTS HAVING A HYSTERECTOMY

Ms. Betty Acker has a history of symptoms due to uterine fibroids. She is admitted the morning of surgery and is scheduled for an abdominal hysterectomy.

12 When obtaining an initial history from Ms. Acker, the nurse should ask questions related to her symptoms. Which one of the following is a more prominent symptom of uterine fibroids?

○ 1. Fever

○ 2. Muscle aching

○ 3. Menorrhagia

○ 4. Amenorrhea

13 The physician orders the insertion of an indwelling catheter prior to surgery. After the labia majora are cleansed, the catheter is inserted into the meatus approximately

○ 1. ½ inch

○ 2. 1 inch

○ 3. 2 to 3 inch

○ 4. 5 to 6 inch

Ms. Acker has an abdominal hysterectomy and returns from the postanesthesia recovery room with an indwelling urethral catheter and antiembolic stockings. Her vital signs are stable.

14 When writing a care plan the nurse should include a notation that the antiembolic stockings should be

○ 1. left in place for 3 days.

○ 2. removed once the client is awake.

○ 3. removed and reapplied daily.

○ 4. removed and reapplied every 8 hours.

15 The nurse is asked to assist with formulating nursing diagnoses for Ms. Acker. Which one of the following is appropriate for this client during the immediate postoperative period?
- ○ 1. Ineffective Airway Clearance related to failure to cough and deep-breathe
- ○ 2. Hypothermia related to infection
- ○ 3. Potential for Infection related to elevated blood glucose levels and intravenous therapy
- ○ 4. Alteration in Nutrition, More than Body Requirements, related to decreased metabolic rate

16 Ten hours postoperatively Ms. Acker complains of severe back pain. At this time the nurse should
- ○ 1. use pillows to support Ms. Acker's back.
- ○ 2. make a notation on Ms. Acker's chart.
- ○ 3. call the physician because pain in this area is unusual.
- ○ 4. change Ms. Acker's position.

17 Three days after surgery Ms. Acker's urethral catheter is removed. Which of the following is the most appropriate nursing task following removal of a urethral catheter?
- ○ 1. Ask the client if she feels more comfortable.
- ○ 2. Measure the urinary output after each voiding.
- ○ 3. Obtain a voided specimen for urinalysis.
- ○ 4. Tell the client to limit her oral fluid intake for the next 12 hours.

Ms. Acker is scheduled to be discharged from the hospital.

18 Which one of the following should the nurse plan to include in a discharge teaching plan for Ms. Acker?
- ○ 1. Douche twice weekly to remove any vaginal discharge.
- ○ 2. Avoid heavy lifting until this is permitted by the physician.
- ○ 3. Avoid walking; sit or lie down most of the day.
- ○ 4. Limit fluids and eat a low salt diet.

NURSING CARE OF CLIENTS WITH BENIGN PROSTATIC HYPERTROPHY

Mr. Stan Richards, age 56, sees his physician because he has difficulty passing urine. A cystoscopy is performed on an outpatient basis, and a diagnosis of benign prostatic hypertrophy is made. He is now scheduled for a suprapubic prostatectomy. When Mr. Richards is admitted to the hospital, he is examined by the physician, who notes that Mr. Richards' bladder is markedly distended. The physician inserts a urethral catheter and orders that Mr. Richards' bladder is to be slowly emptied over a period of 1 hour.

19 To understand the physician's order, the nurse should know that rapid emptying of the bladder could result in
- ○ 1. marked hypertension and diuresis.
- ○ 2. hypernatremia and hyperkalemia.
- ○ 3. damage to the bladder and rectum.
- ○ 4. moderate to severe hypotension and hematuria.

The nurse performs a preoperative assessment of Mr. Richards.

20 The nurse observes Mr. Richard's behavior and determines that he appears extremely frightened and apprehensive. This fact must be immediately reported to the physician because apprehensive clients
- ○ 1. are prone to complications, such as cardiac arrest and shock.
- ○ 2. must be given a larger dose of the preoperative medication.
- ○ 3. are uncooperative after surgery.
- ○ 4. may suddenly refuse to be taken to the operating room.

21 Upon return from surgery the nurse observes that Mr. Richards has two catheters: a cystostomy catheter in the incision and a urethral catheter. When checking the catheters the nurse should
- ○ 1. be sure that both catheters empty into one closed drainage system.
- ○ 2. place the closed drainage systems above the level of the bed.
- ○ 3. be sure that each catheter is connected to a separate closed drainage system.
- ○ 4. apply a clamp to the cystostomy catheter.

22 The nurse is assigned to obtain a temperature on Mr. Richards, who appears to be having profuse diaphoresis. Using a thermometer, which of the following is the most correct method of obtaining a temperature on the client who has had a suprapubic prostatectomy?
- ○ 1. Axillary temperature
- ○ 2. Oral temperature
- ○ 3. Rectal temperature
- ○ 4. Tympanic membrane temperature

23 One problem associated with a prostatectomy is hematuria during the immediate postoperative period. Which one of the following nursing tasks, related to the occurrence of hematuria, is most correct?
- ○ 1. Monitor the client's level of consciousness.
- ○ 2. Keep the client flat in bed.
- ○ 3. Check the patency of all catheters.
- ○ 4. Monitor the rate of the intravenous infusion.

Two days after surgery Mr. Richards complains of severe pain and spasms in his bladder.

24 The nurse can suggest to Mr. Richards that his pain may be relieved if he
○ 1. turns on his side.
○ 2. avoids trying to urinate as a catheter is keeping his bladder empty.
○ 3. takes deep breaths.
○ 4. avoids thinking about his discomfort or pain.

25 The physician orders irrigation of the urethral catheter. Unless the physician orders otherwise, indwelling catheters are irrigated with
○ 1. sterile water.
○ 2. sterile normal saline.
○ 3. tap water.
○ 4. sterile sodium bicarbonate.

26 The physician requests that Mr. Richards' oral fluid intake be increased. To answer any questions Mr. Richards may have the nurse should know that the purpose of drinking extra fluids is to
○ 1. keep the catheters free of blood clots and mucous.
○ 2. remove electrolytes from the bladder.
○ 3. help increase his bladder capacity.
○ 4. prevent incontinence.

27 The nurse is asked to participate in discharge teaching. Which one of the following should be included in a teaching plan for Mr. Richards?
○ 1. Avoid eating foods containing roughage.
○ 2. Avoid heavy lifting and strenuous exercise.
○ 3. Use an enema if constipation occurs.
○ 4. Limit fluid intake to three to four glasses of water per day.

Mr. Richards sees his physician 2 weeks after discharge from the hospital. He states that he is experiencing some urinary incontinence. The physician asks the nurse to explain Kegel exercises to Mr. Richards.

28 Which one of the following is the correct method of performing Kegel exercises?
○ 1. Tighten the perineal muscles for 5 to 20 seconds and then relax them for 5 to 20 seconds.
○ 2. Lie supine, and alternately raise and lower the legs.
○ 3. Tighten the abdominal muscles for 45 seconds.
○ 4. Roll from side to back to side four to six times.

NURSING CARE OF CLIENTS WITH CANCER OF THE PROSTATE GLAND

Mr. Barber has cancer of the prostate and is scheduled for a radical perineal prostatectomy and bilateral orchiectomy.

29 The evening before surgery Mr. Barber is given an enema. He appears nervous and asks the nurse why

an enema is necessary. The most correct response is based on the fact that
○ 1. it is important to prevent constipation during the postoperative period.
○ 2. most surgeons prefer clients have an enema.
○ 3. the enema contains an antibiotic that must be given rectally.
○ 4. it is important to keep the client comfortable the night before surgery.

30 Ms. Barber asks the physician why her husband's testicles must be removed. She then asks the nurse to reexplain the reason for this procedure. The nurses' explanation is based on the fact that
○ 1. the only way the prostate can be safely removed is by first removing the testicles.
○ 2. the testicles also are malignant and must be removed.
○ 3. tumors of this area tend to invade the testicles and bladder.
○ 4. it is necessary to remove the source of male hormones to prevent progression of the tumor.

Mr. Barber is discharged from the hospital and scheduled to see his physician in 2 weeks. At the time of his first visit, the physician prescribes estradiol (Estrace), which is an estrogen. Before he leaves the physician's office the nurse notices that Mr. Barber appears very upset.

31 Mr. Barber asks the nurse why he has to take a female hormone when he is a man. To discuss drug therapy with Mr. Barber the nurse should know that
○ 1. estrogens may help prevent the spread of the tumor.
○ 2. estrogens are used to replace the small amounts of female hormones manufactured by the male.
○ 3. short-term therapy with these drugs prevents incontinence.
○ 4. long-term therapy with these drugs is necessary to prevent urinary retention.

NURSING CARE OF CLIENTS WITH A SEXUALLY TRANSMITTED DISEASE

Mr. Tom Lawrence seeks medical attention because he has symptoms related to his urinary tract. Following an initial examination, the physician tells Mr. Lawrence that he has symptoms of gonorrhea, and further tests will be necessary to confirm the diagnosis. The physician also states that he will examine or test Mr. Lawrence for other sexually transmitted diseases.

32 Mr. Lawrence asks the nurse what tests will be done if the physician is testing him for gonorrhea. The most correct answer is that the physician will

○ 1. obtain a sample of his urethral discharge.
○ 2. schedule him for a cystoscopy.
○ 3. ask him to bring in a urine specimen.
○ 4. draw some blood for a laboratory test for gonorrhea.

The physician tells Mr. Lawrence that his sexual partner(s) also should be tested for gonorrhea.

33 Mr. Lawrence asks the nurse what will happen if his female partner is not treated. The most correct response is based on the fact that women who are not treated may develop
○ 1. encephalitis and kidney failure.
○ 2. urethritis and kidney infections.
○ 3. inflammation of the pelvic organs and sterility.
○ 4. a high fever and bladder infection.

The physician asks the nurse to give Mr. Lawrence 1 g (two tablets) of probenecid (Benemid) one-half hour before the administration of intramuscular penicillin.

34 To explain to Mr. Lawrence the reason for the drug, the nurse should know that the purpose of probenecid administration is to
○ 1. prolong plasma levels of penicillin.
○ 2. relax the client.
○ 3. reduce pain at the injection site.
○ 4. prevent allergic reactions to penicillin.

35 The physician asks the nurse to prepare 4 to 8 million U of aqueous procaine penicillin G (APPG), which will be given intramuscularly. The total fluid volume of penicillin is 8 mL. When preparing this intramuscular injection the nurse should
○ 1. have the client lie down, and have him draw up his knees while the injection is being given.
○ 2. give two intramuscular injections of 4 mL each in two different sites.
○ 3. inject the 8 mL slowly in one injection site.
○ 4. give the injection in the upper arm.

36 When giving an intramuscular injection, the needle is inserted at a
○ 1. 45-degree angle.
○ 2. narrow angle.
○ 3. 30-degree angle.
○ 4. 90-degree angle.

37 The physician asks the nurse to prepare materials for a fluorescent treponemal antibody absorption test, which is a test for diagnosing syphilis. Which of the following is necessary for this test?
○ 1. A fluorescent lamp
○ 2. Needles, syringes, specific blood collection tubes
○ 3. A microscope, slides, pipette
○ 4. Sterile blotters, curette

Mr. Jack Stanley has been recently diagnosed as having acquired immunodeficiency syndrome (AIDS) and is admitted to the hospital for treatment of Pneumocystis carinii pneumonia.

38 The nurse is assigned to help with obtaining materials for his room. The isolation technique usually used for those with AIDS is
○ 1. strict isolation.
○ 2. blood and body fluid precautions.
○ 3. infectious precautions.
○ 4. contact isolation.

39 During a nursing conference a nursing assistant asks the nurse if AIDS can be spread only by means of sexual contact. The most correct answer is based on the fact that, according to present knowledge, AIDS
○ 1. also can be transmitted by exposure to blood or needles infected with the AIDS virus.
○ 2. is sometimes transmitted by casual contact with individuals with AIDS.
○ 3. is transmitted only by sexual contact with an individual infected with the AIDS virus.
○ 4. can be transmitted by exposure to respiratory secretions.

40 During a nursing conference a nursing assistant asks if there is a reason why Mr. Stanley developed pneumonia. The nurse can answer this question based on the fact that those with AIDS
○ 1. take medications that lower their resistance.
○ 2. have an increased white blood cell count.
○ 3. are usually anemic.
○ 4. are susceptible to opportunistic infections.

INDIVIDUAL TEST ITEMS

41 When obtaining a client history, which of the following should the nurse recognize as symptoms of premenstrual syndrome (PMS)?
○ 1. Weight loss, palpitations, decreased blood pressure
○ 2. Headache, nervousness, irritability
○ 3. Dry skin, diarrhea, bradycardia
○ 4. Muscle aching, joint pain, hypertension

42 The nurse working in a physician's office reviews a client's record and notes that the client has a history of menorrhagia. To plan follow-up questions on subsequent office visits, the nurse should know that menorrhagia refers to
○ 1. painful menstruation.
○ 2. bleeding that occurs between regular menstrual periods.
○ 3. excessive menstrual flow.
○ 4. absence of menstruation.

43 The nurse is assigned to teach young women attending a gynecology clinic. The physician suggests

that the nurse include explaining ways to prevent toxic shock syndrome. Which one of the following suggestions can be included in this teaching session?
○ 1. Avoid using super absorbent tampons.
○ 2. Take a diuretic at the onset of menstruation.
○ 3. Avoid the use of large sanitary pads.
○ 4. Use a tampon only during the night.

44 Which of the following are included in the instructions for a client having a pelvic examination?
○ 1. Self-administer an enema or take a laxative for 2 nights prior to the examination.
○ 2. Void immediately before the examination.
○ 3. Douche the day before the examination.
○ 4. Do not eat or drink fluids after midnight.

45 Ms. Dodd has been told by her physician that she has genital warts, which are caused by a human papillomavirus infection. She asks the nurse if there is any danger or problems associated with this condition. The most correct response is based on the fact that genital warts
○ 1. can be treated with an antibiotic, such as penicillin or tetracycline.
○ 2. appear to increase the risk of cancer of the vulva, vagina, and cervix.
○ 3. can be prevented if the individual takes birth control pills.
○ 4. are of no danger and need not be treated.

46 The physician asks the nurse to discuss the use of an oral contraceptive with Ms. Sheppard. The nurse should instruct Ms. Sheppard that oral contraceptives
○ 1. are taken at the same time each day, preferably in the evening.
○ 2. must be taken on an empty stomach.
○ 3. are started on the first day of menstruation.
○ 4. are best taken in the morning before breakfast.

47 The nurse obtains a health history from Ms. Reeves, who states that she usually has symptoms when she ovulates. If Ms. Reeves has a normal menstrual cycle, how many days after ovulation should menstruation begin?
○ 1. 3 days
○ 2. 7 days
○ 3. 14 days
○ 4. 21 days

48 Ms. Manning is scheduled for a Papanicolaou test (Pap smear) at the time of her next visit to the physician's office. Which one of the following instructions should the nurse give to Ms. Manning?
○ 1. Do not douche for 2 to 3 days before this test.
○ 2. Do not drink coffee or alcoholic beverages for 2 days before this test.
○ 3. It will be necessary to fast from midnight the night before the test.

○ 4. Bring a sanitary napkin with you because bleeding usually occurs after this test.

49 The nurse is asked to plan a health teaching program for women of child-bearing age with genital herpes. Which one of the following should the nurse include in a teaching session?
○ 1. The physician will prescribe an antiviral drug as soon as a pregnancy is confirmed.
○ 2. Genital herpes in the mother has no effect on the infant.
○ 3. Wait until the infection has been cured before becoming pregnant.
○ 4. If pregnant, inform the physician of a history of genital herpes.

50 The physician asks the nurse to describe the laparoscopy procedure for sterilization to Ms. Bruce. Which one of the following is part of a *correct* explanation of this procedure?
○ 1. Two small abdominal incisions are made to introduce the instruments.
○ 2. Hospitalization for 4 to 5 days is normally required.
○ 3. This procedure is performed vaginally.
○ 4. This procedure requires the consent of the sexual partner.

51 The nursing assistant is assigned to give Ms. Bailey, who has had an abdominal hysterectomy, a sitz bath. She is instructed to use the special sitz bathtub. She asks the nurse why the regular bathtub cannot be used. The most correct reply is based on the fact that a regular bathtub
○ 1. is more slippery and is dangerous when used for surgical clients.
○ 2. cannot supply water that is of the desired temperature for this procedure.
○ 3. applies heat to the legs and alters the desired effect of heat directed to the pelvic region.
○ 4. cannot be kept as clean as a special sitz bathtub.

52 Ms. Hull has had an electrocauterization of her cervix for chronic cervicitis. Following the procedure the nurse should instruct Ms. Hull to
○ 1. douche the next day to remove debris and blood clots.
○ 2. avoid straining and heavy lifting until the physician permits this activity.
○ 3. stay in bed for the next 5 days.
○ 4. return for a physician's examination in 6 months.

53 The physician asks the nurse to position a client for a vaginal examination. Which one of the following positions is normally used for this type of examination?
○ 1. Lithotomy position
○ 2. Sims' position

○ 3. Dorsal recumbent position
○ 4. Left lateral position

54 Ms. Hodges is being treated for endometriosis and asks the nurse why she has so much pain. The most correct answer is based on the fact that the
○ 1. endometrium does not respond to hormones.
○ 2. ectopic endometrial tissue bleeds into spaces that have no outlet.
○ 3. pituitary gland fails to secrete luteinizing hormone.
○ 4. uterine endometrium fails to develop during puberty.

55 The nurse is assigned to teach health-seeking behaviors to young women. One topic the nurse plans to include is the importance of the Pap test, which is used mainly to detect
○ 1. ovarian cysts.
○ 2. cervical cancer.
○ 3. patency of the fallopian tubes.
○ 4. uterine infections.

56 The nurse is assigned to administer a vaginal irrigation (douche). Which one of the following is *correct*?
○ 1. The irrigation is best administered with the client standing in a bathtub.
○ 2. Before inserting, the nozzle is lubricated with petroleum jelly.
○ 3. The temperature of the solution should be between 80°F and 84°F.
○ 4. The nozzle is inserted downward and backward within the vagina.

57 The nurse is assigned to give Ms. Milton perineal care. When cleansing the perineum, the cotton ball or washcloth is gently directed
○ 1. side to side across the labia majora.
○ 2. downward from the pubic area to the anus.
○ 3. upward from the anus to the pubic area.
○ 4. from the urinary meatus to the vagina.

58 The nurse prepares to give Ms. Edwards a vaginal suppository, which is inserted by means of a special applicator supplied with the drug. Which one of the following is correct?
○ 1. Ask the client to void prior to inserting the suppository.
○ 2. Lubricate the tip of the suppository with petroleum jelly.
○ 3. Insert the applicator tip gently and with an upward and forward motion.
○ 4. Insert the applicator approximately ½ in and depress the plunger.

59 The nurse is asked to discuss the signs and symptoms of vaginitis caused by the fungus *Candida albicans* with Ms. Burrows. Which one of the following is a usual sign and symptom of this infection?

○ 1. Pain high in the abdomen
○ 2. Intense vaginal and perineal itching
○ 3. Decrease in urinary output
○ 4. High fever

60 The nurse is participating in a health class for young women. One subject is cancer of the ovary. Which one of the following statements is *correct*?
○ 1. Early symptoms of cancer of the ovary are vague.
○ 2. This type of cancer has a high cure rate.
○ 3. Chemotherapy is not used for treating ovarian cancer.
○ 4. The most prominent early symptom is an irregular menstrual cycle.

61 A nurse assistant attending a nursing conference hears that one of her clients has a hydrocele. She asks the nurse how this condition is treated. The most correct response is
○ 1. usually the problem requires no medical or surgical intervention.
○ 2. surgery may be necessary to correct the problem.
○ 3. wearing a scrotal support usually corrects the problem.
○ 4. drug therapy usually helps control the collection of fluid.

62 A client is scheduled for a cystoscopy and asks the nurse what the physician will be able to see during the procedure. The most correct reply is the
○ 1. kidneys and ureters.
○ 2. bladder and rectum.
○ 3. prostate and ureters.
○ 4. urethra and bladder.

63 Mr. Dorn has a vasectomy. He asks the nurse why he must use a method of birth control because today he had a sterilization procedure. The most correct answer is
○ 1. the sperm count will not be negative until his testosterone levels decrease.
○ 2. a second minor surgery usually is necessary to ensure sterilization.
○ 3. some live sperm will be present in the ejaculatory fluid for a period of time.
○ 4. even though a vasectomy is performed, a condom is still recommended for 1 to 2 years.

64 A nurse is assigned to instruct a client in the method of testicular self-examination. The instruction should include mention that the best time to perform this task is
○ 1. immediately after getting out of bed in the morning.
○ 2. immediately before going to bed.
○ 3. in the morning after breakfast.
○ 4. after a warm bath or shower.

65 To effectively teach men the importance of testicular self-examination, the nurse should know that testicular carcinoma
○ 1. rarely metastasizes.
○ 2. has a high incidence of early metastasis.
○ 3. cannot be detected by laboratory tests.
○ 4. must first be biopsied to confirm the diagnosis.

66 A client is scheduled for an ultrasound examination of the prostate. To describe the procedure to the client, the nurse should plan to relate that
○ 1. the procedure is performed using a cystoscope.
○ 2. a probe will be inserted into the rectum.
○ 3. a flat disk is placed on the abdomen.
○ 4. this procedure uses x-rays to produce a visual image.

67 A female nurse is assigned to obtain a history from a male client with a urinary tract problem and sexual dysfunction. Which one of the following statements might place the client more at ease and willing to give a history of his problem?
○ 1. "When did you first notice this problem?"
○ 2. "Why do you think you have a problem?"
○ 3. "Do you think your sexual dysfunction is psychologic?"
○ 4. "Does your sexual dysfunction seem to be related to your urinary tract problem?"

68 The nurse is assigned to give perineal care to an uncircumsized male client. Which of the following is correct?
○ 1. The anal area is washed at a separate time.
○ 2. The foreskin is retracted and the area beneath the foreskin cleansed.
○ 3. The foreskin should not be retracted except by a physician.
○ 4. The scrotum is carefully washed with sterile normal saline.

69 The nurse is assigned to teach a class in health behaviors to young men. Which of the following can be stated as a probable cause of cancer of the penis?
○ 1. A diet high in acidic foods
○ 2. Poor personal hygiene
○ 3. Exercise
○ 4. Circumcision

70 When continuous bladder irrigation is used following prostate surgery, the rate of flow is adjusted
○ 1. to run at 60 drops per minute.
○ 2. according to the client's oral intake.
○ 3. to maintain an output of 500 mL every 8 hours.
○ 4. to keep the drainage a light pink.

71 The nurse is assigned to check a client's continuous bladder irrigation. Which one of the following solutions is normally used for continuous or intermittent bladder and catheter irrigations?
○ 1. Hydrogen peroxide
○ 2. Bacteriostatic water
○ 3. Sterile normal saline
○ 4. Plain water

The Nursing Care of Clients with Disorders of the Neurologic System

NURSING CARE OF CLIENTS WITH A SEIZURE DISORDER

Ms. Rita Alden, age 23, has a possible seizure disorder and is admitted to the hospital for diagnostic studies and observation.

72 Ms. Alden is scheduled for an electroencephalogram (EEG). The nurse is assigned to explain the procedure to Ms. Alden. Which one of the following is *correct*?
○ 1. The procedure takes 10 to 15 minutes.
○ 2. An enema will be necessary the night before and the morning of the procedure.
○ 3. The procedure is done in a darkened room.
○ 4. The blood pressure will be taken every 10 to 15 minutes during the procedure.

73 Ms. Alden is placed on seizure precautions because she appears to be having frequent tonic-clonic seizures. Which one of the following safety measures may be used for this client?
○ 1. Keep the side rails down to prevent injury.
○ 2. Keep the room brightly lit day and night.
○ 3. Pad the raised side rails of the bed.
○ 4. Keep the door to the room closed at all times.

74 Ms. Alden tells the nurse that she smells roses, yet there are no flowers in her room. This statement should alert the nurse to the possibility that Ms. Alden
○ 1. is hallucinating.
○ 2. is experiencing an aura.
○ 3. may be imagining she smells roses.
○ 4. may have an allergy.

Ms. Alden lets out a loud cry and begins to have a tonic–clonic seizure while the nurse is in the room.

75 When a client has a tonic-clonic seizure, which one of the following nursing tasks has the highest priority?
○ 1. Remove the top bed sheet.
○ 2. Take the blood pressure and pulse.
○ 3. Give oxygen by nasal cannula.
○ 4. Establish a patent airway.

76 Which of the following actions is *incorrect* when the nurse is present when a client has a tonic-clonic seizure?

○ 1. Restrain the arms and legs to prevent injury.
○ 2. Remove pillows from the bed.
○ 3. Remove restrictive clothing.
○ 4. Suction the oral cavity.

Ms. Alden's medication regimen is discussed during a nursing conference. The nurse in charge discusses the importance of not omitting Ms Alden's anticonvulsant medication.

77 Which one of the following is the most correct reason for *not* omitting an anticonvulsant?
○ 1. Status epilepticus may occur.
○ 2. Seizures may become less frequent.
○ 3. Urinary retention may occur.
○ 4. Petit mal seizures may occur.

78 Which one of the following could the nurse recommend that would most likely provide Ms. Alden with counseling, vocational guidance, and low-cost prescription services?
○ 1. The Red Cross
○ 2. The Salvation Army
○ 3. The Epilepsy Foundation of America
○ 4. The United Way

NURSING CARE OF CLIENTS WITH PARKINSON'S DISEASE

Ms. Sophie Grant, age 72, has Parkinson's disease. She is admitted to a long-term care facility because of a steady deterioration of her condition. The nurse is assigned to evaluate Ms. Grant and assist with developing a plan of care.

79 Which one of the following initial assessments of Ms. Grant is the most important when the nurse is assigned to contribute to a care plan?
○ 1. Ability to carry out activities of daily living (ADL)
○ 2. Evaluation of intelligence
○ 3. Food preferences
○ 4. Financial status

80 Ms. Grant is relatively inactive. Which of the following nursing tasks can be used to prevent muscle contractures?
○ 1. Have the client sit in a chair several times a day.
○ 2. Administer active or passive range-of-motion exercises.
○ 3. Encourage a high-protein diet.
○ 4. Offer fluids at frequent intervals during waking hours.

81 Ms. Grant is to receive levodopa (Dopar) *b.i.d.* The drug is given
○ 1. daily.
○ 2. twice a day.
○ 3. three times a day.
○ 4. four times a day.

82 The pharmacy supplies a capsule form of levodopa. Which one of the following measures may be used to help Ms. Grant swallow her medication?
○ 1. Soak the capsule in water until it is soft.
○ 2. Have Ms. Grant hold the capsule in her mouth to soften the capsule's coating.
○ 3. Puncture holes in the both ends of the capsule to allow saliva to enter.
○ 4. Have Ms. Grant take several sips of water before placing the capsule in her mouth.

83 Ms. Grant has moderately severe tremors and occasionally has difficulty speaking. Which one of the following would *not* be of value in helping Ms. Grant communicate her needs to the medical team?
○ 1. Encourage the use of gestures to answer questions.
○ 2. Use questions to help determine the client's needs.
○ 3. Encourage the client to speak slowly.
○ 4. Supply a pad and pen so the client can communicate in writing.

The nurse is concerned about Ms. Grant's relative immobility and performs an assessment of her skin, especially areas over bony prominences.

84 To prevent skin breakdown, which one of the following may the nurse include in a plan of care for this client?
○ 1. Change her position every 2 hours.
○ 2. Offer her a diet high in minerals and low in protein.
○ 3. Change her position every 4 to 6 hours.
○ 4. Apply lotion and then powder to areas prone to skin breakdown.

85 Which one of the following is the best method of evaluating the effectiveness of skin care given for the prevention of skin breakdown?
○ 1. Ask the client if pain is noted in any area, especially over bony prominences.
○ 2. Check the function of the flotation mattress or pad every 8 hours.
○ 3. Determine if members of the health team are changing the client's position.
○ 4. Check the client's skin at the time of each position change.

NURSING CARE OF CLIENTS WITH ALZHEIMER'S DISEASE

Ms. Loretta Daniels, age 59, is admitted to the hospital for evaluation. Her physician states that she may have early symptoms of Alzheimer's disease but wishes to perform tests to rule out other disorders.

86 During an initial assessment of Ms. Daniels, the nurse should observe this client for early signs and symptoms of Alzheimer's disease, which include

○ 1. hypotension and restlessness.
○ 2. memory loss and behavioral disturbances.
○ 3. periodic episodes of loss of consciousness.
○ 4. periodic episodes of paralysis.

87 The nurse in charge writes a nursing diagnosis of *Anxiety related to the disease process.* Which of the following nursing measures could be used to reduce Ms. Daniels' anxiety?
○ 1. Tell Ms. Daniels that things are done differently in a hospital.
○ 2. Maintain a structured daily routine.
○ 3. Explain to Ms. Daniels that she must follow hospital rules.
○ 4. Assign a nurse assistant rather than a nurse to administer care.

Ms. Daniels at times appears confused, uncooperative, and upset, especially when she is with other clients.

88 Which one of the following could the nurse use to improve or modify the behavior of this client?
○ 1. Have her eat her meals with others and join others for recreation.
○ 2. Provide a diet consisting of food preferences.
○ 3. Encourage a long afternoon nap.
○ 4. Reduce confusing stimuli.

Ms. Daniels needs to void frequently during the night.

89 Which one of the following nursing tasks might decrease Ms. Daniels' need to get up and void during the night?
○ 1. Limit her fluid intake during late evening hours.
○ 2. Have her ambulate during evening hours.
○ 3. Give Ms. Daniels her prescribed sedative late in the evening.
○ 4. Have Ms. Daniels participate in recreational activities.

The nurse assistant reports that Ms. Daniels tries to get out of bed to go to the bathroom.

90 The nurse goes to Ms. Daniels' room and notes that the side rails have been raised when Ms. Daniels is in bed. Which one of the following is the most appropriate action?
○ 1. Restrain Ms. Daniels when she is in bed.
○ 2. Warn Ms. Daniels that she must not get out of bed without help.
○ 3. Answer calls for assistance as soon as possible.
○ 4. Keep Ms. Daniels' room dark so she cannot see to get out of bed.

Ms. Daniels is ready for discharge from the hospital. The physician has told the family that Ms. Daniels has Alzheimer's disease.

91 Which one of the following recommendations should the nurse make to Ms. Daniels' caretakers?

○ 1. A high calorie diet is to be avoided.
○ 2. Do not allow Ms. Daniels to leave home unless someone is with her.
○ 3. Encourage Ms. Daniels to take long afternoon or early evening naps.
○ 4. Because she is confused, do not allow Ms. Daniels to take part in family activities.

NURSING CARE OF CLIENTS WITH A CEREBRAL ANEURYSM

Mr. James Bell, age 33, is admitted to the hospital with a possible ruptured cerebral aneurysm in the circle of Willis.

92 The nurse is assigned to develop a care plan for Mr. Bell. Which one of the following should be included in this care plan?
○ 1. Place Mr. Bell on his affected side.
○ 2. Monitor blood glucose levels.
○ 3. Allow Mr. Bell to ambulate with assistance for brief periods.
○ 4. Keep Mr. Bell as quiet as possible.

93 Which one of the following nursing assessments should be performed when it is suspected that Mr. Bell may be bleeding from his aneurysm and showing signs of increased intracranial pressure?
○ 1. Note the amount of food he consumed at each meal.
○ 2. Look for a change in his level of consciousness.
○ 3. Observe Mr. Bell for signs of anxiety.
○ 4. Measure Mr. Bell's intake and output.

94 The nurse is asked to use the Glasgow Coma Scale to evaluate Mr. Bell. Which one of the following responses is part of this type of assessment?
○ 1. The eye opening response
○ 2. The knee jerk reflex response
○ 3. The value response
○ 4. The testing response

Mr. Bell has a craniotomy for ligation of the aneurysm.

95 Which one of the following positions is usually used for the postoperative craniotomy client?
○ 1. Place the client in a supine position with the foot of the bed elevated.
○ 2. Place the client prone on a flat bed.
○ 3. Elevate the head of the bed.
○ 4. Keep the client turned on the operative side.

96 If moderate amounts of straw-colored fluid are noted on the surgical dressing, this indicates
○ 1. continued bleeding from the aneurysm.
○ 2. an infection.
○ 3. the aneurysm has been effectively sealed off.
○ 4. leakage of cerebrospinal fluid.

97 At a nursing conference a nurse assistant asks why Mr. Bell is receiving only 1000 mL of intravenous

fluid per day and is still not to take anything orally. The most correct answer is based on the fact that

- ○ 1. fluids are limited to reestablish kidney function.
- ○ 2. an intentional fluid volume deficit is ordered to prevent cerebral edema.
- ○ 3. neurosurgical clients are given excessive amounts of intravenous fluids during surgery.
- ○ 4. a fluid volume excess is ordered to prevent further bleeding from the aneurysm.

98 Twelve hours after surgery Mr. Bell develops edema around his eyes and is unable to see. Which one of the following measures might the nurse use to prevent Mr. Bell from becoming confused?

- ○ 1. Keep the lights on in his room day and night.
- ○ 2. Talk to him when entering the room.
- ○ 3. Leave the television or radio on day and night.
- ○ 4. Tell him to listen for things, and he will then know what is going on.

Two days after surgery the nurse is assigned to perform neurologic assessments on Mr. Bell.

99 Which one of the following observations would be considered a neurologic deficit?

- ○ 1. Difficulty swallowing and speaking
- ○ 2. Depression
- ○ 3. Mild headache
- ○ 4. Inability to move both lower extremities

100 Mr. Bell is now receiving 2500 mL of intravenous fluid every 24 hours. How many milliliters of intravenous fluid should the nurse plan to give every 8 hours?

- ○ 1. 255 mL
- ○ 2. 530 mL
- ○ 3. 833 mL
- ○ 4. 1000 mL

NURSING CARE OF CLIENTS WITH A BRAIN TUMOR

Ms. Eva Curtis has been diagnosed as having a large brain tumor in the right parietal lobe. A craniotomy is performed. Ms. Curtis leaves surgery with a head dressing. No tubes or drains have been inserted in the surgical incision. Not all of the tumor could be removed, and Ms. Curtis is scheduled for future radiation and chemotherapy.

101 Following surgery Ms. Curtis is transported to the postanesthesia recovery room. Which one of the following tasks is performed in the recovery room to provide a data base for ongoing assessments of this client?

- ○ 1. Reviewing the client's health history
- ○ 2. Obtaining a complete neurologic assessment
- ○ 3. Reviewing preadmission laboratory tests
- ○ 4. Checking to determine if the client has pain

Ms. Curtis has returned from the postoperative recovery room.

102 Which position is contraindicated for this client?

- ○ 1. Elevation of the head of the bed
- ○ 2. Lying on her right side
- ○ 3. Lying on her left side
- ○ 4. Lying supine

103 The physician orders Ms. Curtis' surgical dressing to be reinforced as needed. Which one of the following techniques is used to reinforce this client's surgical dressing?

- ○ 1. Sterile dressings and aseptic technique
- ○ 2. Sterile dressings and clean technique
- ○ 3. Clean dressings and aseptic technique
- ○ 4. Clean dressings and clean technique

Ms. Curtis has developed cerebral edema, and the physician orders an osmotic diuretic.

104 Which one of the following tasks should be performed when the client receives an osmotic diuretic?

- ○ 1. Observe the client for signs of hypernatremia.
- ○ 2. Turn and position the client every 2 hours.
- ○ 3. Measure spinal fluid pressure.
- ○ 4. Measure the urinary output at more frequent intervals.

105 Ms. Curtis has moderately severe left-sided weakness. Once rehabilitation is allowed, the nurse should

- ○ 1. encourage the client to perform passive exercises for both arms.
- ○ 2. feed the client until both sides are equal in strength.
- ○ 3. encourage the client to exercise her left arm using her right arm and hand.
- ○ 4. encourage the client to ambulate by herself at more frequent intervals.

Ms. Curtis is discharged from the hospital and is receiving radiation therapy on an outpatient basis.

106 On a visit to her physician's office Ms. Curtis states that she has begun to lose her hair. Which one of the following may the nurse recommend to Ms. Curtis?

- ○ 1. Wear a wig.
- ○ 2. Do not go out during daytime hours.
- ○ 3. Apply a skin-softening lotion to the scalp.
- ○ 4. Wash the hair daily.

Ms. Curtis finishes radiation therapy and begins chemotherapy.

107 During a visit to the oncologist's office, Ms. Curtis complains of soreness in her mouth. Which one of the following may the nurse recommend to Ms. Curtis?

○ 1. Use a stiff tooth brush to remove accumulated food from the teeth.

○ 2. Rinse the mouth with mouth wash.

○ 3. Avoid drinking water except at meals.

○ 4. Eat a soft, bland diet.

NURSING CARE OF CLIENTS WITH A CEREBROVASCULAR ACCIDENT

Mr. Robert Cranston, age 79, is admitted to the hospital with a possible cerebrovascular accident (CVA, stroke). Initial examination by the physician detects right-sided weakness and possible right-sided paralysis, an elevated blood pressure, and a decreased level of consciousness.

108 When performing an initial assessment on Mr. Cranston, the nurse should know that if a client has had a CVA,

○ 1. paralysis is always present.

○ 2. the onset of symptoms is almost always gradual.

○ 3. signs and symptoms depend on the area of the brain affected by the CVA.

○ 4. unconsciousness is rarely seen immediately after a CVA.

The nurse is assigned to help develop a plan of care for Mr. Cranston.

109 Which one of the following has the *highest* priority for planning short- and long-term rehabilitation goals for Mr. Cranston?

○ 1. Preventing bowel and bladder incontinence

○ 2. Preventing contractures and joint deformities

○ 3. Establishing bowel regularity

○ 4. Creating a positive atmosphere

110 The nurse in charge enters a nursing diagnosis of *Ineffective airway clearance related to decreased level of consciousness and inability to swallow* on Mr. Cranston's record. When developing a plan of care, the nurse should check to see that

○ 1. Mr. Cranston is kept in a supine position.

○ 2. the pillow is removed from beneath Mr. Cranston's head.

○ 3. Mr. Cranston receives adequate oral fluids.

○ 4. a suction machine is in the room.

111 The physician orders range-of-motion exercises to be performed by the nurse. Unless ordered otherwise, these exercises are performed

○ 1. on the paralyzed side.

○ 2. on the affected and unaffected sides.

○ 3. once daily, after morning care.

○ 4. in the evening.

112 Mr. Cranston begins to respond to his surroundings but at times appears confused and disoriented. Which one of the following nursing tasks may help Mr. Cranston?

○ 1. Give Mr. Cranston a newspaper to read.

○ 2. Tell Mr. Cranston that he will soon know where he is.

○ 3. Encourage family members to talk less to Mr. Cranston because he may become more confused.

○ 4. State the day of the week, month, and year each time a health team member enters Mr. Cranston's room.

113 The nurse assistant asks the nurse why planning special care of Mr. Cranston's skin is so important. The most appropriate reply is based on the fact that Mr. Cranston

○ 1. is unable to move about in bed.

○ 2. most probably has a fluid volume deficit.

○ 3. is older and therefore skin breakdown cannot be avoided.

○ 4. is confused.

Mr. Cranston has difficulty speaking and being understood. He also has some movement in his right arm and leg.

114 When it is necessary to ask Mr. Cranston one or more questions, the nurse may improve communication with Mr. Cranston by

○ 1. asking questions that require a yes or no answer.

○ 2. having the family try to interpret Mr. Cranston's answers to questions.

○ 3. asking Mr. Cranston to think and speak slowly so his responses can be understood.

○ 4. referring Mr. Cranston to a speech therapist.

115 After the acute phase has passed, how may the nurse develop a plan of care that focuses on Mr. Cranston's self-care deficit?

○ 1. Ask Mr. Cranston what he would like to do for himself.

○ 2. Evaluate his ability to perform ADL.

○ 3. Talk to Mr. Cranston's family to determine what they want him to do.

○ 4. Ask the physician if Mr. Cranston needs physical therapy.

116 Mr. Cranston has right-sided weakness and appears to be able to feed himself but has difficulty holding a fork between his fingers. Which one of the following may be used to improve Mr. Cranston's ability to eat?

○ 1. Use a fork with a curved handle placed on the hand below the knuckles.

○ 2. Serve only high-calorie liquid foods.

○ 3. Have Mr. Cranston use a tablespoon instead of a fork.

○ 4. Cut all his food into small pieces.

117 When assisting Mr. Cranston with ADL, he should

○ 1. not be left alone when washing or eating.

○ 2. not be allowed to use his unaffected side.

○ 3. be discouraged from using his affected side.

○ 4. be allowed to do as much as he can.

Mr. Cranston is to be discharged to his home.

118 Which one of the following may the nurse use to help the family adjust to present and future problems that may occur?

○ 1. Provide a list of public and private agencies that may assist with home care.

○ 2. Encourage the family to be totally responsible for Mr. Cranston.

○ 3. Advise Mr. Cranston that he must cooperate with his family.

○ 4. Discuss the average cost of the home improvements necessary to care for Mr. Cranston.

NURSING CARE OF CLIENTS WITH A SPINAL CORD INJURY

Mr. Stanley Everett, age 29, suffered a spinal cord injury and an injury to his chest and right arm in an automobile accident. Emergency medical personnel are called to treat and then transport Mr. Everett to the hospital. He is brought to the hospital and complains of severe pain in his chest and arms and being unable to move his legs.

119 Two nurses are volunteer members of an emergency medical unit. When Mr. Everett is removed from the scene of the accident and placed on an ambulance stretcher, he should be

○ 1. placed in a seated position to prevent airway obstruction.

○ 2. positioned on a firm, hard board that is placed on top of the stretcher.

○ 3. rolled onto the stretcher.

○ 4. lifted by two people onto a stretcher that has a soft mattress.

Following diagnostic x-rays and physicial examination, the physician states that Mr. Everett has had a severe spinal cord injury in the lumbar region.

120 Which one of the following is a *primary* goal when developing a care plan for Mr. Everett?

○ 1. Keep visitors to a minimum.

○ 2. Maintain alignment of his spine.

○ 3. Start him on sips of water to maintain fluid balance.

○ 4. Turn him every 4 hours.

121 The physician orders meperidine (Demerol) 50 mg intramuscularly for pain associated with injuries above the waist. Which one of the following muscles should be used for injecting this medication?

○ 1. Deltoid

○ 2. Dorsogluteal

○ 3. Vastus lateralis

○ 4. Ventrogluteal

122 The nurse is assigned to assess Mr. Everett for evidence of spinal shock. Which of the following may indicate this problem has occurred?

○ 1. Tachycardia, mild hypotension, increased respiratory rate

○ 2. Abdominal distention, hypertension, fever

○ 3. Spastic paralysis, incontinence, mental confusion

○ 4. Bradycardia, pronounced hypotension, decreased respiratory rate

123 Plans for rehabilitation of the client with a spinal cord injury are begun immediately after admission to the hospital and focus primarily on

○ 1. telling the client he must learn to accept the effects of the injury.

○ 2. making the client as comfortable as possible.

○ 3. strengthening and making the most use of unparalyzed areas.

○ 4. finding the type of wheelchair most suited to the client's preinjury activities.

124 During rehabilitation Mr. Everett asks the nurse why drinking extra fluids is important. The most correct answer is based on the fact that an increased fluid intake

○ 1. prevents kidney stones and bladder infections.

○ 2. maintains a normal fluid volume in body cells.

○ 3. prevents diarrhea.

○ 4. prevents skin breakdown at pressure sites.

125 Which one of the following may help Mr. Everett increase physical strength in his arms during rehabilitation following the acute phase of his injury?

○ 1. Encourage movement of the upper extremities.

○ 2. Have him practice isometric exercises of the lower extremities.

○ 3. Have him practice getting in and out of a chair.

○ 4. Encourage the use of an overhead bar or a trapeze.

126 A nurse assistant asks the nurse if normal function is returning to Mr. Everett's legs because she noted that his legs periodically move. The most correct answer is based on the fact that these movements most likely are

○ 1. the result of a flaccid paralysis.

○ 2. an indication that the spinal cord is healing.

○ 3. an indication that the client will regain some movement in the lower extremities.

○ 4. spastic, involuntary muscle spasms.

NURSING CARE OF CLIENTS WITH MULTIPLE SCLEROSIS

Ms. Wilma Jackson, age 31, has had multiple sclerosis for 6 years. She is admitted to the hospital because of

the development of decubitus ulcers on her sacrum and hip.

127 When developing a plan of care, the nurse should know that management of Ms. Jackson will
○ 1. depend on the abilities and skills of all health team members.
○ 2. include total physical care.
○ 3. depend on her symptoms and severity of her disease.
○ 4. include recognition that the disease is curable when diagnosed early.

128 When performing an initial assessment, the nurse notes that Ms. Jackson has footdrop. Which one of the following may be used to prevent further development of this problem?
○ 1. A footboard
○ 2. A trocanter roll
○ 3. Sheepskin boots
○ 4. A knee-to-hip brace

129 Ms. Jackson occasionally is incontinent. The physician orders a bladder training program. Which one of the following is the *first* step in a bladder training program?
○ 1. Ask the client if she wishes to be continent.
○ 2. Keep a record of actual voiding times for a 2- to 3-day period.
○ 3. Obtain an adequate supply of incontinent pads.
○ 4. Place the client on the bedpan every 4 to 6 hours.

130 When a bladder training program is instituted, Ms. Jackson is encouraged to
○ 1. limit her fluid intake.
○ 2. drink 2000 to 3000 mL of fluid daily.
○ 3. eat a diet high in bulk-producing foods.
○ 4. drink fluids only in the morning.

INDIVIDUAL TEST ITEMS

131 The nurse reviews a client's record to develop a care plan. The record states that the client has dysphasia, which should alert the nurse that the client has
○ 1. weakness in one extremity.
○ 2. difficulty speaking.
○ 3. paralysis on one side of the body.
○ 4. difficulty swallowing.

132 A nurse assists the physician performing a lumbar puncture. Which one of the following is the correct procedure for sending the tubes containing spinal fluid to the laboratory?
○ 1. Notify the laboratory, and refrigerate the tubes until they are picked up by laboratory personnel.
○ 2. Notify the laboratory, and place the tubes in a plastic tray at the bedside.

○ 3. Notify the laboratory, and place the tubes in a warming oven until they are picked up by laboratory personnel.
○ 4. Take the tubes to the laboratory immediately.

133 An order is written for 10 mg of morphine intramuscularly for pain. The adult client has meningitis. The nurse should question this order based on the fact that
○ 1. morphine rarely relieves the pain associated with meningitis.
○ 2. this is twice the normal dose of morphine.
○ 3. narcotics usually are contraindicated because they interfere with accurate neurologic assessments.
○ 4. morphine has high addiction potential.

134 The nurse is assigned to help develop a care plan for a client with Guillain-Barré syndrome. When planning care the nurse should know that treatment of this disorder
○ 1. is primarily supportive.
○ 2. involves the administration of large doses of antibiotics.
○ 3. is aimed at preventing spinal cord involvement.
○ 4. involves placing the client on stool and body fluid precautions.

135 Which one of the following should the nurse plan to include in a bowel training program for a client with a neurologic deficit?
○ 1. Administer an enema 1 hour after each meal.
○ 2. Encourage a diet high in foods that produce bulk.
○ 3. Limit the fluid intake to 500 mL/day to avoid diarrhea.
○ 4. Withhold the prescribed stool softener unless the client is constipated.

136 A nurse assistant notes that a client has a history of transient ischemic attacks (TIAs) and during a nursing conference asks the nurse what the symptoms of this disorder are. The most correct answer is
○ 1. fever, rash, and diarrhea.
○ 2. lightheadedness, numbness, and weakness or paralysis of one or more extremities.
○ 3. hypotension, joint pain, and headache.
○ 4. memory loss, depression, and abdominal pain.

137 The nurse participates in a nursing conference about a client with muscular dystrophy. A nurse assistant asks what the signs and symptoms of this disorder are. The most correct answer is
○ 1. joint enlargement and pain.
○ 2. progressive muscular weakness and wasting.
○ 3. muscle enlargement and tenderness.
○ 4. paralysis and fever.

138 Mr. Lake has trigeminal neuralgia. Which one of the following should the nurse include in a care plan for this client?

○ 1. Use care to prevent excessive stimulation of trigger areas.
○ 2. Encourage Mr. Lake to brush his teeth after eating.
○ 3. Encourage Mr. Lake to lie on the affected side.
○ 4. Use a mild, unscented soap for morning care.

139 Ms. James has been diagnosed as having myasthenia gravis. To develop a care plan for Ms. James the nurse should know that the primary symptom of this disease is
○ 1. hypotension.
○ 2. muscle weakness.
○ 3. paralysis on one side of the body.
○ 4. diarrhea.

140 Mr. Atkins has Bell's palsy. Which one of the following is the most correct addition to a care plan for Mr. Atkins?
○ 1. After each meal the inside of the client's mouth is checked for injury or particles of food.
○ 2. The prescribed antibiotic is given parenterally.
○ 3. Range-of-motion exercises are performed on the affected extremity.
○ 4. A clear liquid diet is necessary until movement returns.

Correct Answers and Rationale

Two numbers appear in parentheses following each rationale. The first number identifies the textbook listed in the references, page 451, and the second number identifies the page(s) in that textbook on which the correct answer can be verified. Occasionally, two textbooks are given for verifying the correct answer.

The Nursing Care of Clients with Disorders of the Reproductive System

CARING FOR A CLIENT WITH BREAST CANCER

1 1. An aspiration biopsy is often performed on an outpatient basis. A local anesthetic is injected, and a needle and syringe are used to remove a small sample of tissue. (14:911; 16:665)
Nursing Process—Implementation
Client Need—Safe, effective care environment

2 4. A modified radical mastectomy is the removal of the breast and axillary lymph nodes. A partial mastectomy is the removal of the tumor and a small amount of breast tissue. A radical mastectomy is the removal of the breast, axillary lymph nodes, and pectoral muscle. A subcutaneous mastectomy is the removal of breast tissue while leaving the skin and nipple intact. (16:699)
Nursing Process—Planning
Client Need—Physiological integrity

3 2. Edema (lymphedema) of the arm on the operative side may be seen when the lymph nodes are removed during a modified radical mastectomy. Edema of the lower extremities is normally not seen with this type of surgery. Lymph node enlargement would not be seen because the lymph nodes have been removed. The client will not be able to move her arm on the operative side for several days after surgery because of the extensive surgery and type of postoperative dressing. This is normal. When the wound begins to heal, arm movement is encouraged. (16:701)
Nursing Process—Evaluation
Client Need—Physiological integrity

4 2. The operative side (in this client the left side) is never used to monitor the blood pressure or pulse or start an intravenous infusion. The unoperative side (in this client the right side) may be used to take a pulse and blood pressure and to start an intravenous infusion. (16:701)
Nursing Process—Implementation
Client Need—Physiological integrity

5 2. Clients having a modified radical mastectomy normally have a restrictive (pressure) dressing applied. This type of dressing prevents movement of the chest muscles and thus reduces lung capacity until the dressing is removed. Having the client take deep breaths and encouraging coughing every 2 hours is of major importance in the prevention of respiratory problems, such as atelectasis and hypostatic pneumonia. (16:702)
Nursing Process—Implementation
Client Need—Safe, effective care environment

6 2. The primary purpose of supporting and elevating the arm of the operative side during the immediate postoperative period is to help prevent edema of the arm and fingers. Supporting and elevating the arm is not likely to prevent contractures or hemorrhage during the *immediate* postoperative period. The lymph nodes have been removed. (16:702)
Nursing Process—Implementation
Client Need—Safe, effective care environment

7 3. It is most important that postmastectomy exercises be practiced on a regular basis. These exercises are necessary to prevent contractures and restore function to the operative side. A prosthesis usually is not recommended until full healing takes place. The physician determines when a prosthesis can be fitted and worn. The type of prosthesis the client wears is an individual preference; no one type appears to be superior. Restricting the water intake will not prevent lymphedema. (16:703-704)
Nursing Process—Implementation
Client Need—Safe, effective care environment

8 4. The incision and area around the incision may be gently washed using a soft washcloth and a mild soap and water. Ointments or creams are not applied to the area unless this practice is approved or recommended by the physician. Wearing sterile gloves when washing the operative area is not necessary. (16:703)
Nursing Process—Implementation
Client Need—Safe, effective care environment

9 4. Because the client is 32 years old, BSE is performed every month, 1 week after the end of

menstruation. When a client is past menopause, BSE should be performed on a selected date each month, for example the first day of the month. (3:734-735)
    Nursing Process—Planning
    Client Need—Health promotion/maintenance

10 2. Standing in front of a mirror helps the client detect any physical breast changes, such as redness, changes in the nipple, or dimpling of the skin. This client had a left mastectomy and is being instructed to examine the right breast. Additional parts of the BSE include lying on the back and placing the right arm up with the hand behind the head when palpating the right breast and axilla. For those with both breasts, this is repeated for the left side. Lying on the abdomen, performing the entire examination while lying on the back, or sitting when palpating the breast are not recommended methods of BSE. (3:734-735)
    Nursing Process—Implementation
    Client Need—Health promotion/maintenance

11 4. The pads of the four fingertips are used to feel for breast abnormalities during a BSE. (3:735)
    Nursing Process—Implementation
    Client Need—Health promotion/maintenance

NURSING CARE OF CLIENTS HAVING A HYSTERECTOMY

12 3. Menorrhagia, or heavy bleeding at the time of menstruation, is one of the more common symptoms of uterine fibroids. (16:686)
    Nursing Process—Collecting data
    Client Need—Physiologic integrity

13 3. The female urethra is approximately 1½ to 2 inches long. Inserting the catheter 2 to 3 inches places the tip of the catheter into the bladder and urine should flow. Once urine flows, the catheter is advanced another ½ to 1 in to ensure that the balloon of the indwelling catheter is well past the bladder neck. (18:518-519)
    Nursing Process—Implementation
    Client Need—Physiological integrity

14 4. Antiembolic stockings should be removed and reapplied every 8 hours. (16:694)
    Nursing Process—Planning
    Client Need—Safe, effective care environment

15 1. The most appropriate nursing diagnosis for this client is related to the respiratory system (eg, ineffective airway clearance). Hyperthermia rather than hypothermia is more likely to occur if an infection is present. An elevated blood glucose level would not be seen unless the client has diabetes mellitus. A decreased metabolic

rate is more likely seen in those with hypothyroidism. (16:692-693)
    Nursing Process—Implementation
    Client Need—Safe, effective care environment

16 3. Severe back pain following a hysterectomy is unusual and must be reported to the physician immediately. While the cause is determined by the physician, this type of pain may be due to an accidental ligation of one or both ureters during surgery. If this is the cause of the pain, surgical intervention, which may involve the insertion of a nephrostomy tube, may be necessary. (16:693)
    Nursing Process—Evaluation
    Client Need—Physiological integrity

17 2. Following removal of an indwelling urethral catheter, the client's urine output is measured after each voiding. Failure to void or voiding in frequent, small amounts is brought to the attention of the physician. (16:693)
    Nursing Process—Implementation
    Client Need—Physiological Integrity

18 2. Heavy lifting, sexual intercourse, vigorous activity, and douching are examples of things to avoid after an abdominal hysterectomy. Once the physician gives permission, these activities can be resumed. (16:695)
    Nursing Process—Planning
    Client Need—Safe, effective care environment

NURSING CARE OF CLIENTS WITH BENIGN PROSTATIC HYPERTROPHY

19 4. Many physicians feel that rapid emptying of a markedly distended bladder could result in moderate to severe hypotension, hematuria, and loss of large amounts of sodium in the urine. When the bladder is to be emptied slowly over a prescribed period, a clamp is placed on the catheter and opened at scheduled intervals (such as every 10 minutes) for a brief period of time. (16:710)
    Nursing Process—Implementation
    Client Need—Physiological integrity

20 1. Clients displaying extreme fear and apprehension are poor surgical risks because they are prone to complications, such as cardiac arrest and irreversible shock during or immediately after surgery. (16:157)
    Nursing Process—Collecting data
    Client Need—Safe, effective care environment

21 3. When more than one of any type of urinary drainage catheter is placed in a client, *each* catheter is connected to a separate closed drainage system unless the physician orders a different method of collecting urinary drainage. Urinary

collection devices are always placed below the level of the bed, as urine drains from the bladder by means of gravity. The cystostomy catheter is never clamped unless an order to clamp the tube is written by the physician. (16:711)
Nursing Process—Implementation
Client Need—Physiological integrity

22 2. Rectal temperatures are avoided for the first postoperative week when a client has had prostatic surgery. Inserting a rectal thermometer may result in perforation of the rectal mucosa and damage to the prostatic capsule, which has been left behind when the prostate is removed. The client has profuse diaphoresis; an axillary temperature might not be as accurate as an oral temperature. A thermometer cannot be used to take a tympanic membrane temperature; a special instrument must be used for this procedure. (16:712)
Nursing Process—Implementation
Client Need—Safe, effective care environment

23 3. Hematuria (blood in the urine) can result in the formation of blood clots that range in size from very small to large. The formation of many small clots or the presence of one or more large clots can obstruct the lumen of one or both catheters. It is most important that the nurse checks the patency of the catheters every 1 to 2 hours. More frequent observations may be needed if bleeding is heavy. Obstruction of a catheter results in urinary retention and possible damage to the operative site. (7:577)
Nursing Process—Implementation
Client Need—Safe, effective care environment

24 2. Clients with a urethral catheter in place often have the feeling they have to void even though their bladder is kept empty by a properly functioning urethral catheter. When the client pushes down to void, painful bladder spasms may occur. Turning on the side, taking deep breaths, or avoiding thinking about the discomfort or pain is not likely to relieve pain due to bladder spasms. (16:710)
Nursing Process—Implementation
Client Need—Safe, effective care environment

25 2. Unless the physician orders otherwise, indwelling catheters are irrigated with sterile, normal saline. (18:528)
Nursing Process—Implementation
Client Need—Physiological integrity

26 1. Extra fluids are encouraged when the client has an indwelling catheter. Unless the physician orders otherwise, the nurse should encourage the client to drink small amounts of fluid at frequent intervals. An increased fluid intake increases urinary output. An increased urine output reduces bladder irritation and keeps the catheter free of blood clots and debris. (18:524-525; 16:712)
Nursing Process—Implementation
Client Need—Safe, effective care environment

27 2. Discharge teaching should include the warning to avoid heavy lifting and strenuous exercise until such activities are permitted by the physician. Constipation can be avoided by eating foods high in roughage; enemas are to be avoided. A liberal fluid intake is encouraged. (16:713)
Nursing Process—Implementation
Client Need—Safe, effective care environment

28 1. Kegel exercises may strengthen the perineal muscles and help control urinary incontinence. These exercises involve tightening the perineal muscles for 5 to 20 seconds and then relaxing these muscles for 5 to 20 seconds. These exercises should be performed 4 or more times per day and 5 to 20 times each session. In the beginning these exercises may cause mild discomfort in the operative area, and the client cannot tolerate performing more than one or two exercises each time. (16:713; 18:509)
Nursing Process—Implementation
Client Need—Health promotion/maintenance

NURSING CARE OF CLIENTS WITH CANCER OF THE PROSTATE GLAND

29 1. An enema empties the lower bowel of fecal material and prevents constipation during the immediate postoperative period. During the initial postoperative period, clients having this surgery experience moderate to severe pain, which may be increased with defecation. They have a tendency to try not to have a bowel movement and thus experience constipation. Several days after surgery, the client may attempt to strain when defecating because the stool present in the lower bowel has become hard. Straining may result in hemorrhage in the operative area. Emptying the lower bowel of stool before surgery and the normal restriction of food intake during the immediate postoperative period may eliminate this problem. (3:774)
Nursing Process—Implementation
Client Need—Health promotion/maintenance

30 4. Prostatic carcinomas tend to progress under the influence of the male hormone testosterone. The physician may decide to remove both testicles (bilateral orchiectomy) to reduce hormonal influence on any remaining tumor cells. (16:709)
Nursing Process—Implementation
Client Need—Health promotion/maintenance

31 1. Estrogen administration may not entirely prevent metastasis but may help to slow the development of metastatic lesions in areas such as the bones of the pelvis. Administration of these drugs also may keep the client with metastatic lesions reasonably comfortable for several years. The nurse may wish to explain to Mr. Barber that these drugs will make him feel more comfortable. (16:709)

Nursing Process—Implementation
Client Need—Psychosocial integrity

NURSING CARE OF CLIENTS WITH A SEXUALLY TRANSMITTED DISEASE

32 1. A sample of the urethral discharge from the male is immediately examined microscopically using the Gram's stain method. The diagnosis of gonorrhea cannot be confirmed by a urinalysis or a specimen of urine, laboratory (blood) test, or cystoscopy. A freshly voided urine specimen may be obtained at the time of the examination and examined for pus cells, white blood cells, or other abnormalities. The freshly voided urine specimen also may be stained and examined for the microorganism causing gonorrhea, but a urethral smear is more accurate. (16:85)

Nursing Process—Implementation
Client Need—Safe, effective care environment

33 3. Untreated gonorrhea in the female may result in inflammation of the pelvic organs (pelvic inflammatory disease, or PID) and sterility, plus the possibility of transmitting the disease to others. The other disorders mentioned in this question are not known to occur when gonorrhea is not treated or is treated inadequately. (7:166)

Nursing Process—Implementation
Client Need—Health promotion/maintenance

34 1. Probenecid is used in the treatment of gout, but it also has the ability to prolong the anti-infective activity of penicillin. Because treatment of gonorrhea with penicillin may consist of a one-time injection of 4.5 million U of aqueous procaine penicillin G, prolonging the activity of penicillin usually ensures eradication of the microorganism causing gonorrhea. Clients are told to return in 7 to 14 days for a repeat examination and urethral smear to be sure the microorganism has been eradicated. (15:315)

Nursing Process—Implementation
Client Need—Health promotion/maintenance

35 2. A total of 8 mL should be given in a divided injection (eg, 4 mL is injected into each site). Two syringes are used to withdraw the drug from the vial. Each syringe should contain 4 mL. Two separate sites for injection must be used, for example the left and right gluteus muscles. Injecting more than 5 mL in one injection site is not recommended. Although the deltoid muscle can be used for an intramuscular injection, a large muscle body, such as the gluteus muscle, is recommended when a larger volume, such as 4 mL, is to be injected. (15:19)

Nursing Process—Implementation
Client Need—Physiological integrity

36 4. A 90-degree angle is recommended for intramuscular injections because this places the medication into the muscle. A 45-degree angle is used for subcutaneous injections. (15:18-19)

Nursing Process—Implementation
Client Need—Physiological integrity

37 2. The fluorescent treponemal antibody absorption test requires the drawing of venous blood. The test is performed by a laboratory. (16:86; 5:464-466)

Nursing Process—Implementation
Client Need—Safe, effective care environment

38 2. Blood and body fluid precautions are normally used when caring for a client with AIDS. For this client protective or reverse isolation also may be used because the client is susceptible to any type of infection. Strict isolation is rarely necessary. (14:699; 18:358-360)

Nursing Process—Implementation
Client Need—Safe, effective care environment

39 1. At the present time it is believed that AIDS is spread by sexual contact with an infected individual; exposure to infected blood or blood products, such as human pooled plasma or whole blood; the sharing of (infected) needles among intravenous drug users; and transmission of the virus from an infected mother to her fetus. (7:167)

Nursing Process—Implementation
Client Need—Safe, effective care environment

40 4. Those with AIDS frequently develop opportunistic infections, that is, infections that result from a failure of the immune system. Examples of opportunistic infections include *Pneumocystis carinii* pneumonia, infectious diarrhea, oral fungal infections, cytomegalovirus infections, and other virus infections, such as herpes simplex. These infections occur because of a decrease in the white blood cells that fight infection. Anemia and medications taken for AIDS are not known to cause opportunistic infections. (16:87)

Nursing Process—Implementation
Client Need—Safe, effective care environment

INDIVIDUAL TEST ITEMS

41 2. Headache, nervousness, irritability, weight gain, personality changes, anxiety, increased physical

activity, breast pain or tenderness, swelling in the extremities, and abdominal bloating are examples of the more common symptoms of PMS. The other items in the question usually are not associated with PMS. (16:669)
Nursing Process—Collecting data
Client Need—Physiological integrity

42 3. An excessive menstrual flow is menorrhagia. Painful menstruation is dysmenorrhea. Bleeding that occurs between menstrual periods is metrorrhagia. Absence of menstruation is amenorrhea. (7:545)
Nursing Process—Planning
Client Need—Physiological integrity

43 1. Toxic shock syndrome has been linked to the use of tampons, especially super absorbent tampons. It has been suggested that tampons should be used only during the time of moderate to heavy flow, changed every 1 to 3 hours, and not used when the flow is light. The use of tampons at night also is not recommended. Taking a diuretic and avoiding the use of large sanitary pads are not preventive measures for this disorder. (7:545-546)
Nursing Process—Implementation
Client Need—Health promotion/maintenance

44 2. Clients having a pelvic examination are instructed to void immediately before the examination. An enema or laxative 1 or 2 days before the procedure normally is not necessary. All clothing should be removed, and a disposable examination gown should be worn because a breast examination is often performed at the same time. Douching is avoided for 2 or 3 days before the test. Fasting is not necessary for this examination. (7:547; 16:667)
Nursing Process—Implementation
Client Need—Safe, effective care environment

45 2. Genital warts are a sexually transmitted disease. There appears to be a relationship between genital warts and an increased risk of cancer of the vulva, vagina, and cervix. No treatment is presently available for a cure. The use of a condom is recommended until the warts disappear. (16:88)
Nursing Process—Implementation
Client Need—Health promotion/maintenance

46 1. Oral contraceptives should be taken at approximately the same time each day, preferably in the evening. They do not need to be taken on an empty stomach. An oral contraceptive is started on the fifth day of menstruation and, depending on the type used, is taken for 20 or 21 days. (16:672-673)
Nursing Process—Implementation
Client Need—Health promotion/maintenance

47 3. Normally, menstruation begins approximately 14 days after ovulation. (16:660)
Nursing Process—Collecting data
Client Need—Physiological integrity

48 1. The client is instructed to avoid douching for 2 to 3 days before having a Pap smear because douching would remove cells that are to be examined by a pathologist. The remaining options are not preparations required for this test. (16:667)
Nursing Process—Implementation
Client Need—Safe, effective care environment

49 4. Herpes cannot be cured; only the symptoms may be treated. Once an individual is infected, the virus remains in the body. Individuals with this infection may have periods when they have no symptoms and other periods when symptoms are present. Women with genital herpes must tell the physician caring for them during pregnancy that they have this infection because it can be a major threat to the baby. Some physicians prefer to deliver the newborn by cesarean section because passage of the baby through the birth canal (vagina) can result in infection of the infant. Antiviral drugs may relieve symptoms but cannot be used during pregnancy because of unknown effects on the fetus. (3:785)
Nursing Process—Planning
Client Need—Health promotion/maintenance

50 1. The laparoscopic procedure for sterilization usually is performed on an outpatient basis. Two small incisions are made in the abdomen. One incision is for the laparoscope and the other for the cautery, which will be used to destroy a section of the fallopian tubes and thus prevent the ascent of sperm into the fallopian tube. The consent of the sexual partner normally is not required for this procedure. (3:748-749)
Nursing Process—Implementation
Client Need—Safe, effective care environment

51 3. A regular bathtub can be used for a sitz bath, but a tub constructed for this purpose is more effective. A regular bathtub applies heat to the legs and alters the effect of heat directed primarily to the pelvic region. In a sitz bathtub heat is applied only to the pelvic region because the legs and feet remain outside of the water. (18:495)
Nursing Process—Implementation
Client Need—Safe, effective care environment

52 2. Following electrocauterization the client is told to avoid straining and heavy lifting because these activities may cause bleeding from the cauterized site. The physician usually reexamines the client in 2 to 4 weeks. Absolute bed rest is not necessary, but the client should rest more than usual. Douching is not done until permitted by the physician. (16:677-678)

Nursing Process—Implementation
Client Need—Health promotion/maintenance

53 1. The lithotomy position is normally used for vaginal examinations. (18:306-307)

Nursing Process—Implementation
Client Need—Safe, effective care environment

54 2. Endometriosis tissue resembling the endometrium is found outside of the uterus, such as on the ovaries and elsewhere in the abdominal or pelvic cavity. This tissue responds to hormonal influence and bleeds when the endometrium of the uterus does (eg, at the time of menstruation). Ectopic endometrial tissue bleeds into spaces having no outlet and thus causes irritation, inflammation, and pain. (16:680)

Nursing Process—Implementation
Client Need—Health promotion/maintenance

55 2. The Pap test is used primarily to detect cancer of the cervix. (16:663)

Nursing Process—Planning
Client Need—Health promotion/maintenance

56 4. Vaginal irrigations are performed with the client in bed or lying in a bathtub. In either area the client must be placed in a dorsal recumbent position. The temperature of the solution should be between 100.5°F and 110°F. The nozzle should not be lubricated with petroleum jelly because this or any other substance that is not water soluble can coat the vaginal wall and interfere with the solution flowing over vaginal tissue. (18:480)

Nursing Process—Implementation
Client Need—Physiological integrity

57 2. Directing the moistened cotton ball or washcloth downward from the pubic are to the anus prevents the introduction of bacteria from the anal area being introduced into the vagina or opening through which urine is released (urinary meatus). (18:97)

Nursing Process—Implementation
Client Need—Physiological integrity

58 1. A full bladder may cause discomfort during insertion of a vaginal medication, such as a suppository. The tip of the suppository may be lubricated with a water-soluble lubricant. Petroleum jelly is not water soluble and will coat the vaginal wall and prevent proper absorption of the drug. The applicator is inserted with a downward and backward motion. The applicator should be inserted approximately 3 to 4 inches before the plunger is depressed to release the drug into the vagina. (18:596)

Nursing Process—Implementation
Client Need—Physiological integrity

59 2. Intense vaginal and perineal itching are the most common signs of a vaginitis due to the fungus *Candida albicans*. Additional symptoms include a watery vaginal discharge that may contain cheesy particles. Occasionally urinary symptoms (dysuria, feeling the need to void frequently) may be seen if the mouth of the urethra is affected. (16:676-677)

Nursing Process—Implementation
Client Need—Health promotion/maintenance

60 1. The early symptoms of ovarian cancer usually are vague. Later, as the tumor enlarges, gastrointestinal symptoms and lower abdominal pain may be noted. Chemotherapy and surgery may be used to treat this type of cancer. The prognosis is poor. (7:557-558)

Nursing Process—Implementation
Client Need—Health promotion/maintenance

61 2. A hydrocele is a collection of a larger than normal amount of fluid in the space between the testis and tunica vaginalis. The physician may aspirate the fluid as a temporary measure, but surgery almost always necessary. Drug therapy or the wearing of a scrotal support will not cure the condition. (16:715)

Nursing Process—Implementation
Client Need—Safe, effective care environment

62 4. A cystoscopy enables the physician to visualize the urethra, bladder, and ureteral openings (orifices) into the bladder. The kidneys and ureters cannot be seen unless a radiopaque dye is injected intravenously and radiographs are taken. This procedure is then called a cystoscopy with retrograde pyelograms. (16:666)

Nursing Process—Implementation
Client Need—Safe, effective care environment

63 3. Live sperm may be present in the ejaculatory fluid for a period of time after a vasectomy. Birth control methods must be used until sperm counts are negative. Although the time varies, the ejaculatory fluid usually is negative for live sperm in approximately 1 to 2 months after a vasectomy. A vasectomy has no effect on testosterone production. A second minor surgical procedure is not needed to ensure that no sperm are present in the ejaculatory fluid. (3:777)

Nursing Process—Implementation
Client Need—Health promotion/maintenance

64 4. Testicular self-examination is best performed after a warm bath or shower when the scrotum is more relaxed. (7:574)

Nursing Process—Implementation
Client Need—Health promotion/maintenance

65 2. Testicular carcinoma has a high rate of early metastasis. Laboratory tests that may confirm the diagnosis include alphafetoprotein and total urine estrogens. When a lesion is detected, a biopsy usually is not performed because this procedure risks spreading highly malignant tumor cells. (16:715)

　　Nursing Process—Implementation
　　Client Need—Health promotion/maintenance

66 2. Transrectal ultrasonography is performed to detect cancer of the prostate. A probe that emits ultrasonic waves is introduced into the rectum. The physician observes the visual images projected on a screen similar to a television screen. This procedure is similar to a sonogram performed on a pregnant client. (3:768)

　　Nursing Process—Planning
　　Client Need—Safe, effective care environment

67 1. Male and female clients may experience difficulty talking about a sexual dysfunction, especially when a member of the health team is of the opposite sex. Beginning the conversation with a sensitive question, such as option 3, may create a barrier between the nurse and the client. Beginning the history with a question that is less sensitive (option 1) may create a more positive relationship between the nurse and the client. Options 2 and 4 are asking the client to make a diagnosis. (3:770)

　　Nursing Process—Implementation
　　Client Need—Psychosocial integrity

68 2. Retracting the foreskin is necessary to remove secretions and prevent infection and other problems. The foreskin is replaced after the area is cleansed. The scrotum can be washed with plain water or soap; normal saline is not necessary for this procedure. The anal area is washed after the penis and scrotum are cleansed. (18:97)

　　Nursing Process—Implementation
　　Client Need—Physiological integrity

69 2. Cancer of the penis is thought to be related to poor personal hygiene. When uncircumcised males fail to retract the foreskin and cleanse the area beneath the foreskin, an irritation develops and may predispose the individual to develop cancer in this area. A diet high in acidic foods, circumcision, and exercise are not known causes of penile cancer. (16:718)

　　Nursing Process—Implementation
　　Client Need—Health promotion/maintenance

70 4. Continuous bladder irrigation is used to keep the bladder and catheters free from clots. The color of the drainage from both catheters (urethral and cystostomic) is observed at frequent intervals, and the rate of flow is adjusted to keep the drainage a light pink. (16:712)

　　Nursing Process—Implementation
　　Client Need—Physiological integrity

71 3. Unless the physician orders otherwise, sterile normal saline is used for bladder and catheter irrigations. (16:712; 7:774)

　　Nursing Process—Implementation
　　Client Need—Physiological integrity

The Nursing Care of Clients with Disorders of the Neurologic System

NURSING CARE OF CLIENTS WITH A SEIZURE DISORDER

72 3. An EEG may take 1 to 2 hours and is performed in a quiet and darkened room to avoid distractions and possible interference with test results. The client is kept as quiet as possible. Normally, the blood pressure is not monitored during this procedure because this physical activity may interfere with test results. No physical preparation, for example as an enema or shaving, is necessary. (7:626)

　　Nursing Process—Implementation
　　Client Need—Safe effective care environment

73 3. When a client with known or suspected tonic-clonic (grand mal) seizures is placed on seizure precautions, the side rails are raised whenever the client is in bed. In addition the side rails should be padded with blankets secured to the bars. Other methods of padding the side rails also may be used. Padding the side rails prevents injury to the extremities if the client has a tonic-clonic seizure. This is especially important if seizures are frequent. Keeping the room brightly lit can be disturbing to the client and is not necessary. In some, seizures are precipitated by bright lights and noise. The door to the room should be left open so that the client can be observed at frequent intervals. (16:427)

　　Nursing Process—Implementation
　　Client Need—Safe, effective care environment

74 2. An aura, which is not experienced by all people with epilepsy, may occur shortly before a convulsive seizure. The aura may be sensory (sounds, smells) or a sensation, such as weakness or numbness in a certain part of the body. In those experiencing an aura, the aura is almost always the same. The type of aura experienced by the client is noted on the chart. (16:425)

　　Nursing Process—Collecting data
　　Client Need—Safe, effective care environment

75 4. When a client begins a tonic-clonic seizure while the nurse is in the room, the highest priority is establishing a patent airway. This can most easily be done by turning this client on her side, allowing saliva and vomitus (if present) to drain

from the mouth. Turning also prevents the tongue from blocking the airway. Insertion of an oral airway may be attempted, but when a client has a tonic-clonic seizure the jaw is usually clenched at the beginning of the seizure, making insertion of an airway difficult if not impossible. At no time should force be used to insert an oral airway. (16:427)
> Nursing Process—Implementation
> Client Need—Physiological integrity

76 1. Forcible restraint of the arms and legs can result in injury. Fractures, severe bruising, and damage to tissues under the skin can occur when the extremities are forcibly restrained. The client can be protected from injury by padded side rails. The nurse also can try to move the client's arm or leg gently away from an object that could cause injury or *gently* restrain one or more extremities without using extreme pressure or force. (16:427)
> Nursing Process—Implementation
> Client Need—Safe, effective care environment

77 1. Status epilepticus, a series of tonic-clonic seizures occurring without the client regaining consciousness, is a serious outcome that may occur if an anticonvulsant medication is omitted. (16:426-427)
> Nursing Process—Implementation
> Client Need—Physiological integrity

78 3. The Epilepsy Foundation of America has chapters in most large cities and is of great value in providing services such as counseling, low-cost prescription services, literature, and vocational guidance. While other agencies may offer some services that are of value, the Epilepsy Foundation is completely geared to helping those with this disorder. (16:428)
> Nursing Process—Implementation
> Client Need—Safe, effective care environment

NURSING CARE OF CLIENTS WITH PARKINSON'S DISEASE

79 1. Evaluation of the ability to carry out various ADL allows the nurse to decide which activities, such as dressing, walking, and eating, may or may not require assistance. Evaluation of intelligence and the client's financial status usually does not influence most decisions related to basic care. Food preferences may be of value, especially if the client eats poorly, but are less important than an evaluation of Ms. Grant's ability to carry out ADL. (16:421)
> Nursing Process—Collecting data
> Client Need—Physiological integrity

80 2. Active or passive range-of-motion exercises help prevent contractures that may occur because of

muscle rigidity associated with parkinsonism. Sitting in a chair, a high-protein diet, or an increased fluid intake will not prevent muscle contractures. (16:423)
> Nursing Process—Implementation
> Client Need—Physiological integrity

81 2. The abbreviation for twice a day medication administration is b.i.d. (18:576)
> Nursing Process—Implementation
> Client Need—Physiological integrity

82 4. Advising the client to take a few sips of water before placing the capsule in her mouth moistens the oral cavity and helps in swallowing an oral medication. Capsules are never softened by placing them in water before administration or having the client hold the capsule in the mouth. Capsules should not be punctured; this maneuver increases the absorption rate and may decrease the effectiveness of the drug. (15:17)
> Nursing Process—Implementation
> Client Need—Physiological integrity

83 4. Ms. Grant has moderately severe tremors and therefore would most likely find it very difficult to write. The other methods listed in the question may be of value in improving communication. (16:422-423)
> Nursing Process—Implementation
> Client Need—Safe effective care environment

84 1. Changing the client's position every 2 hours and giving meticulous skin care at the time of each position change may help prevent the formation of decubitus ulcers. A diet high in minerals and low in protein will not prevent skin breakdown. Applying lotion followed by the application of powder may cause caking of the powder and lead to further skin irritation and breakdown. (16:469)
> Nursing Process—Planning
> Client Need—Physiological integrity

85 4. Visually inspecting the skin, especially areas over bony prominences, is the best method of evaluating the effectiveness of skin care and looking for areas of potential or real impaired skin integrity. Some clients may have little or no feeling in areas of skin breakdown; therefore, asking the client if pain is noted would not be effective for these individuals. The function of a flotation pad or mattress should be checked, but this alone is not enough to detect areas of skin breakdown. It is the responsibility of the nurse in charge to determine if members of the health team are changing the client's position, but visual inspection remains the best method of identifying this problem. (16:469)
> Nursing Process—Evaluation
> Client Need—Physiological integrity

NURSING CARE OF CLIENTS WITH ALZHEIMER'S DISEASE

86 2. Memory loss, particularly of recent events and names, and behavioral disturbances are two of the more common early signs of Alzheimer's disease. (16:444)
Nursing Process—Collecting data
Client Need—Physiological integrity

87 2. Maintaining a structured daily routine rather than daily activities that constantly change often helps reduce the anxiety seen in those with Alzheimer's disease. Change often creates anxiety because the client has difficulty remembering events and becomes confused when the daily routine varies. Telling the client that things are different in a hospital or that she must follow hospital rules creates rather than relieves anxiety. Assigning a nurse assistant rather than a nurse to administer care would most likely have no affect on the client's level of anxiety. (16:444-445)
Nursing Process—Implementation
Client Need—Psychosocial integrity

88 4. Clients with Alzheimer's are often confused, have an impaired memory, and adapt poorly to change. By reducing confusing stimuli, such as noise and hurried activities, and using reality orientation, the client may maintain contact with reality. A quiet and pleasant environment, the absence of hurried activities, and a reduction in noise often help improve behavior. Some clients have difficulty with and are confused by being with others; therefore, eating meals with others and joining in recreational activities may cause additional confusion. Taking a nap or eating foods that are liked are not likely to change the client's behavior. (16:445)
Nursing Process—Implementation
Client Need—Psychosocial integrity

89 1. Limiting the fluid intake 1 to 3 hours before the client goes to bed may eliminate the need to rise during the night to void. Ambulating or participating in recreational activities would not decrease the need to void during the night. These clients usually are not given sedatives or hypnotics to help them sleep because administration of these drugs may cause confusion and disorientation. (16:445)
Nursing Process—Implementation
Client Need—Physiological integrity

90 3. Answering calls for assistance as soon as possible may eliminate or change Ms. Daniels' behavior. Warning her not to get out of bed will be of little value because these clients are confused and have short-term memory loss. Restraints may add to confusion and should not be applied unless they are absolutely necessary, and there is a physician's order to do so. Keeping the room dark also adds to confusion and creates a potential risk for the client and health team members. (16:445)
Nursing Process—Planning
Client Need—Safe, effective care environment

91 2. Those with Alzheimer's should not be allowed to leave home alone because they may become confused and lost. A family member must be present at all times because these clients should not be left alone or unsupervised. A high calorie diet is encouraged because many of these individuals eat poorly and lose weight. Short naps can be taken, but long naps during the day may result in the client being awake and confused at night. Those with Alzheimer's should be encouraged to participate in family activities until they are no longer physically able to do so. (16:445)
Nursing Process—Implementation
Client Need—Safe, effective care environment

NURSING CARE OF CLIENTS WITH A CEREBRAL ANEURYSM

92 4. Clients with a cerebral aneurysm are kept as quiet as possible because any activity may cause or increase bleeding. Placing the client on his affected side or monitoring blood glucose levels are not directly related to the management of a client with a cerebral aneurysm. (16:442-443)
Nursing Process—Planning
Client Need—Physiological integrity

93 2. A change in the level of consciousness is an important assessment that may determine an increase in intracranial pressure. The physician is notified immediately when *any* change in the level of consciousness occurs because emergency treatment may be necessary. (16:407-408)
Nursing Process—Collecting data
Client Need—Physiological integrity

94 1. The eye-opening response, best verbal response, and best motor response are the three parts of the Glasgow Coma Scale. (16:407-409)
Nursing Process—Collecting data
Client Need—Physiological integrity

95 3. Unless the physician orders otherwise, the head of the bed is elevated to prevent cerebral edema. (7:658)
Nursing Process—Implementation
Client Need—Physiological integrity

96 4. Cerebrospinal fluid is straw-colored (eg, pale yellow). Leakage of cerebrospinal fluid can be serious because loss of moderate to large amounts of spinal fluid removes the protective cushioning required by the structures (brain, meninges, nerves) in the cranial vault. Spinal fluid leakage also indicates that there is a communication between the subarachnoid space, where spinal fluid circulates, and the outside, which may result in an infection—a serious consequence of cranial surgery. If spinal fluid leakage is noted, the physician is notified immediately. (16:454)

> Nursing Process—Collecting data
> Client Need—Physiological integrity

97 2. An intentional fluid volume deficit, that is, the withholding of oral fluids and a low volume of intravenous fluids, may be ordered by the physician in an attempt to prevent cerebral edema. (16:454)

> Nursing Process—Implementation
> Client Need—Physiological integrity

98 2. Talking to the client when entering the room, touching him when talking to him, and explaining what is going on or what the nurse is doing in the room often helps to reduce confusion when the client is unable to see. Leaving the television or lights on will not reduce confusion and may even cause confusion. Asking the client to listen for sounds to understand what is happening is not appropriate during the immediate postoperative period. Edema around the eyes usually disappears in a few days, and the client should be able to see. (16:454)

> Nursing Process—Implementation
> Client Need—Safe, effective care environment

99 1. A neurologic deficit may be defined as a decrease in or absence of one or more functions of the nervous system. Difficulty swallowing and speaking, sensory impairments, and paralysis are examples of neurologic deficits. A mild headache during the first several days after a craniotomy is not unusual. Depression is most probably not a neurologic deficit; many of these clients become depressed when they think about their possible limitations following surgery. However, the client should be continually assessed for any change in his level of consciousness or any change in his emotional status. (7:658)

> Nursing Process—Collecting data
> Client Need—Physiological integrity

100 3. The total volume for 24 hours is 2500 mL. To determine the amount received in 8 hours, divide 2500 by 8. The answer is 833 (mL). (15:5; 16:134)

> Nursing Process—Planning
> Client Need—Physiological integrity

NURSING CARE OF CLIENTS WITH A BRAIN TUMOR

101 2. A complete neurologic assessment is performed immediately after a neurosurgical procedure and while the client is in the recovery room in order to provide a data base for future neurologic assessments during the postoperative period. This nursing task is extremely important and helps determine any major or minor change in the client's neurologic status. Reviewing the health history or preadmission laboratory tests does not provide a neurologic data base. Determining if the client has pain is only one part of a complete neurologic assessment. (16:452)

> Nursing Process—Collecting data
> Client Need—Physiological integrity

102 2. A craniotomy was performed on the right side because the tumor was located in the right parietal lobe. Because the tumor was large, this client is not positioned on her operative (right) side during the postoperative period because the space left by the removed tumor may cause a shift of the contents of the cranial vault. (7:658)

> Nursing Process—Implementation
> Client Need—Physiological integrity

103 1. Sterile dressing and aseptic technique are used to reinforce the surgical dressing following a craniotomy because the moist area can introduce microorganisms into the meninges. Introduction of microorganisms into the meninges can result in a serious and possibly life-threatening central nervous system infection. (16:454)

> Nursing Process—Implementation
> Client Need—Safe, effective care environment

104 4. An osmotic diruretic given to reduce cerebral edema requires more frequent measurement of the urinary output. The frequency of these measurements may depend on the physician's orders. If no order is written regarding the frequency of measurements, the nurse should measure the urinary output at least every 2 hours. Hyponatremia is more probable than hypernatremia (increased sodium in the blood). While turning and repositioning are necessary to prevent skin breakdown, this task is not related to the administration of an osmotic diuretic. Spinal fluid pressure can be measured only by the use of an intracranial monitoring device. The client description states that no tubes (eg, intracranial monitoring device or other types of equipment) or drains were inserted. (16:454)

> Nursing Process—Implementation
> Client Need—Physiological integrity

105 3. Passive exercises to the affected side can be performed by this client once she has been shown how to perform these exercises. Because the weakness may be permanent, feeding the client until both sides are equal in strength is not appropriate. If the client is right-handed, she may be able to feed herself, provided her food is pre-

pared (eg, cut-up, containers opened). Passive exercises would be performed only on the affected side; active exercises can be performed on the unaffected side. Ambulatory activities can only be performed with assistance, because the left side is weak. (16:472)
Nursing Process—Implementation
Client Need—Physiological integrity

106 1. A wig, cap, or scarf may be used to disguise hair thinning or hair loss. Lotions or frequent hair washing are not recommended and should be used only if permitted by the physician. Unless prohibited by the physician, outside activities during daylight hours are allowed. (16:212)
Nursing Process—Implementation
Client Need—Psychosocial integrity

107 4. Eating a soft, bland diet may decrease irritation and soreness in the mouth. If this condition becomes severe, the physician may prescribe a local anesthetic gel. A soft toothbrush is recommended to clean the teeth. Oral rinses with warm water may be used; mouthwashes may contain alcohol and thus further irritate the mouth. Frequent rinses with water or sips of water may help relieve dryness and soreness. (16:212)
Nursing Process—Implementation
Client Need—Safe, effective care environment

NURSING CARE OF CLIENTS WITH A CEREBROVASCULAR ACCIDENT

108 3. Signs and symptoms of a CVA depend on the area of the brain affected and may include numbness, weakness, paralysis, loss of speech, blurred vision, and tingling. Paralysis occurs when motor areas of the brain are affected and may or may not be present. Symptoms usually occur suddenly and without warning. Unconsciousness may occur and is usually seen after a severe cerebral hemorrhage. (16:437)
Nursing Process—Collecting data
Client Need—Physiological integrity

109 2. This client has weakness and possible paralysis on his right side. Because of a neurologic motor deficit, preventing contractures and joint deformities has the highest priority in the development of short- and long-term rehabilitation goals. If the client is to attain maximum results from a rehabilitation program, contractures and joint deformities, which can become permanent, will interfere with the attainment of these goals. The remaining items in this question also may be goals but usually are of a lesser priority. (16:439)
Nursing Process—Planning
Client Need—Physiological integrity

110 4. The airway of the semicomatose client must be kept clear at all times. One possible symptom of a CVA is difficulty swallowing, with the client unable to handle respiratory and oral secretions. Suctioning may be necessary to maintain a patent airway until the client is more alert and able to handle respiratory and oral secretions. Keeping the client in a supine position may block the oral airway. Removing the pillow beneath the head usually is not necessary, but a smaller pillow can be substituted for the normal-sized pillow. Adequate fluids are necessary, but Mr. Cranston is semicomatose and therefore would probably be unable to swallow oral fluids. Giving oral fluids poses a danger of aspiration. (16:439)
Nursing Process—Planning
Client Need—Physiological integrity

111 2. Range-of-motion exercises are performed on the affected (paralyzed) and unaffected sides, with equal time given to each side. This is especially important when the client is semicomatose or comatose. The number of times per day these exercises are performed varies, but they should be performed at least three times a day. If the client is responsive, he is encouraged to perform active range-of-motion exercises on the unaffected side. (16:439-440)
Nursing Process—Implementation
Client Need—Physiological integrity

112 4. Stating the day of the week, month, and year each time entering the room is part of reality orientation and may help this client become more aware of his surroundings. Giving this client a newspaper to read at this time is inappropriate because he may have visual problems or still may be somewhat disoriented. Telling the client he will soon know where he is or encouraging family members not to engage in conversations with the client is not appropriate. (16:440)
Nursing Process—Implementation
Client Need—Psychosocial integrity

113 1. Being unable to move normally about in bed during waking and sleeping hours increases the possibility that the client will have impaired skin integrity and skin breakdown. Clients of any age will incur skin breakdown if their position is not changed at frequent and regular intervals. A position change is recommended every 2 hours, day and night. (16:468-469, 471-472)
Nursing Process—Planning
Client Need—Physiological integrity

114 1. When a client has difficulty speaking and being understood, an effort must be made to improve communication. One method that may be used is asking questions that require a yes or no answer. The client can then be instructed to nod or shake his head when responding to a question. The family may not be always present when the nurse wishes to ask the client a question. Asking the client to think and speak slowly usually will not improve communication when the client has incurred damage to the speech center of the brain. While the physician may refer the client to a speech therapist, the nurse should attempt to use other methods of improving communication. (16:475)

Nursing Process—Implementation
Client Need—Safe, effective care environment

115   2. The nurse can develop a plan of care focused on the areas of self-care that may be improved by evaluating what the client is or is not able to do. Areas that may be covered are eating with or without assistance, dressing, grooming, washing, and so on. Once it is determined what the client cannot do, an effort is made to improve these areas. Asking the client or his family what he or they would like him to do does not identify areas of strengths and weaknesses. The physician determines if physical therapy will be of value in improving the ability to administer self-care. (16:473)

Nursing Process—Evaluation
Client Need—Safe, effective care environment

116   1. A fork with a curved handle and fitting over the hand below the knuckles eliminates the need to hold a fork with the fingers. This type of device, which can be made or purchased, provides support to the eating utensil. The shoulder muscles are used to raise and lower the fork and pick up food. The remaining items in this question would not be of value in helping this client eat with a fork. (16:472)

Nursing Process—Implementation
Client Need—Health promotion/maintenance

117   4. When performing ADL, clients should be allowed to do as much as they can but also should be assisted with tasks they find difficult. Leaving the client alone often reduces anxiety as he tries to perform those tasks that were once performed without thinking. The client is encouraged to use the unaffected side and encouraged to use his weakened extremity as much as possible. By using the affected (weakened) extremity, the client is performing active range-of-motion exercises. (16:473)

Nursing Process—Implementation
Client Need—Health promotion/maintenance

118   1. Providing a list of agencies that may assist with home care may help the family deal with the emotional and physical conflicts that arise when a disabled family member is cared for at home. When families know that there are others they can turn to for help, they may be more able to accept the responsibilities of home care. (16:475)

Nursing Process—Implementation
Client Need—Safe, effective care environment

NURSING CARE OF CLIENTS WITH A SPINAL CORD INJURY

119   2. Great care must be exercised in moving and lifting those with a known or suspected spinal cord injury. Four to five people are necessary to lift the victim onto a firm, hard board that is then placed on the stretcher. The victim's back, neck, and head are kept in straight alignment. To immobilize the head and neck, a cervical collar usually is applied at this time. (7:651)

Nursing Process—Implementation
Client Need—Physiological integrity

120   2. Of the four options in this question, the most important and thus a primary goal is maintaining alignment of the spine to prevent further injury to the spinal cord. (7:652; 3:345)

Nursing Process—Planning
Client Need—Physiological integrity

121   1. When a medication is administered by the subcutaneous or intramuscular route to the client with paraplegia, the injection is given *above* the level of paralysis. Delayed and erratic absorption may occur when intramuscular injections are given below the waist and into tissue affected by paralysis. The deltoid muscle must be chosen in this question because the other sites listed are below the waist. (16:458; 15:19)

Nursing Process—Implementation
Client Need—Physiological integrity

122   4. Signs and symptoms of spinal shock include bradycardia, pronounced hypotension, decreased respiratory rate, decreased temperature, flaccid paralysis, and warm, dry skin. (16:456-457)

Nursing Process—Collecting data
Client Need—Physiological integrity

123   3. When paralysis is determined to be permanent, management of the client focuses on preventing disabilities and strengthening areas that are not affected by the injury. This client has paralysis below the waist; therefore, rehabilitation is aimed at strengthening areas above the waist, namely the arms, chest muscles, and respiratory and cardiac systems. Those with a spinal injury must be allowed to come to terms with their disability; they cannot be told to do so. Comfort is important but not the focus of rehabilitation. Finding the correct type of wheelchair is part of rehabilitation but not the main focus of this process. (14:789)

Nursing Process—Planning
Client Need—Physiological integrity

124　1. When clients are relatively immobile and additionally have an indwelling urethral catheter, bladder infections and kidney stones may be prevented if the fluid intake is increased. (14:788; 16:470)
　　Nursing Process—Implementation
　　Client Need—Safe, effective care environment

125　4. Using an overhead bar or trapeze to practice lifting the upper and lower body off the bed helps increase upper physical strength. Until such time as strength returns to the upper body, the client often has difficulty moving from the bed to a chair and back. Isometric exercises of the *upper* extremities also may be of value but cannot be performed by the client on the paralyzed lower extremities. The client most probably has been using his upper extremities to eat, brush his teeth, and perform other ADL. (16:458)
　　Nursing Process—Implementation
　　Client Need—Physiological integrity

126　4. Strong, involuntary muscle spasms that may occur after the spinal cord adjusts to the injury may be confused with voluntary movement. The client has no control over these spasms that occur when flaccid paralysis, which occurs immediately after the injury, is replaced by spastic paralysis, which is seen later. In time these muscle spasms may cease. (3:347)
　　Nursing Process—Implementation
　　Client Need—Physiological integrity

NURSING CARE OF CLIENTS WITH MULTIPLE SCLEROSIS

127　3. Care of clients with multiple sclerosis is individualized. Many symptoms are associated with multiple sclerosis. The type and extent of nursing management will depend on the symptoms and severity of the disorder. All health team members caring for a client with multiple sclerosis should be able to perform those tasks necessary for the managment of this client. (3:351)
　　Nursing Process—Planning
　　Client Need—Physiological integrity

128　1. A footboard with the client's feet at right angles to the leg will help prevent footdrop. Sheepskin boots may be used to prevent decubitus formation in the heel. A trocanter roll may be used to prevent outward rotation of the leg but is of no value in preventing footdrop. A knee-to-hip brace is not an appropriate device for the prevention of footdrop when the client is confined to bed. (16:469)
　　Nursing Process—Implementation
　　Client Need—Physiological integrity

129　2. Once the client's voiding pattern has been established, members of the health team can plan to place the client on a bedpan or take her to the bathroom at the anticipated time of voiding. Usually, taking the client to the bathroom or placing the client on a bedpan is begun on a 2-hour schedule. (3:361)
　　Nursing Process—Implementation
　　Client Need—Health promotion/maintenance

130　2. Extra fluids during waking hours are encouraged for those on a bladder training program. An increased fluid intake helps prevent urinary tract complications associated with immobility, namely bladder infection and calculus (stone) formation in the urinary tract. Usually fluids are restricted after 6:00 PM, and the client is taken to the bathroom to void before retiring. Limiting fluids after 6:00 PM may decrease the need to void or eliminate nighttime incontinence. (3:361; 16:470)
　　Nursing Process—Implementation
　　Client Need—Physiological integrity

INDIVIDUAL TEST ITEMS

131　2. Clients with dysphasia have an impairment in speech and therefore cannot make their needs known or communicate effectively with others. Weakness in one extremity is called monoplegia. Paralysis on one side of the body is called hemiplegia. Slurred speech is called dysarthria. Difficulty swallowing is called dysphagia. (3:324)
　　Nursing Process—Planning
　　Client Need—Safe, effective care environment

132　4. Samples of spinal fluid are taken to the laboratory immediately. Laboratory personnel must be made aware that the samples are being delivered and have just been obtained from the client. (3:326)
　　Nursing Process—Implementation
　　Client Need—Safe, effective care environment

133　3. Narcotics, especially the opiate narcotics, are rarely used for pain associated with neurologic disorders because they interfere with accurate neurologic assessments, especially assessment of the level of consciousness and pupil size and reaction to light. (3:333)
　　Nursing Process—Implementation
　　Client Need—Physiological integrity

134　1. Treatment for Guillain-Barré, a disorder of unknown etiology affecting peripheral nerves and spinal nerve roots, is primarily supportive and depends on the symptoms. Management is therefore aimed at preventing complications associated with the symptoms. There is no specific drug therapy for this disorder. Stool and body fluid precautions are not necessary. (16:412)
　　Nursing Process—Planning
　　Client Need—Safe, effective care environment

135 2. A diet high in foods that produce bulk, for example bran, fresh fruits, and vegetables, help in establishing regularity and preventing diarrhea. An enema or suppository may be required early in the program and is given daily. It is not necessary, and at times may be dangerous, to limit the fluid intake. A stool softener may be prescribed for daily use but should be withheld if diarrhea occurs. (16:470)
    Nursing Process—Planning
    Client Need—Health promotion/maintenance

136 2. Light headedness, double vision, loss of vision in one eye, variable changes in the level of consciousness, and numbness, weakness, or paralysis of one or more extremities are symptoms of TIAs. Additional symptoms also may be seen and depend on the area(s) of the brain that temporarily lack oxygen. (16:436)
    Nursing Process—Implementation
    Client Need—Safe, effective care environment

137 2. Muscular dystrophy is a hereditary, progressive, and chronic neuromuscular disorder. The chief symptoms are progressive muscle weakness and wasting. (16:417)
    Nursing Process—Implementation
    Client Need—Safe, effective care environment

138 1. Trigger areas or spots, when stimulated, produce severe pain in those with trigeminal neuralgia. Even the slightest stimulation, such as a breeze or draft touching the trigger area, can cause severe pain. Brushing the teeth, washing the affected side, and lying on the affected side would cause pain in clients with this disorder. (16:417)
    Nursing Process—Implementation
    Client Need—Safe, effective care environment

139 2. Muscle weakness, which can range from mild to severe, is the primary symptom of myasthenia gravis. The area or areas affected depend on the involved muscle groups. Drooping of the eyelids and difficulty swallowing are common early symptoms of this disorder. (16:416)
    Nursing Process—Planning
    Client Need—Physiological integrity

140 1. Clients with Bell's palsy, a disease of the seventh cranial nerve, have weakness or paralysis of the facial muscles, including those involved with chewing. The inside of the mouth is checked after each meal for injury or remaining food particles. Meticulous oral care is essential. Antibiotics are of no value in the treatment of Bell's palsy because the cause of the disorder is unknown. Improvement usually occurs in a few weeks. It is not necessary to give a clear liquid diet, but a soft diet requires less chewing and thus is tolerated better than a regular diet. (16:418-420)
    Nursing Process—Implementation
    Client Need—Physiological integrity

Classification of Test Items

Unit IV Review Test 10

Directions: After each question the correct answer is given as well as a classification of each test question. Compare the correct answer with your answer. If a question has been answered *incorrectly*, draw a line to the end of the four columns. When finished, add up your correct scores and place the results at the bottom of each column.

Score Calculation:

To determine the percentage of the number of questions you answered correctly, divide the **Number Correct** by the **Number Possible**, as example 122 (the number of questions answered correctly) divided by 140 (the number of questions in the test) = .87 or 87%.

NURSING PROCESS

C = Collecting data
P = Planning
I = Implementation
E = Evaluation

CLIENT NEEDS

S = Safe, effective care environment
P = Physiological integrity
M = Psychosocial integrity
H = Health promotion/maintenance

Question #	Answer #	Nursing Process C	Nursing Process P	Nursing Process I	Nursing Process E	Client Needs S	Client Needs P	Client Needs M	Client Needs H
1	1			I		S			
2	4		P				P		
3	2				E		P		
4	2			I			P		
5	2			I		S			
6	2			I		S			
7	3			I		S			
7	4			I		S			
9	4		P						H
10	2			I					H
11	4			I					H
12	3	C					P		
13	3			I			P		
14	4		P			S			
15	1			I		S			
16	3				E		P		
17	2			I			P		
18	2		P			S			
19	4			I			P		

NURSING PROCESS

C = Collecting data
P = Planning
I = Implementation
E = Evaluation

CLIENT NEEDS

S = Safe, effective care environment
P = Physiological integrity
M = Psychosocial integrity
H = Health promotion/maintenance

Question #	Answer #	Nursing Process				Client Needs			
		C	P	I	E	S	P	M	H
20	1	C				S			
21	3			I			P		
22	2			I		S			
23	3			I		S			
24	2			I		S			
25	2			I			P		
26	1			I		S			
27	2			I		S			
28	1			I					H
29	1			I					H
30	4			I					H
31	1			I				M	
32	1			I		S			
33	3			I					H
34	1			I					H
35	2			I			P		
36	4			I			P		
37	2			I		S			
38	2			I		S			
39	1			I		S			
40	4			I		S			
41	2	C					P		
42	3		P				P		
43	1			I					H
44	2			I		S			
45	2			I					H
46	1			I					H
47	3	C					P		
48	1			I		S			
49	4		P						H
50	1			I		S			
51	3			I		S			

NURSING PROCESS

C = Collecting data
P = Planning
I = Implementation
E = Evaluation

CLIENT NEEDS

S = Safe, effective care environment
P = Physiological integrity
M = Psychosocial integrity
H = Health promotion/maintenance

Question #	Answer #	Nursing Process				Client Needs			
		C	P	I	E	S	P	M	H
52	2			I					H
53	1			I		S			
54	2			I					H
55	2		P						H
56	4			I			P		
57	2			I			P		
58	1			I			P		
59	2			I					H
60	1			I					H
61	2			I		S			
62	4			I		S			
63	3			I					H
64	4			I					H
65	2			I					H
66	2		P			S			
67	1			I				M	
68	2			I			P		
69	2			I					H
70	4			I			P		
71	3			I			P		
72	3			I		S			
73	3			I		S			
74	2	C				S			
75	4			I			P		
76	1			I		S			
77	1			I			P		
78	3			I		S			
79	1	C					P		
80	2			I			P		
81	2			I			P		
82	4			I			P		
83	4			I		S			

NURSING PROCESS

C = Collecting data
P = Planning
I = Implementation
E = Evaluation

CLIENT NEEDS

S = Safe, effective care environment
P = Physiological integrity
M = Psychosocial integrity
H = Health promotion/maintenance

Question #	Answer #	Nursing Process				Client Needs			
		C	P	I	E	S	P	M	H
84	1		P				P		
85	4				E		P		
86	2	C					P		
87	2			I				M	
88	4			I				M	
89	1			I			P		
90	3		P			S			
91	2			I		S			
92	4		P				P		
93	2	C					P		
94	1	C					P		
95	3			I			P		
96	4	C					P		
97	2			I			P		
98	2			I		S			
99	1	C					P		
100	3		P				P		
101	2	C					P		
102	2			I			P		
103	1			I		S			
104	4			I			P		
105	3			I			P		
106	1			I				M	
107	4			I		S			
108	3	C					P		
109	2		P				P		
110	4		P				P		
111	2			I			P		
112	4			I				M	
113	1		P				P		
114	1			I		S			

NURSING PROCESS

C = Collecting data
P = Planning
I = Implementation
E = Evaluation

CLIENT NEEDS

S = Safe, effective care environment
P = Physiological integrity
M = Psychosocial integrity
H = Health promotion/maintenance

Question #	Answer #	Nursing Process				Client Needs			
		C	P	I	E	S	P	M	H
115	2				E	S			
116	1			I					H
117	4			I					H
118	1			I		S			
119	2			I			P		
120	2		P				P		
121	1			I			P		
122	4	C					P		
123	3		P				P		
124	1			I		S			
125	4			I			P		
126	4			I			P		
127	3		P				P		
128	1			I			P		
129	2			I					H
130	2			I			P		
131	2		P			S			
132	4			I		S			
133	3			I			P		
134	1		P			S			
135	2		P						H
136	2			I		S			
137	2			I		S			
138	1			I		S			
139	2		P				P		
140	1			I			P		
Number Correct									
Number Possible	140	14	22	100	4	48	61	6	25
Percentage Correct									

REVIEW TEST 11

The Nursing Care of Clients with Disorders of the Cardiovascular System

Nursing Care of Clients with Hypertensive Heart Disease
Nursing Care of Clients with Coronary Artery Disease
Nursing Care of Clients with Myocardial Infarction
Nursing Care of Clients with Congestive Heart Failure
Nursing Care of Clients with Disorders of the Conduction System
Nursing Care of Clients with Inflammatory Disorders of the Heart

Correct Answers and Rationale
Classification of Test Items

Directions: With a pencil, blacken the circle in front of the option you have chosen for your correct answer.

The Nursing Care of Clients with Disorders of the Cardiovascular System

NURSING CARE OF CLIENTS WITH HYPERTENSIVE HEART DISEASE

A nurse volunteers to assess blood pressures on people participating in a local community hospital's annual health fair.

1 A woman who weighs 225 lb approaches the nurse to have her blood pressure checked. What *modification* should the nurse make when taking her blood pressure? The nurse should
   ○ 1. take the blood pressure on her thigh.
   ○ 2. pump the manometer up to 225 mm Hg.
   ○ 3. use an extra large blood pressure cuff.
   ○ 4. have her lie down during the assessment.

2 Which one of the following adult blood pressure recordings would the nurse consider to be hypertensive?
   ○ 1. 138/88 mm Hg
   ○ 2. 132/96 mm Hg
   ○ 3. 120/80 mm Hg
   ○ 4. 90/60 mm Hg

The nurse finds that another person at the health fair has a blood pressure of 146/82.

3 Which of the following recommendations would be most appropriate for the nurse to make based on this blood pressure recording? It would be *best* for the nurse to recommend that the client

   ○ 1. see a physician immediately.
   ○ 2. have it rechecked in 1 month.
   ○ 3. evaluate it again next year.
   ○ 4. delay action at this time.

A person at the health fair hands a notebook containing a record of his blood pressure measurements to the nurse. He points to one entry and asks the nurse what the third number recorded in the blood pressure measurement of 136/72/60 represents.

4 The best explanation for the third number in the series of recorded numbers is that it was at that pressure that
   ○ 1. the sound became muffled.
   ○ 2. the last sound was heard.
   ○ 3. the sound intensified.
   ○ 4. the sound became faint.

5 A client who is being treated for hypertension comes to the health fair. He indicates to the nurse that he performs all of the following listed activities. Avoiding which one would help most to reduce his blood pressure?
   ○ 1. Eating brown rice
   ○ 2. Walking his dog
   ○ 3. Playing the piano
   ○ 4. Smoking cigarettes

6 A client with an elevated blood pressure says to the nurse, "I feel fine even though my blood pressure is elevated. What signs and symptoms should I look for?" The nurse would be most accurate in telling

Timby B, Scherer JC: LIPPINCOTT'S REVIEW FOR NCLEX–PN. © 1994 J.B. Lippincott Company.

this person that some hypertensive people experience
- ○ 1. fatigue.
- ○ 2. nausea.
- ○ 3. anorexia.
- ○ 4. polyuria.

NURSING CARE OF CLIENTS WITH CORONARY ARTERY DISEASE

During an annual physical examination, Mr. Andrew Weaver is found to have borderline hypertension and elevated cholesterol and triglycerides.

7 If the nurse finds all of the following data in Mr. Weaver's health history, which one is the most significant factor in predisposing him to hypertension? The client indicates that
- ○ 1. he is employed as an architect.
- ○ 2. his ethnic origin is British.
- ○ 3. he had chickenpox as a child.
- ○ 4. his father died of a stroke.

The physician tells Mr. Weaver that his high cholesterol and triglyceride levels probably contribute to his elevated blood pressure.

8 When Mr. Weaver asks the nurse to explain how cholesterol leads to hypertension, the best explanation is that excess fat in the blood
- ○ 1. expands the circulating blood volume.
- ○ 2. thickens the lining of the arteries.
- ○ 3. interferes with the excretion of urine.
- ○ 4. stimulates the heart to beat faster.

9 The physician gives Mr. Weaver a copy of a low cholesterol diet. If Mr. Weaver tells the nurse that his usual breakfast is eggs, sausage, and wheat bread and butter, the healthiest change the nurse could *suggest* is to substitute
- ○ 1. wheat toast for bread.
- ○ 2. margarine for butter.
- ○ 3. cereal for eggs.
- ○ 4. ham for sausage.

10 The client asks the nurse if he can still drink buttermilk on his low cholesterol diet. The most accurate information from the nurse is that buttermilk contains about the same calorie and fat content as
- ○ 1. white whole milk.
- ○ 2. 1% lowfat milk.
- ○ 3. condensed milk.
- ○ 4. homogenized milk.

Mr. Weaver receives a prescription for niacin tablets from his physician. The physician explains that niacin, one of the water-soluble B vitamins, is for lowering his triglyceride level.

11 It would be best for the nurse to tell Mr. Weaver that an unpleasant side effect he may experience while taking niacin is
- ○ 1. discolored urine.
- ○ 2. frequent burping.
- ○ 3. flushing of the skin.
- ○ 4. foul-smelling feces.

12 Mr. Weaver also will be taking furosemide (Lasix) 40 mg orally every day for his hypertension. When the nurse instructs him about his medications, at what time of the day would it be best to tell him to take the furosemide?
- ○ 1. Before bedtime
- ○ 2. When arising
- ○ 3. With his main meal
- ○ 4. In the late afternoon

13 If Mr. Weaver likes all of the following fruit in his packed lunch, which one would be best for him to eat?
- ○ 1. Apples
- ○ 2. Grapes
- ○ 3. Bananas
- ○ 4. Pineapple

14 Which of the following seasonings should the nurse tell Mr. Weaver it is best to avoid?
- ○ 1. Pepper
- ○ 2. Garlic
- ○ 3. Salt
- ○ 4. Vinegar

Mr. John Zales, age 42, is interested in enrolling in a fitness program. His physician has scheduled him for a stress electrocardiogram (EKG) as part of his physical evaluation.

15 When Mr. Zales asks of what use the EKG will be, it would be most correct for the nurse to explain that a stress EKG
- ○ 1. shows how the heart performs during exercise.
- ○ 2. determines his potential target heart rate.
- ○ 3. verifies how much he needs to improve his fitness.
- ○ 4. can predict if he will have a heart attack soon.

Mr. Zales experiences chest pain during the stress EKG, and the test is stopped. His physician discusses scheduling a heart catheterization and coronary arteriogram in the near future.

16 When Mr. Zales learns that his condition is serious enough to require a heart catheterization, he appears extremely worried and fearful. At such times it is best for the nurse to
- ○ 1. teach the client how coronary artery disease is best treated.

○ 2. listen to the client express his feelings about his condition.

○ 3. explain to the client how well others have done having this test.

○ 4. avoid discussing the heart catheterization until he has relaxed.

17 The nurse carries out the teaching plan for cardiac catheterization and coronary arteriogram. Which of the following indicates that Mr. Zales understands what will happen during the testing procedure? The client says that he will

○ 1. be able to hear his heart beating in his chest.

○ 2. experience a heavy sensation all over his body.

○ 3. be anesthetized and won't feel any discomfort.

○ 4. feel a warm sensation as the dye is instilled.

18 Prior to the heart catheterization and coronary arteriogram, it is essential that the nurse ask Mr. Zales if he is allergic to iodine or

○ 1. penicillin.

○ 2. morphine.

○ 3. shellfish.

○ 4. eggs.

19 The femoral artery is the site used to thread the heart catheter. When the procedure is completed and he returns to his room, the nurse should keep Mr. Zales flat in bed with the leg used for the catheterization

○ 1. extended.

○ 2. flexed.

○ 3. abducted.

○ 4. adducted.

20 When the client returns to the nursing unit following the heart catheterization and coronary arteriogram, it is especially important for the nurse to

○ 1. palpate the client's distal peripheral pulses.

○ 2. auscultate the client's lung and heart sounds.

○ 3. percuss all four quadrants of the client's abdomen.

○ 4. inspect the skin integrity on the client's back.

Mr. Walter Stewart suffers with periodic chest pain.

21 If Mr. Stewart is typical of others who have angina pectoris, he will tell the nurse that his chest pain is relieved by

○ 1. aspirin.

○ 2. rest.

○ 3. heat.

○ 4. ice.

22 Mr. Stewart takes nitroglycerin sublingual tablets when he experiences angina. Mr. Stewart administers the nitroglycerin correctly if he places the tablet

○ 1. between his gum and cheek.

○ 2. at the back of his throat.

○ 3. under his tongue.

○ 4. between his teeth.

23 If Mr. Stewart experiences all of the following after taking his nitroglycerin, which one would the nurse consider a side effect of his medication?

○ 1. Headache

○ 2. Seizure

○ 3. Diarrhea

○ 4. Rash

24 Nitroglycerin tablets lose their potency if exposed to light and air. The client has a correct understanding of how to assess when the tablets need replacing if he says that they

○ 1. smell like vinegar.

○ 2. become discolored.

○ 3. no longer tingle when used.

○ 4. disintegrate when touched.

25 The nurse should tell Mr. Stewart that if his chest pain is not relieved after taking one nitroglycerin tablet he should

○ 1. take another tablet in 5 minutes.

○ 2. drive to the emergency department.

○ 3. call his physician without delay.

○ 4. swallow two more additional tablets.

Mr. Rodney Clayton has been following a low-fat, reduced-calorie diet and taking a long-acting nitrate, isosorbide dinitrate (Isordil), as treatment for his angina caused by coronary artery disease.

26 Mr. Clayton tells the nurse that he tries to consume foods that are low in saturated fat. Which one of the following would be the best choice for him to use?

○ 1. Margarine

○ 2. Shortening

○ 3. Coconut oil

○ 4. Corn oil

27 Mr. Clayton says he loves those hot apple pies at the fast food restaurant. He wants to know how many calories they contain. The literature supplied by the fast food chain indicates that one hot apple pie contains 2 g of protein, 14 g of fat, and 31 g of carbohydrates. The nurse would be most accurate in telling him that one hot apple pie would be *equal* to

○ 1. 47 calories.

○ 2. 199 calories.

○ 3. 255 calories.

○ 4. 343 calories.

28 Which one of the following symptoms, if identified by Mr. Clayton, is an indication to the nurse that his dosage of isosorbide dinitrate needs to be adjusted? Mr. Clayton says he experiences

○ 1. nausea.
○ 2. anorexia
○ 3. drowsiness.
○ 4. dizziness.

The physician recommends that Mr. Bernard Hoffman undergo percutaneous transluminal coronary angioplasty (PTCA) because his chest pain does not seem to be controlled anymore with medications.

29 If Mr. Hoffman understands his physician's explanation of the PTCA procedure, he will describe that a
○ 1. balloon tipped catheter will be inserted into a coronary artery.
○ 2. teflon graft will be used to replace an area of weakened heart muscle.
○ 3. section of vein from his leg will be grafted around a narrowed coronary artery.
○ 4. battery operated pacemaker will be implanted to maintain his heart rate.

Mr. Hoffman has been taking propranolol hydrochloride (Inderal).

30 When Mr. Hoffman asks the nurse how this drug helps prevent angina, the best explanation is that it
○ 1. reduces the workload of the heart.
○ 2. promotes excretion of body fluid.
○ 3. alters pain receptors in the brain.
○ 4. dilates the major coronary arteries.

31 While Mr. Hoffman takes propranolol hydrochloride, the nurse can expect that his pulse rate will be
○ 1. slow.
○ 2. fast.
○ 3. irregular.
○ 4. weak.

32 On advice of his physician, Mr. Hoffman has been taking one baby aspirin daily. The best explanation for the drug therapy in this situation is that aspirin tends to
○ 1. relieve chest pain.
○ 2. prevent blood clots.
○ 3. reduce muscle spasms.
○ 4. promote well-being.

33 When Mr. Hoffman returns to his room following the PTCA procedure, which one of the following should be reported immediately to the physician?
○ 1. Urine output of 100 mL/h
○ 2. Blood pressure of 108/68
○ 3. Dry mouth
○ 4. Chest pain

Mr. Louis Myers' coronary arteries are narrowed again despite having repeated PTCA procedures. The physician recommends that he have coronary artery bypass graft (CABG) surgery.

34 The care plan indicates that the nurse should use a pulse oximeter to monitor Mr. Myers' oxygenation status following the CABG procedure. The nurse would be *most correct* in attaching the sensor to Mr. Myers'
○ 1. chest.
○ 2. thigh.
○ 3. arm.
○ 4. finger.

35 A nursing assistant is observed taking Mr. Myers' pulse. Which one of the following actions indicates that the nursing assistant needs more instruction? The nursing assistant
○ 1. places her thumb over the radial artery.
○ 2. counts the pulse rate for 1 full minute.
○ 3. rests the client's arm on his abdomen.
○ 4. presses the artery against the bone.

36 Mr. Myers is experiencing acute pain in his incisional area. The nurse could expect that pain may have which one of the following effects on the client's vital signs?
○ 1. The temperature may be elevated.
○ 2. The pulse rate may become rapid.
○ 3. The respiratory rate may slow.
○ 4. The blood pressure may fall.

The physician orders a patient-controlled analgesia (PCA) infuser pump for Mr. Myers.

37 What information would be best for the nurse to provide the client regarding the use of a PCA infuser pump?
○ 1. Press the control button when pain medication is needed.
○ 2. Call the nurse each time the PCA infuser needs to be used.
○ 3. Use the PCA infuser only when the pain is severe.
○ 4. Frequent use of the PCA infuser can cause addiction.

38 Which of the following information about the client's use of a PCA pump infuser would be most important for the nurse to communicate to the staff on the next shift?
○ 1. The name of the client's physician
○ 2. The purpose for using the infuser
○ 3. The number of doses administered
○ 4. The client's sense of independence

39 Which of the following findings observed by the nurse is evidence that collateral circulation at the *donor* graft site is adequate?
○ 1. The client is free of chest pain.
○ 2. The toes are warm and normal size.
○ 3. The client moves his leg easily.
○ 4. The heart rate remains regular.

NURSING CARE OF CLIENTS WITH MYOCARDIAL INFARCTION

Mr. Phillip Roth, a 53-year-old businessman, is admitted to the hospital with severe chest pain. The admitting diagnosis is possible myocardial infarction.

40   As the nurse assesses Mr. Roth, which additional finding often is associated with a myocardial infarction?
- ○ 1. The client is sweating profusely.
- ○ 2. The client's face is flushed.
- ○ 3. The client says he is thirsty.
- ○ 4. The client has a moist cough.

41   Which of the following questions is *least* helpful when assessing Mr. Roth about his pain?
- ○ 1. "How long have you been in pain?"
- ○ 2. "Where is your pain located?"
- ○ 3. "What were you doing when your pain started?"
- ○ 4. "Do you think an injection for pain would help?"

42   If Mr. Roth is typical of other people who experience a myocardial infarction, he is likely to tell the nurse that his discomfort radiates to his
- ○ 1. flank.
- ○ 2. groin.
- ○ 3. abdomen.
- ○ 4. shoulder.

43   Which of the following statements should the nurse expect Mr. Roth to use when describing his pain?
- ○ 1. The pain comes and goes.
- ○ 2. The pain came on slowly.
- ○ 3. The pain is tingling in nature.
- ○ 4. The pain has remained continuous.

44   Which one of the following prescribed medications would the nurse plan to give to relieve Mr. Roth's discomfort?
- ○ 1. A nonsteroid, such as ibuprofen (Advil)
- ○ 2. A nonsalicylate, such as acetaminophen (Tylenol)
- ○ 3. A salicylate, such as acetylsalicylic acid (aspirin)
- ○ 4. A narcotic, such as meperidine hydrochloride (Demerol)

Although Mr. Roth's wife pleaded that he go to the emergency department when his pain began, he delayed seeking medical attention. He said he was not having a heart attack but rather attributed his discomfort to having strained muscles doing yard work.

45   The nurse would be *most correct* in explaining to Mr. Roth's wife that her husband's hesitation in going to the hospital was an example of a coping technique called
- ○ 1. regression.
- ○ 2. projection.
- ○ 3. denial.
- ○ 4. undoing.

46   The nurse continues to gather information about Mr. Roth from his wife while the physician is examining her husband. If she reports all of the following, which one is *least* likely to have predisposed Mr. Roth to having a myocardial infarction?
- ○ 1. Smoking cigarettes
- ○ 2. Eating fatty foods
- ○ 3. Working under emotional stress
- ○ 4. Drinking an occasional cocktail

Mr. Eric Forslund comes to the emergency department for what he says is acute indigestion or food poisoning, which he states began several hours ago.

47   If Mr. Forslund's symptoms are due to an acute myocardial infarction, which one of the following laboratory test results should the nurse expect to be abnormally high?
- ○ 1. Alkaline phosphatase
- ○ 2. Alphafetoprotein (AFP)
- ○ 3. Creatinine phosphokinase (CPK)
- ○ 4. Gamma-glutamyl transferase

Because Mr. Forslund has been experiencing symptoms for only a few hours, the physician plans to administer the drug streptokinase (Streptase).

48   The nurse would be *most correct* in explaining to Mr. Forslund that streptokinase is given to
- ○ 1. dissolve blood clots.
- ○ 2. slow his heart rate.
- ○ 3. improve heart contraction.
- ○ 4. lower his blood pressure.

49   For which adverse effect should the nurse plan to monitor when a client receives streptokinase or another similar drug?
- ○ 1. Hypertension
- ○ 2. Constipation
- ○ 3. Bleeding
- ○ 4. Vomiting

50   Which one of the following findings would indicate to the nurse that Mr. Forslund is having an allergic reaction to the streptokinase (Streptase)?
- ○ 1. Urticaria
- ○ 2. Dysuria
- ○ 3. Hemoptysis
- ○ 4. Dyspepsia

Ms. Gloria Haskins, who works as a secretary, has had hypertension for more than 10 years. A nurse who is taking care of some personal business observes her collapse at her desk.

51 The first action the nurse should take is to
○ 1. open her airway.
○ 2. give two breaths.
○ 3. shake her gently.
○ 4. lay her on the floor.

52 The best method the nurse can use to open Ms. Haskins' airway is to
○ 1. elevate her neck.
○ 2. lift her chin.
○ 3. press on her jaws.
○ 4. clear her mouth.

53 The best method for determining if rescue breathing should be performed is to
○ 1. observe the victim's skin color.
○ 2. feel for pulsations at the neck.
○ 3. listen for spontaneous breathing.
○ 4. blow air into the victim's mouth.

54 To deliver an *optimum* amount of air into the victim's lungs, the nurse should
○ 1. press on the victim's trachea.
○ 2. remove the victim's dentures.
○ 3. pinch the victim's nose shut.
○ 4. squeeze the victim's cheeks.

Ms. Haskins remains unresponsive and pulseless.

55 The correct placement for the nurse's hands before administering cardiac compression is
○ 1. on the lower half of the sternum.
○ 2. below the tip of the xiphoid process.
○ 3. over the costal cartilage.
○ 4. directly above the manubrium.

56 The nurse should compress the chest of an adult victim at a rate no less than
○ 1. 15 compressions per minute.
○ 2. 40 compressions per minute.
○ 3. 60 compressions per minute.
○ 4. 80 compressions per minute.

Eventually, a second person arrives to assist the nurse with cardiopulmonary resuscitation (CPR).

57 When two rescuers perform CPR, the rate of compressions to ventilations should be
○ 1. 15 compressions to two breaths.
○ 2. five compressions to one breath.
○ 3. one compression for each breath.
○ 4. one compression to five breaths.

58 The *best* evidence the nurse can use for determining that the cardiac compressions can be discontinued is that
○ 1. the victim's color improves.
○ 2. the pupils become dilated.
○ 3. a pulse can be palpated.
○ 4. the victim begins to vomit.

Mr. Eldon Miller begins experiencing chest pain in the early evening but waits until morning to be seen by a physician. EKG changes and laboratory tests confirm that Mr. Miller has had a myocardial infarction. EKG leads are attached to his chest to monitor his heart rate and rhythm.

59 Mr. Miller is startled by an alarm that sounds when one of the leads comes loose. The best approach the nurse can use for relieving Mr. Miller's anxiety at this time is to
○ 1. turn off the cardiac monitor.
○ 2. explain why the alarm sounded.
○ 3. give him a prescribed tranquilizer.
○ 4. provide him with a magazine to read.

The physician orders nitroglycerin in a transdermal patch form (Nitrodisc).

60 Which of the following nursing actions is *essential* when applying the transdermal patch?
○ 1. Rotate the site of application.
○ 2. Squeeze the drug reservoir.
○ 3. Tape the patch to the chest.
○ 4. Apply ice to the skin area.

61 The nurse should withhold the application of the nitroglycerin patch and notify the physician based on which one of the following assessment findings? The client's
○ 1. temperature is 99.8°F (37.7°C).
○ 2. respiratory rate is 24 at rest.
○ 3. apical heart rate is 90.
○ 4. blood pressure is 94/62.

Mr. Miller's physician subsequently orders the calcium channel blocker diltiazem hydrochloride (Cardizem).

62 The medication administration record indicates that the nurse should administer the diltiazem hydrochloride *a.c.* This drug would be administered correctly if the nurse brought the medication to Mr. Miller
○ 1. at his bedtime.
○ 2. before his meals.
○ 3. once each day.
○ 4. as necessary.

63 Mr. Miller says to the nurse one day, "This scares me. I'm concerned about what could happen to me." Of the following comments, which one is best for the nurse to make at this time?
○ 1. "What are your concerns?"
○ 2. "Why are you so scared?"
○ 3. "Your doctor says you're doing just fine."
○ 4. "You need to concentrate on getting well."

64 Mr. Miller is on a calorie-restricted, low-fat, low-sodium diet. He appears to understand his diet instructions if he says he should avoid using

○ 1. catsup.
○ 2. vinegar.
○ 3. onions.
○ 4. lemon.

65 If the nurse observes Mr. Miller do all of the following, which one should the nurse caution him to avoid because of its potentially dangerous consequences?
○ 1. Reading a murder mystery
○ 2. Straining to have a stool
○ 3. Washing his hands and face
○ 4. Playing a game of solitaire

To evaluate the damage done to Mr. Miller's heart, the physician orders an echocardiogram.

66 Mr. Miller has a correct understanding of an echocardiogram if he tells the nurse that this examination involves imaging the heart using
○ 1. heat waves.
○ 2. sound waves.
○ 3. radiation waves.
○ 4. electric waves.

NURSING CARE OF CLIENTS WITH CONGESTIVE HEART FAILURE

Ms. Cora Nesbitt is admitted to the hospital with left-sided congestive heart failure.

67 When obtaining a health history from Ms. Nesbitt, the nurse is most likely to find that when her illness began, Ms. Nesbitt *first* noticed that she had dyspnea and
○ 1. anorexia.
○ 2. fatigue.
○ 3. nausea.
○ 4. headaches.

68 When auscultating Ms. Nesbitt's lung sounds, the nurse is *most likely* to hear
○ 1. grating sounds.
○ 2. growling sounds.
○ 3. crackling sounds.
○ 4. rumbling sounds.

69 The care plan for Ms. Nesbitt indicates that her apical–radial pulse rate must be assessed daily. Which one of the following describes the correct technique for performing this assessment?
○ 1. The nurse counts the apical and then the radial pulse rate.
○ 2. The nurse listens to the heart while feeling the pulse.
○ 3. One nurse counts the apical rate at the same time another counts the radial rate.
○ 4. One nurse counts the apical and radial rate, and a second nurse watches the time.

70 The position the nurse should plan to use to help Ms. Nesbitt feel most comfortable would be a
○ 1. back-lying position.
○ 2. face-lying position.
○ 3. side-lying position.
○ 4. semi-sitting position.

71 The nurse would expect that emotionally Ms. Nesbitt would be feeling
○ 1. depressed.
○ 2. anxious.
○ 3. defensive.
○ 4. aggressive.

72 Ms. Nesbitt is to receive oxygen by mask. After attaching the tubing to the oxygen supply, the nurse should start the flow of oxygen to the mask
○ 1. before applying the mask to the client's face.
○ 2. after the mask is secured to the client's face.
○ 3. just as the mask is placed on the client's face.
○ 4. if the client cannot feel the room air on her face.

Mr. Sherman Wilks, a resident in a nursing home, develops severe shortness of breath. After the nurse reports the change in his condition to the physician, he prescribes 80 mg of intramuscular furosemide (Lasix) stat. The physician recommends that Mr. Wilks then be transferred to a nearby hospital to continue treating his congestive heart failure that has been complicated by acute pulmonary edema.

73 If the furosemide comes prepared in an ampule labeled 40 mg/2 mL, the nurse would be accurate in administering
○ 1. 0.25 mL.
○ 2. 0.4 mL.
○ 3. 1 mL.
○ 4. 4 mL.

74 As the nurse prepares to withdraw the furosemide, the best technique for removing the medication from the stem of the glass ampule is to
○ 1. allow the ampule to stand undisturbed for a few minutes.
○ 2. tap the stem of the ampule with the fingernail a few times.
○ 3. hold the ampule upside down then flip it right side up.
○ 4. roll the ampule gently between the palms of the hands.

75 The best evidence that furosemide (Lasix) has had a therapeutic effect is that the client's
○ 1. pulse becomes slower.
○ 2. blood pressure stabilizes.
○ 3. urinary output increases.
○ 4. anxiety is diminished.

While awaiting transport to the hospital, the physician tells the nurse to apply blood pressure cuffs to each of Mr. Wilks' four extremities to simulate the use of rotating tourniquets.

76 What guideline is best for the nurse to use for monitoring that the blood pressure cuffs are properly inflated?
- ○ 1. A distal pulse can be palpated.
- ○ 2. His fingers and toes look pale.
- ○ 3. He can feel the nurse's touch.
- ○ 4. Capillary refill is delayed.

77 If the simulated tourniquets are rotated on a 15-minute schedule, how long in 1 hour is there an inflated blood pressure cuff on each of Mr. Wilks' extremities?
- ○ 1. 15 minutes
- ○ 2. 30 minutes
- ○ 3. 45 minutes
- ○ 4. 60 minutes

Mr. Wilks is transferred by ambulance to the emergency department.

78 As the nurse begins to leave the examining room following a basic physical assessment, Mr. Wilks reaches out toward the nurse. Though he is too breathless to speak, the nurse believes that the client is extremely frightened. What is the *best* action for the nurse to take at this time?
- ○ 1. Stay with the client.
- ○ 2. Call for the physician.
- ○ 3. Tell him he'll be okay.
- ○ 4. Record the collected data.

79 Mr. Wilks continues to receive furosemide daily. It is essential for the nurse to monitor the serum level of which one of the following electrolytes when a client is receiving furosemide?
- ○ 1. Calcium
- ○ 2. Magnesium
- ○ 3. Potassium
- ○ 4. Bicarbonate

80 Which one of the following physical assessments is most important for a nurse to monitor daily on a client with congestive heart failure?
- ○ 1. Pupil response
- ○ 2. Bowel sounds
- ○ 3. Appetite
- ○ 4. Weight

Ms. Lucille Ganser sees her physician, who has been treating her for hypertension.

81 Which one of the following findings should alert the office nurse that Ms. Ganser may be developing right-sided congestive heart failure?
- ○ 1. Her urine contains glucose.
- ○ 2. Her ankles are swollen.
- ○ 3. She has lost weight.
- ○ 4. She seems depressed.

82 An additional finding the nurse is likely to detect during the physical assessment that supports the possibility of right-sided congestive heart failure is
- ○ 1. neck vein distension.
- ○ 2. burning during urination.
- ○ 3. periodic constipation.
- ○ 4. chronic indigestion.

The physician admits Ms. Ganser to the hospital to digitalize her. He leaves written orders for the nurse to administer 0.5 mg of digoxin (Lanoxin) orally every 4 hours during the next 24 hours unless the client develops digitalis toxicity.

83 If Ms. Ganser develops digitalis toxicity, the nurse is most likely to detect
- ○ 1. anorexia and nausea.
- ○ 2. dizziness and insomnia.
- ○ 3. pinpoint pupils and double vision.
- ○ 4. ringing in the ears and itchy skin.

84 Before administering the digoxin to Ms. Ganser it is *essential* that the nurse assess her
- ○ 1. pulse rate.
- ○ 2. blood pressure.
- ○ 3. heart sounds.
- ○ 4. lung sounds.

After the digitalizing loading doses have achieved their therapeutic effect, the physician revises the drug order. Ms. Ganser is now to receive a daily maintenance dose of 0.125 mg of digoxin orally.

85 Each tablet of digoxin contains 0.25 mg. How much should the nurse administer to Ms. Ganser each day?
- ○ 1. ½ tablet
- ○ 2. 1 tablet
- ○ 3. 2 tablets
- ○ 4. 4 tablets

86 The nurse collects all of the following data; which one is an indication that the next dose of digitalis should be withheld until the physician can be consulted?
- ○ 1. The apical heart rate is 56 beats per minute.
- ○ 2. The blood pressure is 134/72/60 while sitting.
- ○ 3. The nurse hears S_1 and S_2 heart sounds.
- ○ 4. The nurse hears vesicular lung sounds.

87 The nurse plans to teach Ms. Ganser how to take her digoxin at home. Which of the following types of information is generally *least* important?
- ○ 1. The purpose for taking the medication
- ○ 2. The name of the drug manufacturer
- ○ 3. The time schedule for taking the drug
- ○ 4. The adverse symptoms that can develop

88 If Ms. Ganser understands the restrictions of a low-sodium diet, she will tell the nurse that of the following list of foods, the *one* that she may consume is
   ○ 1. canned chicken soup.
   ○ 2. frozen sausage pizza.
   ○ 3. fresh garden salad.
   ○ 4. smoked ocean fish.

NURSING CARE OF CLIENTS WITH DISORDERS OF THE CONDUCTION SYSTEM

Mr. Alvin Cook sees his physician because he has been experiencing brief fainting spells lately. When the nurse performs the preexamination assessment, Mr. Cook's pulse rate is 52 beats per minute. The physician attaches a Holter monitor for recording an ambulatory EKG before sending Mr. Cook home.

89 Which one of the following instructions should the nurse give Mr. Cook to best interpret the information being collected by the Holter monitor over the next 24 hours?
   ○ 1. Record the time and type of physical activities performed.
   ○ 2. Take the radial pulse rate every hour during the next day.
   ○ 3. Try to relax and limit exercise as much as possible.
   ○ 4. Eat lightly and avoid hot or spicy foods.

90 Which one of the following should the nurse tell Mr. Cook to avoid for the next 24 hours?
   ○ 1. Bathing
   ○ 2. Sleeping
   ○ 3. Dancing
   ○ 4. Working

The physician admits Mr. Cook for the insertion of an artificial pacemaker.

91 The nurse uses a diagram of the heart to illustrate the heart's conduction system to Mr. Cook. If Mr. Cook understands the nurse's explanation, which one of the following will he identify as the site of the natural pacemaker?
   ○ 1. Purkinje fibers
   ○ 2. Bundle of His
   ○ 3. Atrioventricular (AV) node
   ○ 4. Sinoatrial (SA) node

92 The nurse watches Mr. Cook's cardiac rhythm on a cardiac monitor after the artificial pacemaker has been inserted. Which of the following must be reported *immediately*?
   ○ 1. Sinus rhythm
   ○ 2. Sinus arrhythmia
   ○ 3. Premature ventricular contractions (PVCs)
   ○ 4. Premature atrial contractions (PACs)

93 To assesses the area where the permanent pacemaker battery has been implanted, the nurse would be most correct in examining the skin
   ○ 1. beneath the left nipple.
   ○ 2. near the brachial artery.
   ○ 3. in the midsternum.
   ○ 4. below the clavicle.

The nurse teaches Mr. Cook how to assess his pulse rate and to report any difference of more than 5 beats from the pacemaker's preset rate.

94 Following the discharge teaching, if Mr. Cook has understood the information correctly, he will identify which one of the following symptoms as *most related* to pacemaker battery failure or electric interference?
   ○ 1. Dizziness
   ○ 2. Drowsiness
   ○ 3. Headache
   ○ 4. Hiccupping

Ms. Agnes Cooper has a rapid atrial heart rate. Cardioversion will be performed.

95 Ms. Cooper has a correct understanding of a cardioversion procedure if she tells the nurse that it involves
   ○ 1. administering an electric current to the heart.
   ○ 2. threading a thin, plastic catheter into her heart.
   ○ 3. evaluating blood flow to areas of heart muscle.
   ○ 4. scanning the heart after injecting a radioisotope.

96 Just prior to the cardioversion, it is essential that the nurse
   ○ 1. wear special goggles and gloves.
   ○ 2. perform a surgical hand scrub.
   ○ 3. stand back from the client and bed.
   ○ 4. use a lead apron as a body shield.

97 The best evidence that the cardioversion procedure has been successful is
   ○ 1. the client regains consciousness immediately.
   ○ 2. normal sinus cardiac rhythm is restored.
   ○ 3. the apical heart rate equals the radial rate.
   ○ 4. the pulse pressure is approximately 40 mm Hg.

NURSING CARE OF CLIENTS WITH INFLAMMATORY DISORDERS OF THE HEART

During a routine preemployment physical examination on Greta Schmidt, the physician detects a heart murmur.

98 If Ms. Schmidt's heart murmur is related to valve damage caused by a childhood infection, which of the following diseases would the nurse expect this client to report having?

○ 1. Varicella (chickenpox)
○ 2. Rubella (German measles)
○ 3. Rheumatic fever
○ 4. Whooping cough

After a diagnostic workup, the physician informs Ms. Schmidt that the cause of her heart murmur is mitral stenosis.

99 The nurse would be most correct in explaining to Ms. Schmidt that the mitral valve is located between the
○ 1. right ventricle and the pulmonary artery.
○ 2. left atrium and left ventricle.
○ 3. right atrium and right ventricle.
○ 4. left ventricle and the aorta.

100 Which one of the following symptoms is Ms. Schmidt most likely to experience as a consequence of mitral stenosis?
○ 1. Palpitations
○ 2. Bradycardia
○ 3. Anorexia
○ 4. Dyspnea

101 While auscultating Ms. Schmidt's heart sounds, the nurse is *likely* to hear best the sound from the mitral valve
○ 1. at the fifth intercostal space in the midclavicular line.
○ 2. at the fourth intercostal space to the left of the sternum.
○ 3. at the second intercostal space to the right of the sternum.
○ 4. at the second intercostal space to the left of the sternum.

The physician prescribes 250 mg of nafcillin sodium (Unipen) P.O. q.i.d. for Ms. Schmidt.

102 What is the best explanation the nurse can give Ms. Schmidt for taking this prescribed medication?
○ 1. It will destroy the virus causing her disease.
○ 2. It will reduce the scar tissue on the valve.
○ 3. It will stop blood clots from forming.
○ 4. It will prevent future bacterial infections.

Mr. William Bennett has been taking diuretics and digitalis for the long-term treatment of mitral stenosis. His symptoms have become progressively worse. He plans to have surgery to replace his mitral valve.

103 Which one of the following statements indicates that Mr. Bennett understands the surgical procedure involving mitral valve replacement? Mr. Bennett says
○ 1. his blood will be circulated through a heart-lung machine.
○ 2. the surgeon will enlarge his valve by inserting his finger.

○ 3. his chest will be opened during surgery but not his heart.
○ 4. a piece of his leg vein will be used to replace his valve.

104 Which one of the following signs is most often found in adult clients, such as Mr. Bennett, who have had chronic cardiac or pulmonary disease most of their lifetime?
○ 1. Deviated nasal septum
○ 2. Flushed facial skin
○ 3. Clubbed fingers
○ 4. Hoarse voice

Several weeks ago, Mr. John Sawyer had a mitral valve replaced. A pulmonary artery catheter was used to monitor pressure within his heart. Mr. Sawyer is now suspected of having bacterial endocarditis.

105 Which one of the following findings documented by the nurse is the best evidence that Mr. Sawyer is experiencing an infectious process? The client has
○ 1. chest pain.
○ 2. a dry cough.
○ 3. a fever.
○ 4. dyspnea.

106 Which one of the following cultures would the nurse *expect* the physician to order to identify the presence of the infectious organism causing bacterial endocarditis?
○ 1. Wound culture
○ 2. Blood culture
○ 3. Sputum culture
○ 4. Urine culture

The physician writes an order allowing Mr. Sawyer to be up in the chair if he can tolerate the increased activity.

107 Which of the following criteria is the best evidence that Mr. Sawyer is able to tolerate the activity involved in getting out of bed?
○ 1. His appetite has improved.
○ 2. He has more restful sleep.
○ 3. His heart rate is stable.
○ 4. He says he is very bored.

108 Mr. Sawyer is disappointed that his progress is so slow. One day he pushes away his lunch tray, and it falls to the floor. In this situation, it would be best for the nurse to
○ 1. clean up the floor and say nothing.
○ 2. find out what food he would prefer.
○ 3. let Mr. Sawyer talk about his anger.
○ 4. leave him alone until he feels better.

Ms. Louise Simmons is admitted with pericarditis.

109 The nurse auscultates the client's chest. Which one of the following would help most when listening to the client's heart and lung sounds?

○ 1. Ask the client to hold her breath.
○ 2. Turn the oxygen off momentarily.
○ 3. Give the client sips of water.
○ 4. Locate the point of the xiphoid.

110 While auscultating the chest of a client with pericarditis, which one of the following is the nurse most likely to hear?

○ 1. Expiratory wheezes
○ 2. Inspiratory gurgles
○ 3. A friction rub
○ 4. A clicking murmur

Correct Answers and Rationale

Two numbers appear in parentheses following each rationale. The first number identifies the textbook listed in the references, page 451, and the second number identifies the page(s) in that textbook on which the correct answer can be verified. Occasionally, two textbooks are given for verifying the correct answer.

The Nursing Care of Clients with Disorders of the Cardiovascular System

NURSING CARE OF CLIENTS WITH HYPERTENSIVE HEART DISEASE

1 3. The cuff size should be appropriate for the person being assessed to obtain an accurate measurement. The cuff width should be 40% of the circumference or 20% wider than the diameter of the arm on which it will be applied. One can assume that a person who is obese will need a larger than usual adult cuff. If the cuff is too narrow for the person, the blood pressure will be higher than its true measurement; if too wide, the measurement will be lower than the true pressure. (18:263)
Nursing Process—Implementation
Client Need—Safe, effective care environment

2 2. The Joint National Committee on Detection, Evaluation, and Treatment of High Blood Pressure recommended in 1988 that health care workers consider a systolic pressure of 140 mm Hg or greater in adults 18 years or older and a diastolic pressure of 90 mm Hg or greater to be abnormally high. This standard can be applied when either the systolic or diastolic, or both, exceed the established criteria. (18:261; 14:382)
Nursing Process—Collecting data
Client Need—Safe, effective care environment

3 2. Before a definite diagnosis of hypertension can be made, there must be evidence that the blood pressure remains consistently elevated. Because many factors can affect blood pressure, such as anxiety, activity, and pain, one abnormal reading is inconclusive. However, because untreated hypertension can cause life-threatening consequences, the person should be reassessed within 2 months. A client should see a physician promptly if the systolic pressure is equal to or exceeds 200 mm Hg or if the diastolic pressure equals or exceeds 115 mm Hg. (18:262)
Nursing Process—Implementation
Client Need—Health promotion/maintenance

4 2. A third recorded blood pressure number indicates the pressure at which the last sound was heard before a period of continuous silence. The American Heart Association advises that the second number, which correlates with the pressure where the sound changed from loud tapping to muffled, is the most accurate index of diastolic pressure but recommends recording all three numbers. (18:266; 19:503)
Nursing Process—Implementation
Client Need—Safe, effective care environment

5 4. Eliminating smoking is a positive step in controlling hypertension. Nicotine stimulates the heart rate, promotes irregular heart beats, and causes vasoconstriction. Vasoconstriction narrows the arterioles and raises blood pressure. Moderate, regular exercise helps to lower blood pressure. Playing the piano promotes relaxation, which lowers blood pressure. Brown rice has not had the outer germ layer removed. It is higher in fiber than white rice. Some believe that a high-fiber diet can lower blood cholesterol and reduce the progression of atherosclerosis. (14:791; 3:464)
Nursing Process—Implementation
Client Need—Health promotion/maintenance

6 1. Hypertension is referred to as the "silent killer" because most are unaware that the condition exists until secondary complications occur. One symptom that accompanies hypertension is fatigue. This may occur because the cells are not receiving an adequate supply of oxygenated blood through narrowed and inelastic blood vessels. Another explanation is that the body requires extra energy to overcome the high pressure within the vascular system when pumping blood. Other signs and symptoms associated with hypertension include headaches, dizziness, blurred vision, blackouts, irritability, shortness of breath, nosebleeds, and chest pain. (3:464; 16:337)
Nursing Process—Implementation
Client Need—Health promotion/maintenance

NURSING CARE OF CLIENTS WITH CORONARY ARTERY DISEASE

7 4. The exact cause of primary or essential hypertension is unknown. However, heredity appears to play an important role. Frequently, there is a strong family history of hypertension or secondary complications, such as stroke, heart attack, or kidney failure. Hyperlipidemia also tends to run in families. Other factors that appear to bring on hypertension include obesity, emotional stress, smoking, and high serum sodium levels. African Americans are at higher risk for hypertension. Occupations in which workers experience anxiety, such as air traffic controllers, are known to contribute to hypertension. There is no established correlation between a childhood infection of chickenpox and hypertension as an adult. (16:337; 7:373)

    Nursing Process—Collecting data
    Client Need—Safe, effective care environment

8 2. A buildup of cholesterol causes atherosclerosis. Fat becomes deposited within the lining of arteries. The deposits enlarge to form plaque. The fatty plaque thickens the arterial walls, causing the passageway for blood to become narrowed. Eventually the plaque is infiltrated with calcium, which causes the vessel to become hard and inelastic. When the normal volume of blood is forced to pass through narrow and inelastic vessels, the pressure within the vessels increases. The heart is prone to failure because it must work very hard to pump against the vascular resistance. (16:306; 14:791)

    Nursing Process—Implementation
    Client Need—Health promotion/maintenance

9 3. In keeping with a low-cholesterol diet, the healthiest change would be to eat cereal rather than eggs for breakfast. Egg yolk is a rich source of cholesterol. There would not be much, if any, appreciable change in levels of cholesterol by substituting the foods listed in the other options. (4:423)

    Nursing Process—Implementation
    Client Need—Health promotion/maintenance

10 2. Despite its name, 1 cup of buttermilk contains only 100 total calories with 1.3 g of saturated fat. It is very similar to 1% lowfat milk, which contains 100 calories and 1.6 g of saturated fat. Nonfat skim milk is the best nutritional choice for controlling both calories and saturated fat. It contains 85 calories and 0.3 g of saturated fat per cup. Homogenization does not lower the calories or fat content of whole milk. Rather, it distributes the cream within the watery portion of milk so that these two components do not separate when the milk stands. Condensed milk is prepared by removing a great deal of the water content from milk. This increases the caloric components tremendously when comparing cup for cup measurements. For example, one cup of condensed milk contains 980 calories and 16.8 g of fat. (4:551-552)

    Nursing Process—Implementation
    Client Need—Health promotion/maintenance

11 3. In doses large enough to lower blood fat components, niacin causes relaxation of peripheral vascular smooth muscle. This causes some people to experience flushing of the skin. The flushing, primarily in the head, neck, and ears, is accompanied by a sensation of warmth, tingling, itching, and headache. This effect tends to subside as therapy continues. (4:419)

    Nursing Process—Implementation
    Client Need—Health promotion/maintenance

12 2. To avoid disturbing sleep with a need for urination, a daily dose of a diuretic like furosemide should be administered in the early morning. (7:505)

    Nursing Process—Implementation
    Client Need—Health promotion/maintenance

13 3. People who take potassium-depleting diuretics should be encouraged to eat foods that replace this electrolyte. One banana contains approximately 10 mEq of potassium. Other fruits that are rich sources include oranges and orange juice, cantaloupe, and nectarines. (7:78-80; 4:465)

    Nursing Process—Implementation
    Client Need—Health promotion/maintenance

14 3. Because sodium causes fluid retention, a client with hypertension would benefit from reducing salt as much as possible from the diet. Reducing the water content in the blood volume will help to lower blood pressure. (7:372; 3:465)

    Nursing Process—Implementation
    Client Need—Health promotion/maintenance

15 1. A stress EKG demonstrates the extent to which the heart tolerates and responds to the additional demands placed on it during exercise. The heart's ability to continue adapting is related to the adequacy of blood supplied to the myocardium through the coronary arteries. If the client develops chest pain, dangerous cardiac rhythm changes, or significantly elevated blood pressure, the diagnostic testing is stopped. (18:169; 16:286; 3:471)

    Nursing Process—Implementation
    Client Need—Safe, effective care environment

16 2. When a person is worried and fearful, the nurse should encourage and listen as the client expresses his feelings. Verbalization often lifts the mental burden that a client is experiencing. Most clients feel alone, overwhelmed, and helpless during a crisis. Listening is an active process even if the nurse does not make many verbal contributions. Learning is impaired during times of mild to severe anxiety. How others have done disregards the uniqueness of the situation for this patient. Avoiding the subject may communicate that the nurse does not care. (17:72; 12:249)

Nursing Process—Implementation
Client Need—Psychosocial integrity

17 4. The contrast dye used during the coronary arteriogram causes vasodilation and is experienced as a brief flush or warmth that spreads over the skin surface. It may be possible to feel fluttering or what some describe as "butterflies" as the catheter is passed into the heart, disturbing its rhythm. Chest pain, if it is experienced, is generally treated with nitroglycerin. The client will receive sedation prior to the diagnostic testing but will not be anesthetized. (16:286-287; 3:470-471)

Nursing Process—Evaluation
Client Need—Safe, effective care environment

18 3. People who are allergic to shellfish also may be sensitive to iodine. The radiopaque dye used during the arteriogram is iodine based. The physician should be notified if the client indicates a history of allergies to either of these substances. The physician may cancel the procedure or be prepared to administer an antihistamine or other emergency drugs. (14:792; 3:471)

Nursing Process—Collecting data
Client Need—Safe, effective care environment

19 1. When the femoral artery is the site used for inserting the heart catheter, the nurse should make sure that the client does not bend his leg or flex his hip for 6 to 8 hours. Flexing the hip may lead to bleeding and clot formation. Sandbags may be placed over the pressure dressing to decrease discomfort and control bleeding. (14:793; 3:472)

Nursing Process—Implementation
Client Need—Physiological integrity

20 1. Peripheral pulses distal to the catheter insertion site must be assessed frequently. The injury to the artery and subsequent bleeding can lead to clot formation. The thrombus could totally occlude the flow of oxygenated blood through the vessel. Absence of a distal pulse must be reported immediately because this is an emergency situation. (14:793; 16:287)

Nursing Process—Collecting data
Client Need—Safe, effective care environment

21 2. Angina is generally relieved by rest. The chest pain is caused by an inadequate supply of oxygenated blood to the myocardium due to partially occluded coronary arteries. Once the myocardium's demand for additional oxygen is reduced through inactivity, the chest pain is relieved. Aspirin, heat, or ice are not appropriate measures for relieving the pain of angina pectoris. (14:797; 16:308)

Nursing Process—Collecting data
Client Need—Physiologic integrity

22 3. Sublingual means under the tongue. Clients must be instructed not to chew or swallow the tablets. They should dissolve in the mouth. The drug is absorbed through the rich blood supply beneath the tongue. Tablets for buccal administration are placed between the gum and cheek. A tablet intended for swallowing should be placed on the tongue at the back of the throat. A chewable tablet should be placed between the teeth. (15:110; 18:594)

Nursing Process—Evaluation
Client Need—Physiological integrity

23 1. Side effects of nitroglycerin include headache, flushing, and dizziness. These effects are the direct result of vasodilation. Relief can be obtained by decreasing the dosage of the drug or taking a mild pain reliever. (15:111; 3:494)

Nursing Process—Evaluation
Client Need—Physiological integrity

24 3. The client should experience a fizzing or tingling in the mouth if nitroglycerin tablets are still fresh. Tablets usually need to be replaced approximately every 3 months. Old aspirin tends to smell like vinegar. Nitroglycerin tablets do not become discolored or disintegrate when touched when they have lost their potency. (14:798; 15:111)

Nursing Process—Evaluation
Client Need—Health promotion/maintenance

25 1. The dose of nitroglycerin may be repeated every 5 minutes until pain is relieved. However, the client should be told to call the physician if the pain is not relieved after three doses within 15 minutes because other treatment may be necessary. A person having chest pain should never drive himself to the hospital. Sublingual tablets should not be swallowed. (15:110; 3:494)

Nursing Process—Implementation
Client Need—Health promotion/maintenance

26 4. Corn oil is an example of a polyunsaturated oil. Using unsaturated fats helps lower blood cholesterol. In limited amounts it is healthier to consume polyunsaturated fats than saturated fats, such as grease or lard, or hydrogenated fats, such as solid vegetable shortenings and hard margarines. Coconut and palm oil are more highly saturated than lard. (4:119, 421)

Nursing Process—Implementation
Client Need—Health promotion/maintenance

27 3. Protein and carbohydrate both have 4 calories per gram; fat contains 9 calories per gram. Thus, the total calorie count for a piece of pie containing 2 g of protein, 14 g of fat, and 31 g of carbohydrate is 255 calories. (4:592)

Nursing Process—Implementation
Client Need—Health promotion/maintenance

28 4. Dizziness is a common side effect of nitrate drugs. Nitrates have a direct relaxing effect on the smooth muscle of blood vessels producing vasodilation. When blood vessels dilate, blood pressure falls, and the client experiences vertigo. Isosorbide dinitrate is administered in a range of 5 to 40 mg. Once the data are reported, the physician may wish to lower the dosage the client is receiving or have him take the drug at night before going to sleep. In some instances, the side effects diminish or disappear after taking the drug over a period of time. (15:108; 3:494)

Nursing Process—Evaluation
Client Need—Physiological integrity

29 1. A PTCA procedure involves dilating narrowed or occluded coronary arteries with a double lumen balloon catheter. The pressure from the inflated balloon compresses the fatty plaque that has narrowed the artery. A CABG procedure uses a piece of leg vein to bypass a narrowed area of coronary artery. A pacemaker is used when it is difficult to maintain the heart rate in the normal range with drug therapy. Grafting skeletal muscle, not teflon, over scarred areas of myocardium is just now in experimental stages. (7:391; 16:357)

Nursing Process—Evaluation
Client Need—Health promotion/maintenance

30 1. Propranolol hydrochloride is a beta-blocker. It blocks the sympathetic receptors for epinephrine. Epinephrine speeds the heart rate, which requires a great deal of oxygen. By blocking the effect of epinephrine, the heart rate is slowed, and not as much oxygen is needed by the myocardium. In addition, at a slower rate the heart fills with a greater volume of blood. Thus, each time the heart contracts, it delivers a substantial amount of blood to the coronary arteries. As long as the coronary arteries can deliver an adequate amount of oxygenated blood to the myocardium, chest pain is prevented. (15:44; 3:478)

Nursing Process—Implementation
Client Need—Health promotion/maintenance

31 1. Beta blockers interfere with the action of epinephrine. They reduce heart rate. Therefore, the pulse rate will tend to be on the lower range of normal or may become bradycardic. (3:478; 15:44)

Nursing Process—Collecting data
Client Need—Physiological integrity

32 2. Aspirin is recommended in low daily doses to reduce the potential for forming a blood clot, which could occlude the narrowed opening in a diseased coronary artery. Aspirin interferes with platelet aggregation or clumping; therefore, it acts as a prophylactic antithrombotic agent. Aspirin is more useful in relieving headaches and musculoskeletal pain than chest pain, and it is not a muscle relaxant. There is no scientific evidence that aspirin improves mood or causes euphoria. (15:70)

Nursing Process—Implementation
Client Need—Health promotion/maintenance

33 4. Signs of complications following PTCA include chest pain, bleeding from the catheter insertion site, and abnormal heart rhythms. Chest pain could indicate that the dilated coronary artery has suddenly closed again. If untreated, a myocardial infarction could occur. An hourly urine output of 30 to 50 mL or more is adequate. A blood pressure of 108/68 is in the low ranges of normal. A dry mouth could be a consequence of fluid restriction and medication administered prior to the procedure. As long as the blood pressure continues to remain in normal ranges, the nurse could relieve the discomfort of a dry mouth by giving oral care and administering oral fluids. (7:391; 16:357)

Nursing Process—Implementation
Client Need—Physiological integrity

34 4. The sensor for pulse oximetry can be applied to the fingertip, toe, ear, or tip of the nose. A pulse oximeter measures the oxygen saturation of hemoglobin. It is a convenient, noninvasive monitoring technique of a client's oxygenation. The sensor would not fit on the chest, thigh, or arm. (3:481)

Nursing Process—Implementation
Client Need—Safe, effective care environment

35 1. Using the thumb to obtain a pulse rate can result in inaccurate data. It is possible that the health care worker could feel his or her own pulse rather than the client's. It is best to rest or support the client's arm and compress the artery against the bone using the fingertips. It is not incorrect to count the pulse for 1 full minute; in fact, this would be preferred if the pulse is be-

lieved to be abnormal in any way. (18:257; 14:379)
Nursing Process—Implementation
Client Need—Safe, effective care environment

36 2. A patient in acute pain is most likely to have a rapid pulse rate, rapid respiratory rate, and rising blood pressure. Pain is least likely to influence body temperature. (18:254; 14:466)
Nursing Process—Collecting data
Client Need—Physiological integrity

37 1. Each time a client feels the need for medication he must press a control button releasing a very low dose of narcotic. The low dosage can be administered at frequent intervals. Usually, less total narcotic is actually used because, with frequent use, the discomfort rarely falls below a tolerable range. It is best to use the PCA infuser before pain becomes severe. PCA infusers are used only for a few days postoperatively, making it unlikely that narcotic addiction would occur. Because the client can use the machine independently, it frees the nurse to perform other responsibilities. (18:185; 3:213)
Nursing Process—Implementation
Client Need—Health promotion/maintenance

38 3. The number of doses the client has administered during the current shift is important information to communicate. It indicates how much pain the client is experiencing and his understanding of how best to use the machine. The name of the client's physician is readily available on multiple records. There is only one use for a PCA infuser pump, and that is to relieve pain. Because the client controls the use of the machine, it does promote a sense of independence. However, that is not the most important information for the nurse to report. (18:186)
Nursing Process—Implementation
Client Need—Safe, effective care environment

39 2. The saphenous vein is the most common blood vessel used for coronary artery bypass grafting. Removing a portion of this leg vein can temporarily impair the return of venous blood back to the heart. Impaired venous return would be manifested by edema and cool skin temperature in the toes, foot, or ankle of the operative leg. Therefore, the fact that the toes are warm and of normal size is the best evidence that venous blood is adequately returning to the heart through other blood vessels in the leg. The ability to move the leg is evidence that neurologic function is intact. A regular heart rate and absence of chest pain is evidence that the newly attached graft is supplying the heart muscle with adequate oxygenated blood. (3:497; 7:388)
Nursing Process—Evaluation
Client Need—Physiological integrity

NURSING CARE OF CLIENTS WITH MYOCARDIAL INFARCTION

40 1. The chest pain accompanying a myocardial infarction is often of such severity that the client becomes extremely diaphoretic. Hypotension is apt to make the client's skin appear pale or ashen. Thirst is associated with hypovolemia or diabetes mellitus. A moist cough is more likely found in clients with respiratory disease and congestive heart failure. (3:480; 16:309)
Nursing Process—Collecting data
Client Need—Safe, effective care environment

41 4. The most pertinent data to assess concerning pain are information on its onset, quality, intensity, location, and duration and what makes the pain better or worse. Although it is important to collaborate with the client on treatment approaches, the ultimate decision as to the route and prescribed drug to administer is a decision that is best made on the basis of the nurse's education and experience. (18:178; 14:463)
Nursing Process—Collecting data
Client Need—Physiological integrity

42 4. A client experiencing a myocardial infarction is likely to describe his pain as being substernal or radiating to the shoulder, arm, teeth, jaw, or throat. (16:309; 14:798)
Nursing Process—Collecting data
Client Need—Physiological integrity

43 4. Unlike angina pectoris, the pain caused by an acute myocardial infarction is not relieved by rest, nitroglycerin, or other nitrate drugs. Many describe the pain associated with a myocardial infarction using such terms as squeezing, suffocating, or crushing. The pain comes on suddenly. (14:798; 16:308)
Nursing Process—Collecting data
Client Need—Physiological integrity

44 4. A narcotic analgesic, such as meperidine hydrochloride or morphine sulfate, usually is required to relieve the severe pain associated with a myocardial infarction. Nonsteroidal, nonsalicylate, and salicylate analgesics generally are prescribed for minor pain. (3:480; 7:379)
Nursing Process—Planning
Client Need—Physiological integrity

45 3. Denial is used to shut out the painful awareness of reality. The person refuses to believe that an event is really happening. Regression occurs when a person resorts to a pattern of behavior characteristic of an earlier age. Projection involves blaming a negative situation on someone or something else. Undoing often takes on the form of offering a verbal apology or gift to make up for unacceptable behavior. (1:54; 12:71; 14:798)

Nursing Process—Implementation
Client Need—Psychosocial integrity

46 4. Of the factors listed in this item, having an occasional alcoholic beverage is least likely to predispose a myocardial infarction. Small amounts of alcohol may increase the good kind of cholesterol called high-density lipoprotein. However, alcohol does elevate triglyceride levels. Because the relationship of elevated triglycerides to heart disease has not been conclusively established, consuming small amounts of alcohol generally is not recommended for preventing atherosclerosis and the potential for a heart attack. Smoking, working under stress, and eating a diet high in fat and cholesterol are definite risk factors in developing a myocardial infarction. (4:417; 14:168)

Nursing Process—Collecting data
Client Need—Safe, effective care environment

47 3. CPK is an enzyme found in high concentrations in the heart and skeletal muscles and in much smaller amounts in brain tissue. The CPK blood level, especially its isoenzyme CPK-MB, begins to become elevated within 2 hours after a myocardial infarction. An elevated alkaline phosphatase is associated primarily with liver and bone diseases. AFP is a substance produced and secreted by tumor cells. The presence of AFP indicates that a person has cancer. Gamma-glutamyl transferase is a test used to determine liver cell dysfunction and to detect alcohol-induced liver disease. (5:343; 16:309)

Nursing Process—Collecting data
Client Need—Physiological integrity

48 1. Streptokinase is a thrombolytic enzyme. It is used to dissolve deep vein and arterial thromboemboli. This and other thrombolytic agents, such as urokinase (Abbokinase), anistreplase (Eminase), alteplase (Activase), and tissue plasminogen activator, activate plasminogen and convert it to plasmin. Plasmin breaks down the fibrin of a blood clot. Thrombolytic agents will not slow the heart rate, improve heart contraction, or lower blood pressure. (15:103; 7:379, 3:481)

Nursing Process—Implementation
Client Need—Health promotion/maintenance

49 3. Bleeding is the most common adverse reaction associated with thrombolytic drug therapy. Blood loss may be internal, involving the gastrointestinal or genitourinary tract, or may result in bleeding within the brain. Bleeding also may be external or superficial, manifested as oozing from venipuncture or injection sites, nosebleeds, and skin bruising. Recent trauma, childbirth, or surgery would be a contraindication in the use of a thrombolytic agent. (15:103; 7:379)

Nursing Process—Planning
Client Need—Physiological integrity

50 1. Urticaria is a term for hives. Hives, welts, and skin rashes are common manifestations of an allergic reaction. In addition, the nurse may observe difficulty breathing, wheezing, and hypotension. Dysuria is a term for painful urination. Hemoptysis indicates that the client is coughing bloody sputum. Dyspepsia is another word for indigestion. Neither dysuria, hemoptysis, nor dyspepsia are commonly associated with allergic reactions. (15:104; 14:1102)

Nursing Process—Collecting data
Client Need—Physiological integrity

51 3. To properly assess the need for resuscitation, the first action should be to gently shake the victim and shout, "Are you OK?" If the victim remains unresponsive, it would be important for the rescuer to then call loudly for additional help. If the victim cannot be aroused and is not breathing, the rescuer should give two breaths. The victim should be on a firm, flat surface before giving cardiac compressions. (3:872; 14:428)

Nursing Process—Implementation
Client Need—Physiological integrity

52 2. The nurse should use the chin lift/head tilt method for opening the airway when neck trauma is not suspected. This is performed by using one hand to lift the chin upward. This position is maintained by placing the other hand across the forehead. The jaw thrust method should be used if the chin lift/head tilt method does not open the airway adequately or if there is a possible neck injury. Placing a hand under the neck is no longer a recommended practice. The mouth can be cleared with a fingersweep after opening the airway. (18:735; 14:428-429)

Nursing Process—Implementation
Client Need—Physiological integrity

53 3. Once the airway is open, some victims may begin breathing spontaneously. The nurse can best assess for spontaneous breathing by leaning over the victim's head and listening or feeling for the movement of air from the nose or mouth. The

chest or abdomen also can be observed for rising and falling. Skin color is not a dependable assessment finding because hypotension, for whatever reason, is likely to cause the victim to appear pale or ashen. A carotid pulse is checked to determine the need for performing heart compressions. Administering rescue breathing may be unnecessary if the victim is spontaneously breathing. (18:736; 14:429)
Nursing Process—Collect data
Client Need—Physiological integrity

54 3. Pinching the nose shut allows maximum ventilation with no loss of air through the nostrils. If there has been a mouth injury or it is impossible to prevent air from leaking in an adult victim, the rescuer may use the mouth-to-nose technique for giving ventilations. When resuscitating an infant or small child, it may be helpful to make a seal by covering both the victim's nose and mouth with the rescuer's mouth. Once the breath has been given, the rescuer should allow the air to be exhaled passively. Pressing on the trachea may interfere with the passage of air. Removing dentures and squeezing the victim's cheeks may interfere with maintaining a tight seal during rescue breathing. (18:736; 14:429-430)
Nursing Process—Implementation
Client Need—Physiological integrity

55 1. Both of the rescuer's hands should be on top of one another on the lower half of the sternum two finger breadths above the xiphoid process. Placing the hands below the tip of the xiphoid process could cause the liver to be lacerated. The costal cartilage connects the ribs to the sternum. Compressing over the costal cartilage could fracture the victim's ribs. The manubrium is the upper portion of the sternum. The hands would be placed too high on the chest if positioned above the manubrium. (3:873; 14:430)
Nursing Process—Implementation
Client Need—Physiological integrity

56 4. The adult chest should be compressed during CPR at a rate between 80 to 100 times per minute. The sternum should be depressed approximately 1½ to 2 inches with each compression. Rates below 80 per minute are not likely to circulate blood adequately. (18:739; 7:395)
Nursing Process—Implementation
Client Need—Physiological integrity

57 2. The American Heart Association recommends that when two rescuers perform CPR, they administer five compressions and then a breath. The ratio for a single rescuer is 15 compressions

to two breaths. CPR should never be interrupted longer than 7 seconds. (18:739)
Nursing Process—Implementation
Client Need—Physiological integrity

58 3. If the pulse returns, cardiac compressions can be stopped. The carotid pulse should be assessed for a full 5 seconds after the first minute of resuscitation and thereafter every 4 to 5 minutes unless consciousness is restored. The victim's color may improve as a consequence of effective resuscitation efforts. Dilated and fixed pupils are an indication that the brain is not adequately oxygenated. Vomiting can occur in a nonbreathing and pulseless victim. It can occur from distending the stomach with air. (18:739; 7:395; 14:431)
Nursing Process—Evaluation
Client Need—Physiological integrity

59 2. Hospitalization, for most people, is a unique experience. Anxiety can be relieved by providing people in an unfamiliar environment with information about hospital equipment, clinical procedures, and agency routines. All explanations should be given in simple, understandable terms. Once informed, the client has a basis for interpreting the reality of his experiences. It would be unsafe to turn off the cardiac monitor because this equipment is used to detect life-threatening changes in his condition. Administering a tranquilizer at this time or distracting him with a magazine would not help prevent a similar reaction in the future. (7:380; 18:26; 17:270-271)
Nursing Process—Implementation
Client Need—Psychosocial integrity

60 1. Application sites should be rotated when topical nitroglycerin ointment or transdermal patches are used. The drug reservoir should not be touched or manipulated in any way. The patch is self-adhering once the adhesive backing is removed. Ointment application papers should be covered with kitchen plastic wrap and taped in place to prevent soiling clothing and to promote drug absorption. The patch can be placed on the chest, back, upper abdomen, or arms. It is not necessary to apply ice to the skin. (15:111; 18:590)
Nursing Process—Implementation
Client Need—Physiological integrity

61 4. Nitroglycerin dilates arterial vessels. This action lowers the blood pressure. Therefore, if the client's blood pressure is already low, as in 94/62, the nurse should check with the physician before applying the patch. It is not uncommon for the temperature of a client with a myocardial infarction to be slightly elevated. This is probably due to the inflammatory response from the injury to the myocardium. A respiratory rate of 24 and an apical heart rate of 90 are within normal limits. (15:108; 14:801)

    Nursing Process—Evaluation
    Client Need—Physiological integrity

62 2. The abbreviation *a.c.* means that a medication should be administered before meals. The abbreviation for a bedtime administration is *h.s.* For giving medication once each day, the physician would use the abbreviation *q.d.* Administering a drug as necessary or as needed is indicated with the abbreviation *p.r.n.* (18:576; 14:279)

    Nursing Process—Implementation
    Client Need—Physiological integrity

63 1. Encouraging a client to talk about his concerns helps him to relieve emotional tension. The best approach is to listen actively, remain nonjudgmental, and avoid offering any personal opinions. Asking a client a "why" question is often nontherapeutic, because the client may not be consciously aware of what is motivating his feelings or behavior. Telling the client that his physician believes he is doing fine implies that his fears are unfounded. A nonempathetic response may cause the client to terminate further discussion. Giving advice, as in "You need to concentrate on getting well," also is nontherapeutic because it blocks continued communication on the subject. (17:79; 9:139)

    Nursing Process—Implementation
    Client Need—Psychosocial integrity

64 1. One tablespoon of catsup contains 156 mg of sodium. Its use is generally omitted on a sodium-controlled diet. Vinegar, onions, and lemons may be used freely by a person on a low-calorie, low-fat, low-sodium diet. (4:443, 447)

    Nursing Process—Evaluation
    Client Need—Health promotion/maintenance

65 2. Straining involves holding one's breath and bearing down against a closed glottis. This action, sometimes called Valsalva's maneuver, increases abdominal and arterial pressure. The increase in arterial pressure acts as resistance to the pumping action of the heart. The flow of blood through the coronary arteries could be temporarily reduced, causing ischemia and chest pain. If the wall of the heart is necrotic, the increase in pressure could cause the weakened muscle to rupture, and the client could hemorrhage to death. Stool softeners generally are ordered prophylactically to eliminate straining when having a stool. Reading a murder mystery and playing solitaire are passive activities that ought not to

affect the cardiovascular system. People who experience heart attacks may participate in their own self-care provided that they do not develop signs of activity intolerance. Signs that indicate that the client should rest include becoming short of breath, developing a rapid or irregular heart rate, and experiencing increased blood pressure. (7:379; 14:800; 16:311)

    Nursing Process—Implementation
    Client Need—Health promotion/maintenance

66 2. An echocardiogram uses ultrasonic (sound) waves to image the heart's structure. The sound waves are reflected back in various ways, depending on the density of the tissues, to produce a replication of the heart that later can be evaluated. An x-ray uses radiation. An EKG picks up electric activity from the heart muscle. Thermography tests sense heat and variations in temperature to formulate images from body structures. (7:370; 3:471; 18:315)

    Nursing Process—Evaluation
    Client Need—Safe, effective care environment

NURSING CARE OF CLIENTS WITH CONGESTIVE HEART FAILURE

67 2. Early left-sided congestive heart failure is manifested by dyspnea and fatigue. Other classic signs and symptoms include a moist cough, orthopnea, tachycardia, restlessness, and confusion. (16:343; 14:803)

    Nursing Process—Collecting data
    Client Need—Safe, effective care environment

68 3. A complication of congestive heart failure is pulmonary edema. In this condition fluid occupies space within the small airways. As air is moved through the fluid-filled airways, the examiner is likely to hear crackles, also called rales. Crackles are high-pitched sounds heard in distant lung areas during inspiration. Some compare this abnormal sound to that made by a popular rice cereal as it comes in contact with milk. (16:345; 18:289)

    Nursing Process—Collecting data
    Client Need—Physiological integrity

69 3. When taking an apical–radial pulse, one nurse listens to the heart and counts the beats while the second one is counting the pulsations in the radial artery. If there is a difference in the two rates, it is called the pulse deficit. The apical rate is always the more accurate. (18:257; 14:380)

    Nursing Process—Implementation
    Client Need—Physiological integrity

70 4. A client with dyspnea usually is most comfortable and has the least amount of difficulty with breathing when placed in either a semisitting

(semi- or mid-Fowler's), sitting (high-Fowler's), or a standing position. Sitting and standing positions cause organs to fall away from the diaphragm, giving more room for the lungs to expand. (18:384, 395; 16:345)
Nursing Process—Planning
Client Need—Physiological integrity

71 2. People who are having difficulty breathing, a common symptom in left-sided congestive heart failure, typically feel anxious, apprehensive, and fearful. They are much less likely to feel depressed, defensive, or aggressive. (16:343; 14:804)
Nursing Process—Collecting data
Client Need—Psychosocial integrity

72 1. Oxygen should be started before applying a mask to the client's face. Flooding the mask with oxygen provides a readily available supply for the client to begin breathing immediately. If the flow of oxygen is begun after the mask is in place, it can intensify the client's breathless feeling. (18:730; 14:822)
Nursing Process—Implementation
Client Need—Physiological integrity

73 4. The correct volume needed to administer 80 mg of furosemide when the dosage strength is 40 mg/2 mL is 4 mL. A common formula to compute proper dosage is as follows: (15:12; 18:574)

$$\frac{\text{dosage desired}}{\text{dosage on hand}} \times \text{quantity} = \text{amount to administer}$$

$$\frac{80 \text{ mg}}{40 \text{ mg}} \times 2 \text{ mL} = \frac{160}{40} = 4 \text{ mL}$$

Nursing Process—Implementation
Client Need—Physiological integrity

74 2. The best technique for bringing medication to the base of an ampule is to tap the stem several times with a fingernail. Allowing the ampule to stand, flipping it back and forth, or rolling the ampule will not bring medication trapped in the stem of an ampule into the base of the container. (18:605; 14:489)
Nursing Process—Implementation
Client Need—Physiological integrity

75 3. An increase in the urinary output indicates that the drug furosemide is achieving its desired effect. By eliminating excessive water from the blood volume, the work of the heart is reduced. Less fluid will accumulate in the lungs. Furosemide may lower the blood pressure due to the change in fluid volume. The pulse rate should not change appreciably when furosemide is given. Once breathing is improved, anxiety should be reduced. However, this is not the best

evidence for assessing the effectiveness of furosemide. (15:125)
Nursing Process—Evaluation
Client Need—Physiological integrity

76 1. Palpating a distal pulse is the best guideline for determining that the blood pressure cuffs being used for rotating tourniquets have been properly inflated. The purpose for using this treatment approach is to create enough pressure to decrease the return of venous blood to the heart yet maintain arterial flow. Feeling a pulse indicates that arterial blood is continuing to move through the extremity. Pale fingers and slow capillary refill indicate reduced arterial blood flow. If a client can perceive sensation, it is an indication that his sensory nerves are intact. (16:349; 7:381)
Nursing Process—Implementation
Client Need—Safe, effective care environment

77 3. In 1 hour, each extremity has a cuff that remains inflated for 45 minutes. One of the four cuffs is deflated in a cyclical fashion every 15 minutes. At the end of 15 minutes, the deflated cuff is reinflated. Then the adjacent cuff is deflated. The pattern progresses in either a clockwise or counterclockwise direction. (7:381; 16:349)
Nursing Process—Implementation
Client Need—Safe, effective care environment

78 1. The presence of another person can do much to relieve anxiety. This is especially true when a person perceives himself or herself in a helpless and powerless situation. It is essential that a fearful person not be left alone. The physician could not do anything more than the nurse in this situation. Telling him he'll be OK is perhaps false reassurance because the outcome of his condition is not predictable. Recording the data can be postponed temporarily or reported verbally if it is needed. (12:355; 14:295)
Nursing Process—Implementation
Client Need—Psychosocial integrity

79 3. It is essential that the nurse monitor the serum potassium level of clients for whom a loop diuretic, like furosemide, is prescribed. A loop diuretic increases the excretion of sodium, chloride, and potassium. Low levels of potassium can cause a disturbance in the conduction system of the heart. Many clients who take a loop diuretic replace the lost potassium by eating foods that contain appreciable amounts of this electrolyte, or potassium supplements are prescribed. (14:513; 15:117)
Nursing Process—Collecting data
Client Need—Physiological integrity

80 4. Significant weight gain or loss, such as a difference of 2 lb or more in 24 hours, indicates major changes in body fluid distribution. Weight gain indicates fluid retention and impaired renal excretion. Weight loss indicates a therapeutic response to medical and drug therapy. Pupil response, bowel sounds, and appetite are appropriate to monitor in the daily assessments, but congestive heart failure is not likely to cause major changes in these findings. (7:383; 16:347)

Nursing Process—Collecting data
Client Need—Physiological integrity

81 2. Swelling of the feet and ankles accompanies right-sided congestive heart failure. Dependent edema occurs because the pumping action of the heart is impaired, decreasing blood flow to the kidneys. The combination of the heart and kidney impairments causes fluid to be retained. Excess fluid builds up in the lower extremities and abdomen. Glucose in the urine is associated with diabetes mellitus. A person with congestive heart failure has a tendency to gain weight due to the retention of fluid. A client with congestive heart failure may coincidentally be depressed. However, this is not a common finding among all people with congestive heart failure. (14:803; 16:344)

Nursing Process—Collecting data
Client Need—Safe, effective care environment

82 1. If neck veins distend with the head elevated 45 degrees or more, it is an indication that an increased volume of blood is not being circulated well through the right side of the heart. Burning on urination is a symptom of a bladder infection or trauma to the urethra. Periodic constipation and chronic indigestion may be due to any number of factors. These are not common findings associated with congestive heart failure. (14:803; 16:345)

Nursing Process—Collecting data
Client Need—Safe, effective care environment

83 1. Gastrointestinal symptoms associated with digitalis toxicity include anorexia, nausea, vomiting, and diarrhea. The client may become drowsy and confused. There may be visual changes, such as blurred vision, disturbance in seeing yellow and green colors, and a halo effect around dark objects. Toxic doses of digitalis drugs also can increase cardiac automaticity, causing a rapid heart rate, or depress the conduction of cardiac impulses, causing a slow heart rate. Serum drug levels can be used to monitor the client's metabolism of digitalis. Pinpoint pupils are associated with opiate toxicity. Ringing in the ears is a symptom of salicylate toxicity. (15:88)

Nursing Process—Collecting data
Client Need—Safe, effective care environment

84 1. Because digitalis preparations affect cardiac automaticity and the conduction system, it is es-

sential that the nurse monitor the client's apical or radial pulse before each administration of the drug. Assessing blood pressure, heart sounds, and lung sounds is part of a comprehensive cardiopulmonary assessment, but they are not directly affected by the administration of digitalis. (15:89, 91; 3:493)

Nursing Process—Implementation
Client Need—Physiological integrity

85 1. Half of a 0.25-mg tablet would be the correct amount of drug to administer to give 0.125 mg. The formula for determining the correct number of tablets is as follows: (15:12; 18:574)

$$\frac{\text{dosage desired}}{\text{dosage on hand}} \times \text{quantity} = \text{amount}$$
$$\text{to administer}$$

$$\frac{0.125 \text{ mg}}{0.25 \text{ mg}} \times 1 \text{ tablet} = \frac{0.125}{0.25}$$
$$= 0.5 \text{ or } 1/2 \text{ tablet}$$

Nursing Process—Implementation
Client Need—Physiological integrity

86 1. Any drug that slows the heart rate, such as digitalis, should be withheld, and the physician should be contacted if the apical heart rate is 60 beats per minute or less. The blood pressure measurement of 134/72/60 is within normal limits. S_1 and S_2 heart sounds are the normal "lub" and "dub" sounds made by the heart during contraction. Vesicular lung sounds are the normal, soft, rustling sounds heard in the periphery of all areas of the lungs. (15:91; 14:804)

Nursing Process—Implementation
Client Need—Physiological integrity

87 2. In general, it is least important to tell a client the name of the drug manufacturer. It is important to explain the purpose of the medication, when to use it, and symptoms associated with an adverse reaction. Noncompliance is greatest when people have been poorly taught concerning their drug regimens. (18:600; 15:32-35)

Nursing Process—Planning
Client Need—Health promotion/maintenance

88 3. People who are on sodium-restricted diets may consume fresh vegetables or vegetables that are canned or frozen without salt. Canned and dehydrated soups contain between 630 and 1300 mg of sodium per cup. Pizza and other convenience foods have sodium added to the crust and sauce. Sodium also is present in the cheese topping. In addition, salt is used when preparing sausage. Smoked fish are salted prior to smoking to promote their preservation. (4:439-445)

Nursing Process—Evaluation
Client Need—Health promotion/maintenance

NURSING CARE OF CLIENTS WITH DISORDERS OF THE CONDUCTION SYSTEM

89 1. A Holter monitor is used to collect data on a person's heart rhythm patterns during normal daily activity. The client should be told to keep a diary or record of the activities he performs and the time at which that activity began and ended. The monitor automatically records the time on a rhythm strip. For an accurate interpretation it is important to correlate the heart rhythm pattern with the performance of physical activity. The client need not assess his radial pulse; the heart rate can be determined from the rhythm strip. The client should perform his usual activities of daily living to obtain pertinent data. There are no dietary restrictions when using a Holter monitor. (3:471; 16:286)

Nursing Process—Implementation
Client Need—Safe, effective care environment

90 1. The nurse should caution a client with a Holter monitor to refrain from bathing, showering, or swimming to keep the electric wires from getting wet. Sleeping, dancing, and working are not contraindicated while a Holter monitor is being used. (3:471; 5:892)

Nursing Process—Implementation
Client Need—Safe, effective care environment

91 4. The SA node is the site of the heart's natural pacemaker. The SA node is called the pacemaker of the heart because it creates the electric impulses that cause the heart to contract. This specialized tissue is located in the wall of the right atrium between the openings for the inferior and superior vena cavae. A properly functioning SA node initiates regular impulses at a rate of 60 to 100 beats per minute. Once an impulse is sent from the SA node, it then travels down several internodal pathways to the AV node, the Bundle of His, the right and left bundle branches, and the Purkinje fibers. (11:203; 16:280)

Nursing Process—Evaluation
Client Need—Health promotion/maintenance

92 3. PVCs are potentially life-threatening. They often precede ventricular tachycardia or ventricular fibrillation. Drug therapy using lidocaine hydrochloride (Xylocaine) is prescribed when dangerous PVCs are noted. Sinus rhythm is the goal after a pacemaker is inserted. Sinus rhythm is a regular pattern of impulses initiated by the SA node or the artificial pacemaker through the conduction system at a rate between 60 and 100 beats per minute. Sinus arrhythmia, although more common in children, is not a dangerous abnormality. Sinus arrhythmia is a regular variation in the heart rate due to changes in the rate and depth of breathing. PACs are impulses initiated in the atrium earlier than usual. Usually the early impulse comes from tissue close by, but not directly from, the SA node. PACs are not particularly dangerous; usually, no treatment is given when they occur. (16:329; 3:488; 7:361-365)

Nursing Process—Collecting data
Client Need—Physiological integrity

93 4. A permanent pacemaker battery is usually implanted beneath the skin below the right clavicle. However, sometimes the area below the left clavicle may be used. The wire for a temporary pacemaker is inserted through a peripheral vein. It is then threaded into the right atrium and the right ventricle. Pacemaker wires may be placed during cardiac surgery in case a client needs pacing postoperatively. The wires can be seen externally from the skin on the chest. (16:329-330; 14:801-802)

Nursing Process—Collecting data
Client Need—Physiological integrity

94 1. Symptoms of battery failure or electric interference include dizziness, fainting, chest pain, dyspnea, confusion, and peripheral edema. These symptoms occur when the pulse rate drops and the cardiac output is decreased. Clients should be taught to move away from microwave ovens, arc welders, or power transformers if these symptoms occur. Some pacemakers have been found to be poorly manufactured, leading to their malfunction. Ordinarily pacemaker batteries do not need to be replaced for many years. Neither drowsiness nor headaches are common symptoms of battery failure or electric interference. Sometimes a client with a pacemaker can develop hiccups if the electric wire makes contact with the diaphragm. (7:366; 14:802)

Nursing Process—Evaluation
Client Need—Health promotion/maintenance

95 1. Cardioversion is similar to defibrillation. It involves administering a mild electric shock to the heart. Cardiac catheterization and angiography involve threading a catheter into the heart. Several types of cardiac imaging can be used to assess blood flow to the heart muscle, such as multigated acquisition and thallium-201 scans. (16:327-328; 3:473)

Nursing Process—Evaluation
Client Need—Safe, effective care environment

96 3. The nurse must avoid contact with the client or bed when the electric current is administered. The person administering the electric current should shout "stand back" or "all clear" just prior to pushing the button that discharges electricity. If there is contact with the client or bed, the nurse also will receive the electric current. Because there is no potential contact with blood, goggles and gloves do not need to be worn. Cardioversion is not an invasive procedure, so surgical asepsis practices do not need to be performed. There is no danger of radiation when a cardioversion is performed, so no lead apron need be worn. (14:803)

> Nursing Process—Implementation
> Client Need—Safe, effective care environment

97   2. The purpose of cardioversion is to stop the rapid cardiac rhythm and reestablish the SA node as the pacemaker. If this occurs, the heart will beat regularly at a rate between 60 to 100 beats per minute. Drugs such as diazepam (Valium) or midazolam (Versed) are used to produce conscious sedation. The client remains awake but usually will not have any memory of what was experienced. Equal apical and radial pulse rates are desirable, but this is not an indication of successful cardioversion. The normal difference between the systolic and diastolic blood pressures, also known as the pulse pressure, is approximately 40 mm Hg. Adequate cardiac output is generally reflected in a normal blood pressure measurement. However, the primary expected outcome of cardioversion is the restoration of normal cardiac rhythm. (16:328; 3:488)

> Nursing Process—Collect data
> Client Need—Safe, effective care environment

NURSING CARE OF CLIENTS WITH INFLAMMATORY DISORDERS OF THE CLIENT

98   3. Rheumatic fever often causes permanent damage to the heart and valves. About half of those people who have had rheumatic fever have narrowed mitral valves. Varicella, rubella, and whooping cough are acute infections, but they are not known to cause damage to heart valves. Intrauterine rubella infection can cause congenital heart defects, deafness, blindness, and mental retardation. (16:293; 7:28, 374)

> Nursing Process—Collecting data
> Client Need—Safe, effective care environment

99   2. The mitral valve is an atrioventricular valve. It is located between the left atrium and left ventricle. The pulmonic valve is between the right ventricle and the pulmonary artery. The tricuspid valve is between the right atrium and right ventricle. The aortic valve is located between the left ventricle and the aorta. (11:199-200; 3:490)

> Nursing Process—Implementation
> Client Need—Health promotion/maintenance

100   4. Dyspnea is the most prominent symptom of mitral stenosis. Stenosis, or narrowing of the mitral valve predisposes a person to left-sided congestive heart failure. Blood that cannot move through the small opening of the mitral valve collects in the left atrium. The accumulating blood eventually backs up into the pulmonary system causing congestion because it cannot be adequately circulated. (14:805; 16:293)

> Nursing Process—Collecting data
> Client Need—Safe, effective care environment

101   1. The sound from the mitral valve is best heard by auscultating the apical area, which is at the fifth intercostal space in the midclavicular line. When assessing heart sounds, the auscultatory areas are not directly over the anatomic locations of the heart valves. The aortic valve is best heard at the second intercostal space to the right of the sternum. The pulmonic valve is best heard at the second intercostal space to the left of the sternum. The tricuspid valve is best heard at the fourth intercostal space to the left of the sternum. (18:291; 3:476)

> Nursing Process—Implementation
> Client Need—Safe, effective care environment

102   4. Some people take a daily maintenance dose of penicillin, like nafcillin sodium, to prevent future streptococcal infections. The heart continues to be damaged by each subsequent infection. If daily doses of antibiotic are not taken, they are prescribed before oral surgery, tooth extractions, or other invasive procedures are performed. Nafcillin sodium will not destroy a virus, reduce scar tissue, or stop blood clots from forming. (14:805; 16:294)

> Nursing Process—Implementation
> Client Need—Health promotion/maintenance

103   1. To maintain adequate perfusion of all the cells in the body during any open heart surgery, blood is oxygenated and circulated by cardiopulmonary bypass using a heart-lung machine. A mitral commissurotomy is a procedure in which the surgeon blindly inserts a finger into the narrowed valve and dilates the opening. When a mitral commissurotomy is performed, the damaged valve is not replaced. Porcine (pork) valves and mechanical valves are used for replacing diseased valvular tissue. (16:356; 3:496)

> Nursing Process—Evaluation
> Client Need—Safe, effective care environment

104   3. Clubbing of the fingers and toes is a sign that occurs after years of poor oxygenation. It is found in people who have had long-term cardiopulmonary diseases. As the name suggests, the fingers appear like clubs; they are wider than normal at the distal end. The angle at the base of the nail is greater than the normal 160 degrees. A deviated nasal septum is most often congenital or caused by trauma. Flushed facial skin is seen in people who are feverish, have hypertension, or excess blood volume. A hoarse voice is symptomatic of diseased or inflamed vocal cords. (16:291; 3:393)

  Nursing Process—Collecting data
  Client Need—Safe, effective care environment

105 3. A fever is one of the classic ways that the body fights an infection. An elevated body temperature tends to destroy or inhibit the growth and reproduction of microorganisms. Chemicals present in white blood cells, which fight infection, trigger a heat-producing response in the hypothalamus. Chest pain usually is caused by inadequate blood supply to the myocardium. Pneumonia is more likely to cause a moist cough. Dyspnea is a common finding in many cardiopulmonary diseases. (14:374; 3:101; 7:375)

  Nursing Process—Collecting data
  Client Need—Physiological integrity

106 2. The diagnosis of bacterial endocarditis is usually made on the basis of the clinical symptoms and finding a pathogen, such as *Streptococcus viridans* or *Staphylococcus aureus*, in the blood. The organism enters through some distant portal of entry, such as the insertion site of the pulmonary artery catheter. The microbes then travel through the bloodstream and eventually invade the heart valves or endocardium. The surgical wound has likely healed by this time. A skin culture would not reveal systemic pathogens. The sputum and urine are not likely to contain pathogens that would be causing cardiac symptoms. (7:375; 16:292; 3:491)

  Nursing Process—Collect data
  Client Need—Physiological integrity

107 3. Evidence of activity intolerance includes rapid or irregular heart rate, hypotension, chest pain, dyspnea, and severe fatigue. If any of these are noted, the nurse would be correct in limiting any further activity. An improved appetite, restful sleep, and an interest in further activity are all positive signs, but they are not appropriate physiologic criteria of a person's ability to tolerate activity. (3:491; 14:805)

  Nursing Process—Collecting data
  Client Need—Physiological integrity

108 3. When a person is emotionally upset, it is most therapeutic to allow the person an opportunity to express his feelings. Saying nothing or leaving the room are of little help because these actions do not provide any support. The client, in this case, is not unhappy with the food. Rather, he is displacing his anger and frustration onto an inanimate object. Finding out a food preference avoids dealing with the emotional issues. (18:26)

  Nursing Process—Implementation
  Client Need—Psychosocial integrity

109 2. To enhance the ability to hear auscultated sounds, it would be best to reduce or eliminate sources of noise in the room. The humidifier attached to the flow meter of the oxygen is likely to cause extra noise, which may interfere with identifying normal and abnormal sounds. Holding the breath may aggravate a client's already compromised ventilation. Giving sips of water and locating the xiphoid will not promote the auscultation of heart or lung sounds. (18:288)

  Nursing Process—Implementation
  Client Need—Safe, effective care environment

110 3. A pericardial friction rub is a grating or leathery sound most often heard in people with pericarditis. It is caused by two layers of tissue moving roughly over one another. Wheezes and gurgles are evidence of pulmonary problems, such as asthma or pneumonia. A clicking sound is associated with the opening of the pulmonic and aortic valves. This is considered a normal sound. A murmur is an abnormal sound made by the turbulent flow of blood through narrow or incompetent valves. (14:805; 16:292-293)

  Nursing Process—Collecting data
  Client Need—Physiological integrity

Classification of Test Items

Unit IV Review Test 11

Directions: After each question the correct answer is given as well as a classification of each test question. Compare the correct answer with your answer. If a question has been answered *incorrectly*, draw a line to the end of the four columns. When finished, add up your correct scores and place the results at the bottom of each column.

Score Calculation:

To determine the percentage of the number of questions you answered correctly, divide the **Number Correct** by the **Number Possible**, as example 97 (the number of questions answered correctly) divided by 110 (the number of questions in the test) = .88 or 88%.

NURSING PROCESS

C = Collecting data
P = Planning
I = Implementation
E = Evaluation

CLIENT NEEDS

S = Safe, effective care environment
P = Physiological integrity
M = Psychosocial integrity
H = Health promotion/maintenance

Question #	Answer #	\multicolumn{4}{c} Nursing Process				\multicolumn{4}{c} Client Needs			
		C	P	I	E	S	P	M	H
1	3			I		S			
2	2	C				S			
3	2			I					H
4	2			I		S			
5	4			I					H
6	1			I					H
7	4	C				S			
8	2			I					H
9	3			I					H
10	2			I					H
11	3			I					H
12	2			I					H
13	3			I					H
14	3			I					H
15	1			I		S			
16	2			I				M	
17	4				E	S			
18	3	C				S			
19	1			I			P		
20	1	C				S			

NURSING PROCESS

C = Collecting data
P = Planning
I = Implementation
E = Evaluation

CLIENT NEEDS

S = Safe, effective care environment
P = Physiological integrity
M = Psychosocial integrity
H = Health promotion/maintenance

Question #	Answer #	Nursing Process				Client Needs			
		C	P	I	E	S	P	M	H
21	2	C					P		
22	3				E		P		
23	1				E		P		
24	3				E				H
25	1			I					H
26	4			I					H
27	3			I					H
28	4				E		P		
29	1				E				H
30	1			I					H
31	1	C					P		
32	2			I					H
33	4			I			P		
34	4			I		S			
35	1			I		S			
36	2	C					P		
37	1			I					H
38	3			I		S			
39	2				E		P		
40	1	C				S			
41	4	C					P		
42	4	C					P		
43	4	C					P		
44	4		P				P		
45	3			I				M	
46	4	C				S			
47	3	C					P		
48	1			I					H
49	3		P				P		
50	1	C					P		
51	3			I			P		
52	2			I			P		

NURSING PROCESS

C = Collecting data
P = Planning
I = Implementation
E = Evaluation

CLIENT NEEDS

S = Safe, effective care environment
P = Physiological integrity
M = Psychosocial integrity
H = Health promotion/maintenance

Question #	Answer #	Nursing Process				Client Needs			
		C	P	I	E	S	P	M	H
53	3	C					P		
54	3			I			P		
55	1			I			P		
56	4			I			P		
57	2			I			P		
58	3				E		P		
59	2			I				M	
60	1			I			P		
61	4				E		P		
62	2			I			P		
63	1			I				M	
64	1				E				H
65	2			I					H
66	2				E	S			
67	2	C				S			
68	3	C					P		
69	3			I			P		
70	4		P				P		
71	2	C						M	
72	1			I			P		
73	4			I			P		
74	2			I			P		
75	3				E		P		
76	1			I		S			
77	3			I		S			
78	1			I				M	
79	3	C					P		
80	4	C					P		
81	2	C				S			
82	1	C				S			
83	1	C				S			
84	1			I			P		

NURSING PROCESS

C = Collecting data
P = Planning
I = Implementation
E = Evaluation

CLIENT NEEDS

S = Safe, effective care environment
P = Physiological integrity
M = Psychosocial integrity
H = Health promotion/maintenance

Question #	Answer #	Nursing Process				Client Needs			
		C	P	I	E	S	P	M	H
85	1			I			P		
86	1			I			P		
87	2		P						H
88	3				E				H
89	1			I		S			
90	1			I		S			
91	4				E				H
92	3	C					P		
93	4	C					P		
94	1				E				H
95	1				E	S			
96	3			I		S			
97	2	C				S			
98	3	C				S			
99	2			I					H
100	4	C				S			
101	1			I		S			
102	4			I					H
103	1				E	S			
104	3	C				S			
105	3	C					P		
106	2	C					P		
107	3	C					P		
108	3			I				M	
109	2			I		S			
110	3	C					P		
Number Correct									
Number Possible	110	33	4	56	17	31	45	7	27
Percentage Correct									

Care of Clients with Disorders of the Endocrine System

Care of Clients with Hyperthyroidism (Exophthalmic Goiter)
Care of Clients with Diabetes Mellitus
g Care of Clients with Addison's Disease
ng Care of Clients with Cushing's Syndrome
vidual Test Items

Correct Answers and Rationale
Classification of Test Items

Directions: With a pencil, blacken the circle in front of the option you have chosen for your correct answer.

The Nursing Care of Clients with Disorders of the Endocrine System

NURSING CARE OF CLIENTS WITH HYPERTHYROIDISM (EXOPHTHALMIC GOITER)

Ms. Hattie Green, age 34, has had mild symptoms of hyperthyroidism for 1 year. Recently, her symptoms have become worse, and her physician has determined that a thyroidectomy will be necessary to treat her disorder. The nurse working in a physician's office records the client's symptoms, problems, and response to medications.

1 Which one of the following may indicate that Ms. Green is not responding to her medication?
   ○ 1. Constipation
   ○ 2. Continued anxiety and restlessness
   ○ 3. Anorexia
   ○ 4. Cool, dry skin

2 Ms. Green asks the nurse where her thyroid gland is located. The *most correct* reply is that the thyroid is
   ○ 1. in the neck behind the trachea.
   ○ 2. in front of the upper half of the sternum.
   ○ 3. behind the upper third of the sternum.
   ○ 4. in the neck in front of the trachea.

3 Ms. Green also asks "What is the purpose of the thyroid gland? What does it do?" The *most correct* response is based on the fact that the thyroid gland
   ○ 1. manufactures iodine.
   ○ 2. helps regulate the production and use of energy by the body.
   ○ 3. uses the hormone thyroxine to manufacture thyroid hormones.
   ○ 4. regulates the production of epinephrine and norepinephrine.

4 Two weeks prior to thyroid surgery, Ms. Green is prescribed an antithyroid drug. The nurse should instruct Ms. Green to complete the prescribed course of therapy because the drug will
   ○ 1. increase the size of the thyroid gland.
   ○ 2. decrease postoperative recovery time.
   ○ 3. decrease bleeding during surgery.
   ○ 4. increase the manufacture of thyroid hormones.

5 When performing an initial physical assessment on Ms. Green at the time of admission to the hospital for surgery the nurse should
   ○ 1. not take her vital signs.
   ○ 2. determine the size of the thyroid gland.
   ○ 3. keep the client on complete bed rest.
   ○ 4. avoid palpating the thyroid gland.

6 Which one of the following should the nurse place in Ms. Green's room before she returns from surgery?
   ○ 1. An ampule of intravenous iodine
   ○ 2. A dressing tray
   ○ 3. A tracheostomy tray
   ○ 4. An ampule of potassium chloride

7 When Ms. Green returns to her room after surgery the nurse should place her in a Fowler's position to
   ○ 1. make it easier for her to talk and eat.
   ○ 2. allow her to watch television without straining her neck.

○ 3. increase blood flow to the operative site.

○ 4. reduce edema in the operative area.

8 As soon as Ms. Green is awake and responding, the nurse should ask her to swallow several times and say a few words. This task is performed to determine if

  ○ 1. there is edema in or around the operative site.

  ○ 2. the surgical dressing adequately covers the incision.

  ○ 3. there is separation of the surgical incision.

  ○ 4. the thyroid gland has been totally removed.

9 The nurse is assigned to observe Ms. Green for signs of hypocalcemia. Which one of the following is *not* a sign of hypocalcemia?

  ○ 1. Carpopedal spasms

  ○ 2. Laryngeal spasm

  ○ 3. Muscle cramps

  ○ 4. Bone pain

10 Which one of the following complaints offered by Ms. Green may indicate hypocalcemia?

  ○ 1. "I think I have lost my appetite."

  ○ 2. "I feel tingling in my arms and legs."

  ○ 3. "It bothers my eyes to watch television."

  ○ 4. "I'm excited about going home soon."

The nurse is asked to check Ms. Green's dressing for bleeding.

11 Which one of the following methods best determines whether bleeding has occurred?

  ○ 1. Use a flashlight to visualize the dressing.

  ○ 2. Pass a hand around the back of the neck and feel for dampness.

  ○ 3. Ask Ms. Green if her dressing feels damp.

  ○ 4. Remove the top layer of the dressing to inspect the dressing closest to the surgical incision.

12 At a nursing conference a nurse assistant asks why the physician does not want Ms. Green to cough every 2 hours because it is the day after her surgery. The *most correct* answer is based on the fact that

  ○ 1. these clients do not encounter respiratory problems.

  ○ 2. coughing may cause bleeding in or around the surgical area.

  ○ 3. most thyroidectomies are performed under local anesthesia.

  ○ 4. coughing may cause a rupture of the larynx.

13 The nurse is assigned to observe Ms. Green for signs of hypoparathyroidism, which include

  ○ 1. numbness and tingling of the extremities and muscle cramping.

  ○ 2. anorexia and weight loss.

  ○ 3. flushing of the skin and fever.

  ○ 4. skin rash and muscle weakness.

14 Ms. Green is to be discharged. Which one of the following should the nurse plan to include in the discharge teaching?

  ○ 1. Liquid and soft foods must be eaten for 2 to 3 weeks.

  ○ 2. Apply an emollient such as petroleum jelly to the incision.

  ○ 3. Do not sleep on your side for 2 to 3 weeks.

  ○ 4. Care should be taken to avoid excessive strain on the incision.

NURSING CARE OF CLIENTS WITH DIABETES MELLITUS

Ms. Carla Davidson, who is 32 years old, had a preemployment physical examination and was found to have elevated blood glucose. She is referred to her primary physician for further tests.

15 The nurse working in a physician's office is asked by the physician to take an initial health history. Which of the following signs and symptoms might Ms. Davidson have if she has diabetes mellitus?

  ○ 1. Diarrhea, anorexia, and weight gain

  ○ 2. Polycholia, polyemia, and polyplegia

  ○ 3. Polyuria, polydipsia, and polyphagia

  ○ 4. Constipation, weight loss, and fever

Ms. Davidson is scheduled for a postprandial glucose test and a glucose tolerance test.

16 When explaining the postprandial glucose test, the nurse can tell Ms. Davidson that this test is performed

  ○ 1. in the evening, 2 hours after the last meal of the day.

  ○ 2. 2 hours after eating a normal meal.

  ○ 3. immediately before the noon meal.

  ○ 4. after fasting since midnight.

17 When explaining the glucose tolerance test, the nurse should inform Ms. Davidson that this test is performed

  ○ 1. early in the morning after fasting from midnight.

  ○ 2. in midafternoon after a meal high in carbohydrates.

  ○ 3. 1 hour after the evening meal.

  ○ 4. in midmorning after a light breakfast.

The physician determines that Ms. Davidson has diabetes mellitus.

18 When told of the diagnosis Ms. Davidson tells the nurse she is afraid that she will not be able to follow the prescribed treatment program. At this time the nurse could

  ○ 1. tell Ms. Davidson that she must comply or suffer serious consequences.

   ○ 2. assure Ms. Davidson that it is very easy to give insulin injections.

   ○ 3. give Ms. Davidson booklets explaining how to give insulin injections.

   ○ 4. allow Ms. Davidson time to express her anxiety and fears.

The physician determines that Ms. Davidson will require insulin. The nurse is asked to participate in a diabetic teaching program for Ms. Davidson.

19 Which of the following should the nurse plan to include when discussing the symptoms of hypoglycemia?

   ○ 1. Muscle soreness, leg cramps, and double vision

   ○ 2. Vomiting, diarrhea, and anorexia

   ○ 3. Weakness, excessive perspiration, and drowsiness

   ○ 4. Tinnitus, dizziness, and constipation

20 The nurse plans to discuss the importance of exercise in the control of diabetes. Which one of the following is correct and should be included in a discussion about exercise?

   ○ 1. Physical exercise improves the use of glucose by the body and improves circulation.

   ○ 2. Exercising for 1 hour three times a week allows for a wider range of food selections in the diet.

   ○ 3. Exercise will require an increase in the dose of insulin.

   ○ 4. When exercising, an extra dose of regular insulin will be required.

The physician prescribes Humulin L (human insulin from recombinant DNA) for Ms. Davidson.

21 Ms. Davidson has been reading literature about insulin and asks the nurse why human insulin sometimes is preferred over insulin obtained from animals. The *most correct* answer is based on the fact that human insulin

   ○ 1. is cheaper.

   ○ 2. appears to cause fewer allergies.

   ○ 3. requires smaller doses than other types of insulin.

   ○ 4. has a longer shelf life.

22 The nurse can emphasize the importance of rotating injection sites by planning to explain that this technique is used to prevent lipodystrophy, which may

   ○ 1. increase the rate of insulin absorption.

   ○ 2. decrease blood glucose values.

   ○ 3. interfere with the absorption of insulin at the affected site.

   ○ 4. interfere with obtaining venous blood for blood glucose tests.

23 The nurse also plans to discuss with Ms. Davidson the importance of personal hygiene because people with diabetes

   ○ 1. are believed to have a lowered resistance to infection.

   ○ 2. often do not feel like engaging in strict personal cleanliness.

   ○ 3. are resistant to most infections.

   ○ 4. require continuous low-dose antibiotic therapy.

24 Ms. Davidson tells the nurse that she never eats breakfast. The nurse should explain to Ms. Davidson that

   ○ 1. if she drinks skim milk in the morning, this will satisfy her need for breakfast.

   ○ 2. she must plan regular times for meals and snacks.

   ○ 3. she can omit breakfast and eat a midmorning high-calorie snack.

   ○ 4. breakfast can be skipped providing she takes her insulin before lunch.

Mr. Ken Edison, age 52, is admitted to the hospital with a tentative diagnosis of diabetic ketoacidosis (DKA). Ms. Edison states that her husband has not seen a physician in several years and has no known medical disorders.

25 The nurse is assigned to perform an initial assessment of Mr. Edison. Which of the following signs and symptoms may be observed by the nurse or described by a client with DKA?

   ○ 1. Hypertension and tachycardia

   ○ 2. Bradycardia and dyspnea

   ○ 3. Double vision and rapid weight gain

   ○ 4. Kussmaul respirations and acetone odor to breath

It is determined that Mr. Edison has DKA.

26 The nurse should observe Mr. Edison for signs of

   ○ 1. fluid volume excess.

   ○ 2. calcium excess (hypercalcemia).

   ○ 3. fluid volume deficit.

   ○ 4. magnesium excess (hypermagnesemia).

27 Mr. Edison, who is now semicomatose, is unable to handle his oral secretions and requires suctioning of his upper airway. Which of the following positions aids in the insertion of a suction catheter?

   ○ 1. Supine

   ○ 2. Recumbent

   ○ 3. Left lateral

   ○ 4. Semi-Fowler's

28 When inserting the suction catheter into Mr. Edison's mouth, the nurse should

   ○ 1. apply suction.

  ○ 2. squeeze the suction tip between the thumb and forefinger.

  ○ 3. not apply suction until the catheter is in the desired area.

  ○ 4. not turn the suction machine on until ready to withdraw the catheter.

29 During a nursing conference the nurse states that on admission Mr. Edison had Kussmaul respirations. A nurse assistant asks what this term means. The *most correct* description of Kussmaul respirations is respirations that are

  ○ 1. slow, deep, and sighing.

  ○ 2. rapid and shallow.

  ○ 3. rapid, deep, and labored.

  ○ 4. slow and shallow, accompanied by retraction of the sternum.

30 To develop an appropriate short-term plan of care, the nurse should know that DKA is treated with

  ○ 1. an oral hypoglycemic agent.

  ○ 2. intravenous glucose.

  ○ 3. intramuscular antibiotics.

  ○ 4. insulin.

Mr. Edison begins to respond to treatment and is more alert.

31 The physician orders Mr. Edison's urine to be tested for glucose and ketones (acetone). When collecting a urine specimen, the nurse should test a second voided specimen, which involves having Mr. Edison

  ○ 1. empty his bladder approximately ½ hour before the specimen to be tested is obtained.

  ○ 2. void into two containers.

  ○ 3. void a small amount of urine, stop, and then void again into a specimen container.

  ○ 4. empty his bladder 2 to 3 hours before obtaining a specimen for testing.

32 The nurse is assigned to check Mr. Edison's urine for glucose and ketones. If Mr. Edison has ketoacidosis, urine test results would be

  ○ 1. negative for ketones (acetone) and negative for glucose.

  ○ 2. positive for ketones (acetone) and positive for glucose.

  ○ 3. negative for ketones (acetone) and positive for glucose.

  ○ 4. positive for ketones (acetone) and negative for glucose.

33 A fasting blood glucose level is drawn on Mr. Edison. To immediately report abnormal results to the physician the nurse should know that a normal fasting blood glucose level is between

  ○ 1. 20 and 40 mg/dL

  ○ 2. 50 and 80 mg/dL

  ○ 3. 80 and 120 mg/dL

  ○ 4. 100 and 160 mg/dL

The physician prescribes regular insulin 20 U stat. for Mr. Edison.

34 How soon after administration of regular insulin should the nurse observe Mr. Edison for possible signs of hypoglycemia?

  ○ 1. 3 to 5 minutes

  ○ 2. 5 to 8 minutes

  ○ 3. Approximately 30 minutes

  ○ 4. Approximately 2 hours

35 The nurse is asked to check the stocked supply of intravenous glucose used to terminate an insulin reaction when the client is unconscious. The glucose used in this situation is labeled as

  ○ 1. 10%.

  ○ 2. 20%.

  ○ 3. 50%.

  ○ 4. 75%.

36 Ms. Edison asks the nurse what caused her husband's illness. The *most correct* reply is based on the fact that DKA results from

  ○ 1. an acute deficiency of insulin.

  ○ 2. receiving too much insulin.

  ○ 3. kidney failure.

  ○ 4. eating a diet high in protein.

Mr. Ralph Williams, age 69, has had diabetes mellitus for many years. Occasionally he cheats on his diet and forgets to take his insulin. He is presently admitted for treatment of an infection in his left foot.

37 Mr. Williams wears a hearing aid in his left ear. When giving daily care to Mr. Williams, the nurse should remove his hearing aid and

  ○ 1. soak it in a warm saline solution for 20 minutes.

  ○ 2. place it in a warmed container until daily care is completed.

  ○ 3. wipe it off with a soft dry tissue before reinsertion.

  ○ 4. wipe off the outside with alcohol before reinsertion.

38 Mr. Williams also has a removable bridge, which is used to replace missing lower front teeth. When giving daily care, the nurse should clean the bridge

  ○ 1. in a sink holding the bridge under running water.

  ○ 2. with a brush while holding the bridge over a soft surface or a basin of water.

  ○ 3. by soaking it in alcohol for 20 minutes.

  ○ 4. by immersing it in hot water for 5 minutes.

The nurse is asked to participate in a diabetic teaching program and is assigned to discuss hyperinsulism, hypoinsulinism, and the importance of diet with Mr. and Ms. Williams.

39 Which of the following would be included in a discussion of how to terminate a hypoglycemic (hyperinsulinism) reaction?
  ○ 1. Allow a tablet of an oral hypoglycemic agent to dissolve slowly in the mouth.
  ○ 2. Eat a high-protein substance, such as cheese.
  ○ 3. Drink a glass of milk.
  ○ 4. Eat or drink a quick-acting carbohydrate, such as orange juice, candy, or a dextrose solution.

40 The nurse also explains to Ms. Williams that if a hypoglycemic reaction should occur, eating or drinking an oral substance to terminate the reaction should not be used if Mr. Williams.
  ○ 1. has had a dose of insulin.
  ○ 2. is unable to swallow.
  ○ 3. has eaten a meal.
  ○ 4. is at work.

41 Mr. Williams is receiving NPH insulin, which is in a suspension. The correct technique for ensuring adequate mixing of the suspension before withdrawing insulin from the vial is to
  ○ 1. shake the vial vigorously.
  ○ 2. rotate the vial between the palms.
  ○ 3. invert the vial for 20 minutes.
  ○ 4. refrigerate the vial for 1 hour before use.

42 Mr. Williams is now prescribed NPH insulin (isophane insulin suspension) and regular insulin, both of which are to be administered in the same syringe. When preparing these two insulins for administration in a single syringe, the insulin syringe is first
  ○ 1. filled with NPH insulin.
  ○ 2. filled with half the dose of the NPH insulin and half the dose of the regular insulin.
  ○ 3. filled with 5 mL of air.
  ○ 4. filled with regular insulin.

43 Mr. Williams is taught the method of withdrawing two insulins in the same syringe for self-administration but has trouble with the accuracy of measuring each dose. The nurse can then suggest that he
  ○ 1. use two separate syringes for administration of his insulin.
  ○ 2. have a visiting nurse administer his insulin.
  ○ 3. have a home health care aide administer his insulin.
  ○ 4. ask his physician if can change the insulin dose.

Mr. Williams has been taught the technique of insulin injection. The nurse is assigned to evaluate Mr. Williams' ability to give his own insulin.

44 Mr. Williams, who weighs 139 pounds, is giving his insulin correctly if he inserts the needle at a
  ○ 1. 15-degree angle.
  ○ 2. 45-degree angle.
  ○ 3. 60-degree angle.
  ○ 4. 120-degree angle.

45 The nurse plans to discuss with Mr. Williams how and where to store insulin when he is home. Which one of the following is correct?
  ○ 1. Insulin is best kept in an area where the temperature is above 60°F.
  ○ 2. Insulin can be safely stored under any temperature.
  ○ 3. Insulin is stored in a cool place or in the refrigerator.
  ○ 4. Insulin should be kept in the freezer.

Mr. Allen Carter, age 44, is a new diabetic who requires insulin. The physician asks the nurse to begin diabetic teaching.

46 When discussing the control of diabetes, the nurse plans to include the fact that severe emotional stress requires contacting the physician because he may
  ○ 1. need to reduce the number of calories in his diet.
  ○ 2. require an increase in his insulin dosage.
  ○ 3. require a decrease in his insulin dosage.
  ○ 4. need to increase his fat intake.

47 The nurse tells Mr. Carter that visual problems due to diabetes mellitus can be prevented or minimized by
  ○ 1. wearing glasses when reading.
  ○ 2. eating more vegetables.
  ○ 3. taking vitamin supplements.
  ○ 4. controlling his blood glucose levels.

48 The nurse also plans to explain to Mr. Carter that a planned and regular program of exercise may
  ○ 1. reduce his daily insulin dosage.
  ○ 2. prevent episodes of hypoglycemia.
  ○ 3. enable him to do without daily insulin injections.
  ○ 4. require that he increase his insulin dosage.

49 The nurse discusses foot care with Mr. Carter, who states that his feet perspire freely. The nurse can recommend that he
  ○ 1. wash his feet only every 2 or 3 days.
  ○ 2. change his socks daily.
  ○ 3. use a preparation to remove any calluses on his feet.
  ○ 4. not soak his feet before trimming his toenails.

50 When discussing the purchase of insulin, Mr. Carter asks if any trade name (brand name) of insulin may be used as long as it is NPH. The most correct answer should include the fact that one brand of insulin should not be substituted for another because
  ○ 1. some people are sensitive to changes in brands of insulin.
  ○ 2. drug companies vary in the number of units per milliliter.

○ 3. a different type needle and syringe must be used.

○ 4. some brands are more expensive than others.

NURSING CARE OF CLIENTS WITH ADDISON'S DISEASE

Mr. William Harding, a 43-year-old who appears acutely ill, is admitted to the hospital with a diagnosis of cholecystitis and is scheduled for a cholecystectomy. He also has Addison's disease (adrenal cortical insufficiency), which was diagnosed approximately 4 years ago.

51 One part of the nurse's initial assessment of Mr. Harding is focused on his history of Addison's disease. Which of one of the following should be obtained from the client during an initial history?

○ 1. The daily dose of corticosteroid replacement therapy

○ 2. The daily dose of pituitary hormone

○ 3. The approximate amount of urine passed daily

○ 4. The cause of his disorder

52 Which one of the following signs might the nurse recognize as a *symptom* of Addison's disease when a physical assessment is performed on Mr. Harding?

○ 1. Excessive weight gain, especially in the trunk of the body

○ 2. Abnormally dark pigmentation of the skin and mucous membranes

○ 3. Multiple bruises on the trunk and extremities

○ 4. Excessive hair growth on the face

53 Before and after gallbladder surgery, the nurse should observe Mr. Harding for signs of acute adrenal crisis, which include

○ 1. dysuria, edema, and bradycardia.

○ 2. hypertension, hypothermia, and weight gain.

○ 3. hypotension, restlessness, nausea, and vomiting.

○ 4. pale skin, constipation, and heartburn.

54 A nursing conference is used to plan Mr. Harding's postoperative care. Which of the following errors could result in acute adrenal crisis when a client has Addison's disease?

○ 1. Inadvertent increase in the flow rate of intravenous fluids from 20 to 30 drops/min

○ 2. Failure to obtain the blood pressure hourly for 3 hours

○ 3. Omission of a daily vitamin and mineral supplement

○ 4. Failure to administer the prescribed corticosteroid

55 The nurse is assigned to observe Mr. Harding for fluid and electrolyte disorders for the next 7 hours. Which of the following fluid and electrolyte problems may be seen in those with Addison's disease?

○ 1. Hyponatremia and dehydration

○ 2. Hypernatremia and edema

○ 3. Fluid volume excess and hyperglycemia

○ 4. Hypervolemia and hypokalemia

NURSING CARE OF CLIENTS WITH CUSHING'S SYNDROME

Ms. Althea Gibson, age 48, sees her physician because she has noted many changes in her appearance over the past several months. After examining Ms. Gibson the physician suspects Cushing's syndrome (adrenal cortical hyperfunction).

56 Which one of the following might the nurse recognize as a symptom of Cushing's syndrome when an initial physical assessment is performed on Ms. Gibson?

○ 1. Signs of extreme weight loss

○ 2. Hypotension

○ 3. Muscle wasting and weakness

○ 4. Fever

57 The physician admits Ms. Gibson to the hospital for further diagnostic tests. When developing a plan of care for Ms. Gibson, the nurse should include

○ 1. a schedule of increased exercise to improve muscle tone.

○ 2. between-meal feedings that are high in protein and calories.

○ 3. frequent rest periods between activities.

○ 4. encouraging extra fluids.

58 The physician determines that Ms. Gibson requires an adrenalectomy. At a nursing conference a nurse assistant asks the nurse why Ms. Gibson's adrenal glands must be removed. The most correct answer is based on the fact that Cushing's syndrome

○ 1. can be due to a lack of adrenal cortical hormones.

○ 2. causes pain in the adrenal glands.

○ 3. results in a decrease in size of the kidneys.

○ 4. can be due to an increase in adrenal cortical hormones.

59 Ms. Gibson is scheduled for a bilateral adrenalectomy. The nurse is assigned to develop a postoperative plan of care. Which one of the following care plan entries assumes the highest priority?

○ 1. Turning, coughing, and deep breathing every 2 hours

○ 2. Making sure the medical team knows that corticosteroid therapy must never be omitted

○ 3. Accurately measuring intake and output

○ 4. Monitoring vital signs

60 Which one of the following should the nurse consider as the most essential addition to a care plan for Ms. Gibson?

○ 1. Observing the client for signs of adrenal crisis
○ 2. Contacting the physician if hypertension develops
○ 3. Testing the urine for glucose and ketones (acetone)
○ 4. Observing the client for an increase in the signs and symptoms of Cushing's syndrome

61 Two nurses are assigned to develop a discharge teaching plan for Ms. Gibson. Which one of the following discharge teaching plan entries is *incorrect*?
○ 1. Immediately contact the physician if unable to take the prescribed medication orally.
○ 2. Obtain adequate rest.
○ 3. Eat a well-balanced diet.
○ 4. If nausea and vomiting should occur, omit the next dose of the medication and contact the physician within 24 hours.

INDIVIDUAL TEST ITEMS

62 When reviewing Ms. Everett's chart, the diagnosis is stated as myxedema. To develop an effective plan of care, the nurse should know that myxedema may be defined as
○ 1. severe hypothryroidism.
○ 2. failure of the adrenal glands to secrete epinephrine.
○ 3. total pituitary failure.
○ 4. a form of diabetes mellitus.

63 Ms. Coleman, who has hyperthyroidism, is scheduled to receive radioactive iodine (^{131}I). To develop an effective plan of care, the nurse should know that
○ 1. Ms. Coleman will need to be placed on radiation precautions for 21 days.
○ 2. radioactive iodine increases the manufacture of thyroid hormones.
○ 3. this treatment attempts to destroy thyroid tissue.
○ 4. other tissues of the body usually are affected by this radioactive preparation.

64 A client is receiving strong iodine solution (Lugol's solution). The dose is ordered as 15 gtt. The nurse correctly interprets this order as meaning 15
○ 1. grams.
○ 2. drams.
○ 3. drops.
○ 4. grains.

65 When giving strong iodine solution (Lugol's solution), the nurse may add the drug to fruit juice to
○ 1. disguise the taste.
○ 2. increase the absorption of the drug.
○ 3. prevent the drug from being absorbed rapidly.
○ 4. enhance the taste.

66 Which one of the following questions should the nurse include in a history obtained from a client with an enlarged thyroid?
○ 1. "Do you think you are hyperthyroid?"
○ 2. "Have you ever had x-ray treatment for acne when you were young?"
○ 3. "What makes you think you have a problem with your thyroid gland?"
○ 4. "Are you prepared to have surgery on your thyroid gland?"

67 A nurse is assigned to care for a client with diabetes insipidus. Which one of the following should be included in a plan of care for this client?
○ 1. Oral temperature every 2 hours
○ 2. Weekly weight
○ 3. Accurate measurement of the intake and output
○ 4. Low-calorie diet

68 A nurse is assigned to assist in the development of a plan of care for a client with hyperparathyroidism. Which one of the following symptoms of this disorder should be considered when developing a plan of care?
○ 1. Bone pain
○ 2. Excessive weight gain
○ 3. Hyperactivity
○ 4. Increase in muscle size

Correct Answers and Rationale

Two numbers appear in parentheses following each rationale. The first number identifies the textbook listed in the references, page 451, and the second number identifies the page(s) in that textbook on which the correct answer can be verified. Occasionally, two textbooks are given for verifying the correct answer.

1 2. Anxiety and restlessness are two symptoms of hyperthyroidism. Additional symptoms may include weight loss; increased appetite; diarrhea; warm, flushed skin; tachycardia; and insomnia. If the client has continued anxiety and restlessness, she still has symptoms of hyperthyroidism; this should be brought to the attention of the physician. (16:628)
　　Nursing Process—Evaluation
　　Client Need—Physiological integrity

2 4. The thyroid gland is located anteriorly (in front of) to the trachea. (16:622)
　　Nursing Process—Implementation
　　Client Need—Health promotion/maintenance

3 2. The thyroid gland controls many body processes, including metabolic cellular functions, stimulation of the synthesis of proteins, activation of the cellular production of heat, stimulation of the manufacture of coenzymes from vitamins, and regulation of carbohydrate metabolism. (16:622; 3:682)
　　Nursing Process—Implementation
　　Client Need—Health promotion/maintenance

4 3. The surgeon may prescribe an antithyroid drug, such as propylthiouracil or methimazole (Tapazole) 2 or more weeks prior to surgery to decrease bleeding during surgery. An antithyroid drug does not increase the size of the thyroid or increase the manufacture of thyroid hormones. Postoperative recovery time is not likely to be directly affected by the administration of an antithyroid preparation. (16:632-633)
　　Nursing Process—Implementation
　　Client Need—Health promotion/maintenance

5 4. When the client is hyperthyroid, palpation of the thyroid gland may release additional thyroid hormones, which in turn could result in severe and sometimes dangerous symptoms of hyperthyroidism. The physician may palpate the thyroid during an initial physical examination, but great care is required for this task, which should be performed only by an experienced examiner. Vital signs can be taken. Unless the physician or-

ders otherwise, complete bed rest is not necessary. (16:632-633)
　　Nursing Process—Collecting data
　　Client Need—Physiological integrity

6 3. Respiratory difficulty due to edema or bleeding in or around the operative site must be reported immediately to the physician because an emergency trachesotomy may be necessary. When a client has a thyroidectomy, a tracheostomy tray should be placed in the client's room or kept in the clinical area. If thyroid crisis should occur, sodium iodide and not intravenous iodine may be administered. Calcium chloride may be used to treat tetany resulting from inadvertent removal of the parathyroid glands. A dressing tray usually is not required because the postoperative dressing is small and rarely requires reinforcement. (3:688)
　　Nursing Process—Implementation
　　Client Need—Physiological integrity

7 4. The primary purpose of placing the postoperative thyroidectomy client in a Fowler's position is to facilitate breathing and reduce edema in the operative area. (3:688)
　　Nursing Process—Implementation
　　Client Need—Physiological integrity

8 1. Asking the client to say a few words and swallow a few times may help identify the presence of edema in or around the operative site, which may produce severe hoarseness or difficulty in talking or swallowing. Edema can be potentially serious because its occurrence can obstruct the airway and cause difficulty in breathing. This task also determines if there has been any damage to the recurrent laryngeal nerve resulting in vocal cord paralysis. (16:634-635)
　　Nursing Process—Collecting data
　　Client Need—Physiological integrity

9 4. Of the four options of this question, bone pain is normally not associated with hypocalcemia. Bone pain may be seen in those with hypercalcemia. (16:634, 121-123)
　　Nursing Process—Collecting data
　　Client Need—Physiological integrity

10 2. Tingling and numbness of the extremities is one symptom of hypocalcemia. Often this may be the first symptom noted by the client. The remaining complaints listed in this question normally are not associated with hypocalcemia. (16:122)

> Nursing Process—Evaluation
> Client Need—Physiological integrity

11 2. Gently passing the hand behind the client's neck and feeling for dampness determines if blood is oozing around to the back of the client's neck. The bed linen also is inspected for drainage each time the client is turned. (16:634)

> Nursing Process—Collecting data
> Client Need—Physiological integrity

12 2. During the immediate postoperative period, some surgeons do not want the client to cough every 2 hours; deep breathing and leg exercises usually are permitted. Coughing may precipitate bleeding in and around the surgical area, which can result in airway obstruction. (16:634)

> Nursing Process—Implementation
> Client Need—Physiological integrity

13 1. Thyroid surgery may result in accidental removal of the parathyroid glands. Clients having a thyroidectomy should be observed for signs of hypoparathyroidism. Numbness and tingling of the extremities or around the lips usually are early signs of hypoparathyroidism. Additional signs and symptoms may include tetany, muscle cramping, continuous contraction of an arm or finger, a positive Chvostek's sign, and laryngeal spasm. Hypoparathyroidism following thyroid surgery must be immediately recognized and treated. (16:636-637)

> Nursing Process—Collecting data
> Client Need—Physiological integrity

14 4. Excessive strain on the incision should be avoided until it is healed. It is not necessary to eat a liquid or soft diet or avoid sleeping on the left or right side unless ordered to do so by the physician. Nothing should be applied to the incision unless recommended by the physician. (16:634-635)

> Nursing Process—Planning
> Client Need—Safe, effective care environment

NURSING CARE OF CLIENTS WITH DIABETES MELLITUS

15 3. Polyuria (excessive secretion and voiding of urine), polydipsia (excessive thirst), and polyphagia (increased appetite) are the classic signs and symptoms of diabetes mellitus. Polycholia (increased secretion of bile), polyemia (increased amount of circulating blood), polyplegia

(paralysis of several muscles), diarrhea, constipation, anorexia, and fever usually are not considered signs and symptoms of this endocrine disorder. Weight gain or loss may be seen in some people. (3:700)

> Nursing Process—Collecting data
> Client Need—Physiological integrity

16 2. Postprandial means after eating. A postprandial glucose test requires the drawing of blood 2 hours after eating a normal meal. A result above 140 mg/dL is considered abnormal. A postprandial glucose test may be performed to determine the need for performing a glucose tolerance test. (3:699)

> Nursing Process—Implementation
> Client Need—Safe, effective care environment

17 1. A glucose tolerance test is performed early in the morning after the client has had nothing to eat or drink after midnight. The client is given a large, measured amount of liquid glucose. Normally, blood and urine samples are taken at 30 minutes and then at 1, 2, and 3 hours. Hospitals or laboratories may slightly vary on the times blood and urine samples are taken. (3:699)

> Nursing Process—Implementation
> Client Need—Safe, effective care environment

18 4. Clients need time to accept their diagnosis and to talk about their disorder and express any fears or concerns they may have. Telling the client that she must comply, assuring her that injections are easy to give, and giving the client booklets to read may make the client feel that the nurse is not interested or does not have the time to listen. (16:652-654)

> Nursing Process—Implementation
> Client Need—Psychosocial integrity

19 3. In addition to weakness, excessive perspiration, and drowsiness, the client experiencing an episode of hypoglycemia also may note symptoms such as personality changes, headache, nausea, hunger, tremors, visual problems (double or blurred vision), and malaise. (16:649)

> Nursing Process—Planning
> Client Need—Physiological integrity

20 1. Physical exercise plays an important part in the management of diabetes mellitus. Exercise improves circulation and the use of glucose by the body; thus, it reduces insulin requirements. (3:702; 16:647)

> Nursing Process—Planning
> Client Need—Physiological integrity

21 2. Human insulin is obtained in one of two ways. One is by a process of genetic engineering using strains of *Escherichia coli*, a microorganism found in the gastrointestinal tract. The other is by chemical modification of pork insulin. Human insulin is not cheaper and does not have a longer shelf life, and its use does not reduce the dose of insulin. Human insulin appears to cause a lower incidence of allergies than insulin obtained from animal sources. (3:702; 15:139)

    Nursing Process—Implementation
    Client Need—Health promotion/maintenance

22 3. Lipodystrophy is a change in subcutaneous fat at the site of previous insulin injections and often occurs when the same site is used repeatedly. Lipodystrophy may interfere with the absorption of insulin when the affected area is used for insulin administration. Localized abscesses also may be seen. This condition can be prevented by rotating injection sites. Lipodystrophy does not decrease blood glucose values or increase the rate of insulin absorption. Lipodystrophy, when it does occur, is not located at sites where venous blood samples normally are obtained. (7:604)

    Nursing Process—Planning
    Client Need—Physiological integrity

23 1. The cause of a lowered resistance to infection in the diabetic client is not fully understood but may be due to high blood glucose levels in uncontrolled diabetes, a suppression of the immune system, or some other factor. (7:605)

    Nursing Process—Planning
    Client Need—Health promotion/maintenance

24 2. Those with diabetes mellitus should not skip or omit meals because it is necessary to maintain a relatively constant and normal blood glucose level by means of diet and insulin administration. (20:319)

    Nursing Process—Implementation
    Client Need—Health promotion/maintenance

25 4. Early signs and symptoms of DKA may be vague. Later, an acetone odor to the breath, weakness, thirst, anorexia, vomiting, drowsiness, abdominal pain, rapid and weak pulse, hypotension, flushed skin, and Kussmaul respirations may be seen. In severe cases the client may be comatose or semicomatose. (16:648)

    Nursing Process—Collecting data
    Client Need—Physiological integrity

26 3. Clients with DKA should be closely observed for signs of a fluid volume deficit (dehydration) and electrolyte imbalances. (16:653)

    Nursing Process—Collecting data
    Client Need—Physiological integrity

27 4. When possible, a client is placed in a semi-Fowler's postion when upper airway suctioning is necessary. (18:710-712)

    Nursing Process—Implementation
    Client Need—Physiological integrity

28 3. Applying suction when inserting a catheter may result in damage to the oral mucosa. The finger does not cover the vent on the suction catheter until the tip of the catheter is in the desired area. The suction machine can be on while the catheter is being inserted but the nurse's finger does not cover the vent (covering the vent allows suction to occur) until the catheter is in place. The tip of the suction catheter is not touched. Depending on hospital policy, oral suctioning is carried out with either aseptic or clean technique. (18:710-712)

    Nursing Process—Implementation
    Client Need—Physiological integrity

29 3. Kussmaul respirations may be described as rapid, deep, labored respirations. (16:648)

    Nursing Process—Implementation
    Client Need—Safe, effective care environment

30 4. The treatment of DKA includes the administration of insulin, usually intravenously. Insulin administration reduces the production of ketones by making carbohydrates available for oxidation by tissues. An oral hypoglycemic agent would be of no value in treating this serious disorder because these drugs are used for those with some pancreatic insulin-secreting activity. Glucose would not be given because blood glucose levels are already elevated. Antibiotics are not indicated because this is not an infectious disorder. (16:648-649)

    Nursing Process—Planning
    Client Need—Physiological integrity

31 1. When testing the urine for glucose and ketones (acetone) the most accurate results are obtained when the client produces urine recently excreted by the kidneys. Having the client empty his bladder ½ hour before the anticipated time and then suggesting that the client drink one to two glasses of water often produces a "fresh" specimen in approximately 30 minutes. (18:537)

    Nursing Process—Implementation
    Client Need—Physiological integrity

32 2. With DKA the urine is positive for glucose and ketones (acetone). (3:711)

    Nursing Process—Implementation
    Client Need—Physiological integrity

33 3. The normal fasting blood glucose level is between 80 and 120 mg/dL. Results significantly below 80 or above 120 mg/dL usually indicate hypoglycemia or hyperglycemia. Significantly abnormal results are immediately reported to the physician. (16:646)

    Nursing Process—Collecting data
    Client Need—Physiological integrity

34 3. Regular insulin is a rapid-acting insulin, which has an onset of action in 30 to 60 minutes. Clients receiving regular insulin should be closely observed for signs of hypoglycemia starting in 30 minutes and then observed at 10- to 15-minute intervals for the next hour. This is especially important when the client is first placed on insulin therapy, is a brittle diabetic, or receives insulin for the correction of DKA. (15:139)
Nursing Process—Collecting data
Client Need—Physiological integrity

35 3. 50% glucose is given intravenously when the client has hyperinsulinism (hypoglycemia) and is unable to take an easily absorbed carbohydrate by mouth. (7:608)
Nursing Process—Implementation
Client Need—Safe, effective care environment

36 1. DKA results when there is an acute deficiency of insulin. When there is an insulin deficiency, the body cannot use glucose and therefore uses fats and proteins for a source of energy, which, when metabolized, result in an abundance of ketones. DKA may be seen when the client, who is a known diabetic and taking insulin, receives or takes an inadequate amount of insulin or omits doses. DKA also may occur when the client is taking the prescribed dose of insulin but radically departs from the prescribed diet for several or more days. The client who has not been diagnosed as having diabetes may develop DKA. (16:648; 3:711)
Nursing Process—Implementation
Client Need—Health promotion/maintenance

37 3. The outside of the hearing aid is cleaned with a soft, dry tissue or cloth to remove any wax (cerumen) that may have accumulated on the outside of the appliance. Alcohol or other liquids should not be used to clean the external surface of the hearing aid. (18:113-114)
Nursing Process—Implementation
Client Need—Physiological integrity

38 2. A brush (toothbrush or partial brush) is used to clean removable bridges. The bridge should be held over a soft surface or basin of water and cleaned with water or diluted oral mouthwash solution. Toothpaste can be used if the bridge has food particles stuck to the denture. Holding the bridge over a sink can result in damage to the dental appliance if it is dropped. Soaking it in alcohol may leave an alcohol residue, which can irritate gum tissue. Dental appliances should not be washed in hot water because this may soften the appliance and lead to breakage or loosening. (18:99-101, 106)
Nursing Process—Implementation
Client Need—Physiological integrity

39 4. Hypoglycemic reactions must be terminated as soon as possible. The ingestion of a quick-acting carbohydrate, such as candy, orange juice, or water with sugar added usually terminates a hypoglycemic reaction. An oral hypoglycemic agent is used to treat diabetes mellitus when the client's pancreas has some insulin-producing ability. High-protein food or a glass of milk would not quickly terminate a hypoglycemic reaction because very little or no sugar may be available in these substances. (16:650)
Nursing Process—Implementation
Client Need—Health promotion/maintenance

40 2. Oral fluids, for whatever reason, are contraindicated if the client is unable to swallow. Aspiration of an oral fluid may be followed by aspiration pneumonia or other serious problems. If the client is at home or work, has a hypoglycemic reaction, and is unconscious, emergency medical help is necessary because intravenous glucose must be administered. (16:650)
Nursing Process—Implementation
Client Need—Health promotion/maintenance

41 2. Suspensions settle on standing. Insulin suspensions such as NPH require mixing before withdrawing the drug from the vial. It is recommended that the vial be rotated between the palms of the hands to ensure a proper mixture. Insulin suspensions must not be shaken vigorously. Inverting the vial for 20 minutes or refrigeration of the vial does not mix the substances contained in the suspension. (7:602)
Nursing Process—Implementation
Client Need—Physiological integrity

42 4. When combining regular insulin and an insulin suspension, such as NPH, the regular insulin, which is a clear solution, is withdrawn from the regular insulin bottle first. Filling the insulin syringe first with the suspension, which is cloudy, does not allow for clear visibility of the regular insulin as it is added to the syringe. (18:622; 7:602-603)
Nursing Process—Implementation
Client Need—Physiological integrity

43 1. Some clients are unable to accurately measure the dose of two insulins when using one syringe. Having the client repeatedly try and then fail to perform this task leads to frustration and discouragement. Two syringes can be used to administer the two insulins whenever there is a problem with accuracy of measurement. (7:603)
Nursing Process—Implementation
Client Need—Physiological integrity

44 2. Insulin is given by the subcutaneous route. Subcutaneous injections are given at a 45-degree angle. Clients who are heavier (180 lb or more) or

who appear to have excessive body fat may require a longer needle. In these people the needle may need to be inserted at a 90-degree angle to reach subcutaneous tissue. (15:18, 141; 18:623)
　　Nursing Process—Evaluation
　　Client Need—Physiological integrity

45 3. Insulin should be stored in a cool place or in the refrigerator. Insulin should not be exposed to warm temperatures, freezing, or excessive heat. (15:144)
　　Nursing Process—Planning
　　Client Need—Health promotion/maintenance

46 2. Severe stress, such as surgery, trauma, illness, or prolonged or intense emotional upset, may require an increase in the insulin dosage. Diabetic clients should be advised to contact their physician if severe stress occurs. (3:711)
　　Nursing Process—Implementation
　　Client Need—Health promotion/maintenance

47 4. Control of the blood glucose level and frequent eye examinations may prevent or minimize the retinal changes (retinopathy) that are often seen in those with diabetes. (3:713)
　　Nursing Process—Implementation
　　Client Need—Health promotion/maintenance

48 1. Planned and regular exercise is an important component in the treatment of diabetes mellitus. Exercise can reduce the daily insulin requirement but does not eliminate the need for insulin in the insulin-dependent diabetic. Exercise must be regular and not sporadic, for example, engaging in a sport activity only on weekends. Hypoglycemia may occur if the client engages in sudden strenuous physical activity. (7:606)
　　Nursing Process—Implementation
　　Client Need—Health promotion/maintenance

49 2. Changing the socks daily, or more often if needed, helps keep the feet dry. The client also can be instructed to rotate his shoes on a daily basis so that moisture has a chance to evaporate. The feet should be washed daily (or more often, if needed) and dried well before putting on socks and shoes. Calluses should not be removed except by a physician or podiatrist. The toenails should be trimmed carefully and the feet soaked before trimming to soften the nails. Nails are trimmed straight across. If the client has a problem cutting his toenails, a podiatrist can be recommended. (18:114-115)
　　Nursing Process—Implementation
　　Client Need—Health promotion/maintenance

50 1. Some diabetics are sensitive to changes in brands of insulin; therefore, clients should be advised to purchase the brand recommended by the physician. Brands should not be changed un-

less the physician approves of the change. If a change in brands is approved by the physician, a different type of needle and syringe is not necessary. The client should purchase the units per milliliter (eg, 40 U or 100 U/mL) recommended by the physician. Most insulin brands are available in both strengths, that is, 40 U/mL or 100 U/mL. Insulin bottles are labeled as to the number of units per milliliter. Insulin does not require a prescription, but needles and syringes do require a prescription. (15:141)
　　Nursing Process—Implementation
　　Client Need—Health promotion/maintenance

NURSING CARE OF CLIENTS WITH ADDISON'S DISEASE

51 1. Clients with Addison's disease require lifetime daily replacement of corticosteroids. Usually, fludrocortisone (Florinef), a synthetic corticosteroid with glucocorticoid and mineralocorticoid properties, is prescribed for this disorder. The nurse should obtain the name of the corticosteroid preparation and the prescribed daily dose during an initial client interview. The approximate amount of urine passed daily is not a relevant question for those with Addison's. The cause of primary Addison's disease often is unknown. (16:638)
　　Nursing Process—Collecting data
　　Client Need—Physiological integrity

52 2. Clients with Addison's disease often have abnormally dark pigmentation of the skin and mucous membranes. The remaining options are signs of Cushing's syndrome (adrenal cortical hyperfunction). (16:638)
　　Nursing Process—Collecting data
　　Client Need—Physiological integrity

53 3. Hypotension, restlessness, nausea, vomiting, fever, and abdominal pain are examples of symptoms of acute adrenal crisis. Acute adrenal crisis is an emergency, and death may occur from severe hypotension and vasomotor collapse. (16:639-639)
　　Nursing Process—Collecting data
　　Client Need—Physiological integrity

54 4. Failure to administer a prescribed corticosteroid preparation one or more times can result in acute adrenal crisis and death of the client. The remaining items in this question would not cause acute adrenal crisis, but failure to monitor the blood pressure hourly could delay recognition of this event. (16:639)
　　Nursing Process—Planning
　　Client Need—Physiological integrity

55 1. Fluid and electrolyte disturbances may occur in those with adrenal cortical insufficiency (Addison's disease) because the adrenal glands are closely related to the regulation of body water and electrolytes. Hyponatremia (decrease in sodium), dehydration (hypovolemia), and mild to severe hyperkalemia (increase in potassium) are the fluid and electrolyte disturbances that may be seen. (16:640)

    Nursing Process—Collecting data
    Client Need—Physiological integrity

NURSING CARE OF CLIENTS WITH CUSHING'S SYNDROME

56 3. Muscle wasting and weakness; moon face; buffalo hump; ruddy face; thin, fragile skin; bruising; striae; peripheral edema; hypertension; hirsutism (females); mood changes; depression; and psychosis are examples of the signs and symptoms of Cushing's syndrome. The remaining options usually are not associated with this disorder. (16:641)

    Nursing Process—Collecting data
    Client Need—Physiological integrity

57 3. Clients with Cushing's syndrome often tire easily and may require rest periods between activities such as bathing, showering, shaving, eating, and walking. The nurse should plan to evaluate daily the client's ability to tolerate activity and adjust activities according to the client's tolerance. Between-meal feedings normally are not necessary because the client may be overweight due to the disease process. Some clients may have latent or overt diabetes mellitus due to a decreased tolerance to carbohydrates, which may be due to Cushing's syndrome. In most hospitals, between-meal feedings are usually ordered by the physician and not the nurse. Extra fluids are not necessary because many people with this disorder have peripheral edema and hypertension, which appears to be due to sodium retention (hypernatremia). (16:642)

    Nursing Process—Planning
    Client Need—Physiological integrity

58 4. Cushing's syndrome results because of an increase in the adrenal cortical hormones, namely corticosteroids and mineralocorticoids. The increase in the corticosteroids causes the clinical manifestations of the disorder. Overproduction of adrenal cortical hormones usually does not affect the size of the kidneys or cause pain. Cushing's syndrome also may be seen in those receiving large doses of corticosteroids for a prolonged period. (16:641)

    Nursing Process—Implementing
    Client Need—Safe, effective care environment

59 2. Two of the hormones produced by the adrenal gland—the corticosteroids and mineralocorticoids—are essential to life. When a client has a bilateral adrenalectomy, oral or intravenous corticosteroid replacement therapy is absolutely essential and must never be omitted. The client may experience acute adrenal crisis if the prescribed corticosteroid is not administered at the correct time and in the correct dose. The remaining options in this question are important, but the administration of a corticosteroid assumes the highest priority. (16:643)

    Nursing Process—Planning
    Client Need—Physiological integrity

60 1. Following an adrenalectomy the client is no longer producing corticosteroids and mineralocorticoids. The development of adrenal crisis can occur even when the prescribed dose of corticosteroid replacement therapy is administered. Early recognition of the signs and symptoms of adrenal crisis is imperative because this may develop into a life-threatening situation. Hypotension may be an early sign of adrenal crisis; hypertension is not likely to occur. An increase in the signs and symptoms of Cushing's syndrome is not likely to occur because the adrenal glands have been removed. Testing the urine for glucose and ketones usually is not necessary but, if ordered is not as essential as observing for signs of adrenal crisis. (16:644)

    Nursing Process—Collecting data
    Client Need—Physiological integrity

61 4. Corticosteroid replacement therapy is essential to life. Advising a client to omit a dose if nausea and vomiting occur is incorrect. The client should be advised to contact the physician immediately if nausea and vomiting occur because the next dose of corticosteroid would have to be administered by the parenteral route. The remaining options in this question are correct. (16:644)

    Nursing Process—Planning
    Client Need—Health promotion/maintenance

INDIVIDUAL TEST ITEMS

62 1. Severe hypothyroidism is also called myxedema. (16:629)

    Nursing Process—Planning
    Client Need—Physiological integrity

63 3. Radioactive iodine (^{131}I) is used to destroy hyperplastic thyroid tissue and thus reduce the activity of the thyroid gland and create a euthyroid (normal thyroid) state. Radioactive iodine does not increase the manufacture of thyroid hormones or affect other tissues of the body.

Radiation precautions usually are not necessary. (16:628)

Nursing Process—Planning

Client Need—Health promotion/maintenance

64 3. Abbreviations for drops, drams, and grains are not recommended. Some references and physicians may use dr for drams, gr for grains, and gtt or gtts for drops. The abbreviation for grams is g. (18:574)

Nursing Process—Implementation

Client Need—Physiological integrity

65 1. Strong iodine solution (Lugol's solution) has a strong taste. Although some people do not mind the taste when the drug is added to water, others find that adding the drug to fruit juice rather than water makes the medication more palatable. (15:222)

Nursing Process—Implementation

Client Need—Physiological integrity

66 2. Enlargement of the thyroid gland may be seen in those with thyroiditis, hyperthyroidism, hypothyroidism, and a thyroid malignancy. The use of x-rays to treat facial acne and enlarged tonsils during early childhood and young adult years has been associated with an increased incidence of thyroid malignancies, which can cause enlargement of the thyroid gland. Inquiring into a history of x-ray treatment to the head or neck is appropriate when the client has an enlarged thyroid gland. The client cannot be expected to know if there is a problem with the thyroid gland or what the problem may be. Surgery may not be indicated if the client can be treated medically. (16:630)

Nursing Process—Collecting data

Client Need—Physiological integrity

67 3. The client with treated or untreated diabetes insipidus requires accurate intake and output measurement. When the disorder is untreated, 15 to 20 L of urine may be passed in a 24-hour period. Treatment with antidiuretic hormone usually reduces the urine output. The dose of the antidiuretic hormone may be based on the urinary output; therefore, accurate measurement is necessary. Weights are usually obtained daily until urine output is normal. The temperature should be monitored at least daily; every 2 hours usually is not necessary. The diet prescribed by the physician depends on the client's needs. (16:626-627)

Nursing Process—Planning

Client Need—Physiological integrity

68 1. Symptoms of hyperparathyroidism include bone pain, spontaneous fractures, constipation, weight loss, poor appetite, fatigue, and depression. When developing a plan of care, the possibility of bone pain and spontaneous fractures should be taken into consideration. (7:611)

Nursing Process—Planning

Client Need—Safe, effective care environment

Classification of Test Items

Unit IV Review Test 12

Directions: After each question the correct answer is given as well as a classification of each test question. Compare the correct answer with your answer. If a question has been answered *incorrectly*, draw a line to the end of the four columns. When finished, add up your correct scores and place the results at the bottom of each column.

Score Calculation:

To determine the percentage of the number of questions you answered correctly, divide the **Number Correct** by the **Number Possible**, as example 63 (the number of questions answered correctly) divided by 68 (the number of questions in the test) = .92 or 92%.

NURSING PROCESS

C = Collecting data
P = Planning
I = Implementation
E = Evaluation

CLIENT NEEDS

S = Safe, effective care environment
P = Physiological integrity
M = Psychosocial integrity
H = Health promotion/maintenance

Question #	Answer #	Nursing Process C	Nursing Process P	Nursing Process I	Nursing Process E	Client Needs S	Client Needs P	Client Needs M	Client Needs H
1	2				E		P		
2	4			I					H
3	2			I					H
4	3			I					H
5	4	C					P		
6	3			I			P		
7	4			I			P		
8	1	C					P		
9	4	C					P		
10	2				E		P		
11	2	C					P		
12	2			I			P		
13	1	C					P		
14	4		P			S			
15	3	C					P		
16	2			I		S			
17	1			I		S			
18	4			I				M	
19	3		P				P		

NURSING PROCESS

C = Collecting data
P = Planning
I = Implementation
E = Evaluation

CLIENT NEEDS

S = Safe, effective care environment
P = Physiological integrity
M = Psychosocial integrity
H = Health promotion/maintenance

Question #	Answer #	Nursing Process				Client Needs			
		C	P	I	E	S	P	M	H
20	1		P				P		
21	2			I					H
22	3		P				P		
23	1		P						H
24	2			I					H
25	4	C					P		
26	3	C					P		
27	4			I			P		
28	3			I			P		
29	3			I		S			
30	4		P				P		
31	1			I			P		
32	2			I			P		
33	3	C					P		
34	3	C					P		
35	3			I		S			
36	1			I					H
37	3			I			P		
38	2			I			P		
39	4			I					H
40	2			I					H
41	2			I			P		
42	4			I			P		
43	1			I			P		
44	2				E		P		
45	3		P						H
46	2			I					H
47	4			I					H
48	1			I					H
49	2			I					H
50	1			I					H
51	1	C					P		

NURSING PROCESS

C = Collecting data
P = Planning
I = Implementation
E = Evaluation

CLIENT NEEDS

S = Safe, effective care environment
P = Physiological integrity
M = Psychosocial integrity
H = Health promotion/maintenance

Question #	Answer #	Nursing Process				Client Needs			
		C	P	I	E	S	P	M	H
52	2	C					P		
53	3	C					P		
54	4		P				P		
55	1	C					P		
56	3	C					P		
57	3		P				P		
58	4			I		S			
59	1		P				P		
60	1	C					P		
61	4		P						H
62	1		P				P		
63	3		P						H
64	3			I			P		
65	1			I			P		
66	2	C					P		
67	3		P				P		
68	1		P			S			
Number Correct									
Number Possible	68	17	15	33	3	7	43	1	17
Percentage Correct									

REVIEW TEST 13

The Nursing Care of Clients with Disorders of the Urologic System

Correct Answers and Rationale
Classification of Test Items

Directions: With a pencil, blacken the circle in front of the option you have chosen for your correct answer.

The Nursing Care of Clients with Disorders of the Urologic System

NURSING CARE OF CLIENTS WITH URETHRITIS

The nurse makes an office appointment for Gordon Brunner because he describes having a slight tickling sensation during urination and a watery discharge from his penis.

1 When obtaining a sexual history from the client, which one of the following questions is *most* important for the nurse to ask?
  ○ 1. Have you had a painless sore on your penis that has now healed?
  ○ 2. Does anyone with whom you have had sex have similar symptoms?
  ○ 3. At what age did you first have intercourse?
  ○ 4. When did you last have sexual intercourse?

2 Because of the sensitive nature of sexual information, which one of the following attitudes would it be *most* important for the nurse to convey to obtain truthful information from the client?
  ○ 1. Sympathetic
  ○ 2. Nonjudgmental
  ○ 3. Encouraging
  ○ 4. Optimistic

The physician informs the nurse that during the examination he will need to obtain a culture of urethral secretions.

3 While assisting the physician, besides furnishing a sterile swab and culture tube, it would be *most* important for the nurse to provide the physician with
  ○ 1. antiseptic.
  ○ 2. lubricant.
  ○ 3. a mask.
  ○ 4. gloves.

The result of the culture indicates Mr. Brunner has nonspecific urethritis from a nongonococcal organism, Chlamydia trachomatis. The physician tells the nurse to phone in a prescription for doxycycline (Vibramycin) 100 mg b.i.d. with a sufficient number of capsules for 7 days of treatment.

4 When the nurse calls Mr. Brunner to ask at which pharmacy he prefers to fill his prescription, which of the following information is *most* important to provide?
  ○ 1. Take the medication until the symptoms clear.
  ○ 2. Refill the prescription again in 1 week.
  ○ 3. Take the medication for the full amount of time.

○ 4. Treatment of this infection is likely to be life-long.

5 One of the *best* methods for the nurse to stress to prevent a recurrence of the chlamydial infection is
○ 1. showering or bathing after intercourse.
○ 2. good handwashing with an antiseptic soap.
○ 3. testing and treating sexual partners.
○ 4. adequate nutrition and fluid intake.

NURSING CARE OF CLIENTS WITH CYSTITIS

Ms. Anne Mitchell calls her physician's office because she has recognized the recurrence of symptoms of cystitis for which she has been treated several times before.

6 When the nurse asks Ms. Mitchell to describe her symptoms, the client will *most likely* report
○ 1. burning on urination.
○ 2. sharp flank pain.
○ 3. purulent discharge.
○ 4. strong smelling urine.

When Ms. Mitchell arrives for her appointment, the nurse instructs her on how to obtain a clean-catch voided urine specimen.

7 After the nurse explains how to cleanse and expose the urethra, which one of the following instructions is *most* accurate?
○ 1. Deposit a sample of the urine from the start of voiding.
○ 2. Collect some urine after voiding a little in the toilet.
○ 3. Hold the specimen container against the external labia.
○ 4. Mix a small amount of antiseptic with the urine sample.

8 When Ms. Mitchell asks the office nurse why women have so many more bladder infections than men, the *most* accurate answer is that
○ 1. the male urethra is straighter, which facilitates the elimination of pathogens.
○ 2. the male urethra is lined with a layer of mucous membrane, which traps microorganisms.
○ 3. the female urethra is shorter, and pathogens enter the bladder more quickly.
○ 4. the female urethra has a larger diameter and is more easily contaminated.

9 Which one of the following instructions from the nurse would be *most* effective for the client to follow to reduce the growth of bacteria in the bladder at this time?
○ 1. Drink a large quantity of fluid.
○ 2. Change underclothing each day.
○ 3. Avoid using public restrooms.
○ 4. Use only white toilet tissue.

The physician prescribes a urinary antiinfective combination of trimethoprim and sulfamethoxazole (Bactrim), one tablet, b.i.d.

10 If the client understands the nurse's directions for taking this prescribed medication, she will indicate that the drug should be taken
○ 1. once a day.
○ 2. twice daily.
○ 3. three times a day.
○ 4. four times a day.

The nurse plans to review prior health teaching to help the client prevent future urinary tract infections.

11 If the client says she does all of the following, which one indicates the best measure for preventing cystitis? The client states that following bowel or bladder elimination, it is important to
○ 1. wipe away from the urinary meatus.
○ 2. perform appropriate handwashing.
○ 3. use a feminine hygiene spray.
○ 4. dry the perineum thoroughly.

NURSING CARE OF CLIENTS WITH PYELONEPHRITIS

Ms. Angela Payne, who has type I diabetes mellitus, is being seen for a routine physical examination. A routine urinalysis is ordered.

12 Which one of the following findings is most suggestive that this client has a urinary tract infection? The urinalysis report shows
○ 1. glycosuria.
○ 2. hematuria.
○ 3. pyuria.
○ 4. proteinuria.

To validate the findings on the routine urinalysis, the physician asks the nurse to obtain a urine specimen by catheterization.

13 It would be best for the nurse to plan to place a female client in which one of the following positions prior to inserting a catheter?
○ 1. Lithotomy position
○ 2. Recumbent position
○ 3. Knee–chest position
○ 4. Prone position

14 The nurse inserts the catheter into the vagina rather than the urinary meatus. Which one of the following actions is *correct* at this time?
○ 1. Wipe the catheter tip with an alcohol swab.
○ 2. Cleanse the catheter tip with Betadine solution.
○ 3. Discard the catheter, and use another sterile one.
○ 4. withdraw the catheter, and insert it in the urethra.

To relieve Ms. Payne's symptoms, the physician orders phenazopyridine (Pyridium), a urinary antiseptic.

15 It would be most important for the nurse to inform Ms. Payne that this drug will cause the urine to
○ 1. look cloudy.
○ 2. appear orange.
○ 3. become scant.
○ 4. smell strong.

Ms. Payne is to have an intravenous pyelogram (IVP). The physician orders a laxative for Ms. Payne the night before the x-ray.

16 When preparing Ms. Payne for the IVP, the nurse should plan to explain that the reason for the laxative is that emptying the bowel
○ 1. also aids in examining the lower gastrointestinal tract.
○ 2. prevents accidental stool incontinence during the x-ray.
○ 3. reduces the potential for constipation or impaction.
○ 4. improves the ability to visualize the urinary structures.

17 The nurse inquires about Ms. Payne's allergies before the IVP. Besides iodine, which one of the following allergies should be reported before Ms. Payne's x-ray?
○ 1. An allergy to eggs
○ 2. An allergy to wheat
○ 3. An allergy to milk
○ 4. An allergy to shellfish

NURSING CARE OF CLIENTS WITH URINARY INCONTINENCE

18 The most important nursing assessment before beginning bladder retraining with an incontinent person is
○ 1. recording the times at which he or she is incontinent.
○ 2. checking the specific gravity of the urine.
○ 3. monitoring the extent of bladder distention.
○ 4. observing the color of the client's urine.

According to the standards of care in the obstetric department of a hospital, all postpartum clients are taught how to perform Kegel exercises to strengthen the pubococcygeal muscles and prevent future problems with urinary stress incontinence.

19 Which one of the following instructions is *correct* when the nurse teaches a client to perform Kegel exercises?
○ 1. Contract and relax the muscles in the vagina.
○ 2. Stand and rock the pelvis back and forth.
○ 3. Push down with the feet and elevate the hips.

○ 4. Pull the abdominal muscles inward and ease off.

During bladder retraining, a client tells the nurse that he intends to restrict his intake of fluid to just the liquids at meals to remain dry for longer periods of time.

20 The *best* response from the nurse in this situation would be to
○ 1. encourage the practice because it shows evidence of client cooperation.
○ 2. encourage the practice because it will lead to accomplishing the goal.
○ 3. discourage the practice because it contributes to constipation.
○ 4. discourage the practice because it potentiates fluid imbalance.

21 An elderly nursing home resident who is incontinent of urine says "What's the sense in living? I'm just a baby nowadays." The *best* response the nurse can offer at this time would be
○ 1. "You're a very nice gentleman."
○ 2. "Cheer up. You can't be serious."
○ 3. "You should expect this at your age."
○ 4. "You're discouraged right now."

Following a stroke, the nursing team has been using an external catheter to prevent skin breakdown in an incontinent male client.

22 When applying an external catheter, which one of the following is *essential*?
○ 1. Lubricate the penis before applying the catheter.
○ 2. Measure the length and circumference of the penis.
○ 3. Leave space between the end of the penis and drainage end of the catheter.
○ 4. Retract the foreskin before rolling the catheter sheath over the penis.

23 After inserting an indwelling catheter into a male client, which one of the following describes an appropriate technique for stabilizing the catheter to avoid a penoscrotal fistula?
○ 1. Tape the catheter to the abdomen.
○ 2. Pass the catheter under the client's leg.
○ 3. Fasten the drainage tubing to the bed with a safety pin.
○ 4. Insert the catheter into the tubing of a collecting bag.

NURSING CARE OF CLIENTS WITH BENIGN PROSTATIC HYPERTROPHY

As a requirement for obtaining a life insurance policy, Mr. Charles Durand has made an appointment with his physician for a physical examination.

24 While obtaining Mr. Durand's history, which one of the following statements would best indicate to the nurse that Mr. Durand has benign prostatic hypertrophy? Mr. Durand says
○ 1. "There is some burning when I urinate."
○ 2. "I wake up nightly needing to urinate."
○ 3. "I feel pressure in my back before voiding."
○ 4. "My urine is almost colorless, like water."

25 To gather more information about symptoms associated with benign prostatic hypertrophy, which one of the following questions would be *most* important for the nurse to ask next?
○ 1. "Have you noticed any changes in sexual function?"
○ 2. "Have you felt any lumps in your scrotum recently?"
○ 3. "Do you have difficulty starting to void?"
○ 4. "Do you have problems controlling urination?"

Mr. Frank Monroe, who has a history of benign prostatic hypertrophy, comes to the emergency department because he has not been able to urinate in 18 hours. The physician instructs the nurse to insert a urethral catheter.

26 Which one of the following techniques may facilitate inserting the tip of the catheter past the enlarged prostate gland?
○ 1. Angle the penis in the direction of the toes.
○ 2. Massage the tissue below the base of the penis.
○ 3. Push the catheter with additional force.
○ 4. Grasp the penis firmly within the hand.

The attempt to insert the urethral catheter is unsuccessful. Mr. Monroe is admitted for insertion of a suprapubic catheter.

27 The written plan for care following the insertion of the suprapubic catheter includes all of the following instructions. Which one is *essential* for evaluating the patency of the catheter?
○ 1. Inspect the skin around the insertion site.
○ 2. Monitor urinary volume every hour.
○ 3. Attach the catheter to a leg bag when up.
○ 4. Encourage oral fluid intake hourly.

Mr. Dale Royce has been scheduled to undergo a transurethral resection of the prostate (TURP) to relieve his urinary symptoms caused by an enlarging prostate gland.

28 Which one of the following findings would the nurse *expect* to observe during the immediate postoperative period?
○ 1. The urine is light pink to clear.
○ 2. The urine contains mucoid sediment.
○ 3. The urine volume is decreased.
○ 4. The urine appears grossly bloody.

The nurse is told in report that Mr. Royce is to receive continuous bladder irrigation through a three-way catheter following his transurethral prostatectomy.

29 Which one of the following will the nurse need to obtain when planning to implement this procedure?
○ 1. An intravenous pole
○ 2. An Asepto (bulb) syringe
○ 3. A round sterile basin
○ 4. Antiseptic solution

30 Postoperatively Mr. Royce tells the nurse that he is having a great deal of discomfort in the area of his bladder. In this situation, before administering an analgesic, it would be *most appropriate* for the nurse to assess that the
○ 1. client's pulse rate is normal.
○ 2. dressing is dry and intact.
○ 3. catheter is draining well.
○ 4. client is coughing adequately.

31 The physician has ordered all of the following medications for the postoperative care of the TURP client. Which one would be the *most appropriate* drug for the nurse to administer for bladder spasms?
○ 1. Acetylsalicylic acid (aspirin) by mouth
○ 2. Propoxyphene napsylate (Darvocet) by mouth
○ 3. Meperidine hydrochloride (Demerol) intramuscularly
○ 4. Belladonna and opium (B & O) rectal suppository

The nurse is assigned to care for a client following a suprapubic prostatectomy. The client has a catheter in the urethra and another in an abdominal incision.

32 Which one of the following is the best action when the nurse records the output for the shift? It would be *most correct* for the nurse to
○ 1. record only the output from the urethral catheter.
○ 2. record only the output from the wound catheter.
○ 3. record the output from each catheter separately.
○ 4. record the combined total output from both catheters.

Several days following a suprapubic prostatectomy, the physician removes the catheter from the abdominal incision.

33 Which one of the following nursing interventions would be important to add to the plan for care following the removal of the suprapubic catheter?
○ 1. Reposition the client every 2 hours.
○ 2. Ambulate the client with assistance.
○ 3. Change abdominal dressing when wet.
○ 4. Encourage deep breathing hourly.

NURSING CARE OF CLIENTS WITH RENAL CALCULI

Following a hospitalization of 6 weeks recuperating from multiple trauma in a motor vehicle accident, Ms. Roberta Green's traction is discontinued, and a long leg cast is applied.

34 If Ms. Green describes all of the following, which one is *most likely* to be associated with renal calculi?
○ 1. Feeling extremely tired and weak
○ 2. Having waves of agonizing flank pain
○ 3. Voiding with frequency and urgency
○ 4. Experiencing chills and fever

35 Which one of the following measures should the nurse plan to implement at this time if kidney stones are suspected?
○ 1. Insert an indwelling catheter.
○ 2. Test the urine for glucose.
○ 3. Apply an abdominal binder.
○ 4. Strain all voided urine.

36 It would be *essential* at this time for the nurse to
○ 1. provide a liberal fluid intake.
○ 2. maintain strict bed rest.
○ 3. restrict further intake of food.
○ 4. encourage diversional activity.

An IVP reveals a large stone in the right ureter. The physician intends to try grabbing the stone with an instrument during cystoscopy.

37 After a cystoscopy, the nurse can expect that the client will experience
○ 1. polyuria.
○ 2. dysuria.
○ 3. anuria.
○ 4. pyuria.

The ureteral stone proves to be too large to grasp and crush during the cystoscopy. Extracorporeal shock wave lithotripsy (ESWL) is planned.

38 Which of the following instructions would be *most correct* for the nurse to provide when preparing a client for ESWL?
○ 1. "Your body will be immersed in a tub of water."
○ 2. "You will have a small abdominal incision."
○ 3. "You will be placed in a pressure chamber."
○ 4. "An electrode will be attached to your flank."

NURSING CARE OF CLIENTS WITH BLADDER CANCER

39 Which one of the following is a common early symptom among people who develop bladder cancer?
○ 1. Difficulty voiding
○ 2. Persistent oliguria

○ 3. Painless hematuria
○ 4. Unusual discharge

40 When asked about factors that are linked to causing cancerous changes in the bladder, the nurse would be *most correct* in identifying which one of the following?
○ 1. Stress incontinence
○ 2. Frequent intercourse
○ 3. Sexual promiscuity
○ 4. Cigarette smoking

The physician recommends that a client's bladder cancer be treated conservatively by instilling an antineoplastic drug within the bladder.

41 When administering the bladder instillation containing the chemotherapeutic drug, it would be *important*, in the interest of safety, for the nurse to
○ 1. wear a double pair of latex gloves.
○ 2. use a glass syringe for the drug.
○ 3. avoid clothing with long sleeves.
○ 4. limit contact time with the client.

NURSING CARE OF CLIENTS WITH URINARY DIVERSIONS

Mr. John Holland's bladder cancer has been unresponsive to treatment. The physician has discussed removing Mr. Holland's bladder and performing a procedure for urinary diversion called an ileal conduit.

42 When Mr. Holland asks the nurse additional questions about the procedure the surgeon discussed, which one of the following is most correct? Your urine will be eliminated
○ 1. into your small intestine.
○ 2. into your large intestine.
○ 3. through an abdominal opening.
○ 4. through a special catheter.

It was reported that during the night Mr. Holland was awake much of the time. When he slept, he was restless. The team leader suggests that Mr. Holland may be anxious.

43 Which one of the following assessments obtained by the nursing assistant assigned to his care would support the team leader's conclusion?
○ 1. Temperature is 98.9°F (37.1°C).
○ 2. Blood pressure is 132/88 mm Hg.
○ 3. Pulse rate is 106 beats per minute at rest.
○ 4. Pulse pressure is 44 mm Hg.

44 The nursing assistant asks the staff nurse for suggestions on how to help Mr. Holland deal with his anxiety. Which statement will help Mr. Holland *most* at this time?
○ 1. "It must be difficult facing this type of surgery."

    ○ 2. "You have one of the best surgeons at this hospital."

    ○ 3. "You'll see; everything will turn out OK for you."

    ○ 4. "Others with your diagnosis have done just fine."

45 Mr. Holland says, "Imagine being unable to control urination." The *most* therapeutic response from the nurse would be

    ○ 1. "Tell me what that means to you."

    ○ 2. "I know just how you're feeling."

    ○ 3. "Well, it's not quite as bad as that."

    ○ 4. "You need to think more positively."

46 Postoperatively, Mr. Holland wears an appliance that collects his urine. He tells the nurse that his skin feels raw and irritated near the stoma. Which nursing action is *appropriate* at this time?

    ○ 1. Increase oral fluids to dilute the urine.

    ○ 2. Remove the appliance and inspect the skin.

    ○ 3. Empty the appliance at more frequent intervals.

    ○ 4. Leave the appliance off for 1 or 2 days.

Mr. Holland is learning to change his ostomy appliance before being discharged. The appliance frequently comes loose from his skin.

47 The nurse notes that urine leaks onto Mr. Holland's skin before he can replace his appliance. Which of the following suggestions would be most helpful? When preparing to apply a new appliance,

    ○ 1. let the urine drip into the toilet.

    ○ 2. insert a tampon into the stoma.

    ○ 3. press a gloved finger over the stoma.

    ○ 4. pinch the stoma with two fingers.

48 Which of the following suggestions would be *most helpful* for ensuring that the appliance remains attached?

    ○ 1. Empty the collection bag frequently.

    ○ 2. Limit fluid intake throughout the day.

    ○ 3. Change the appliance each morning.

    ○ 4. Avoid eating gas-forming vegetables.

NURSING CARE OF CLIENTS WITH GLOMERULONEPHRITIS

49 When the nurse reviews the medical history of a client, which one of the following would the nurse find commonly precedes the symptoms associated with glomerulonephritis?

    ○ 1. Trauma to the lower abdomen

    ○ 2. An upper respiratory infection

    ○ 3. Treatment with an antibiotic

    ○ 4. An allergic reaction to x-ray dye

50 The nurse conducts a head-to-toe physical assessment on a person with acute glomerulonephritis. If this person is similar to most with this disease,

which one of the following is the nurse likely to observe?

    ○ 1. Skin hemorrhages

    ○ 2. Absence of body hair

    ○ 3. Flushed appearance

    ○ 4. Facial puffiness

51 Which one of the following nursing actions would be most essential when planning the care of a person with acute glomerulonephritis?

    ○ 1. Ambulate twice daily.

    ○ 2. Assist with mouth care.

    ○ 3. Monitor weight daily.

    ○ 4. Encourage fluid intake.

52 Which one of the following laboratory tests would be most essential for the nurse to monitor when caring for a person with glomerulonephritis?

    ○ 1. Serum amylase

    ○ 2. Blood glucose

    ○ 3. Blood urea nitrogen (BUN)

    ○ 4. Complete blood count (CBC)

53 When a client with glomerulonephritis complains of a headache, which nursing action should be performed first?

    ○ 1. Administer a prescribed analgesic.

    ○ 2. Assess the client's blood pressure.

    ○ 3. Reduce environmental stimuli.

    ○ 4. Change the client's position.

54 The nurse is informed that a 24-hour urine collection for creatinine clearance is to be started at 8:00 AM. Which of the following actions is correct? The nurse has the client void at 8:00 AM and

    ○ 1. refrigerates the specimen.

    ○ 2. disposes of the specimen.

    ○ 3. sends the specimen to the laboratory.

    ○ 4. places the specimen in preservative.

55 A nurse uses a color reagent strip (dipstick) to test a voided specimen for all of the following. Which one can the nurse expect to be present in the urine of a client with glomerulonephritis?

    ○ 1. Glucose

    ○ 2. Bilirubin

    ○ 3. Albumin

    ○ 4. Acetone

56 The nurse inspects the urine of a client with glomerulonephritis. Which one of the following suggests that the urine contains red blood cells?

    ○ 1. The urine appears cloudy.

    ○ 2. The urine appears smoky.

    ○ 3. The urine appears bright orange.

    ○ 4. The urine appears dark yellow.

57 A client with glomerulonephritis is on a low-sodium diet. Which one of the following menu choices would it be *best* for the nurse to recommend?

    ○ 1. Hot dog with potato salad

○ 2. Beef bullion and crackers
○ 3. Chicken salad on lettuce wedge
○ 4. Cheese pizza with thin crust

58 A client with glomerulonephritis is being treated with the steroid methylprednisolone (Medrol) by oral administration. To reduce the potential for peptic ulcer, it would be *best* for the nurse to administer the medication
○ 1. with fresh tap water.
○ 2. with food or meals.
○ 3. on an empty stomach.
○ 4. between meal times.

NURSING CARE OF CLIENTS WITH RENAL FAILURE

Olive Martin has chronic glomerulonephritis and is now being cared for in the early stages of renal failure.

59 Which one of the following urinary patterns would the nurse most accurately associate with this client's diagnosis? Renal failure is characterized by
○ 1. oliguria.
○ 2. ketonuria.
○ 3. hematuria.
○ 4. dysuria.

A team conference is held to discuss the care of Ms. Martin.

60 Which one of the following planned nursing assessments is a priority in the management of Ms. Martin's care?
○ 1. Monitoring body temperature
○ 2. Measuring intake and output
○ 3. Checking for urinary retention
○ 4. Listening for bowel sounds

The physician orders a fluid challenge of 500 mL of intravenous fluid to be infused at a rapid rate, followed by the administration of a loop diuretic intravenously to sustain or improve renal function.

61 While the fluid is being administered, which one of the following is most important for the nurse to assess?
○ 1. Pedal edema
○ 2. Skin integrity
○ 3. Oral mucosa
○ 4. Lung sounds

62 Because of impaired urine elimination, which one of the following skin problems will require *additional* team planning?
○ 1. Reduced perspiration
○ 2. Extreme oiliness
○ 3. Loss of skin turgor
○ 4. Pronounced itching

63 Ms. Martin is on a sodium-restricted diet. When she complains about the bland taste of her food, which one of the following would be best for the nurse to recommend *instead* of salt?
○ 1. Catsup
○ 2. Mustard
○ 3. Soy sauce
○ 4. Lemon juice

64 Ms. Martin complains about being thirsty due to fluid restrictions. Which one of the following nursing actions would be most appropriate?
○ 1. Give her hard candy to suck.
○ 2. Provide her with ice chips.
○ 3. Offer her an ice cream bar.
○ 4. Supply her with fresh fruit.

65 The care plan indicates that Ms. Martin should be weighed regularly. Which one of the following should the nurse consider when planning to weigh this client?
○ 1. When the client has been weighed before
○ 2. When the client last took a drink of fluid
○ 3. How much the client has eaten so far today
○ 4. Whether the client feels like being weighed today

When it becomes evident that Ms. Martin will need long-term dialysis, an internal arteriovenous fistula is created for hemodialysis.

66 Which one of the following assessments is it *most* important for the nurse to perform regularly on the client with an arteriovenous fistula?
○ 1. Check the color and temperature of the hand.
○ 2. Monitor wrist and finger range of motion.
○ 3. Observe tone and coordination of arm muscles.
○ 4. Inspect forearm skin integrity and turgor.

Another person with advanced renal failure is being prepared for peritoneal dialysis.

67 Immediately after the dialysate solution has been instilled, which one of the following nursing actions is correct?
○ 1. Clamp the tubing from the infusion.
○ 2. Drain the infused dialysate solution.
○ 3. Restrict movement as much as possible.
○ 4. Encourage the client to drink fluids.

68 Which one of the following should be reported *immediately* when caring for a client undergoing peritoneal dialysis?
○ 1. Loss of body weight
○ 2. Even, deep breathing
○ 3. Elevated body temperature
○ 4. Output that exceeds intake

69 Which one of the following findings is the *best* evidence that peritoneal dialysis was effective?
○ 1. The client's urine output increases.
○ 2. The client's appetite improves.

○ 3. The client's potassium level falls.
○ 4. The client's red cell count is lower.

INDIVIDUAL TEST ITEMS

70 When should the nurse plan to catheterize a client to measure residual urine?
○ 1. Immediately after the person voids
○ 2. Shortly after arising in the morning
○ 3. When the bladder feels uncomfortably full
○ 4. Approximately 1 hour after drinking 1 quart of water

71 A nurse determines that a client's bladder is distended, but he is unable to void. Which one of the following actions would be *most helpful* after the person is positioned on the toilet?
○ 1. Encouraging the client to drink a full glass of water
○ 2. Instructing the client to take rapid, shallow breaths
○ 3. Suggesting that the client press inward and downward over the bladder
○ 4. Advising the client to hold his breath and forcefully bear down

72 Which one of the following is the *best* technique for obtaining a urine specimen for a culture when the client has an indwelling catheter?
○ 1. Remove the catheter and have the client void.

○ 2. Aspirate urine from the port on the drainage tubing.
○ 3. Drain a sample of urine from the collection bag.
○ 4. Obtain a specimen when the catheter is replaced.

73 Which solution should the nurse plan to use for irrigating an indwelling catheter?
○ 1. Sterile distilled water
○ 2. Sterile povidone iodine
○ 3. Sterile hydrogen peroxide
○ 4. Sterile normal saline

74 A client returns from surgery with a flank incision after undergoing a nephrectomy. This type of client is at high risk for developing the following postoperative problems. Which one is it *essential* to plan measures to detect and prevent?
○ 1. Hypoventilation
○ 2. Bradycardia
○ 3. Abdominal distention
○ 4. Incisional hernia

75 Which one of the following is the *best* indication to the nurse that a client's renal function is adequate?
○ 1. The heart rate is 88 beats per minute.
○ 2. The systolic blood pressure is 136 mm Hg.
○ 3. Urine output for today totals 645 mL.
○ 4. Respirations are 22 breaths per minute.

Correct Answers and Rationale

Two numbers appear in parentheses following each rationale. The first number identifies the textbook listed in the references, page 451, and the second number identifies the page(s) in that textbook on which the correct answer can be verified. Occasionally, two textbooks are given for verifying the correct answer.

The Nursing Care of Clients with Disorders of the Urologic System

NURSING CARE OF CLIENTS WITH URETHRITIS

1 2. Asking a person if any sexual partner has had similar symptoms would help to determine if the cause of the symptoms is due to a sexually transmitted disease. A painless sore is more likely a symptom of syphilis infection, which would not commonly cause the symptoms this patient describes. The age at which a person first had sexual intercourse would be unrelated to the present symptoms. Incubation periods vary among sexually transmitted diseases; identifying the most recent date of intercourse would not provide significant information. (3:523; 14:930)
  Nursing Process—Collecting data
  Client Need—Safe, effective care environment

2 2. Conveying a nonjudgmental attitude will facilitate obtaining truthful information from the person who may feel uncomfortable discussing sexual information. Being sympathetic, encouraging, and optimistic are all positive attributes, but none of these is as important as being nonjudgmental. (16:89-90)
  Nursing Process—Implementation
  Client Need—Psychosocial integrity

3 4. Because body secretions potentially contain microorganisms that can be transmitted to caregivers, it is important to wear gloves as a barrier against direct contact with infectious material. The use of an antiseptic or lubricant would interfere with obtaining an adequate specimen. Wearing a mask would not be as important as wearing gloves, because the urethral secretions are not apt to splash or spray areas such as the nose or mouth. Sexually transmitted diseases are spread by direct contact rather than droplet or air transmission. (16:89; 5:409)
  Nursing Process—Implementation
  Client Need—Safe, effective care environment

4 3. To ensure adequate treatment, the client with a sexually transmitted disease should be told to continue taking the prescribed medication for the full amount of time. Symptoms may clear in a short time after initial treatment, but the organisms may not be totally destroyed. The infection may persist without adequate treatment. The need for a refill should be at the discretion of the health professional. Long-term or repeated use of an antibiotic can cause an organism to develop resistance. Aggressive and appropriate short-term treatment should be adequate for the present infection. Further treatment should not be required unless reinfection occurs. (16:91, 740)
  Nursing Process—Implementation
  Client Need—Health promotion/maintenance

5 3. Although all of the measures listed are important health practices in preventing infections, the most important method for preventing a recurrence of a sexually transmitted disease is to eliminate the infection in other sex partners. Unless this occurs, the pathogenic organism will be transmitted again. (14:930; 16:89, 91)
  Nursing Process—Implementation
  Client Need—Health promotion/maintenance

NURSING CARE OF CLIENTS WITH CYSTITIS

6 1. One of the classic symptoms of cystitis is pain or burning on urination. Other symptoms include frequency and urgency. Flank pain is more often experienced by people who have pyelonephritis. The urine may contain white blood cells, causing it to appear cloudy, but a purulent discharge is not a common complaint. Concentrated urine has a strong odor, but this is not usually the case among people who develop cystitis. People with cystitis may report foul-smelling urine rather than urine that smells strongly of ammonia. (16:739; 7:512)
  Nursing Process—Collecting data
  Client Need—Safe, effective care environment

7 2. The client should collect urine from midstream. The first portion of voided urine is wasted because it may contain organisms present at the distal urethra. Voiding clears them from the urethra. The urine collected in midstream will more likely reflect the status of conditions within the bladder. The mouth of the container and inside of the specimen container must be kept sterile. Holding the container against the labia will transfer organisms and contaminate the specimen. The antiseptic should be used to cleanse the external genitalia and not be mixed with the collected urine. (18:535; 7:500)

> Nursing Process—Implementation
> Client Need—Safe, effective care environment

8   3. Because the female urethra is shorter than the male's, pathogens can travel to the bladder at a much faster rate. Also the female urethra is more easily contaminated with organisms about the rectum if hygiene is not adequate. Pathogens have to travel further in the longer male urethra. The male urethra is more curved, which tends to act as a barrier to the progression of pathogens toward the bladder. Both the male and female urethra are lined with mucous membrane. The diameter of the urethra is similar in both sexes. (3:532; 16:739)

> Nursing Process—Implementation
> Client Need—Health promotion/maintenance

9   1. Consuming a large intake of fluid will promote frequent urinary elimination. Frequent voiding causes pathogens to pass out of the bladder with the urine. Decreasing the numbers of pathogens present in the urinary tract can reduce the rate of growth. Changing underclothing regularly is an appropriate hygiene measure; however, it is not the most effective measure for reducing bacteria in the bladder. Personal hygiene measures rather than the sanitary conditions of a restroom, regardless of whether it is public or private, are more important in reducing bladder infections. The color of toilet tissue does not contribute to or prevent cystitis. (14:891; 16:740)

> Nursing Process—Implementation
> Client Need—Health promotion/maintenance

10   2. The abbreviation *b.i.d.* means two times per day. The abbreviation for once a day is *q.d.* Three times a day is indicated by the abbreviation *t.i.d.* When *q.i.d.* is written, it means four times a day. (18:576)

> Nursing Process—Evaluation
> Client Need—Health promotion/maintenance

11   1. The most important technique for preventing future urinary tract infections is to eliminate introducing organisms from the rectum or vagina through improper wiping. Handwashing following elimination assists in reducing the transmission of pathogens to other body structures such as the eyes and mouth. However, handwashing is not as likely to reduce the risk of cystitis as much as correct wiping. The use of chemicals like those in feminine hygiene sprays should be avoided because they often contain substances to which many people are sensitive. Drying the perineum is a comfort measure and is appropriate in eliminating moisture that may facilitate bacterial growth, but it is not as significant as the manner in which the perineum is wiped. (7:513; 14:891)

> Nursing Process—Evaluation
> Client Need—Health promotion/maintenance

NURSING CARE OF CLIENTS WITH PYELONEPHRITIS

12   3. Pyuria means there is pus in the urine. Pus is formed from white blood cells and dead bacteria. Glycosuria means there is sugar in the urine, which is common among diabetics. Blood in the urine, or hematuria, also may be found in people with pyelonephritis, but it is not as significant as identifying pus in the urine. Proteinuria refers to the fact that a plasma protein, usually albumin, is being excreted in the urine. (7:513; 16:741)

> Nursing Process—Collecting data
> Client Need—Physiological integrity

13   2. When it is necessary to insert a catheter, the recumbent position is best for the majority of female clients. This position involves placing the client on the back with the knees flexed and the soles of the feet flat on the bed. For females who may have arthritis of the hips or another condition that would interfere with recumbent positioning, a side-lying position may be used as an alternative. The lithotomy position involves supporting the feet in stirrups. It is used when a female undergoes a pelvic examination. The knee–chest position is used for rectal or lower bowel examinations. The prone position is used when examining the spine and back. (14:400; 18:516)

> Nursing Process—Implementation
> Client Need—Safe, effective care environment

14   3. A contaminated catheter should be discarded. Before proceeding, the nurse should obtain a second, sterile catheter. Sterility cannot be ensured by wiping the contaminated catheter with an alcohol swab or cleansing with Betadine solution. If the contaminated catheter is reinserted from the vagina into the urethra, there is a potential for transferring pathogens to the urinary tract. (14:453; 18:342)

> Nursing Process—Implementation
> Client Need—Safe, effective care environment

15   2. People who receive phenazopyridine should be informed that the drug will change the color of the urine to orange. Phenazopyridine does not

cause the urine to look cloudy, decrease in volume, or smell strong. (3:533)
Nursing Process—Implementation
Client Need—Health promotion/maintenance

16 4. A laxative is given the evening before an IVP to empty the bowel of gas and stool, which, if present, could obstruct the view of the urinary structures during the x-ray. An IVP is not used to examine the lower gastrointestinal tract. Stool incontinence is not generally a problem associated with an IVP. Laxatives are generally given to treat constipation, not to prevent it. (14:885; 16:726)
Nursing Process—Planning
Client Need—Safe, effective care environment

17 4. People who have an allergy to shellfish also may be allergic to iodine-based dyes or antiseptics. During an IVP an iodine-based dye is used. However, nonionic contrast agents, which produce fewer allergic reactions, are available as a substitute. Sensitivity to eggs, wheat, or milk generally will not cause any life-threatening consequences to a person undergoing an IVP. (3:523; 14:885)
Nursing Process—Implementation
Client Need—Physiological integrity

NURSING CARE OF CLIENTS WITH URINARY INCONTINENCE

18 1. Keeping a log of incontinence can help the nurse identify patterns in the frequency of urination. The data can then be used to schedule toileting activities to correspond to the filling and emptying patterns demonstrated by the client. Checking the urine's specific gravity, monitoring bladder distention, and observing the color of urine are all appropriate assessments when caring for clients having problems with urinary elimination. However, these assessments are not necessarily as pertinent to planning a successful bladder retraining program as identifying urinary elimination patterns. (16:735; 18:506)
Nursing Process—Collecting data
Client Need—Physiological integrity

19 1. Kegel exercises are performed by contracting and relaxing the muscles in the vagina. Pelvic rocking helps to relieve backache associated with dysmenorrhea and is considered a good conditioning exercise during the prenatal period. The other options describe exercises for improving muscle tone but are not specific to the pubococcygeal muscles. (14:920; 19:192)
Nursing Process—Implementation
Client Need—Physiological integrity

20 4. Restricting fluid intake should be discouraged because it can potentially lead to fluid imbalance. Concentrated urine also is more likely to foster stone formation. Inadequate fluid intake does contribute to constipation, but that is not the main reason for discouraging the client from limiting his fluid intake. Although the client is invested in the plan, it would be unsafe to encourage him in his plan to restrict his fluid intake. (16:735; 18:509)
Nursing Process—Implementation
Client Need—Health promotion/maintenance

21 4. Reflecting feelings demonstrates empathy. It is a useful therapeutic communication technique. It lets the client know that the nurse has recognized the emotion underlying the spoken words in the verbal statement. Disagreeing with the client by saying that he is a "nice gentleman" often blocks further communication. Belittling the client's feelings by challenging the seriousness of his statement also interferes with communication. Giving advice is a nontherapeutic form of interaction; it is demonstrated in the examples in which the nurse says "Cheer up" and "You should expect this at your age." (9:139; 12:262)
Nursing Process—Implementation
Client Need—Psychosocial integrity

22 3. A space should be provided between the end of the penis and the drainage end of the catheter. This prevents irritation to the urinary meatus and promotes drainage of urine. Lubrication is not appropriate because it would interfere with maintaining the catheter in place. External catheters are similar to latex condoms. They stretch to fit. Therefore measuring the penis is unnecessary. The foreskin of an uncircumcised male should never be left in a retracted position because it could have a tourniquet effect and interfere with circulation of blood to the tissue. (18:513)
Nursing Process—Implementation
Client Need—Physiological integrity

23 1. Anchoring the indwelling catheter in a male client to the abdomen eliminates pressure and irritation at the penoscrotal angle. Pressure in this area can predispose to fistula formation. The catheter and tubing are passed over a client's leg to prevent obstruction of drainage from body weight. It is appropriate to fasten the drainage tubing to the bed so that there is a straight line from the bed to the collection bag and to insert the catheter into the tubing of the collection bag. However, neither of these nursing actions will prevent a penoscrotal fistula from forming. (7:653; 18:525)
Nursing Process—Implementation
Client Need—Physiological integrity

NURSING CARE OF CLIENTS WITH BENIGN PROSTATIC HYPERTROPHY

24 2. Nocturia, being awakened by a need to urinate, is a common finding among people with benign prostatic hypertrophy. Burning on urination is more likely a sign of a bladder infection, which could be secondary to benign prostatic hypertrophy. Feeling pressure in the back would more likely indicate pathology involving the kidney. Colorless or very light yellow urine indicates that the urine is dilute. This could be caused from an endocrine disturbance, such as diabetes insipidus, or from some other dysfunction in renal tubular reabsorption. (16:708; 14:895)
  Nursing Process—Collecting data
  Client Need—Physiological integrity

25 3. Due to obstruction of the urethra from an enlarging prostate gland, men with benign prostatic hypertrophy often describe hesitancy when initiating urination. That is, they feel the need to urinate, but it takes some time before urine is released. The stream of urine also is diminished. Benign prostatic hypertrophy usually does not cause sexual dysfunction or incontinence. The prostate gland is not located in the scrotum. It is palpated by rectal examination. (3:773; 7:576)
  Nursing Process—Collecting data
  Client Need—Physiological integrity

26 1. Lowering the penis from an upright position to one in which the penis is pointed in the direction of the toes sometimes helps to pass a catheter beyond the narrowing caused by an enlarged prostate gland. The penis should be grasped firmly whenever a catheter is inserted. If resistance is met when inserting a catheter, it should never be forced. Massaging the tissue below the base of the penis is not a technique that will facilitate passage through an enlarged prostate gland. (14:459; 18:521)
  Nursing Process—Implementation
  Client Need—Physiological integrity

27 2. Ensuring that there is adequate urinary output from the suprapubic catheter would be the best evidence that the catheter is patent. Inspecting the skin is essential for detecting skin breakdown or infection. Attaching the catheter to a leg bag promotes the ability of the client to move about. Encouraging oral intake would promote the formation of urine, but an increased fluid intake is not a measure of catheter patency. (3:531; 16:710-711)
  Nursing Process—Evaluation
  Client Need—Physiological integrity

28 4. Hematuria generally is present following a TURP for at least 24 hours. Vital signs should be monitored to evaluate if the volume of blood loss is causing shock. It may take 24 to 48 hours for the urine to become light pink and transparent. The volume of urine should be within normal range unless complications, such as hypovolemic shock or obstruction of the catheter, occur. Sediment may be present in the urine due to the remnants of prostatic tissue; however, the blood that is mixed with the urine initially would obscure the ability of the nurse to identify the presence of tissue or mucoid debris. (7:578)
  Nursing Process—Collecting data
  Client Need—Physiological integrity

29 1. A continuous bladder irrigation is performed by instilling normal saline solution hung from an intravenous pole through one lumen of the urinary catheter. The solution flows into the bladder, dilutes the urine and sediment, and drains out the catheter into a gravity drainage bag. An Asepto syringe and sterile container for irrigation solution would be used for performing an intermittent catheter irrigation. Sterile normal saline, not an antiseptic solution, is used for a continuous bladder irrigation and intermittent catheter irrigation. (14:896; 7:578)
  Nursing Process—Planning
  Client Need—Safe, effective care environment

30 3. The nurse should assess if the catheter is draining well before administering an analgesic for bladder discomfort. Obstruction of the catheter can cause bladder spasms. Restoring patency would be more appropriate in the case of catheter obstruction than administering an analgesic. Administering an analgesic is not necessarily contingent on a normal pulse rate. There is no dressing following a TURP; the surgery is performed through the urethra. A narcotic analgesic may depress the respiratory center, but assessing the client's ability to cough would not affect the decision to withhold or administer an analgesic. (3:774; 16:712)
  Nursing Process—Collecting data
  Client Need—Physiological integrity

31 4. Belladonna and opium rectal suppositories are considered the most effective drugs for relieving bladder spasms following a TURP. Aspirin should be avoided because it may increase the tendency to bleed. Darvocet and Demerol are synthetic narcotic analgesics. Narcotics alone do not seem to lessen the spasms; they may decrease the pain. (3:774; 16:712)
  Nursing Process—Implementation
  Client Need—Physiological integrity

32 3. The best method for recording output when a client has more than one catheter is to record the volume that drained from each catheter as a separate entry in the medical record. Recording only the output from the urethral catheter or the output from the wound catheter would not provide accurate data on total output. If the two volumes are added together and recorded as a single entry, it is difficult to evaluate the status of urinary drainage from each catheter. (3:774; 14:896)

> Nursing Process—Implementation
> Client Need—Physiological integrity

33 3. After a suprapubic catheter is removed, urine may leak from the incisional area and saturate the sterile dressing. A wet dressing provides a "wicking" action by which microorganisms are attracted in the direction of the impaired tissue. A dressing saturated with urine also can lead to skin breakdown. If standards of care are being followed, the postoperative care plan should already indicate nursing orders for repositioning the client, ambulating with assistance, and encouraging deep breathing. (3:774)

> Nursing Process—Planning
> Client Need—Physiological integrity

NURSING CARE OF CLIENTS WITH RENAL CALCULI

34 2. When kidney stones move, they cause renal or ureteral colic, which is experienced as episodic waves of excruciating pain. The pain may begin in the flank area and radiate to the inguinal ring, the inner aspect of the thigh, and the external genitals. Feeling tired and weak, frequency and urgency, and chills and fever generally are not experienced by people with kidney stones unless they are due to secondary complications. (3:544; 16:747)

> Nursing Process—Collecting data
> Client Need—Physiological integrity

35 4. Because the diagnosis and treatment of renal calculi is enhanced by examining the components of the stone itself, the nurse should strain all urine. Remnants of the stone may appear as minute pieces of gravel. Because voiding is not necessarily affected, a catheter would be unnecessary. Testing for the presence and amount of glucose in the urine would not provide significant information about kidney stones. Applying an abdominal binder may be a comfort measure for some; however, it is likely to be ineffective, considering the severity of pain experienced by clients with renal calculi. (7:515; 14:893)

> Nursing Process—Planning
> Client Need—Physiological integrity

36 1. When a kidney stone is suspected, fluid volume intake should be increased to 3000 mL or more per 24 hours. By increasing oral fluids, the po-

tential for passing the stone during urination is increased. Frequent urination of dilute urine also may prevent a secondary urinary tract infection. Bed rest would be inappropriate; in fact, it may contribute to additional stone formation. Activity, if comfort allows, may promote movement of the stone into the bladder, where it may be passed. Diversional activity may relieve boredom and improve sensory deprivation, but it is not the most essential nursing measure from among the options provided. (7:514; 16:749)

> Nursing Process—Implementation
> Client Need—Physiological integrity

37 2. Due to the instrumentation and dilation of the urethra, it is common for people to complain of burning when urinating following a cystoscopy. The nurse can reduce or relieve the discomfort by promoting a liberal fluid intake, providing sitz baths, and administering a prescribed mild analgesic. Polyuria, anuria, and pyuria would indicate other complications or conditions affecting the renal system. (3:525; 14:886)

> Nursing Process—Collecting data
> Client Need—Safe, effective care environment

38 1. When ESWL is performed, the client is immersed in a tub of water. The water promotes localization and transmission of the shock waves. As an alternative, ESWL may be administered with the client sitting in a chair equipped with a water cushion. No incision is made, and the client is not placed in a pressure chamber when ESWL is performed. The shock wave is a form of ultrasound, not electricity. Although the client's heart rate and rhythm are assessed during the procedure with a cardiac monitor, the leads are attached to the chest and not the flank. (14:894; 16:747)

> Nursing Process—Planning
> Client Need—Safe, effective care environment

NURSING CARE OF CLIENTS WITH BLADDER CANCER

39 3. The most common symptom of bladder cancer is painless hematuria. Dysuria, if present, generally is due to a concurrent urinary tract infection secondary to obstruction of urine. Oliguria may occur later as the disease becomes more advanced and obstruction occurs. Bladder cancer, which has not spread to adjacent pelvic structures, usually is not associated with an unusual discharge from any body orifice. (16:754; 3:546)

> Nursing Process—Collecting data
> Client Need—Safe, effective care environment

40 4. There is a correlation between cigarette smoking, even being exposed passively to cigarette smoke, and the development of bladder cancer. Other carcinogenic factors include long-term exposure to chemical solvents and dyes. Neither stress incontinence nor sexual activities seem to be implicated as a causal agent in bladder cancer. (3:546; 7:515)

Nursing Process—Implementation
Client Need—Health promotion/maintenance

41 1. Recommendations for promoting safety when handling toxic chemotherapeutic agents include wearing two pairs of surgical latex gloves, which are less permeable than polyvinyl gloves. A gown with cuffs and a mask or goggles also should be worn to prevent direct contact with the drug. There is no particular advantage in using a glass syringe. In fact, there would be a greater potential hazard if a glass syringe were dropped and broken. The uncontained drug would be considered a toxic spill. Time in contact with the client is not a safety hazard with chemotherapy, but it is a factor in radiation therapy involving sealed and unsealed implants. (14:710; 15:238; 18:633)

Nursing Process—Implementation
Client Need—Safe, effective care environment

NURSING CARE OF CLIENTS WITH URINARY DIVERSIONS

42 3. An ileal conduit, or ileal loop procedure, involves implanting the ureters into a section of the ileum that has been removed from the rest of the small intestine. The section of ileum is fashioned into a stoma that opens onto the abdomen. When a ureterosigmoidostomy is performed, the ureters are attached to the sigmoid colon, and urine is eliminated with stool by way of the rectum. Currently there are no procedures in which the ureters are implanted directly into the small intestine. If a Koch pouch, or continent urostomy, is performed, urine is siphoned with a catheter from an internal collection pouch. (3:547, 616; 16:755)

Nursing Process—Implementation
Client Need—Health promotion/maintenance

43 3. A pulse rate of more than 100 in the absence of activity or some accompanying pathology suggests that the sympathetic nervous system is stimulated. The sympathetic nervous system responds when a person is experiencing a real or perceived threat to his well-being. The data in the other options are generally within normal limits. (17:271; 18:26)

Nursing Process—Collecting data
Client Need—Physiological integrity

44 1. Sharing perceptions with the client by stating that "it must be difficult" shows empathy. It gives the person permission to unburden himself. Telling the client that he has one of the best surgeons may not encourage the client to verbalize further because it is unlikely that he will disagree. Offering a reassuring cliché that "everything will turn out OK" cannot be guaranteed. It would indicate that the nursing assistant feels uncomfortable discussing any problems with which Mr. Holland currently is concerned. Saying that "others have done just fine" minimizes and belittles the uniqueness of the situation from the client's perspective. (9:138-139; 12:354-355)

Nursing Process—Implementation
Client Need—Psychosocial integrity

45 1. Encouraging the client to verbalize more and express his feelings is a therapeutic communication technique. Because it is impossible for a nurse to know how a client is feeling, this statement diminishes the nurse's credibility. The client may lose faith in the ability of the nurse to be truly empathetic. Minimizing the despair that he is feeling by saying "it's not as bad as that" is likely to interfere with any further discussion. Giving the client the advice to "think more positively" is likely to be interpreted as disapproval for the way the client is currently feeling. (9:139; 12:262)

Nursing Process—Implementation
Client Need—Psychosocial integrity

46 2. It is important for the nurse to assess the condition of the skin to plan appropriate interventions. If the skin is excoriated, it will probably take more than just diluting the urine or emptying the appliance more frequently to restore skin integrity. It is impossible to leave the appliance off because urine is released constantly. (18:534)

Nursing Process—Implementation
Client Need—Physiological integrity

47 2. Inserting a tampon or a gauze square into the stoma will momentarily absorb the urine and keep the skin dry. Leaning over the toilet would put the client in an awkward position during the time the appliance is being changed. It generally takes two hands to manipulate the appliance during its application; therefore, pressing a finger over the stoma or pinching the stoma would interfere with the coordination that is needed. (7:524; 18:534)

Nursing Process—Implementation
Client Need—Health promotion/maintenance

48 1. Emptying the collection bag would decrease the weight and pull on the skin to which the appliance is attached. Fluids should not be restricted; this would concentrate the urine and increase the risk for dehydration, skin irritation, and infection. To avoid skin impairment, an appliance generally is not changed on a daily basis. However, it must be changed if it becomes loose or uncomfortable. It is unlikely that avoiding gas-forming food would have any affect at all on a person with a urostomy. (18:534)

> Nursing Process—Implementation
> Client Need—Health promotion/maintenance

NURSING CARE OF CLIENTS WITH GLOMERULONEPHRITIS

49 2. Although definite evidence linking a streptococcal infection with glomerulonephritis has not been established, many identify that they experienced an upper respiratory infection or sore throat 2 to 3 weeks before the onset of glomerulonephritis. There has been no correlation with trauma, antibiotic therapy, or an allergy specific to x-ray dye. (14:892; 16:741)

> Nursing Process—Collecting data
> Client Need—Safe, effective care environment

50 4. A common sign associated with glomerulonephritis is that the face often appears puffy, especially around the eyes. The skin is pale, not flushed. Skin hemorrhages are a common finding in liver disease and blood dyscrasias. The distribution of body hair is not directly related to glomerulonephritis. (3:534; 7:510)

> Nursing Process—Collecting data
> Client Need—Physiological integrity

51 3. Because glomerulonephritis impairs renal function, monitoring weight on a daily basis is essential for evaluating how much fluid the person is retaining. Ambulation is not usually impaired; however, if the client is hypertensive or has other circulatory complications, activity may be restricted. Mouth care is important for all who cannot attend to their own self-care; it is not a common problem among people with glomerulonephritis. Owing to fluid retention, many people who have glomerulonephritis will be on fluid restrictions. (7:511; 14:892)

> Nursing Process—Planning
> Client Need—Physiological integrity

52 3. The results of a BUN test indicate how efficiently the glomeruli are removing nitrogen wastes from the blood. An elevation indicates glomerular dysfunction. Serum amylase levels aid in diagnosing and monitoring pancreatitis. A blood glucose test is used for monitoring people with diabetes mellitus. A complete blood count is helpful for baseline information, but it is not as

essential in evaluating the course of glomerulonephritis as the BUN. (7:501; 14:884)

> Nursing Process—Collecting data
> Client Need—Physiological integrity

53 2. It would be important for the nurse to first assess the client's blood pressure. People with glomerulonephritis often are hypertensive; hypertension can be accompanied by a headache. Hypertension also may be an indication of increased intracranial pressure. If the headache is caused by hypertension, a priority intervention would be to reduce the blood pressure and treat the cause. Implementing comfort measures, such as reducing environmental stimuli, administering a prescribed analgesic, and changing the client's position, all may be appropriate, but assessing the client should take place first. (3:534; 16:742)

> Nursing Process—Implementation
> Client Need—Physiological integrity

54 2. Urine that has been formed before the time a 24-hour urine collection starts should not be included with the collected urine. Valid results require that the urine collected be produced within the 24-hour period. Properly collected urine may be refrigerated in a large container, or the container may be kept in a basin of ice. After all of the urine from the 24-hour period is collected, the entire specimen is sent to the laboratory. Laboratory policy should be consulted as to whether urine from a 24-hour collection should be mixed with a preservative rather than refrigerated. (14:368; 18:535)

> Nursing Process—Implementation
> Client Need—Safe, effective care environment

55 3. People with glomerulonephritis generally manifest albuminuria. Glucose and acetone would be expected in a person with uncontrolled diabetes mellitus. Bilirubin may be present in the urine of a person with liver or gallbladder disease. (7:510; 16:742-743)

> Nursing Process—Collecting data
> Client Need—Physiological integrity

56 2. The presence of blood can give a smoky appearance to urine. Cloudy urine suggests the presence of white blood cells. If the urine appears bright orange, the nurse might investigate if the client has ingested a substance containing a water-soluble dye. Concentrated urine is likely to appear dark yellow. (3:534; 18:503)

> Nursing Process—Collecting data
> Client Need—Physiological integrity

57 3. Chicken salad on a lettuce wedge is the menu item that contains the least amount of sodium among the options provided. Processed meats are highly salted. Bouillon and other canned soups generally contain a great deal of salt. Dairy products are high in sodium. Baked goods, such as crackers and pizza crust, also contain sodium bicarbonate or salt. (4:443, 610)

> Nursing Process—Implementation
> Client Need—Health promotion/maintenance

58 2. Medications that irritate stomach mucosa or cause nausea should be administered with food. The presence of food in the stomach dilutes the acidity level and protects the mucous membrane from erosion. The mucous membrane of the stomach is more susceptible to irritation if the medication is given on an empty stomach or between meals. Taking the medication with water is not as beneficial as taking the drug when food is present in the stomach. (15:25)

> Nursing Process—Implementation
> Client Need—Physiological integrity

NURSING CARE OF CLIENTS WITH RENAL FAILURE

59 1. The first stage of renal failure is generally characterized by oliguria; that is, a urine output of less than 400 to 500 mL in 24 hours. The nurse may observe a diuretic phase following a period of oliguria or anuria as the client's condition improves. People in renal failure do not experience pain or discomfort with urination. The urine of a person in renal failure does not contain abnormal amounts of ketones or red blood cells. (16:762; 7:515)

> Nursing Process—Collecting data
> Client Need—Physiological integrity

60 2. Measuring intake and output accurately is a priority when planning the care of a client with renal failure. This information aids in evaluating fluid balance and adjusting fluid restrictions. Urinary retention is not common in renal failure because the client is not producing much urine. Generally, a urinary catheter is inserted to aid in monitoring the output of a person in renal failure. The body temperature may be monitored to assess for signs of infection or other complications; however, it is not likely to be affected by the primary condition. The nurse would not expect any abnormalities in bowel sounds in clients with renal failure. (14:537; 16:765)

> Nursing Process—Planning
> Client Need—Physiological integrity

61 4. It is most important to assess lung sounds because administering fluid in the presence of oliguria or anuria may lead to congestive heart failure and pulmonary edema. Fluid overload can be manifested by pedal edema, but that is not a life-threatening consequence. Skin integrity may

become impaired due to inactivity, edema, and elimination of nitrogenous wastes through the skin. Skin impairment would not be an immediate problem with fluid therapy. The oral mucosa would not undergo adverse changes with the administration of fluid. (3:538; 16:765)

> Nursing Process—Collecting data
> Client Need—Physiological integrity

62 4. The skin of a client in renal failure becomes dry and intensely itchy due to the excretion and evaporation of nitrogenous wastes through the skin. The skin should be wiped frequently with plain, warm water and patted dry. The nurse may choose to apply a lubricating skin cream or lotion. Owing to edema, the skin is taut and puffy. (7:516-517; 16:764-765)

> Nursing Process—Planning
> Client Need—Physiological integrity

63 4. Lemon juice can be used to enhance the flavor of fish, eggs, and some vegetables. Other seasonings that could be recommended include fresh herbs such as parsley, dill, oregano, and so forth. Fresh onion also is acceptable. Catsup, prepared mustard, and soy sauce are high in sodium and should be avoided. (5:447)

> Nursing Process—Implementation
> Client Need—Health promotion/maintenance

64 1. Hard candy, especially if it is sour or tart flavored, will increase salivation and reduce the sensation of thirst without increasing fluid intake. People in renal failure, unless they are diabetic, are not generally restricted in the amount of carbohydrate they may consume. Ice chips, ice cream, and fresh fruit all contain fluid, which must be considered in the fluid restriction. (3:538; 7:518)

> Nursing Process—Implementation
> Client Need—Physiological integrity

65 1. To evaluate trends in weight, the nurse should weigh the client at the same time daily using the same scale each time. The amount of clothing should be similar at each weighing. If the time of weighing is consistent, the amount of food or liquids that the client has been consuming is not likely to vary considerably. It is important to collaborate with the client, but obtaining the weight should not be omitted or postponed for frivolous reasons. (7:518; 18:651)

> Nursing Process—Planning
> Client Need—Physiological integrity

66 1. The color and temperature of the hand should be assessed regularly for signs of inadequate circulation. Blood clots may form in the joined vessels and occlude tissue perfusion. Joint range of

motion, muscle tone and coordination, and skin integrity are not likely to be affected. (3:539)
Nursing Process—Collecting data
Client Need—Physiological integrity

67 1. The infusion tubing should be clamped, usually for 15 to 45 minutes, to allow osmosis and diffusion to take place between the dialysate and the peritoneum. The peritoneal cavity is drained after the dwell time. The client is free to ambulate, change positions, or remain in bed during peritoneal dialysis. The amount of activity would depend on the safety needs of each client. The client may eat and drink during peritoneal dialysis; however, oral fluids continue to be restricted throughout dialysis and for as long as the client is in renal failure. (3:541; 16:768)
Nursing Process—Implementation
Client Need—Safe, effective care environment

68 3. An elevated temperature is unexpected. Its presence indicates that an infection may be occurring. It is expected that a client undergoing peritoneal dialysis will lose weight and have an output that exceeds intake. Regular, deep breathing generally indicates that ventilation is adequate. Rapid, shallow breathing may indicate that the volume of instilled fluid is interfering with chest excursion. If shortness of breath occurs, the nurse may try elevating the head of the bed or changing positions while evaluating the response of the client before notifying the charge nurse or physician. Shortness of breath, although uncomfortable, may be short-lived. Relief is likely to coincide with the drainage of infused dialysate solution. (14:899; 16:768)
Nursing Process—Implementation
Client Need—Physiological integrity

69 3. One of the beneficial effects of dialysis is the lowering of the elevated serum potassium. A lower red cell count is not a desired effect. Most people with renal failure become anemic because the kidney's ability to produce erythropoietin is impaired. Blood transfusions or injections of genetically engineered erythropoietin are often necessary. Peritoneal dialysis is not expected to improve renal output. If renal function improves, it is rather due to accompanying therapy or healing on the cellular level. Improvement of appetite is far too subjective to be used as an indicator of a therapeutic response to peritoneal dialysis. (14:899; 16:766)
Nursing Process—Evaluation
Client Need—Safe, effective care environment

70 1. A person should be catheterized immediately after voiding to measure residual urine. This measurement indicates if the person is emptying his or her bladder during urination. If the residual urine volume is 150 mL or more, it indicates that the bladder is not being completely emptied. Determining the volume of residual urine can be performed at any time as long as voiding has taken place just prior to the catheterization. Waiting until the bladder feels full or 1 hour after drinking water would not ensure an accurate measurement of residual urine volume. (14:883; 18:514)
Nursing Process—Planning
Client Need—Physiological integrity

71 3. Urinary retention may be relieved by pressing inward and downward over the bladder in what is referred to as Credé's maneuver. This technique facilitates bladder emptying by increasing intraabdominal pressure above urethral pressure, thus allowing urine to be expelled. Drinking a full glass of water would not help the situation immediately and may contribute to greater distention of the bladder. Taking rapid, shallow breaths would not aid relaxation of the internal urinary sphincter. Performing Valsalva's maneuver by holding the breath and bearing down is more helpful when trying to eliminate stool. (14:889; 18:510)
Nursing Process—Implementation
Client Need—Physiological integrity

72 2. It is best to obtain a urine specimen for culture without opening the drainage system. Most companies now manufacture drainage tubing that has a self-sealing port near where the catheter is connected. The port should be cleansed with an antiseptic before piercing the port with a needle and syringe. It is not necessary to remove the catheter. The specimen should be fresh; it should not be obtained from urine that has been collecting for some time in the drainage bag. It would be inappropriate to delay obtaining the urine specimen until the next time the catheter is replaced. (18:535-536)
Nursing Process—Implementation
Client Need—Safe, effective care environment

73 4. The standard of care is to use 30 to 60 mL of sterile normal saline when irrigating an indwelling catheter. If for some reason another solution would be substituted, a medical order would be written specifying the solution, its strength, and volume. (18:528-529)
Nursing Process—Planning
Client Need—Safe, effective care environment

74 1. Clients with a flank incision tend to take shallow breaths because deep breathing increases pain. Hypoventilation places these clients at risk for pulmonary complications postoperatively. There would be no correlation between a flank incision and the potential for bradycardia. In fact, tachycardia would more likely accompany hypoxemia. People undergoing intestinal surgery or who have abdominal incisions are more likely to develop abdominal distention. Obesity is a predisposing factor in the development of an incisional hernia. (7:527-528; 14:894; 16:753)

Nursing Process—Planning
Client Need—Physiological integrity

75 3. All of the assessments in the options are within normal limits. However, the best indication that renal function is adequate is an output of at least 400 to 500 mL in 24 hours. If renal failure occurs, the client will manifest oliguria with a 24-hour output less than 400 mL, or the client will be anuric. (14:898; 16:762)

Nursing Process—Evaluation
Client Need—Physiological integrity

Classification of Test Items

Unit IV Review Test 13

Directions: After each question the correct answer is given as well as a classification of each test question. Compare the correct answer with your answer. If a question has been answered *incorrectly*, draw a line to the end of the four columns. When finished, add up your correct scores and place the results at the bottom of each column.

Score Calculation:

To determine the percentage of the number of questions you answered correctly, divide the **Number Correct** by the **Number Possible**, as example 65 (the number of questions answered correctly) divided by 75 (the number of questions in the test) = .86 or 86%.

NURSING PROCESS

C = Collecting data
P = Planning
I = Implementation
E = Evaluation

CLIENT NEEDS

S = Safe, effective care environment
P = Physiological integrity
M = Psychosocial integrity
H = Health promotion/maintenance

Question #	Answer #	Nursing Process				Client Needs			
		C	P	I	E	S	P	M	H
1	2	C				S			
2	2			I				M	
3	4			I		S			
4	3			I					H
5	3			I					H
6	1	C				S			
7	2			I		S			
8	3			I					H
9	1			I					H
10	2				E				H
11	1				E				H
12	3	C					P		
13	2			I		S			
14	3			I		S			
15	2			I					H
16	4		P			S			
17	4			I			P		
18	1	C					P		
19	1			I			P		

NURSING PROCESS

C = Collecting data
P = Planning
I = Implementation
E = Evaluation

CLIENT NEEDS

S = Safe, effective care environment
P = Physiological integrity
M = Psychosocial integrity
H = Health promotion/maintenance

Question #	Answer #	Nursing Process				Client Needs			
		C	P	I	E	S	P	M	H
20	4			I					H
21	4			I				M	
22	3			I			P		
23	1			I			P		
24	2	C					P		
25	3	C					P		
26	1			I			P		
27	2				E		P		
28	4	C					P		
29	1		P			S			
30	3	C					P		
31	4			I			P		
32	3			I			P		
33	3		P				P		
34	2	C					P		
35	4		P				P		
36	1			I			P		
37	2	C				S			
38	1		P			S			
39	3	C				S			
40	4			I					H
41	1			I		S			
42	3			I					H
43	3	C					P		
44	1			I				M	
45	1			I				M	
46	2			I			P		
47	2			I					H
48	1			I					H
49	2	C				S			
50	4	C					P		

NURSING PROCESS

C = Collecting data
P = Planning
I = Implementation
E = Evaluation

CLIENT NEEDS

S = Safe, effective care environment
P = Physiological integrity
M = Psychosocial integrity
H = Health promotion/maintenance

Question #	Answer #	Nursing Process				Client Needs			
		C	P	I	E	S	P	M	H
51	3		P				P		
52	3	C					P		
53	2			I			P		
54	2			I		S			
55	3	C					P		
56	2	C					P		
57	3			I					H
58	2			I			P		
59	1	C					P		
60	2		P				P		
61	4	C					P		
62	4		P				P		
63	4			I					H
64	1			I			P		
65	1		P				P		
66	1	C					P		
67	1			I		S			
68	3			I			P		
69	3				E	S			
70	1		P				P		
71	3			I			P		
72	2			I		S			
73	4		P			S			
74	1		P				P		
75	3				E		P		
Number Correct									
Number Possible	75	20	12	38	5	18	39	4	14
Percentage Correct									

REVIEW TEST 14

The Nursing Care of Clients with Disorders of the Eye, Ear, Nose, and Throat

Nursing Care of Clients with Eye Injuries
Nursing Care of Clients with Visual Acuity Problems
Nursing Care of Clients with Impaired Vision
Nursing Care of Clients with Cataracts
Nursing Care of Clients with Glaucoma
Nursing Care of Clients with a Detached Retina
Nursing Care of Clients Undergoing Assessment of the Ears and Auditory System
Nursing Care of Clients with Disorders of the External Ear
Nursing Care of Clients with Otitis Media
Nursing Care of Clients with Otosclerosis
Nursing Care of Clients with Meniere's Disease
Nursing Care of Clients with a Nosebleed
Nursing Care of Clients with Sinusitis
Nursing Care of Clients with Nasal Surgery
Individual Test Items
Nursing Care of Clients with Pharyngitis
Nursing Care of Clients with Laryngitis
Nursing Care of Clients with Cancer of the Larynx
Nursing Care of Clients Having a Tonsillectomy
Nursing Care of Clients with an Occluded Airway

Correct Answers and Rationale
Classification of Test Items

Directions: With a pencil, blacken the circle in front of the option you have chosen for your correct answer.

The Nursing Care of Clients with Disorders of the Eye, Ear, Nose, and Throat

NURSING CARE OF CLIENTS WITH EYE INJURIES

Ms. Robertson, the high school chemistry teacher, sends her student, Ben, to be seen by the school nurse. Ben has been performing a chemistry laboratory experiment, and his eye has been splashed with a chemical.

1 Which one of the following is the *most* important information for the nurse to obtain at this time?

○ 1. If safety glasses were worn
○ 2. The names of the chemicals
○ 3. The treatment already given
○ 4. If Ben's vision is impaired

2 The nurse plans to irrigate the student's irritated eye. Which one of the following solutions would be *best* to use?

○ 1. Tap water
○ 2. Sodium bicarbonate
○ 3. Acetic acid
○ 4. Magnesium sulfate

Timby B, Scherer JC: LIPPINCOTT'S REVIEW FOR NCLEX–PN. © 1994 J.B. Lippincott Company.

3 It is *essential* for the nurse to direct the flow of the irrigating solution
- ○ 1. directly onto the cornea.
- ○ 2. away from the inner canthus.
- ○ 3. within the anterior chamber.
- ○ 4. toward the nasolacrimal duct.

4 After providing emergency treatment of the chemical splash, it would be *best* that the nurse refer the student to a(n)
- ○ 1. optician.
- ○ 2. ophthalmologist.
- ○ 3. optometrist.
- ○ 4. podiatrist.

NURSING CARE OF CLIENTS WITH VISUAL ACUITY PROBLEMS

A nurse is working in a physician's office. Several clients have been scheduled to be examined for problems with their vision.

5 A client asks the nurse to tell her the technical name the doctor used for nearsightedness. The *most* accurate response is
- ○ 1. presbyopia.
- ○ 2. amblyopia.
- ○ 3. hyperopia.
- ○ 4. myopia.

6 A nursing assistant confides to the nurse that her father is in need of eyeglasses, but he cannot afford them. To which one of the following organizations could the nurse refer them for help?
- ○ 1. The Loyal Order of the Moose
- ○ 2. The American Legion
- ○ 3. Lions International
- ○ 4. The Knights of Columbus

7 The nurse reads in the medical record that a client has astigmatism. The nurse would expect that when assessing this person the client would *most likely* describe that without his glasses
- ○ 1. objects appear blurred and distorted.
- ○ 2. he cannot see near objects clearly.
- ○ 3. he cannot see far objects clearly.
- ○ 4. objects appear unusually small.

8 A Snellen chart will be used to assess a client's visual acuity. Before his examination the nurse would be *most* correct in explaining that he will be asked to
- ○ 1. read words that are the size of newsprint.
- ○ 2. read letters from a distance of 20 feet.
- ○ 3. look at a colored picture and identify an image.
- ○ 4. look at a screen and say when he sees an object.

9 One of the clients being examined today is legally blind. The chart indicates that the person has 20/ 200 vision. The nurse explains that this means the person
- ○ 1. sees at 20 ft what normal people see at 200 ft.
- ○ 2. sees only $^{20}/_{200\text{ths}}$ of what normal people see.
- ○ 3. sees 20-ft high objects when they are 200 ft away.
- ○ 4. sees 20% of what others see at 200 ft.

10 A client asks the nurse about the best way to clean his new prescription glasses. The *best* recommendation is that he wash the lenses with soap and warm water or commercial glass cleaner and dry them
- ○ 1. with a paper tissue.
- ○ 2. with a soft cloth.
- ○ 3. using a paper towel.
- ○ 4. by air evaporation.

11 A client is having difficulty removing a hard contact lens before his eye examination. The nurse could use a suction plunger or manually remove it by
- ○ 1. sliding the lens under the upper or lower eyelid.
- ○ 2. lifting an edge of the lens with a finger nail.
- ○ 3. pressing on the center of the lens to break the adhesion.
- ○ 4. bringing the eyelid margins toward the edges of the lens.

12 The nurse discusses a client's routine for caring for his hard contact lenses. Which one of the following indicates a need for more teaching? The client says that she
- ○ 1. removes her contacts before going to sleep.
- ○ 2. wets them with saliva if they slip out of place.
- ○ 3. stores the lenses in solution when not being worn.
- ○ 4. cleans her contacts in the palm of her hand.

NURSING CARE OF CLIENTS WITH IMPAIRED VISION

13 The nurse is caring for a client who has both eyes patched. Which addition to the care plan would be the *best* method for reducing the client's anxiety?
- ○ 1. Touch the client before speaking.
- ○ 2. Explain what you plan to do beforehand.
- ○ 3. Shut the room door to decrease noise.
- ○ 4. Leave the room lights on all the time.

14 The nurse observes the nursing assistant ambulating Mr. Freeman, a blind client, in the hall. Which of the following instructions is appropriate?
- ○ 1. Let Mr. Freeman take your arm while walking.
- ○ 2. Take Mr. Freeman's arm while walking with him.
- ○ 3. Position Mr. Freeman in front and to your side.
- ○ 4. Have Mr. Freeman walk independently by your side.

15 Trauma has caused the tissue around the eyes of a client to swell, occluding his vision. He is despondent over his temporary dependence on the nursing staff. Which of the following would be the *best* plan for promoting this client's feeling of self-reliance when it is time to eat?
- ○ 1. Help him locate his food by comparing its placement to clock positions.
- ○ 2. Ask a hospital volunteer to feed the client so he does not have to ask for help.
- ○ 3. Order food that can be sipped from containers rather than those that require eating utensils.
- ○ 4. Ask the dietary department to serve his food using paper plates and cups.

16 Mr. Myer uses an artificial eye. When removing Mr. Myer's artificial eye, it is best to do so by
- ○ 1. lifting the upper eyelid.
- ○ 2. inverting the upper eyelid.
- ○ 3. separating the two eyelids.
- ○ 4. depressing the lower eyelid.

NURSING CARE OF CLIENTS WITH CATARACTS

The nurse is assigned to care for Mr. Smoker, age 68, who has bilateral senile cataracts.

17 When assessing Mr. Smoker, which one of the following is the client *most* likely to describe to the nurse?
- ○ 1. Gradually failing eyesight
- ○ 2. Fullness within the eye
- ○ 3. Ocular pain or discomfort
- ○ 4. Flashes of light

18 As the nurse inspects Mr. Smoker's eyes, she is *most* likely to observe
- ○ 1. ruptured blood vessels on the eye.
- ○ 2. an irregularly shaped iris.
- ○ 3. a white spot behind the pupil.
- ○ 4. a painless corneal lesion.

19 The physician has informed Mr. Smoker that he will eventually need surgery. When scheduling his next appointment, which one of the following statements indicates that the client understands the treatment plan? Mr. Smoker says that he will need surgery when
- ○ 1. his loss of vision interferes with his activities of daily living.
- ○ 2. the pain can no longer be controlled through the use of eye drops.
- ○ 3. the changes are obvious to others and make him feel self-conscious.
- ○ 4. his cataracts reach maximum maturity, and no further changes are observed.

20 Mr. Smoker is scheduled for surgery. Which one of the following is the *most* important nursing action at the time of his admission?

- ○ 1. Informing his family where to wait
- ○ 2. Orienting him to his room environment
- ○ 3. Checking his height and weight
- ○ 4. Explaining how to use the television

21 Mr. Smoker is scheduled to have the cataract removed from his right eye. Preoperative orders include the following: (1) Scrub face with povidone iodine for 10 minutes on the morning of surgery. (2) Clip eyelashes on the right eye after admission. (3) Instill tropicamide (Mydriacil) 1% 2 gtt O.S. 30 minutes before surgery. It would be *essential* that the nurse
- ○ 1. carry out the physician's orders as written.
- ○ 2. question the directions for giving eye drops.
- ○ 3. let the operating room nurse clip the lashes.
- ○ 4. encourage the client to scrub his own face.

22 When instilling eye drops, the nurse instructs the client to look up and drops the medication
- ○ 1. onto the cornea.
- ○ 2. at the inner canthus.
- ○ 3. at the outer canthus.
- ○ 4. in the lower conjunctival sac.

23 Mr. Smoker returns from surgery. Four hours later he tells the nurse that he is experiencing severe pain in his operative eye. Which one of the following nursing actions is *most* appropriate.
- ○ 1. Report the finding to the nurse in charge.
- ○ 2. Give the client a prescribed analgesic.
- ○ 3. Assess his pupil response with a penlight.
- ○ 4. Reposition him on his operative side.

24 The nursing team meets to individualize a standardized nursing care plan for Mr. Smoker. Which one of the following nursing orders should be *eliminated* when planning the care of a postoperative client who has had a cataract extraction?
- ○ 1. Keep bed in low position at all times.
- ○ 2. Reapply antiembolic stockings b.i.d.
- ○ 3. Urge to cough every 2 hours while awake.
- ○ 4. Assist when ambulating in hall or room.

25 Before Mr. Smoker is discharged, which one of the following is *essential* for the nurse to teach him to ensure the success of his surgery?
- ○ 1. He can resume a normal diet.
- ○ 2. He should avoid bending over.
- ○ 3. His eye may feel scratchy.
- ○ 4. He may wear dark glasses.

NURSING CARE OF CLIENTS WITH GLAUCOMA

The nurse is assigned to care for Ms. Lake, a client with chronic glaucoma.

26 One of the chief characteristics of glaucoma that Ms. Lake and clients like her are *likely* to report is
- ○ 1. itching and burning eyes.
- ○ 2. headaches while reading.

○ 3. seeing halos around lights.
○ 4. loss of central vision.

27 The nurse prepares to assist the physician while he examines Ms. Lake. Which one of the following instruments would be *most* important to have ready?
○ 1. Ophthalmoscope
○ 2. Tonometer
○ 3. Tuning fork
○ 4. Speculum

28 Which one of the following is the patient with untreated glaucoma *likely* to experience as a result of his disease?
○ 1. Tunnel vision
○ 2. Double vision
○ 3. Bulging eyes
○ 4. Bloodshot eyes

29 Ms. Lake is to administer timolol maleate (Timoptic) 1 gtt in each eye daily. Which of the following comments indicates to the nurse that Ms. Lake needs more teaching?
○ 1. "I must wash my hands before instilling the drops."
○ 2. "This drug decreases the formation of fluid in my eye."
○ 3. "I'll need to take this until my eye pressure is normal."
○ 4. "The cap on the container should be replaced immediately."

30 It would be essential for the nurse to withhold the administration and notify the physician if which one of the following drugs were ordered for a client with glaucoma?
○ 1. Atropine sulfate
○ 2. Morphine sulfate
○ 3. Magnesium sulfate
○ 4. Ferrous sulfate

31 Drug therapy is no longer effective in controlling the pressure in Mr. Smoker's left eye. The physician performs an iridectomy. When the nurse assesses Mr. Smoker's operative eye following surgery, which one of the following should be observed?
○ 1. The pupil will appear cloudy and gray.
○ 2. The pupil will be a fixed size and shape.
○ 3. The colored area of the iris will be gone.
○ 4. A section of the iris will appear black.

NURSING CARE OF CLIENTS WITH A DETACHED RETINA

32 When the nurse takes the client's health history, which one of the following is *most* likely to be a cause for a retinal detachment?
○ 1. The client is younger than 40 years old.
○ 2. The client fell within the last day.
○ 3. The client has a history of hypertension.
○ 4. The client is recovering from pneumonia.

33 The physician orders that the nurse patch both of the client's eyes. The patches should be applied so
○ 1. the eyelids are partially open.
○ 2. that tight pressure is exerted.
○ 3. the eyelids cannot be opened.
○ 4. that the client can still see.

34 The nurse brings the client fresh water. To maintain the client's dignity, the *most* important nursing action before leaving would be to
○ 1. straighten the client's linen.
○ 2. tell the client you are going.
○ 3. offer to give the client a back rub.
○ 4. share some current events with her.

35 The client is on strict bed rest with the head of her bed slightly elevated. One day she says, "I'm not having any pain, and I'm not dying. Why can't I just get up once to go to the bathroom?" The *best* response from the nurse would be
○ 1. "Gravity may help to reattach the separated retina."
○ 2. "You don't want to be permanently blind, do you?"
○ 3. "I can get you a sedative if it's hard to lay still."
○ 4. "It sounds like you're getting tired of being here."

36 The client undergoes a scleral buckling procedure. Postoperatively the client experiences all of the following problems. Which one has the *highest* priority for the nurse's attention at this time?
○ 1. Pain
○ 2. Vomiting
○ 3. Anxiety
○ 4. Boredom

NURSING CARE OF CLIENTS UNDERGOING ASSESSMENT OF THE EARS AND AUDITORY SYSTEM

A nurse has been asked to help with the admission of several clients on a busy medical-surgical unit. The items that follow relate to the assessment of these people.

37 The nurse inspects Mr. Ziker's ears. She notes the presence of crystalline deposits within the auricle known as *tophi*. The nurse can expect that this client is *likely* to also have a history of
○ 1. lymphadenitis.
○ 2. pancreatitis.
○ 3. gouty arthritis.
○ 4. bacterial endocarditis.

38 The client asks that questions be repeated during the nursing admission interview. If the client worked at all of the following occupations, which one is *most likely* to have contributed to his hearing loss?

○ 1. Telephone operator
○ 2. Computer programmer
○ 3. Musician
○ 4. Accountant

39 The client is embarrassed when the nurse inspects his ear canal. He says, "Please bring me something so I can clean my ears." The *best* response would be
○ 1. "It is best to use the corner of a soapy wash cloth."
○ 2. "Do you prefer a short or long cotton applicator?"
○ 3. "Have you ever tried removing ear wax with a hairpin?"
○ 4. "I can refer you to a doctor who will clean them."

40 Which one of the following instruments would the nurse use to test the hearing of a client?
○ 1. Otoscope
○ 2. Tuning fork
○ 3. Reflex hammer
○ 4. Stethoscope

41 A client complains of ringing in his ears. Which one of the following questions would be important to ask at this time?
○ 1. "What childhood diseases have you had?"
○ 2. "Were you born prematurely?"
○ 3. "Do you eat a well-balanced diet?"
○ 4. "How much aspirin do you take?"

42 A client who is being admitted wears a hearing aid. The client is frustrated by the loud, shrill noise called feedback that he hears occasionally. Which of the following nursing actions will *most likely* reduce or eliminate the problem with feedback?
○ 1. Repositioning the hearing aid within the ear
○ 2. Cleaning the hearing aid with a soft cloth
○ 3. Replacing the battery in the hearing aid
○ 4. Turning the volume in the hearing aid down

43 A client states he has experienced diminished hearing lately. He takes all of the following drugs. Which one could be affecting the client's hearing?
○ 1. Acetaminophen (Tylenol)
○ 2. Propranolol (Inderal)
○ 3. Gentamicin (Garamycin)
○ 4. Cimetidine (Tagamet)

NURSING CARE OF CLIENTS WITH DISORDERS OF THE EXTERNAL EAR

44 The nurse is about to instill a prescribed medication for softening cerumen in the ear of an adult. Which one of the following is the *correct* technique for straightening the ear canal of this client?
○ 1. Pull the ear upward and backward.
○ 2. Pull the ear downward and forward.
○ 3. Pull the ear upward and forward.
○ 4. Pull the ear downward and backward.

45 After instilling the ear drops, which of the following should the nurse tell the client?
○ 1. Remain in position for at least 5 minutes.
○ 2. Pack a cotton pledget tightly in the ear.
○ 3. Don't blow your nose for at least 1 hour.
○ 4. Avoid drinking very warm or cold beverages.

46 A client is being seen at his physician's office. His ear canal is red, swollen, and tender. The tympanic membrane is intact. Which other finding during the nursing assessment indicates that his symptoms probably are due to an infection in the external ear?
○ 1. There is foul smelling drainage present.
○ 2. His hearing is diminished in that ear.
○ 3. He hurt his head in a fall from a bicycle.
○ 4. The nurse notes the presence of dandruff.

NURSING CARE OF CLIENTS WITH OTITIS MEDIA

47 A client asks the nurse why adults do not experience middle ear infections as frequently as children. The nurse would be most correct in explaining that, in a child, organisms travel more easily from the nasopharynx to the middle ear because the eustachian tube is
○ 1. shorter and straighter.
○ 2. longer and straighter.
○ 3. shorter and more curved.
○ 4. longer and more curved.

48 Which one of the following instructions would be best to prevent acquiring a middle ear infection?
○ 1. When chewing food, keep your mouth closed.
○ 2. When blowing the nose, keep your mouth open.
○ 3. When sneezing, cover your mouth.
○ 4. When coughing, turn your head.

49 Which one of the following is the best evidence that the antibiotic prescribed for acute otitis media is having a therapeutic effect?
○ 1. The ear feels less warm to the touch.
○ 2. Ringing sounds within the ear stops.
○ 3. Ear drainage is watery.
○ 4. Ear discomfort is relieved.

50 If a client with a middle ear infection described all of the following, which one is *most* indicative that the infection has spread to the inner ear? The client indicates that he is experiencing
○ 1. headaches.
○ 2. sore throat.
○ 3. nasal congestion.
○ 4. dizziness.

The physician intends to perform a myringotomy in which the eardrum will be incised.

51 When planning the preparation of the client for a myringotomy, the *best* explanation from the nurse as to its purpose is that this procedure will
○ 1. prevent permanent hearing loss.
○ 2. provide a pathway for drainage.
○ 3. aid in administering medications.
○ 4. maintain motion of the ear bones.

52 Following the myringotomy, it would be *best* for the nurse to instruct the client that the cotton pledget in his ear canal should be
○ 1. left in place until it is saturated.
○ 2. loosely placed within the ear canal.
○ 3. soaked in peroxide before insertion.
○ 4. removed when the cotton becomes dry.

NURSING CARE OF CLIENTS WITH OTOSCLEROSIS

Ms. Anne Jordan is being seen in the doctor's office for diminished hearing due to otosclerosis.

53 As the nurse acquires the client's health history, which one of the following is *common* among people with otosclerosis?
○ 1. The onset of their hearing loss started in childhood.
○ 2. They have high fevers with upper respiratory infections.
○ 3. They have had their tonsils and adenoids removed.
○ 4. One or more relatives have been similarly diagnosed.

54 Ms. Jordan asks the nurse to explain what the doctor meant by saying that she had a conductive hearing loss. The nurse would be *most* correct in explaining that this type of hearing loss results when
○ 1. sound waves do not travel to the inner ear.
○ 2. the structures in the inner ear malfunction.
○ 3. the eighth cranial nerve is permanently damaged.
○ 4. electric conversion of sound is not produced

55 The team leader prepares the initial nursing care plan on Ms. Jordan. She makes a nursing diagnosis of *High Risk for Impaired Verbal Communication related to hearing loss.* She asks the admitting nurse to assist with identifying an appropriate goal for this problem. The best goal would be that
○ 1. Ms. Jordan states that she is able to understand staff communication.
○ 2. the staff will improve communication techniques.
○ 3. Ms. Jordan demonstrates an ability to express herself to staff.
○ 4. Ms. Jordan will be able to communicate basic needs.

56 The nurse helps the team leader plan measures to promote effective communication with Ms. Jordan.

Which one of the following nursing measures is *essential* to the care of this client?
○ 1. Speak directly into the client's ear.
○ 2. Face the client when speaking to her.
○ 3. Drop voice at the end of each sentence.
○ 4. Raise pitch of voice one octave higher.

57 Ms. Jordan is scheduled for a stapedectomy. She does not seem to be able to understand the technical words and information the doctor provided about the surgery. The *best* alternative method for helping her comprehend the details of the procedure would be to
○ 1. provide her with a printed pamphlet on the topic.
○ 2. ask another stapedectomy client to talk with her.
○ 3. refer the communication to someone who can sign.
○ 4. write all of the information out in long hand.

58 Ms. Jordan says to the nurse, "There are so many awful complications that can happen with this surgery." The *best* response from the nurse would be
○ 1. "You've got the best surgeon on the staff."
○ 2. "Tell me more about how you're feeling."
○ 3. "Don't worry; those things hardly ever happen."
○ 4. "Let's think about something more pleasant."

59 During the stapedectomy Ms. Jordan was thrilled that her hearing was suddenly restored. However, postoperatively her hearing is less acute. Which one of the following would be most accurate as an explanation to reassure Ms. Jordan? The full extent of hearing may not be evident until
○ 1. edema and packing in the operative area are gone.
○ 2. several years following the operative procedure.
○ 3. she is fitted with a molded plastic hearing aid.
○ 4. the prosthesis becomes stabilized with new bone.

60 The nurse tells the staff person assigned to Ms. Jordan that she is at high risk for injury postoperatively owing to
○ 1. fatigue.
○ 2. diplopia.
○ 3. vertigo.
○ 4. pain.

61 Postoperatively, the nurse assesses Ms. Jordan for possible facial nerve paralysis. The *best* technique for assessing this nerve's function is to
○ 1. ask her to say, "ah."
○ 2. identify a familiar odor.
○ 3. touch the cornea with cotton.
○ 4. ask the client to smile.

62 For the first 24 hours, which body position must be specified on the nursing care plan of a client with a stapedectomy?
○ 1. Flat with the operative ear uppermost
○ 2. Trendelenburg with the knees gatched
○ 3. Supine with the head of the bed elevated
○ 4. Prone with the head on the operated side

63 The nurse gives instructions to the nursing assistant who will be caring for Ms. Jordan. Which one of the following is *not* contraindicated following a stapedectomy?
○ 1. Blowing the nose
○ 2. Sneezing
○ 3. Straining to have a stool
○ 4. Chewing food

64 The nurse provides Ms. Jordan with discharge instructions. Which one of the following indicates that she understands what activity is contraindicated for the next 6 months? Ms. Jordan says she should avoid
○ 1. listening to music.
○ 2. flying in an airplane.
○ 3. driving an automobile.
○ 4. reading for long periods.

NURSING CARE OF CLIENTS WITH MENIERE'S DISEASE

65 Mr. Forrest has been admitted to the hospital for possible Meniere's disease. The subjective symptom this client is *most likely* to describe is
○ 1. burning.
○ 2. pressure.
○ 3. vertigo.
○ 4. pain.

66 Mr. Forrest will undergo a caloric test. The teaching plan for preparing the client for this diagnostic test should include the explanation that
○ 1. cold and warm water will be instilled within his ears.
○ 2. he will wear earphones through which he will hear sounds.
○ 3. electrodes will be attached to his head in a dark room.
○ 4. blood will be drawn and refrigerated before examination.

67 During the caloric test, if Mr. Forrest has Meniere's disease, the nurse is *most likely* to observe
○ 1. the onset of severe symptoms.
○ 2. no response or change in symptoms.
○ 3. nystagmus and slight dizziness.
○ 4. aphasia and loss of consciousness.

68 The nurse observes that Mr. Forrest seems anxious whenever a member of the nursing staff enters his room. If Mr. Forrest's anxiety is due to fear that nursing care will intensify his symptoms, which one

of the following nursing measures would be *most* appropriate to add to his plan for care?
○ 1. Let the client suggest ways to carry out his care.
○ 2. Discontinue all nursing care measures at this time.
○ 3. Restrict care to just nutrition and elimination needs.
○ 4. Carry out nursing activities quickly and efficiently.

69 The client asks the nurse to clarify his doctor's explanation about the cause of Meniere's disease. The nurse would be most accurate in stating that the cause of the disease is unknown but that the symptoms are related to a(n)
○ 1. electrolyte deficit.
○ 2. excess of fluid.
○ 3. vitamin deficiency.
○ 4. genetic defect.

70 While caring for a client with Meniere's disease, which one of the following nursing actions would help most in preventing nausea and vomiting?
○ 1. Increase oral fluids.
○ 2. Change positions often.
○ 3. Keep room lights dim.
○ 4. Avoid jarring the bed.

71 The client with Meniere's disease responds to conservative treatment at this time. He is talking about being discharged. Which one of the following statements indicates that the client needs additional information? The client says
○ 1. "I should stop salting my food so much."
○ 2. "Future attacks may last minutes or days."
○ 3. "My hearing will gradually improve."
○ 4. "Meniere's disease is not curable."

NURSING CARE OF CLIENTS WITH A NOSEBLEED

Mr. Clark, age 53, comes to the emergency department with a nosebleed.

72 While assessing Mr. Clark, the nurse obtains all of the following data. Which may be a *causative* factor in his nosebleed?
○ 1. His pulse rate is 110 beats per minute.
○ 2. His blood pressure is 200/104 lying down.
○ 3. His temperature is 97.6°F (36.7°C) orally.
○ 4. His respirations are 24 per minute.

73 Mr. Clark is frightened by seeing the amount of blood that has collected on his shirt. Which one of the following actions would be *most* helpful to Mr. Clark at this time?
○ 1. Lay Mr. Clark down so he won't see his clothes.
○ 2. Give Mr. Clark a popular magazine to read.
○ 3. Replace his clothing with a hospital gown.
○ 4. Cover Mr. Clark's eyes with a bath towel.

74 Which of the following would be *most* helpful in controlling the nosebleed? Have Mr. Clark
    ○ 1. lie down and swallow frequently.
    ○ 2. lie down and breathe through his mouth.
    ○ 3. sit forward and apply direct pressure.
    ○ 4. sit forward and clench his teeth.

75 The bleeding area is chemically cauterized with silver nitrate. Before Mr. Clark leaves the emergency department it is *essential* that the nurse tell the patient to
    ○ 1. limit his dietary intake to just fluids.
    ○ 2. sleep in a recliner or with his head up.
    ○ 3. take his carotid pulse at hourly intervals.
    ○ 4. avoid blowing his nose for several hours.

NURSING CARE OF CLIENTS WITH SINUSITIS

76 Susan Aster has had a prolonged upper respiratory infection. She is seeing the doctor today because she continues to have a low-grade fever, poor appetite, and malaise. If Susan has sinusitis in the maxillary sinuses, it is *likely* she will tell the nurse that she feels pain
    ○ 1. over her eyes.
    ○ 2. near her eyebrows.
    ○ 3. in her cheeks.
    ○ 4. above her ears.

77 The physician recommends that Susan purchase an over-the-counter nasal spray. Before leaving the office, the nurse stresses that Susan follow the directions exactly as they are stated on the container. This information is essential because overuse of nasal decongestants will
    ○ 1. lead to physical addiction in a very short time.
    ○ 2. offer shorter and shorter periods of symptomatic relief.
    ○ 3. thin the mucous membranes, causing them to bleed.
    ○ 4. lower a person's resistance to various pathogens.

78 The nurse should instruct a client that the *best* position for instilling nose drops is to
    ○ 1. bend the head forward.
    ○ 2. push the nose laterally.
    ○ 3. tilt the head backward.
    ○ 4. open the mouth wide.

79 A nurse observes a colleague administering nasal medications. If the medication nurse performs all of these actions, which one indicates *inappropriate* care? The nurse
    ○ 1. reads the drug label three times.
    ○ 2. asks a client to state his name.
    ○ 3. uses another client's container.
    ○ 4. washes her hands at the bedside.

NURSING CARE OF CLIENTS WITH NASAL SURGERY

Ms. Janet Smallcombe is having a rhinoplasty procedure to improve the appearance of her nose cosmetically.

80 Gauze has been packed within Ms. Smallcombe's nose postoperatively. Which one of the following techniques is *best* for detecting postoperative hemorrhage?
    ○ 1. Observing the gauze for bleeding
    ○ 2. Inspecting the back of the throat
    ○ 3. Removing and replacing the packing
    ○ 4. Looking for bleeding from the nostrils

81 The nurse collects all of the following data. Which one indicates that the client who has had nasal surgery should receive frequent oral care?
    ○ 1. The client says her throat is sore.
    ○ 2. The client's dressing is bloody.
    ○ 3. The client is slightly nauseated.
    ○ 4. The client is mouth breathing.

82 Ms. Smallcombe asks the nurse postoperatively what she looks like. The *best* response from the nurse would be,
    ○ 1. "I'm sure you will look absolutely gorgeous."
    ○ 2. "I didn't think you were unattractive before."
    ○ 3. "Your face is swollen with bruises around the eyes."
    ○ 4. "Your personality is more important than your looks."

INDIVIDUAL TEST ITEMS

83 A client at a clinic tells the nurse that she has an old-fashioned steam vaporizer at home. She plans to use it to help relieve her child's nasal congestion. It is best to discourage the client from using this equipment because its use can cause
    ○ 1. a fire if the water reservoir runs dry.
    ○ 2. excess moisture saturation in the room.
    ○ 3. burns from contact with heated water vapor.
    ○ 4. rapid growth of environmental pathogens.

84 The nurse assesses a newly admitted client. Which one of the following findings suggests that the client may have had a fractured nose at some earlier time?
    ○ 1. Multiple polyps are noted on the nasal mucous membranes.
    ○ 2. The client's nose is red, unusually large, and bulbous.
    ○ 3. The septum deviates to the side, narrowing one naris.
    ○ 4. Serous drainage is noted within the nares and pharynx.

NURSING CARE OF CLIENTS WITH PHARYNGITIS

85 The physician orders a throat culture on a client with pharyngitis. Which one of the following describes the best technique for carrying out this procedure? The nurse

○ 1. asks the client to expectorate sputum in a jar.
○ 2. wipes the inner mouth and tongue with gauze.
○ 3. swabs the throat with a sterile cotton applicator.
○ 4. collects saliva in a sterile culture tube.

86 A physician prescribes penicillin for a client whose throat culture indicated that beta hemolytic *Streptococcus* was present in the specimen. The nurse stresses that the client take all of the medication prescribed because if the infection is untreated or undertreated, it may be followed by

○ 1. glomerulonephritis.
○ 2. chickenpox.
○ 3. shingles.
○ 4. whooping cough.

NURSING CARE OF CLIENTS WITH LARYNGITIS

87 A campaigning politician's wife calls his doctor's office and asks what she might do to treat her husband's onset of laryngitis. The nurse would be acting appropriately by telling her that until the client is examined, it would be best to

○ 1. take a multivitamin.
○ 2. rest the voice.
○ 3. maintain bedrest.
○ 4. massage the throat.

88 The client's hoarseness is still present after 2 weeks of symptomatic treatment. The physician schedules the client for a direct laryngoscopy. Which one of the following statements indicates to the nurse that the client understands the reason the test was ordered? "This test is done because chronic or prolonged hoarseness is associated with

○ 1. emphysema."
○ 2. bronchitis."
○ 3. laryngeal cancer."
○ 4. enlarged adenoids."

89 Following a direct laryngoscopy, which of the following assessments is *most* important for the nurse to monitor?

○ 1. Respiratory effort
○ 2. Color of the skin
○ 3. Urinary output
○ 4. Body temperature

90 Which one of the following assessment techniques should the nurse perform before allowing a client food or fluids following a direct laryngoscopy?

○ 1. Touch the arch of the palate with a tongue blade.
○ 2. Listen to the abdomen for active bowel sounds.
○ 3. Inspect the oral mucous membranes for moisture.
○ 4. Palpate the throat while the client swallows.

NURSING CARE OF CLIENTS WITH CANCER OF THE LARYNX

91 A client is undergoing a total laryngectomy. The team gathers to develop a nursing care plan. Which one of the following nursing actions is the *most* appropriate plan for dealing with the client's impaired verbal communication?

○ 1. Lip-read client's attempts at communication.
○ 2. Inform client to speak slowly when talking.
○ 3. Listen attentively to the client's vocalizations.
○ 4. Provide the client with paper and pencil.

92 The nurse prepares to suction the laryngectomy client's tracheostomy tube. To avoid hypoxemia, the *maximum* amount of time the nurse should apply suction is no more than

○ 1. 5 seconds.
○ 2. 15 seconds.
○ 3. 20 seconds.
○ 4. 30 seconds.

93 The nursing team discusses a client's angry and depressed reaction to his diagnosis of cancer, the change in his body image, and the loss of speech following a laryngectomy. Which one of the following *best* indicates that the client is now beginning to resolve his grief? The client

○ 1. requests only his wife be allowed to visit.
○ 2. says his doctor made an incorrect diagnosis.
○ 3. looks at the tracheostomy tube in a mirror.
○ 4. asks the nurse to help him bathe and shave.

NURSING CARE OF CLIENTS HAVING A TONSILLECTOMY

94 The nurse is assigned to care for a client immediately following a tonsillectomy. Besides monitoring the vital signs, the nurse should look for which one of the following clues that indicates postoperative bleeding?

○ 1. Frequent swallowing
○ 2. Periodic belching
○ 3. Occasional coughing
○ 4. Grinding of teeth

95 Until the tonsillectomy client regains consciousness, the best body position to maintain is

○ 1. dorsal recumbent.
○ 2. side-lying.
○ 3. high Fowler's.
○ 4. horizontal recumbent.

NURSING CARE OF CLIENTS WITH AN OCCLUDED AIRWAY

96 A frantic businessman calls his physician's office because a client has choked on a piece of hard candy. What information in the following list would the nurse need to know *first* before recommending further action?
○ 1. Is the person able to walk?
○ 2. Is the person able to cough?
○ 3. In what position is the person?
○ 4. Can the person still swallow?

97 During a school banquet a piece of meat becomes lodged in a person's airway. He cannot talk. He uses the universal sign to indicate that he cannot breathe. A guest who is a nurse prepares to perform the Heimlich maneuver. The most accurate placement for the hands is to place the thumb-side of the fist
○ 1. on the manubrium.
○ 2. on the xiphoid process.
○ 3. below the navel.
○ 4. below the sternum.

Correct Answers and Rationale

Two numbers appear in parentheses following each rationale. The first number identifies the textbook listed in the references, page 451, and the second number identifies the page(s) in that textbook on which the correct answer can be verified. Occasionally, two textbooks are given for verifying the correct answer.

The Nursing Care of Clients with Disorders of the Eye, Ear, Nose, and Throat

NURSING CARE OF CLIENTS WITH EYE INJURIES

1 3. A chemical splash to the eye should be treated immediately. The longer the chemical is in contact with the eye, the greater the potential damage. Although the names of the chemicals would be important, time should not be lost in determining an agent that will neutralize them. Safety glasses should be required when working with chemicals. However, the priority is still treating the chemical splash if that has not already been done. It is too soon to evaluate the extent of sensory damage. (16:492; 14:969)
Nursing Process—Collecting data
Client Need—Physiological integrity

2 1. Any type of available water can be used in an emergency to flush the eye and dilute the chemical. Tap water from a faucet or shower is generally available. The other chemical solutions may be appropriate depending on the specific chemical that caused the trauma, but they may need to be diluted to a specific strength to prevent additional damage to the eye. (7:690; 16:492)
Nursing Process—Planning
Client Need—Physiological integrity

3 2. The irrigating solution should flow from the inner canthus toward the outer canthus. This is an especially important principle to follow so that substances in one eye do not come in contact with tissue of the other eye. It would be best to instill the force of the water on the conjunctiva rather than onto the sensitive cornea, causing discomfort or reflex blinking. The anterior chamber is not an external eye structure. The nasolacrimal duct lies in the area of the inner canthus. (16:492; 18:478)
Nursing Process—Implementation
Client Need—Physiological integrity

4 2. An ophthalmologist is a physician who is trained to diagnose and treat eye diseases and traumatic injuries. An optician fills prescriptions for corrective lenses. An optometrist tests vision and prescribes glasses or contact lenses to correct visual acuity. A podiatrist is trained in the care of feet. (16:487; 14:958)
Nursing Process—Implementation
Client Need—Safe, effective care environment

NURSING CARE OF CLIENTS WITH VISUAL ACUITY PROBLEMS

5 4. The term for nearsightedness is myopia. Presbyopia is a type of farsightedness associated with aging. It is caused by loss of elasticity in the lenses. Amblyopia is commonly referred to as "lazy eye." Untreated amblyopia results in the loss of vision in one eye due to lack of use. Hyperopia is farsightedness. (16:487; 14:959)
Nursing Process—Implementation
Client Need—Health promotion/maintenance

6 3. Lions International is an organization that has vision and hearing improvement as its major goal. Local or state chapters can provide information and assistance to those who need glasses, a guide dog, hearing aid, or surgery but cannot afford it. The other organizations are both fraternal and philanthropic, but they have not named vision or hearing assistance as their project. (14:962)
Nursing Process—Implementation
Client Need—Health promotion/maintenance

7 1. Astigmatism is caused by an irregularly shaped cornea or lens. Objects may appear blurred and wider or taller than they actually are. People with hyperopia cannot see near objects clearly. People with myopia cannot see far objects clearly. No visual acuity disorder will cause objects to appear unusually small. (14:959; 16:487)
Nursing Process—Collecting data
Client Need—Safe, effective care environment

8 2. A Snellen chart is used to test far vision. The client stands 20 ft from the chart and is asked to read letters that progressively become smaller. A Jaeger chart, with samples of small-sized print, is used to test near vision. Ishihara plates are used to test color vision. A tangent screen is used to assess the peripheral visual field. This test requires that the client indicate when he sees a stimulus in his peripheral vision. (14:958-959; 6:297-298)

Nursing Process—Planning
Client Need—Safe, effective care environment

9 1. Normal vision is 20/20. This means that a person sees at 20 ft what other people normally see at 20 ft. The larger the denominator in the fraction, the less acute the vision. Thus, a person who has 20/200 vision sees at 20 ft what people normally would see at 200 feet. (16:483-484; 14:958)

Nursing Process—Implementation
Client Need—Health promotion/maintenance

10 2. Glasses should be washed first before wiping to avoid scratching the surface with dirt and dust. Paper products should not be used for drying because they are made from wood pulp, which could scratch the lenses, especially if they are made of plastic. Air drying would be tedious and likely to leave the glasses streaked. (18:106)

Nursing Process—Planning
Client Need—Health promotion/maintenance

11 4. Contact lenses remain in position owing to the surface tension created by moisture between them and the cornea of the eye. Techniques for removing a lens involve breaking the seal by allowing air beneath the edge of the lens. A suction cup should not be used to remove soft contact lenses. Sliding the lens under an eyelid only changes its location. The fingernails should never be used because they may damage the cornea. Pressing the center of the lens will not break the adhesion. (18:109; 7:675)

Nursing Process—Implementation
Client Need—Physiological integrity

12 2. Saliva contains organisms that can be transferred to the eye, resulting in an infection and possibly permanent eye damage. Hard lenses should not be worn while sleeping. Storing the lenses in solution prevents scratching from contact with the surface of a dry container. The palm of a washed hand provides a convenient area for cleaning. (18:111; 14:961)

Nursing Process—Evaluation
Client Need—Health promotion/maintenance

NURSING CARE OF CLIENTS WITH IMPAIRED VISION

13 2. Anxiety occurs because a person feels threatened by an unexpected or unfamiliar situation. Having care explained before it is performed prepares a person for what is about to take place. A sightless client should always be spoken to before being touched. Shutting the door would increase a client's feeling of isolation and fear that

he will not receive help if needed. Having adequate light would help the partially sighted but not someone who cannot see. (18:29-30; 7:672)

Nursing Process—Planning
Client Need—Psychosocial integrity

14 1. A blind person feels safer and more secure by following the lead of someone who is sighted. This is best accomplished by having the blind person stand slightly behind and to the side while taking the sighted person's arm. Safety is a higher priority in an unfamiliar environment than total independence. (7:672; 14:965)

Nursing Process—Evaluation
Client Need—Safe, effective care environment

15 1. Using the imagery of a clock can help the sightless person locate food and feed himself. Feeding a client would not promote self-reliance. Ordering liquid forms of nourishment without collaborating first with the client may imply that he is not capable of eating like an adult and may lower his self-esteem. Beverages in paper cups are more likely to spill during the client's attempts at eating independently, which may reinforce his feelings of inadequacy. (18:156; 14:965)

Nursing Process—Planning
Client Need—Psychosocial integrity

16 4. The best way to remove an artificial eye is to depress the lower eyelid. The prosthesis should then drop from the socket into the nurse's hand. Lifting or everting the upper eyelids and separating the two eyelids are not recommended techniques for removing an artificial eye. (18:107; 3:840)

Nursing Process—Implementation
Client Need—Physiological integrity

NURSING CARE OF CLIENTS WITH CATARACTS

17 1. As senile cataracts form, they cause progressively diminished vision. The visual change is due to degeneration of the lenses of the eye due to aging. Fullness and ocular pain or discomfort are more likely due to trauma or an inflammatory process. Seeing flashes of light is a symptom described by someone with a detached retina. (16:499; 7:684)

Nursing Process—Collecting data
Client Need—Safe, effective care environment

18 3. A cataract results in an opacity of the lens. The lens lies behind the iris. The center of the iris is the pupil. When the eye is examined, the usual black pupil now appears white, gray, or yellow. Ruptured blood vessels on the eye are associated with conditions in which the blood pressure has been suddenly elevated, such as when perform-

ing Valsalva's maneuver while vomiting or defecating. An irregularly shaped iris can be the result of surgery performed for the treatment of glaucoma. A pterygium may appear as a growth on the cornea. (16:498; 3:831)
Nursing Process—Collecting data
Client Need—Physiological integrity

19 1. The time for cataract removal is usually left to the client. It largely depends on the person and when the impaired vision interferes with the quality of his life. Cataracts are painless. The opinions of others should not influence the timing of surgery. Postponing surgery until a cataract "ripens" is no longer considered a standard for care. (14:972; 7:684-685)
Nursing Process—Evaluation
Client Need—Safe, effective care environment

20 2. The client with cataracts has poor vision. Familiarizing him with his surroundings is essential in preventing accidental injuries. Informing his family where to wait and checking his height and weight are important but are not the highest priority at this time. Because a person with cataracts cannot see very well, he is not likely to be interested in watching television. (7:685; 3:827)
Nursing Process—Planning
Client Need—Safe, effective care environment

21 2. The nurse should clarify any aspect of the drug order that may seem inaccurate. The physician wrote the abbreviation for left eye, but the cataract from the right eye is scheduled to be removed. Therefore, the order should be questioned. The client or the nurse can scrub the skin. It is not essential that the client do this himself. Usually, the nurse preparing the client for surgery would be responsible for clipping the eyelashes on the operative eye. (18:575)
Nursing Process—Implementation
Client Need—Safe, effective care environment

22 4. Eye drops and ointments should be placed in the exposed lower conjunctival sac. If they are placed on the cornea, they may cause discomfort and reflex blinking. Medication may be systemically absorbed when instilled at the inner canthus. Placing eye drops and ointments at the outer canthus makes it difficult to distribute them in the eye. (18:588; 14:965)
Nursing Process—Implementation
Client Need—Safe, effective care environment

23 1. It is not normal to have severe pain following cataract surgery. Severe pain is an indication that intraocular hemorrhage may be occurring. It is essential to report these data to the nurse in charge who may then contact the client's surgeon. Giving an analgesic can mask the symptom

and thereby decrease the perception of its significance. Assessing pupils will not reveal the cause of the symptom. The pupils will most likely be dilated and not respond to light. Postoperatively, cataract clients usually are not allowed to lie on their operative side. (14:972; 16:502)
Nursing Process—Implementation
Client Need—Physiological integrity

24 3. Coughing, straining, or squeezing the eyelids together can increase intraocular pressure. These activities should be avoided to prevent strain on the delicate sutures or dislodging an intraocular lens implant. The client should deep-breathe to prevent postoperative respiratory complications. All the other orders are appropriate for this patient. (14:972; 3:832)
Nursing Process—Planning
Client Need—Physiological integrity

25 2. Stooping, bending over, and heavy lifting can increase intraocular pressure. These types of activities should be avoided for at least 4 to 6 weeks postoperatively. The client can eat similarly to his preoperative routine without any harmful effects. His eye may feel scratchy from the eye sutures, but this is not an indication of a postoperative complication. Postoperatively, most clients experience discomfort in bright light. Wearing dark glasses can reduce this temporary sensitivity. (16:503; 7:685-686)
Nursing Process—Implementation
Client Need—Safe, effective care environment

NURSING CARE OF CLIENTS WITH GLAUCOMA

26 3. People with both chronic and acute glaucoma generally describe the appearance of rainbow halos or rings, particularly around lights. Itching and burning are likely due to an allergic response. Headaches may occur when a client who is in need of corrective lenses strains to read. The loss of central vision is a symptom of macular degeneration. (16:496-497; 7:682)
Nursing Process—Collecting data
Client Need—Safe, effective care environment

27 2. The symptoms of glaucoma occur as a result of increased intraocular pressure. This condition is diagnosed using an instrument called a tonometer. An ophthalmoscope is an instrument used for viewing the fundus or back portion of the eye. A tuning fork is used to assess hearing and vibratory sense. A speculum is an instrument that widens a cavity. (14:960; 3:835)
Nursing Process—Implementation
Client Need—Safe, effective care environment

28 1. The person with glaucoma experiences a loss of peripheral vision. If left untreated, the client may eventually be able to see only what is focused directly on the macula. Patients describe this as looking through a tube or tunnel. Double vision can be due to neurologic diseases or a weakness in eye muscles. Bulging eyes, also called exophthalmos, can accompany hyperthyroidism. Inflamed eyes can be due to various irritating substances. (16:497; 7:682)
Nursing Process—Collecting data
Client Need—Physiological integrity

29 3. Glaucoma is a chronic disease and will require daily administration of medication until the client is treated surgically. Handwashing and replacing the cap are aseptic measures to prevent the transmission of organisms within the eye. Timolol maleate is a beta adrenergic blocking agent that decreases aqueous humor formation without constricting the pupil. (14:971)
Nursing Process—Evaluation
Client Need—Safe, effective care environment

30 1. Atropine sulfate and other anticholinergic drugs dilate the pupil. This blocks the drainage of aqueous humor. It could cause an acute attack due to extremely high intraocular pressure. If untreated, the client may become permanently blind. Morphine sulfate is a narcotic analgesic. Magnesium sulfate is known as epsom salts. Ferrous sulfate is an iron preparation. None of these last three substances is contraindicated for clients with glaucoma. (16:498; 14:971)
Nursing Process—Implementation
Client Need—Physiological integrity

31 4. An iridectomy involves removing a piece of the iris to allow aqueous humor to flow from the posterior chamber into the anterior chamber and out Schlemm's canal. The iris will no longer appear perfectly round. The section that was removed will appear black. (16:496; 3:835)
Nursing Process—Collecting data
Client Need—Physiological integrity

NURSING CARE OF CLIENTS WITH A DETACHED RETINA

32 2. Retinal detachment can have multiple etiologies. The more common etiologies include trauma, such as a blow to the head, myopia, and degenerative changes. Aging is a factor. The most common period for retinal detachment is between the ages of 50 and 60 years. There is no relationship between infection and hypertension as a cause for a detached retina. (14:972: 16:500)
Nursing Process—Collecting data
Client Need—Safe, effective care environment

33 3. Keeping the eyelids closed protects them from contact with dust or fibers. It also prevents the eye from becoming dry because blinking would be prohibited. Pressure should be applied only if it was specifically ordered. The intent is to keep the eyes at rest. Being able to see would contradict this purpose. (14:964)
Nursing Process—Implementation
Client Need—Physiological integrity

34 2. Because the client whose eyes are patched has no visual cue as to whether the nurse is still in the room, it is important to indicate when he is being left alone. It can be frustrating and embarrassing to carry on a conversation when no one is there to respond. (3:826; 18:29)
Nursing Process—Implementation
Client Need—Psychosocial integrity

35 1. Most people are willing to comply with the prescribed therapy if they understand its purpose. Bed rest and bilateral patching are frequently the initial conservative treatments for a detached retina before surgical alternatives are considered. Asking the client if he wants to be permanently blind may heighten his anxiety. Sedatives often are prescribed. However, in this case the situation does not warrant the added risks from sedation. Responding in a superficial manner, as in the last example, treats the client's question as frivolous. (14:972)
Nursing Process—Implementation
Client Need—Psychosocial integrity

36 2. Vomiting raises intraocular pressure and should be treated immediately. If an antiemetic is not ordered, the nurse should notify the charge nurse or the physician. Pain can be expected following surgery for a detached retina. Although pain causes discomfort, its treatment, or lack thereof, will not affect the outcome of the surgical procedure. Anxiety and boredom are not physiologic problems and therefore do not rank as high on the list of priorities. (14:972; 7:690; 16:503)
Nursing Process—Evaluation
Client Need—Safe, effective care environment

NURSING CARE OF CLIENTS UNDERGOING ASSESSMENT OF THE EARS AND AUDITORY SYSTEM

37 3. Gout is caused by high serum levels of uric acid. The uric acid precipitates and migrates to joints and connective tissue. Tophi are subcutaneous deposits of uric acid crystals that are common among people with gout. Lymphadenitis would cause an enlargement of lymph nodes, but these would feel like soft tissue and be found behind the ear, in the throat, or in the occipital area. Pancreatitis is unrelated to any joint or connective tissue abnormalities. Bacterial endocarditis is a complication of a streptococcal infection. The primary streptococcal infection can cause enlarged painful joints, but the ear would be unaffected. (3:665; 16:803)

    Nursing Process—Collecting data
    Client Need—Physiological integrity

38 3. Musicians can be exposed to excessively high levels of sound, which can contribute to hearing loss. People who listen to amplified music or who work around noisy environments also are susceptible to decreased hearing. There is no significant evidence that the other occupations are associated with impaired hearing. (3:853)

    Nursing Process—Collecting data
    Client Need—Physiological integrity

39 1. The accumulation of normal cerumen is best removed by washing the ears with soapy water and a soft cloth. Hard and sharp objects can injure the ear canal or tympanic membrane. A referral would be appropriate only if the cerumen is excessively hard or impacted within the ear. (3:852; 18:108)

    Nursing Process—Implementation
    Client Need—Health promotion/maintenance

40 2. A tuning fork is used to test for conductive and sensorineural hearing loss. The Weber test is performed by striking the tuning fork and placing it centrally on the forehead. The Rinne test is performed by striking the tuning fork and placing it on the mastoid bone and beside the ear. An otoscope is used to inspect the physical structures in the external ear. A reflex hammer is used to test deep tendon responses. A stethoscope is used to auscultate body sounds. (14:853; 7:692)

    Nursing Process—Collecting data
    Client Need—Safe, effective care environment

41 4. Tinnitus, ringing or buzzing in the ears, can be associated with many ear disorders. It is a common symptom experienced by people who take repeated, high dosages of aspirin. The other questions in this item will not necessarily help to establish a cause-and-effect relationship with the client's symptom. (15:71; 14:974)

    Nursing Process—Collecting data
    Client Need—Physiological integrity

42 1. Feedback, a loud shrill noise, occurs when a hearing aid is not positioned correctly within the ear. Cleaning, replacing the battery, and regulating the volume are important to the care of a client with a hearing aid, but they will not affect feedback. (18:114; 7:694)

    Nursing Process—Implementation
    Client Need—Physiological integrity

43 3. The aminoglycoside family of antibiotics, of which gentamicin is one example, is considered to be ototoxic and nephrotoxic. Propranolol can cause vertigo but does not affect hearing acuity. Neither cimetidine nor acetaminophen is known to be ototoxic. (15:164)

    Nursing Process—Evaluation
    Client Need—Physiological integrity

NURSING CARE OF CLIENTS WITH DISORDERS OF THE EXTERNAL EAR

44 1. The correct technique for straightening the ear canal of an adult is by pulling the ear upward and backward. For a child, the ear is pulled downward and backward. (18:593; 14:977)

    Nursing Process—Implementation
    Client Need—Physiological integrity

45 1. Maintaining a position, such as the head tilted to the side, or a side-lying position will facilitate the movement of the medication to the lowest area of the ear canal. Cotton may be loosely inserted within the ear to collect drainage and any excess volume of medication. The eustachian tube does connect the middle ear with the pharynx. However, if the tympanic membrane is intact, blowing the nose should not displace the medication. The temperature of beverages will not affect the instillation of ear drops. (18:594; 14:976)

    Nursing Process—Implementation
    Client Need—Physiological integrity

46 1. Cerumen should be the only substance found in the ear on inspection. The presence of drainage, called otorrhea, suggests that an inflammatory process is the underlying problem. Because the drainage is foul smelling, the likelihood that the inflammation is due to a pathogen should be suspected. Hearing can be diminished owing to the swelling. Trauma could rupture the eardrum, but injuring the head is most likely unrelated to an infection. Dandruff suggests a dry, flaky dermatitis of the scalp and not something that would contribute to the ear symptoms. (14:979; 3:855)

    Nursing Process—Collecting data
    Client Need—Safe, effective care environment

NURSING CARE OF CLIENTS WITH OTITIS MEDIA

47 1. Organisms travel more easily through a pathway that is short and straight. With growth, the eustachian tube changes to a 45-degree angle. This natural curve provides a barrier against ascending pathogens. (16:508; 19:552)

    Nursing Process—Implementation
    Client Need—Health promotion/maintenance

48 2. To avoid forcing infectious organisms from the nasopharynx into the eustachian tube leading to the middle ear, it would be best when blowing the nose to keep the mouth open. Esthetically, chewing food with the mouth closed shows good table manners. To prevent transmitting infectious organisms to others when sneezing, it is helpful to cover the mouth. The same principle applies to turning the head while coughing. (7:696)

    Nursing Process—Implementation
    Client Need—Health promotion/maintenance

49 4. As the collection of fluid behind the tympanic membrane is decreased, ear discomfort becomes relieved. The inflamed area in the middle ear is beyond the reach of the fingers. Hearing is diminished because sound conduction is impaired. Tinnitus, or disturbing sounds, is not generally a problem for a person during the acute phase of the infection. Watery or purulent drainage is an indication that the eardrum has become perforated. (7:697-689)

    Nursing Process—Evaluation
    Client Need—Physiological integrity

50 4. Signs of labyrinthitis (inflammation of the labyrinth of the inner ear) are characterized by dizziness, nausea, vomiting, and nystagmus. Headaches may indicate the infection has extended to the meningeal area of the brain. Sore throat and nasal congestion are more likely to be caused by the primary upper respiratory infection, which often precedes a middle ear infection. (7:699; 16:509)

    Nursing Process—Collecting data
    Client Need—Physiological integrity

51 2. A myringotomy provides a pathway for drainage, which relieves pain. A surgical incision heals more efficiently than a spontaneous rupture of the eardrum. Although hearing may be diminished, it is less so with an incised tympanic membrane. Systemic drugs rather than topical drugs are more effective in treating a middle ear infection. Incising the eardrum will not generally preserve motion of the ossicles in the middle ear. (7:696; 16:509)

    Nursing Process—Planning
    Client Need—Safe, effective care environment

52 2. Loosely packed cotton is more likely to absorb drainage than tightly packed cotton. The cotton pledget should be replaced on a scheduled basis or as it becomes moist. It would be incorrect to wait until the cotton is totally saturated. The ear canal is generally cleansed before inserting the dry cotton. (7:697; 16:509)

    Nursing Process—Implementation
    Client Need—Health promotion/maintenance

NURSING CARE OF CLIENTS WITH OTOSCLEROSIS

53 4. Although the cause of otosclerosis is unknown, most have a family history of this condition. The onset of this disorder usually becomes apparent when clients are in their 20s or 30s. High fevers are known to cause sensorineural hearing loss due to damage to the acoustic nerve. Otosclerosis is caused by an ankylosing of the bones in the middle ear. Having the tonsils or adenoids removed can reduce the incidence of chronic otitis media, but removal has not been found to influence the development of otosclerosis. (16:510; 14:980)

    Nursing Process—Collecting data
    Client Need—Physiological integrity

54 1. A conductive hearing loss occurs when there is a barrier in the transmission of vibrating sound waves from the external and middle ear to the inner ear. Common causes of conductive hearing loss include otosclerosis, otitis media, and a ruptured tympanic membrane. The other options in this item describe the causes of sensorineural hearing loss. (16:504; 14:973)

    Nursing Process—Implementation
    Client Need—Health promotion/maintenance

55 1. The ability to understand staff is a client-centered goal. Accomplishing this goal indicates that the approaches used by staff to communicate with the hearing-impaired client are effective. The goal should not indicate what the nursing team hopes to accomplish. The client with normal speech but decreased hearing should not have difficulty verbally communicating to staff. (16:506; 2:257)

    Nursing Process—Planning
    Client Need—Safe, effective care environment

56 2. Most hearing-impaired people have learned to adapt by lip reading or speech reading. To use this skill others need to face the client so that lip movements and facial expressions can be seen. Speaking into the client's ear can distort the words and mask the visual cues. Dropping the voice may cause some of the words to be missed. Raising or lowering the pitch of the voice would help only a person with a hearing loss in one or the other vocal registers. High tones are generally more difficult to hear. (16:504-505; 3:861; 7:694)

    Nursing Process—Planning
    Client Need—Safe, effective care environment

57 1. As long as the client is literate and is not visually impaired, reading a descriptive pamphlet is an appropriate alternative. Another stapedectomy client should not be the primary resource for explaining technical information. A client with otosclerosis is probably not so profoundly deaf that he would have learned sign language himself. Hand-writing short sentences or words is appropriate, but writing lengthy technical information would be tedious and time consuming. (16:506; 2:253)

Nursing Process—Implementation
Client Need—Safe, effective care environment

58 2. Encouraging the client to discuss her feelings is a therapeutic intervention. Endorsing or defending the expertise of the surgeon will not relieve the client's fears about the risks she is facing. Giving advice, offering a reassuring cliché, and changing the subject are nontherapeutic communication techniques. (12:262; 9:139)

Nursing Process—Implementation
Client Need—Psychosocial integrity

59 1. There is usually rebound swelling immediately after the surgery. The ear is packed and covered with a dressing. Both contribute to a temporary decrease in hearing acuity. This setback is only temporary and should eventually subside in the absence of any complications. The success of the surgery will be known in a matter of weeks. If the surgery is successful, the client should not need a hearing aid. The prosthetic stapes is secured to the incus by a fine wire loop or hook. It will move immediately without any bone formation around it. (3:858; 7:699)

Nursing Process—Implementation
Client Need—Psychosocial integrity

60 3. Vertigo is often experienced by the stapedectomy client postoperatively owing to a loss of perilymph or labrynthitis. Side rails should be raised and the client assisted with ambulation. The client undergoing stapedectomy is generally young or middle-aged and is not likely to feel exceptionally tired. Diplopia is not associated with the effects of this surgery. There is some discomfort, but it is not a major postoperative problem predisposing the client to injury. (3:857;7:698)

Nursing Process—Implementation
Client Need—Safe, effective care environment

61 4. The facial nerve can be assessed by asking the client to perform facial motor movements, such as smiling, frowning, wrinkling the forehead, whistling, or puffing the cheeks. If the facial nerve is intact, the nurse will observe that both sides of the face move symmetrically. Opening the mouth and saying "ah" is a method of testing the function of the glossopharyngeal nerve. The olfactory nerve is assessed by identifying a familiar odor, the source of which cannot be seen. Touching the cornea with a wisp of cotton or an

applicator assesses the trigeminal nerve. (7:699; 14:151)

Nursing Process—Collecting data
Client Need—Physiological integrity

62 1. Keeping the client flat and the operative ear up helps to maintain the placement of the prosthetic stapes and reduce the occurrence of vertigo. None of the other positional choices would accomplish this goal. (3:858; 7:699)

Nursing Process—Planning
Client Need—Safe, effective care environment

63 4. Raising the pressure within the eustachian tube and the middle ear increases the potential for displacing the prosthetic stapes. Blowing the nose, especially with the nares compressed; sneezing; coughing; vomiting; straining to have a stool; bending; and heavy lifting should be avoided postoperatively. Chewing food generally will not increase the pressure within the eustachian tube and middle ear. A liquid diet is usually ordered immediately postoperatively because it is more easily consumed in a flat position. Raising the head can cause dizziness and nausea. (16:514; 3:858)

Nursing Process—Planning
Client Need—Safe, effective care environment

64 2. Situations in which air pressure changes are likely to occur, such as flying and diving, should be avoided. None of the other activities are specifically contraindicated for a client who has had a stapedectomy. (3:858; 7:699)

Nursing Process—Evaluation
Client Need—Health promotion/maintenance

NURSING CARE OF CLIENTS WITH MENIERE'S DISEASE

65 3. The major symptom of Meniere's disease is severe vertigo. This is not described as simply dizziness, but rather a sensation of seeing and feeling motion or rotation. The other symptoms are not related to Meniere's disease. (16:511; 7:699; 14:981)

Nursing Process—Collecting data
Client Need—Safe, effective care environment

66 1. A caloric test involves instilling cold and warm solution separately into each ear. An audiometric test requires that headphones be worn. Electrodes are used for electroencephalography and electronystagmography. A refrigerated blood sample is not used for a caloric test. (3:854)

Nursing Process—Planning
Client Need—Safe, effective care environment

67 1. A client with Meniere's disease will develop a sudden onset of severe symptoms associated with his disease, such as vertigo, nausea, vomiting, and tinnitus. If there is no response to the instillation of warm or cold solution within the ear, it indicates an auditory nerve tumor. Normal people may experience slight dizziness and nystagmus during a caloric test. Aphasia and loss of consciousness would be unrelated to the mechanics or physiology of a caloric test. (3:854, 856)
Nursing Process—Collecting data
Client Need—Safe, effective care environment

68 1. Allowing the client to participate in the planning and implementation of nursing activities will maintain his locus of control. The client, more so than anyone else, knows what movement will cause him the least discomfort. Discontinuing or restricting nursing activities would not reflect a high standard of care. Performing nursing activities quickly may heighten the client's anxiety because unexpected movements can induce or aggravate his symptoms. (7:699; 14:981)
Nursing Process—Planning
Client Need—Psychosocial integrity

69 2. Meniere's disease seems to be related to an increase in endolymphatic fluid within the spaces of the labyrinth in the inner ear. Neither electrolyte or vitamin deficiency nor genetics has been implicated as a cause of Meniere's disease. (3:856; 7:699)
Nursing Process—Implementation
Client Need—Health promotion/maintenance

70 4. Sudden movement of the client's head or making sudden movements may precipitate an attack that includes nausea and vomiting. Decreasing fluid intake may be beneficial. Changing positions frequently should be avoided. The intensity of room lights is not a factor in controlling the symptoms of Meniere's disease. (14:980; 3:856)
Nursing Process—Implementation
Client Need—Physiological integrity

71 3. Hearing loss becomes progressively worse with each subsequent attack. Low-sodium diets are prescribed to control the volume of endolymph. The period of time that symptoms will last is unpredictable. Surgery may be performed in advanced cases to eliminate the vertigo, nausea, and vomiting. However, permanent deafness is a consequence of most surgical procedures. (14:981; 3:857)
Nursing Process—Evaluation
Client Need—Health promotion/maintenance

NURSING CARE OF CLIENTS WITH A NOSEBLEED

72 2. Nosebleeds can result when the arterial blood pressure becomes high. The hypertension causes capillaries in the nasal membrane to rupture, causing bleeding. A pulse rate of 110 may be the result, rather than cause, of the blood loss. Anxiety can cause a transient elevation in both heart and respiratory rate. An oral temperature of 97.6°F (36.7°C) is slightly lower than normal. However, a low temperature is not likely to cause the nose to bleed. (3:378; 7:328)
Nursing Process—Evaluation
Client Need—Physiological integrity

73 3. Fear is an emotional response to a real or imagined danger. It occurs when a person feels helpless or powerless to control the situation in which he is involved. Eliminating or reducing the fear-provoking stimulus, in this case the bloody clothing, will probably diminish his fear. Laying the client down would not be appropriate because the first aid treatment for a nosebleed involves having the client sit forward. A towel would not likely stay in place without laying the client down. An anxious or fearful person probably will not be able to concentrate on reading. (12:355-356)
Nursing Process—Implementation
Client Need—Psychosocial integrity

74 3. The best first aid measure for controlling a nosebleed is to apply direct pressure. The client should sit forward to allow the blood to drain from his nose rather than down his nasopharynx into his throat. An upright position also tends to lower the blood pressure. Swallowing, mouth-breathing, and clenching the teeth will not control bleeding. (7:328; 3:378; 14:416)
Nursing Process—Implementation
Client Need—Physiological integrity

75 4. Blowing the nose may retraumatize the ruptured nasal capillaries, causing bleeding to recur. There is no need to restrict his intake to liquids. Taking his carotid pulse is unnecessary. Keeping his head up may help lower his blood pressure, but it is not the most essential information that the client should receive. (3:378; 16:328)
Nursing Process—Implementation
Client Need—Health promotion/maintenance

NURSING CARE OF CLIENTS WITH SINUSITIS

76 3. When a client has an inhalant type of allergy, upper respiratory infection, or nasal obstruction,

the maxillary sinuses are the most frequently infected. The maxillary sinuses are located in the cheek. Pain from maxillary sinusitis is described as being in the cheek or the upper teeth. If the frontal sinuses are infected, the pain is felt near the eyes. (14:830; 16:227)
Nursing Process—Collecting data
Client Need—Safe, effective care environment

77 2. Overuse of nasal decongestants leads to "rebound phenomenon." This means that the congestion becomes worse and recurs in less time after using the drug. Discontinuing the use of the drug causes the client to experience the original nasal congestion, but systemic withdrawal symptoms typical of addiction do not occur. Most decongestants are adrenergic drugs, which cause vasoconstriction, not bleeding. The mucous membrane may sting, burn, or feel dry. The immune system is unaffected by nasal decongestants. (15:263; 14:817)
Nursing Process—Implementation
Client Need—Health promotion/maintenance

78 3. Gravity and head positioning can facilitate movement of the medication within the nasal passages rather than down toward the pharynx. None of the other described positions will help distribute nasal medications where they are intended for use. (18:595; 14:817)
Nursing Process—Implementation
Client Need—Health promotion/maintenance

79 3. Even though the same drug and dosage strength are prescribed, each client should have his medication dispensed from a separate container. This is especially important because contact between the nasal mucosa and administrative dropper can transmit organisms to another client. Reading the label three times, asking the client to state his name, and handwashing are all important principles to follow when administering medications. (14:817)
Nursing Process—Evaluation
Client Need—Safe, effective care environment

NURSING CARE OF CLIENTS WITH NASAL SURGERY

80 2. At frequent intervals, the nurse should use a flashlight and tongue depressor to inspect the back of the throat for draining blood. A "mustache dressing" usually is applied beneath the nostrils and held in place with strips of adhesive. This external dressing is applied to absorb drainage that saturates the packing. However, bleeding already may be excessive before it is noticed externally. The packing is not removed until 24 to 48 hours following surgery. Blood would be

lost in the posterior pharynx before it would be evident from the nostrils. (14:831)
Nursing Process—Implementation
Client Need—Physiological integrity

81 4. Breathing through the mouth is very drying to the oral mucous membranes. A sore throat can be relieved by offering cool or warm liquids or by using a medicated gargle. A bloody dressing indicates a need to change or reinforce the dressing. Many people are nauseated from swallowing blood; mouth care will not relieve this discomfort. (14:831)
Nursing Process—Evaluation
Client Need—Physiological integrity

82 3. It is best for the nurse to remain objective and limit her response to describing the client's external appearance. Predicting that the client will look gorgeous could be false reassurance because body image is a personal concept. The client most likely felt unattractive prior to the surgery; contradicting the client's opinion may cause her to lose faith in future things the nurse says. Telling the client that personality is more important also is the nurse's subjective opinion. It borders on giving advice, which is a nontherapeutic communication technique. (14:722; 9:140-141)
Nursing Process—Implementation
Client Need—Psychosocial integrity

INDIVIDUAL TEST ITEMS ON NURSING CARE INVOLVING DISORDERS OF THE NOSE

83 3. Steam vaporizers produce humidification by heating water to a boiling state. Machines of this type, however, pose the potential for accidental scalding. Use of this type of machine is virtually obsolete. Cool mist humidifiers are now preferred. (18:706; 7:175)
Nursing Process—Implementation
Client Need—Safe, effective care environment

84 3. Injuries to the nose, such as a fracture, if not cared for, can bend the septum to one side or the other. Nasal polyps generally are due to chronic inflammation. An enlarged, red, bulbous nose may be from a skin condition, such as acne rosacea. Serous drainage indicates concurrent irritation from an allergen or pathogen. (7:341; 14:830)
Nursing Process—Collecting data
Client Need—Safe, effective care environment

NURSING CARE OF CLIENTS WITH PHARYNGITIS

85 3. A throat culture is obtained by touching a sterile applicator to the inflamed tissue. A sputum spec-

imen is obtained by expectoration. A throat culture is obtained from the posterior pharynx rather than the mouth and tongue. Organisms in saliva would not necessarily indicate the pathogen causing pharyngitis. (16:66; 14:813)
    Nursing Process—Implementation
    Client Need—Safe, effective care environment

86 1. Rheumatic fever, rheumatic heart disease, and glomerulonephritis are but a few of the consequences following untreated or undertreated infections caused by the beta hemolytic *Streptococcus* organism. To ensure that the organism is destroyed, the American Heart Association recommends that streptococcal infections be treated with penicillin or erythromycin for a full 10 days. The other three diseases are infectious but are not caused by this particular organism. (16:229; 3:377; 8:710)
    Nursing Process—Implementation
    Client Need—Health promotion/maintenance

NURSING CARE OF CLIENTS WITH LARYNGITIS

87 2. Speaking in a normal voice or whispering should be avoided. This will rest swollen vocal cords and allow the local edema to subside. Laryngitis is not associated with a vitamin deficiency. Simple laryngitis does not usually require bed rest. Massaging the throat may provide comfort for some people, but it will not relieve hoarseness. (16:231)
    Nursing Process—Implementation
    Client Need—Health promotion/maintenance

88 3. Persistent hoarseness is the earliest symptom of cancer of the larynx. Nagging cough or hoarseness is one of the seven early warning signs of cancer identified by the American Cancer Society. The other diseases cause respiratory symptoms, none of which is hoarseness. (3:275; 16:233; 7:343)
    Nursing Process—Evaluation
    Client Need—Safe, effective care environment

89 1. Any sign of airway obstruction must be reported immediately. Labored respirations would precede cyanosis, which is a *late* sign of impaired gas exchange. All of the listed physical assessments are important. However, an obstructed airway would be the most life-threatening. (3:377)
    Nursing Process—Collecting data
    Client Need—Physiological integrity

90 1. The nurse should establish that the gag reflex is present before the client is given food or oral fluids. Stimulating the palatal arch should cause the client to gag if the effects of the local anesthetic have worn off. The other choices are techniques of physical assessment but are unlikely to be affected by a laryngoscopy. (3:377; 6:329)
    Nursing Process—Collecting data
    Client Need—Safe, effective care environment

NURSING CARE OF CLIENTS WITH CANCER OF THE LARYNX

91 4. Until the laryngectomy client learns esophageal speech or the use of a mechanical vibrator, providing paper and pencil or a magic slate is the best alternative for communication. Lip reading is often frustrating for nursing personnel who are unaccustomed to this technique. The client has a permanent loss of natural voice as a result of a total laryngectomy. (16:234; 14:833)
    Nursing Process—Planning
    Client Need—Safe, effective care environment

92 2. Suctioning removes oxygen along with liquid secretions. Even though the client is preoxygenated before removing secretions, suctioning longer than 15 seconds can cause hypoxemia. To simulate what the client is experiencing, the nurse can refrain from breathing while applying suction. (18:719; 14:826)
    Nursing Process—Implementation
    Client Need—Physiological integrity

93 3. Looking at the tracheostomy tube can be interpreted as dealing with the reality of the loss. This is a positive step toward acceptance and adaptation. Grieving follows a cycle of denial or disbelief, anger, depression, bargaining, and acceptance. Believing that there has been a misdiagnosis is an example of denial. Social isolation indicates a state of depression characterized by withdrawal from human interaction. Asking the nurse to help him bathe and shave suggests that the client perceives himself as helpless. (9:314; 12:362; 2:722)
    Nursing Process—Evaluation
    Client Need—Psychosocial integrity

NURSING CARE OF CLIENTS HAVING A TONSILLECTOMY

94 1. Frequent swallowing often accompanies hemorrhage following nasal or oral surgery. The incorrect items are not associated with blood loss. (14:653; 3:379)
    Nursing Process—Collecting data
    Client Need—Physiological integrity

95 2. Following a tonsillectomy the client should be maintained in a side-lying or prone position. This position enables blood to drain from the mouth rather than be swallowed or aspirated. Once the client is alert and can control his own secretions, a semi-Fowler's position is appropriate. (3:379; 14:653)

> Nursing Process—Implementation
> Client Need—Physiological integrity

NURSING CARE OF CLIENTS WITH AN OCCLUDED AIRWAY

96 2. The ability to cough indicates that the foreign object in the airway has not totally obstructed the passage of air. As long as the person has only a partial obstruction, he should be allowed to cough to clear his own airway. The ability to walk is not important except to verify that the person's brain is still receiving oxygen and he has not lost consciousness. The position of the victim is not the most important data to obtain at this time. The ability to swallow will not relieve the lodged object if it is in the airway. (8:702; 18:742)

> Nursing Process—Collecting data
> Client Need—Physiological integrity

97 4. The thumb side of the fist should be placed against the abdomen above the navel and below the xiphoid process. The xiphoid process is the tip of the sternum. The manubrium is the upper portion of the sternum. (18:714; 14:432)

> Nursing Process—Implementation
> Client Need—Physiological integrity

Classification of Test Items

Unit IV Review Test 14

Directions: After each question the correct answer is given as well as a classification of each test question. Compare the correct answer with your answer. If a question has been answered *incorrectly*, draw a line to the end of the four columns. When finished, add up your correct scores and place the results at the bottom of each column.

Score Calculation:

To determine the percentage of the number of questions you answered correctly, divide the **Number Correct** by the **Number Possible**, as example 88 (the number of questions answered correctly) divided by 97 (the number of questions in the test) = .90 or 90%.

NURSING PROCESS

C = Collecting data
P = Planning
I = Implementation
E = Evaluation

CLIENT NEEDS

S = Safe, effective care environment
P = Physiological integrity
M = Psychosocial integrity
H = Health promotion/maintenance

Question #	Answer #	Nursing Process				Client Needs			
		C	P	I	E	S	P	M	H
1	3	C					P		
2	1			I			P		
3	2			I			P		
4	2			I		S			
5	4			I					H
6	3			I					H
7	1	C				S			
8	2		P			S			
9	1			I					H
10	2		P						H
11	4			I			P		
12	2				E				H
13	2		P					M	
14	1				E	S			
15	1		P					M	
16	4			I			P		
17	1	C				S			
18	3	C					P		
19	1				E	S			

NURSING PROCESS

C = Collecting data
P = Planning
I = Implementation
E = Evaluation

CLIENT NEEDS

S = Safe, effective care environment
P = Physiological integrity
M = Psychosocial integrity
H = Health promotion/maintenance

Question #	Answer #	Nursing Process				Client Needs			
		C	P	I	E	S	P	M	H
20	2		P			S			
21	2			I		S			
22	4			I		S			
23	1			I			P		
24	3		P				P		
25	2			I		S			
26	3	C				S			
27	2			I		S			
28	1	C					P		
29	3				E	S			
30	1			I			P		
31	4	C					P		
32	2	C				S			
33	3			I			P		
34	2			I				M	
35	1			I				M	
36	2				E	S			
37	3	C					P		
38	3	C					P		
39	1			I					H
40	2	C				S			
41	4	C					P		
42	1			I			P		
43	3				E		P		
44	1			I			P		
45	1			I			P		
46	1	C				S			
47	1			I					H
48	2			I					H
49	4				E		P		
50	4	C					P		

NURSING PROCESS

C = Collecting data
P = Planning
I = Implementation
E = Evaluation

CLIENT NEEDS

S = Safe, effective care environment
P = Physiological integrity
M = Psychosocial integrity
H = Health promotion/maintenance

Question #	Answer #	Nursing Process				Client Needs			
		C	P	I	E	S	P	M	H
51	2		P			S			
52	2			I					H
53	4	C					P		
54	1			I					H
55	1		P			S			
56	2		P			S			
57	1			I		S			
58	2			I				M	
59	1			I				M	
60	3			I		S			
61	4	C					P		
62	1		P			S			
63	4		P			S			
64	2				E				H
65	3	C				S			
66	1		P			S			
67	1	C				S			
68	1		P					M	
69	2			I					H
70	4			I			P		
71	3				E				H
72	2				E		P		
73	3			I				M	
74	3			I			P		
75	4			I					H
76	3	C				S			
77	2			I					H
78	3			I					H
79	3				E	S			
80	2			I			P		
81	4				E		P		

NURSING PROCESS

C = Collecting data
P = Planning
I = Implementation
E = Evaluation

CLIENT NEEDS

S = Safe, effective care environment
P = Physiological integrity
M = Psychosocial integrity
H = Health promotion/maintenance

Question #	Answer #	Nursing Process				Client Needs			
		C	P	I	E	S	P	M	H
82	3			I				M	
83	3			I		S			
84	3	C				S			
85	3			I		S			
86	1			I					H
87	2			I					H
88	3				E	S			
89	1	C					P		
90	1	C				S			
91	4		P			S			
92	2			I			P		
93	3				E			M	
94	1	C					P		
95	2			I			P		
96	2	C					P		
97	4			I			P		
Number Correct									
Number Possible	97	24	14	45	14	35	34	10	18
Percentage Correct									

COMPREHENSIVE EXAMINATION

Parts I and II

GENERAL INSTRUCTIONS FOR THE COMPREHENSIVE EXAMINATION

A two-part comprehensive examination that resembles NCLEX-PN as closely as possible is presented next. Each part consists of 120 items. Follow these instructions for both parts of the comprehensive examination:

Each item consists of four possible answers or options. (Items are described more fully on page XX in the Introduction.) Read each item carefully, and then select the one correct or best answer for each item.

Indicate your choice for the correct or best answer on the appropriate answer sheets at the end of this book. The answer sheets are perforated and may be removed for convenience of use.

There is only one correct answer for each item. If you think the correct answer for an item is not among the options, choose the option that you believe is the best possible answer.

Work systematically, and proceed steadily. Do not spend too much time on any one item.

Time your progress occasionally so that you know you will finish the entire part on which you are working in 2 hours.

Correct answers and rationale are provided for both parts of the comprehensive examination so that you can determine how well you scored. If you gave correct answers to approximately 180 to 190 items or more of the 240 items in the examination (75% to 80%), you are probably prepared for the national licensing examination. However, if you answered fewer than 180 to 190 items correctly, it is suggested that you continue with your reviewing. It is also suggested that you concentrate your review on subject matter on which you tested poorly in the review tests. The tables on pages 422 and 447, when completed, will help you identify your areas of weakness and strength.

Proceed to the next page for Part I of the comprehensive examination.

PART I OF THE COMPREHENSIVE EXAMINATION

Allow yourself 2 hours to complete Part I. Start this part now.

1 Which one of the following signs is the *best* indication that a client's tracheostomy needs suctioning?
   ○ 1. The pulse rate is decreased.
   ○ 2. The skin is cool and moist.
   ○ 3. The respirations are noisy.
   ○ 4. The client is lethargic.

2 Before suctioning a patient with a tracheostomy, which one of the following nursing actions should the nurse plan to perform *first*?
   ○ 1. Insert the suction catheter within the tracheostomy.
   ○ 2. Instill 5 mL of saline within the tracheostomy.
   ○ 3. Administer 100% oxygen for 1 to 2 minutes.
   ○ 4. Occlude the vent on the catheter for 15 seconds.

3 A physician has tested and recommended that a hospital employee use a hearing aid. The employee asks the nurse how the hearing aid will help him. The nurse would be *most* accurate in telling this person that a hearing aid will
   ○ 1. amplify what is currently heard.
   ○ 2. make sounds sharper and clearer.
   ○ 3. produce more distinct, crisp speech.
   ○ 4. eliminate hearing garbled sounds.

4 The nurse observes a colleague caring for a client who just returned to his room following a bronchoscopy. The nurse should intervene if which one of the following actions is seen? The nurse giving care
   ○ 1. takes the client's radial pulse.
   ○ 2. offers the client some water.
   ○ 3. raises the head of the bed.
   ○ 4. provides an additional blanket.

5 A client becomes angry and shouts at the nurse when a meal that was served is not to his liking. In this situation it would be *best* for the nurse to
   ○ 1. say something humorous and promise to call the dietitian.
   ○ 2. listen attentively and allow the client to express himself.
   ○ 3. leave the room and allow the client a period of privacy.
   ○ 4. explain that although it is tasteless, it is nutritious.

6 The client with a retinal detachment is most likely to describe which one of the following symptoms?
   ○ 1. Seeing flashes of light
   ○ 2. Being unable to see light
   ○ 3. Feeling discomfort in light
   ○ 4. Seeing more poorly in daylight

7 A nurse notes that a 2-year-old boy has evidence of tooth decay in the upper anterior teeth. When discussing this finding with the child's mother, which one of the following is the *most* likely contributing cause?
   ○ 1. The child does not brush his teeth regularly each morning.
   ○ 2. The child goes to bed with a bottle of fruit juice at night.
   ○ 3. The child takes a sweetened chewable vitamin each day.
   ○ 4. The child sucks his thumb whenever he is tired or bored.

8 Which one of the following indicates that Bryant's traction is applied properly to a small child?
   ○ 1. The child can sit up without experiencing discomfort.
   ○ 2. The child can reach the trapeze hanging above the bed.
   ○ 3. The child's buttocks are raised slightly off the mattress.
   ○ 4. The child's legs are pulled toward the bottom of the bed.

9 When the nursing team plans the care of the client in sickle cell crisis, one of the priorities *must* include
   ○ 1. promoting self-care.
   ○ 2. preventing immobility.
   ○ 3. relieving discomfort.
   ○ 4. improving self-esteem.

10 It is *essential* for the nurse to tell a client receiving external radiation therapy that when he bathes he should
   ○ 1. avoid getting this area of skin wet.
   ○ 2. use alcohol instead of soap in this area.
   ○ 3. cover the reddened area with clear plastic.
   ○ 4. use tepid water and soft wash cloth.

11 If a pregnant client in her third trimester tells the nurse that a severe headache has lasted for 2 days,

the best plan of action would be to tell the client to

- ○ 1. increase her rest and leisure activities.
- ○ 2. eliminate coffee or other sources of caffeine.
- ○ 3. take two aspirin and lie down for 1 hour.
- ○ 4. be checked in the physician's office today.

12 A client with peripheral vascular disease asks the nurse to trim her toenails. Which of the following is the *best* action the nurse can take at this time?

- ○ 1. Cut the nails straight across the edge.
- ○ 2. Use special clippers or cuticle scissors.
- ○ 3. Consult the client's physician about this.
- ○ 4. Soak the client's feet in warm water first.

13 The nurse is examining a toddler in the pediatric clinic. Which one of the following statements made by the mother should make the nurse suspect that the child may have cystic fibrosis? The mother says her

- ○ 1. child's perspiration is very salty.
- ○ 2. child vomits immediately after eating.
- ○ 3. child's stools are soft and bright yellow.
- ○ 4. child's urine is very light colored.

14 A 72-year-old client tells the nurse that he would like to donate his corneas when he dies. The *most* accurate response is

- ○ 1. "Your next of kin must charge a fair price for them."
- ○ 2. "There currently is no longer a need for corneas."
- ○ 3. "Corneas are accepted regardless of the donor's age."
- ○ 4. "Corneas are not harvested from donors older than age 30."

15 Which one of the following statements indicates that the client who will be taking long-term corticosteroid medication understands the danger in their use? The client says

- ○ 1. "I should never suddenly stop taking my medication."
- ○ 2. "My reaction time will be slowed while taking this drug."
- ○ 3. "If I forget to take one dose, I should double the next."
- ○ 4. "I should not take this drug for more than 6 months."

16 A client has returned from a bronchoscopy. Which one of the following assessments is *most* indicative that the client is developing an airway obstruction?

- ○ 1. The client's voice is hoarse.
- ○ 2. The client has a weak cough.
- ○ 3. Each breath produces a squeaky sound.
- ○ 4. Each respiration is slow and deep.

17 A home health care nurse visits a client who takes a prescribed diuretic. The *best* evidence the nurse could use for evaluating the drug's effectiveness is checking the client's

- ○ 1. weight.
- ○ 2. pulse.
- ○ 3. appetite.
- ○ 4. reflexes.

18 When applying nitroglycerin ointment, which is the *best* technique for the nurse to use?

- ○ 1. Squeeze a ribbon of ointment onto paper.
- ○ 2. Rub the ointment thoroughly into the skin.
- ○ 3. Press the mouth of the tube to the chest.
- ○ 4. Spread the ointment over the heart area.

19 When teaching mothers of newborns how to administer rescue breathing to an infant, it would be *best* for the nurse to tell them to cover the nose and mouth of the infant and blow

- ○ 1. very forcefully.
- ○ 2. to fill the cheeks.
- ○ 3. a small puff of air.
- ○ 4. as much air as possible.

20 When helping to plan the nursing care of a client with an acute respiratory infection, such as pneumonia, the *primary* focus should be on

- ○ 1. relieving the cough.
- ○ 2. improving oxygenation.
- ○ 3. providing nourishment.
- ○ 4. encouraging self-care.

21 All of the following are normal findings the nurse can expect when assessing a client who has just undergone hemodialysis. Which one is the *best* evidence that the client can safely resume his routine activities?

- ○ 1. The client's skin is warm and dry.
- ○ 2. The client's blood pressure is stable.
- ○ 3. The client has lost several pounds.
- ○ 4. The client feels less fatigued.

22 Which one of the following questions would be most important for the nurse to ask *first* when assessing a client who has attempted suicide by taking an overdose of medication?

- ○ 1. How many pills were taken?
- ○ 2. Why did you take the pills?
- ○ 3. What is the name of the drug?
- ○ 4. Where were the pills obtained?

23 A 6-year-old child has had chronic serous otitis media and has just had polyethylene tubes inserted through the eardrum into the middle ear. The nurse is working with the team leader to develop a teaching plan for discharge instructions. Which of the following is essential to include on the teaching plan?

- ○ 1. Allow the child to eat only soft or liquid food.
- ○ 2. Raise your voice when speaking to the child.
- ○ 3. Insert ear plugs whenever the child swims or showers.
- ○ 4. Irrigate the ears daily while the tubes are in place.

24 When suctioning a tracheostomy, which one of the following techniques is correct?
- ○ 1. The nurse lubricates the catheter tip with K-Y jelly.
- ○ 2. The nurse instructs the client to take panting breaths.
- ○ 3. The nurse applies suction while inserting the catheter.
- ○ 4. The nurse uses a sterile glove to insert the catheter.

25 What technique would be *best* for the nurse to use to assess the neurologic function of an extremity that is covered with a cast? The nurse should
- ○ 1. ask the client to wiggle his fingers or toes.
- ○ 2. depress the nail bed and observe the color return.
- ○ 3. feel the temperature of the fingers or toes.
- ○ 4. compare the sizes of fingers or toes bilaterally.

26 During a nursing interview of a teenager with extreme weight loss, which of the following information best correlates with the profile of a person with anorexia nervosa?
- ○ 1. The client is the middle child of three siblings.
- ○ 2. The client is a high achiever in school and activities.
- ○ 3. The client thinks her classmates do not like her.
- ○ 4. The client experienced many illnesses during childhood.

27 Which one of the following behaviors creates the *highest* risk to both the infant and the mother during pregnancy?
- ○ 1. Restricting food intake to avoid gaining weight
- ○ 2. Remaining sexually active throughout the pregnancy
- ○ 3. Participating regularly in an aerobic exercise program
- ○ 4. Becoming pregnant for the first time after age 25

28 A client who weighs 88 lb is to receive 2 mg of a drug per kilogram of body weight. This client should receive
- ○ 1. 0.4 mg
- ○ 2. 44 mg
- ○ 3. 8 mg
- ○ 4. 80 mg

29 The nurse administers oxytocin (Pitocin) following the delivery of the placenta. The *best* evidence that the drug has achieved its intended effect is
- ○ 1. postpartal pain is relieved.
- ○ 2. the uterus becomes firm.
- ○ 3. lactation is suppressed.
- ○ 4. uterine contractions cease.

30 A moderately obese adult discusses all of the following approaches for reestablishing weight loss when a plateau weight has been reached. Which plan would be *best* for the nurse to support?
- ○ 1. Taking an appetite suppressant
- ○ 2. Performing more physical exercise
- ○ 3. Fasting for 24 hours each week
- ○ 4. Eating less than 1000 calories per day

31 A depressed client says to the nurse, "No one really cares what happens to me." The *best* response from the nurse would be
- ○ 1. "You're exaggerating! Lots of people care about you."
- ○ 2. "Talking like that will only make you feel more sad."
- ○ 3. "Tell me why you think no one cares what happens to you."
- ○ 4. "It sounds like you're feeling ignored or abandoned."

32 A client has had surgery for a detached retina. Unless orders to the contrary are given, it is *essential* that the care plan indicate that this client
- ○ 1. rest quietly in bed.
- ○ 2. restrict his fluids.
- ○ 3. elevate his head.
- ○ 4. have bright light.

33 When the tonsillectomy client asks the nurse why his physician told him to avoid taking aspirin or aspirin products temporarily, the *best* explanation is that aspirin
- ○ 1. lowers the temperature and therefore can mask a fever.
- ○ 2. interferes with clotting and promotes bleeding.
- ○ 3. irritates the stomach and could cause an ulcer.
- ○ 4. reduces inflammation and conceals symptoms of infection.

34 The *best* evidence that Kegel exercises are being performed correctly is that the client can
- ○ 1. perform deep knee bends without back discomfort.
- ○ 2. touch the toes without abdominal discomfort.
- ○ 3. sit in a tailor position and fill the lungs deeply.
- ○ 4. stop and restart the flow of urine during voiding.

35 A 3-year-old child is admitted with a diagnosis of laryngotracheobronchitis (croup). As the nurse examines the client, which one of the following is *most* characteristic of this condition?
- ○ 1. Barking cough
- ○ 2. Mild lethargy
- ○ 3. Nasal discharge
- ○ 4. Severe vomiting

36 The nurse is to apply acyclovir (Zovirax) ointment to a herpes simplex type I lesion. Which of the following actions is appropriate?
- ○ 1. The nurse touches the tube to the lesion.
- ○ 2. The nurse dons a gown, mask, and goggles.
- ○ 3. The nurse wears a glove during application.
- ○ 4. The nurse covers the center of the lesion.

37 The nurse observes all of the following when assessing a newborn. Which one is a criterion used for Apgar scoring?
- ○ 1. Presence of vernix
- ○ 2. Urine elimination
- ○ 3. Skin color
- ○ 4. Birth weight

38 Which is the best documentation for the nurse to record in the medical record of a schizophrenic client who claims to be seeing demons in his room?
- ○ 1. Experiencing hallucinations
- ○ 2. Frightened by hallucinations
- ○ 3. States seeing "demons in my room"
- ○ 4. Having distorted sensory perceptions

39 Owing to profuse diarrhea, a male client with ulcerative colitis frequently soils his hospital linen and himself. The best plan for the nursing team to follow to protect the client's self-esteem is to
- ○ 1. assign only male nurses to clean and care for the client.
- ○ 2. ask the client's wife to help clean him when possible.
- ○ 3. hold the client responsible for all of his own hygiene.
- ○ 4. clean the client of stool in a nonjudgmental manner.

40 A mother says her child inserted a dry pea into her ear yesterday. She instilled water within the ear and thought the pea came out. After the physician removes the pea, which information should the nurse plan to provide to prevent a future recurrence?
- ○ 1. Alcohol would have been a better substance to use.
- ○ 2. Pounding the side of the head could loosen the pea.
- ○ 3. Moisture causes vegetative matter, such as a pea, to swell.
- ○ 4. Using a blow dryer at the ear could dehydrate a pea.

41 To remove an object that completely obstructs the airway of an unconscious adult, the nurse should plan to position the hands correctly and administer
- ○ 1. six to ten abdominal thrusts.
- ○ 2. two quick ventilations of air.
- ○ 3. five chest thrusts and a breath.
- ○ 4. fifteen chest compressions.

42 Which of the following is the best evidence that a client with a colostomy is adjusting to his change in body image?
- ○ 1. The client wears loose-fitting garments.
- ○ 2. The client applies cologne heavily.
- ○ 3. The client empties his own appliance.
- ○ 4. The client asks to see a clergyman.

43 Following an upper gastrointestinal x-ray, sometimes referred to as a barium swallow, which nursing assessment is *essential* to monitor?
- ○ 1. The ability to eat
- ○ 2. The passage of stool
- ○ 3. The color of urine
- ○ 4. The feeling of hunger

44 A mother calls the pediatrician's office and describes her 2-year-old's symptoms as a tight cough, low-grade fever, flushed skin, and anorexia. Which temporary measure could the nurse suggest to promote expectoration?
- ○ 1. Give the child plenty of milk to drink.
- ○ 2. Hold the child in a steamy bathroom.
- ○ 3. Keep the child confined to his crib.
- ○ 4. Administer liquid aspirin as directed.

45 A hospitalized client has a sealed source of radiation inserted within her vagina to treat cancer. What information should be discussed before a nurse cares for this client?
- ○ 1. Is the nurse sensitive to radiation?
- ○ 2. Could the nurse possibly be pregnant?
- ○ 3. Does the nurse have a chronic disease?
- ○ 4. How long has the nurse been employed?

46 To best determine the emotional needs of an unmarried pregnant teenager, the nurse should assess
- ○ 1. the age and identity of the baby's father.
- ○ 2. the client's understanding of contraception.
- ○ 3. why the client became sexually active.
- ○ 4. how the family feels about the pregnancy.

47 When caring for a client following postreduction of a fractured mandible in which the lower jaw and upper jaw have been immobilized together, which piece of equipment should the nurse plan to have available at the bedside?
- ○ 1. A rubber tourniquet
- ○ 2. A tracheostomy set
- ○ 3. Wire-cutting scissors
- ○ 4. A flexible gastric tube

48 The best technique the nurse can use for detecting thrombophlebitis postoperatively is to
- ○ 1. have the client dorsiflex his feet.
- ○ 2. palpate the dorsalis pedis pulses.
- ○ 3. observe his gait while walking.
- ○ 4. monitor the client's temperature.

49 Prior to discharge, a client with a colostomy says, "There is so much to remember about my care. I don't know who to contact if I have questions or problems." The best person to whom the nurse could plan to refer this client would be a(n)
- ○ 1. enterostomal therapist.
- ○ 2. gastroenterologist.

○ 3. gastronomer.
○ 4. entomologist.

50 Which of the following statements made by an alcoholic client who is to start taking disulfiram (Antabuse) indicates a need for *more* health teaching?
○ 1. "If I miss one dose of the drug, I'll experience nausea, vomiting, and fainting."
○ 2. "I can get very sick if I consume alcohol in any form while taking this drug."
○ 3. "I can have a reaction even 2 weeks after I stop taking this drug."
○ 4. "I shouldn't apply after-shave lotion or cologne to my skin while taking this drug."

51 The team leader asks the practical nurse to discontinue the administration of intravenous fluid on an assigned client. Which one of the following nursing actions is *essential* at that time? The nurse must
○ 1. pull the curtain.
○ 2. don latex gloves.
○ 3. lower the side rail.
○ 4. weigh the client.

52 A few days before a client is to have a malignant growth removed from his colon, he says to the nurse, "I am scared. This operation worries me." In this situation, it would be *best* for the nurse to say
○ 1. "There is no need for fear and worry; trust me."
○ 2. "Tell me more specifically about your concerns."
○ 3. "You know as well as I that you have an excellent surgeon."
○ 4. "Try to relax. Worrying will only make matters worse."

53 While assisting with a physical examination, the nurse should plan to have topical anesthesia ready for use when the physician wishes to
○ 1. test deep tendon reflexes.
○ 2. remove vaginal secretions.
○ 3. measure intraocular pressure.
○ 4. examine the tympanic membranes.

54 A nurse caring for a 45-year-old client would be *most* correct in attributing which one of the following behaviors to generativity, a typical developmental task of middle adulthood. The client
○ 1. expresses fear of having further illnesses.
○ 2. wishes to know the purpose of his medications.
○ 3. wants to resume writing a book about his boyhood.
○ 4. desires to learn more about using a computer.

55 To plan care with respect to cultural values, the best method for determining if a hospitalized client of the Jewish faith follows the strict orthodox customs of his religion is to
○ 1. ask if he speaks the Hebrew language.
○ 2. inquire as to his dietary preferences.

○ 3. question if he wears a skull cap.
○ 4. see if the client has been circumcised.

56 Which one of the following nursing actions would be *most* correct if a chest tube was pulled from its insertion site?
○ 1. Cover the opening to keep out air.
○ 2. Reinsert the displaced chest tube.
○ 3. Apply suction with a thin catheter.
○ 4. Tell the client to hold his breath.

57 A nursing student asks how to help his wife, a victim of sexual abuse as a child, with posttraumatic stress disorder. The *best* plan the nurse can recommend is to
○ 1. always act happy and enthusiastic around her.
○ 2. prevent her from isolating herself from people.
○ 3. encourage her to talk about her traumatic experience.
○ 4. take frequent vacations or do pleasurable activities.

58 Which of the following is the *best* evidence that the client who has experienced a cerebrovascular accident has adjusted to the perceptual problems associated with his stroke?
○ 1. The client talks in a normal tone of voice.
○ 2. The client participates in his self-care.
○ 3. The client shares feelings about his altered health status.
○ 4. The client visually checks the position of his extremities.

59 An indication that a client with nephrotic syndrome is experiencing a therapeutic effect from corticosteroid therapy is an increase in the client's
○ 1. body weight.
○ 2. muscle mass.
○ 3. urinary output.
○ 4. blood pressure.

60 When a nasogastric tube is removed, which one of the following nursing measures should the nurse plan to carry out first?
○ 1. Providing the client oral hygiene
○ 2. Giving the client some soft food
○ 3. Offering a nonnarcotic analgesic
○ 4. Discontinuing intake and output

61 The nursing team has been trying to prepare the spouse of a terminally ill client for his death. Which of the following is the *best* indication that the nursing interventions have been effective? The spouse
○ 1. controls her emotions when visiting her husband.
○ 2. asks friends to come along during visiting hours.
○ 3. discusses plans for living with a widowed sister.
○ 4. researches information about her husband's illness.

62 A client is startled and continues to worry about an alarm that sounded from his intravenous infusion pump. The *best* plan the nurse can implement for relieving the patient's anxiety at this time is to
○ 1. infuse the solution by gravity.
○ 2. explain why the alarm sounded.
○ 3. give a prescribed tranquilizer.
○ 4. provide a magazine for reading.

63 The nurse obtains all of the following findings when assessing a newborn immediately after delivery. Which one is considered the *most* ominous sign?
○ 1. Heart rate over 100
○ 2. Flaccid muscle tone
○ 3. Loud, vigorous cry
○ 4. Flushed skin color

64 One hour after delivery the nurse notes that a postpartum mother has pronounced vaginal bleeding. The action the nurse should take *first* would be to
○ 1. call the physician.
○ 2. massage the uterus.
○ 3. count the pulse rate.
○ 4. elevate the legs.

65 A surgical client asks the nurse why leg exercises are important to perform. The *best* explanation is that leg movement, which involves contracting and relaxing leg muscles, helps to prevent
○ 1. loss of muscle strength.
○ 2. formation of blood clots.
○ 3. swelling of the extremities.
○ 4. developing varicose veins.

66 When removing an indwelling retention catheter, the *first* step the nurse should take is to
○ 1. clamp the tubing.
○ 2. deflate the balloon.
○ 3. irrigate the catheter.
○ 4. cleanse the meatus.

67 A depressed client makes all of the following comments. Which one *best* indicates a need to assess her more closely for suicide?
○ 1. "You don't let me get any rest."
○ 2. "I can't stand my roommate."
○ 3. "I'd like you to have my grandmother's locket."
○ 4. "When do you think the doctor will discharge me?"

68 The physician prescribes an antibiotic to treat a child's otitis media. Which antibiotic in the list below, if prescribed, should the nurse question because it can permanently discolor teeth when used before 8 years of age?
○ 1. cefazolin (Kefzol)
○ 2. amoxicillin (Amoxil)
○ 3. oxytetracycline (Terramycin)
○ 4. gentamicin (Garamycin)

69 Which is the best response to the 82-year-old Alzheimer's patient who says she must leave the extended care facility to be home when her children return from school?
○ 1. "Nonsense! You're too old to have children that young."
○ 2. "I'm sure a neighbor will take care of them for awhile."
○ 3. "I'll call the school and tell them to expect you later."
○ 4. "You're in a nursing home. I'm your nurse."

70 A 3-year-old child is hospitalized with laryngotracheobronchitis (croup). The nursing care plan indicates that the assigned nurse should provide oral fluids frequently. Which one of the following should be *avoided* for a child with this diagnosis?
○ 1. Ginger ale
○ 2. Apple juice
○ 3. Whole milk
○ 4. Cold water

71 When resuscitating an unresponsive infant, where is the *best* location for checking a pulse?
○ 1. Over the radial artery
○ 2. Over the femoral artery
○ 3. Over the brachial artery
○ 4. Over the carotid artery

72 A nurse finds a client who appears to have fallen out of the hospital bed. Which action should the nurse perform *first*?
○ 1. Report the accident to the proper person.
○ 2. Move the person back to bed or a chair.
○ 3. Call for assistance to help the client.
○ 4. Check the client's physical condition.

73 Which one of the following is the *best* evidence of healthy parent–newborn interaction?
○ 1. The parents observe the care of their newborn.
○ 2. The parents are pleased with the baby's gender.
○ 3. The parents watch and listen to their newborn.
○ 4. The parents touch and talk to the newborn.

74 The nursing team meets for a conference to plan the care of a client with anorexia nervosa. Which of the following has the *highest* priority at this time?
○ 1. Changing the client's distorted body image
○ 2. Improving the client's coping techniques
○ 3. Restoring adequate nutrition
○ 4. Developing assertiveness

75 A postoperative client is to have a clear liquid diet. Which one of the following items could the nurse plan to provide?
○ 1. A glass of milk
○ 2. A bowl of ice cream
○ 3. A dish of gelatin
○ 4. A cup of creamed soup

76 The nursing team reviews the effectiveness of interventions being used to promote a confused client's orientation. Which one of the following is the *best* evidence of progress in accomplishing the goal?

○ 1. The client walks with others to the dining room.

○ 2. The client dresses himself without difficulty.

○ 3. The client locates his room without assistance.

○ 4. The client talks on the telephone to his family.

77 A child recovering from rheumatic fever has bathroom privileges. The nurse observes that he experiences shortness of breath walking to the bathroom. Which of the following changes in the nursing care plan would be *best* for the nurse to suggest?

○ 1. Use a bedside commode for elimination.

○ 2. Administer oxygen after elimination.

○ 3. Ambulate with assistance to the bathroom.

○ 4. Provide a walker when using the bathroom.

78 A nurse teaches an asthmatic client how to use a hand-held aerosol inhaler. Which one of the following is *correct* information? Inhale slowly and deeply while depressing the cartridge, and then

○ 1. immediately exhale the aerosol.

○ 2. briefly hold the inhaled breath.

○ 3. quickly swallow the bubble of air.

○ 4. intermittently cough and breathe.

79 A client brings her 2-year-old son to the physician's office. She tells the nurse that the child has been irritable, feels warm, and has not been eating or drinking as usual. As the nurse observes the child, what additional finding is *most* suggestive that the child may have a middle ear infection?

○ 1. The child wants to be held.

○ 2. The child is cutting teeth.

○ 3. The child swallows frequently.

○ 4. The child tugs at his ear.

80 All of the following medications are ordered for a client with Meniere's disease. Which one would be *most* appropriate for the nurse to administer to the client during an acute attack?

○ 1. acetaminophen (Tylenol)

○ 2. meclizine (Antivert)

○ 3. meperidine (Demerol)

○ 4. triazolam (Halcion)

81 Assuming that none of the following nursing measures is contraindicated, which one would be *best* for helping a postoperative male client void?

○ 1. Encourage the client to use a bedpan rather than a urinal.

○ 2. Help the client to stand to void using a urinal.

○ 3. Increase the client's fluid intake until he voids.

○ 4. Teach him perineal exercises to improve sphincter tone.

82 The nurse notes that a client with jaundice has been scratching his skin. Which one of the following nursing actions would be the best plan for preventing skin impairment?

○ 1. Bathe him with very warm water.

○ 2. Dust his body with cornstarch.

○ 3. Trim the client's fingernails.

○ 4. Use hypoallergenic bed linen.

83 A client with a history of substance abuse tells the nurse that he is experiencing a "racing heart" and chest pain. Which one of the following questions would be *most* appropriate at this time? When was the last time you used

○ 1. heroin?

○ 2. cocaine?

○ 3. barbiturates?

○ 4. marijuana?

84 Which one of the following is the best evidence that a client with a tracheostomy has remained adequately oxygenated while being suctioned?

○ 1. The heart rate stays within 88 to 92 beats per minute.

○ 2. A moderate amount of tracheal secretions is removed.

○ 3. The client remains alert during suctioning.

○ 4. The client's skin is warm and dry.

85 A neighbor tells a nurse that her child has been exposed to chickenpox. Which drug should the nurse warn the mother to avoid using if the child develops a fever or discomfort?

○ 1. acetaminophen (Tylenol)

○ 2. ibuprofen (Advil)

○ 3. aspirin (Anacin)

○ 4. indomethacin (Indocin)

86 During the first stage of labor the nurse finds that the fetal heart rate gradually slows and reaches its lowest point during a contraction; it returns to normal near the end of the contraction. Which of the following is *most* appropriate based on this assessment?

○ 1. No action is indicated at this time.

○ 2. Notify the obstetrician immediately.

○ 3. Turn the client onto her back in bed.

○ 4. Elevate the head of the client's bed.

87 A client in labor tells the nurse that her contractions are occurring every 10 minutes. The correct method for timing the frequency of contractions is to count the time interval between the

○ 1. beginning of one contraction to the end of the contraction.

○ 2. end of one contraction and the beginning of the next one.

○ 3. beginning of one contraction and the end of the next one.

○ 4. beginning of one contraction and the beginning of the next.

88 While irrigating a colostomy, the client complains of severe cramping. The nurse's *best* course of action in this situation is to
- ○ 1. remove the irrigating cone for a few minutes.
- ○ 2. instruct the client to bear down and grunt.
- ○ 3. stop administering the solution temporarily.
- ○ 4. increase the rate of fluid instillation.

89 Which one of the following comments made by a client who is taking aspirin is *most* likely due to the effects of the drug therapy?
- ○ 1. "My thoughts are racing."
- ○ 2. "I'm urinating a lot."
- ○ 3. "I've developed diarrhea."
- ○ 4. "I hear buzzing in my ears."

90 A patient is given a prescription for the benzodiazepine alprazolam (Xanax). Which of the following indicates that the client understands the implications of taking this drug? The client says
- ○ 1. he should not drink alcohol while taking this drug.
- ○ 2. he will need to continue taking this drug lifelong.
- ○ 3. this drug can cause insomnia in some people.
- ○ 4. a blood test will be required periodically.

91 A nurse observes all of the following behaviors in a hospitalized toddler. Which is the *best* evidence that the child is reacting severely to being separated from his parents?
- ○ 1. The child prefers to play with toys by himself.
- ○ 2. The child ignores his parents when they visit.
- ○ 3. The child experiences anorexia and weight loss.
- ○ 4. The child takes a morning and afternoon nap.

92 A nursing assistant asks what she can give a client to drink who just returned from a tonsillectomy. The *best* recommendation is
- ○ 1. hot tea.
- ○ 2. warm bullion.
- ○ 3. cold water.
- ○ 4. orange juice.

93 A child ingests an unknown quantity of pills. When the child eventually vomits after the administration of syrup of ipecac, the *most* important nursing action would be to
- ○ 1. provide mouth care.
- ○ 2. examine the emesis.
- ○ 3. measure the emesis.
- ○ 4. document the effect.

94 Immediately following an injury to the musculoskeletal system, the *best* measure the nurse can use to relieve swelling is to
- ○ 1. wrap the part in a warm compress.
- ○ 2. soak the part in warm running water.
- ○ 3. apply an ice bag to the injured area.
- ○ 4. bind the area tightly with a firm support.

95 Which one of the following is the *best* plan the nurse can use to facilitate drying a plaster cast?
- ○ 1. Increase the temperature of the room.
- ○ 2. Turn the client every 1 to 2 hours.
- ○ 3. Fan the wet cast with folded newspaper.
- ○ 4. Take the client outside in the sun.

96 Which one of the following statements made by a primigravida would indicate to the nurse that "lightening" has occurred?
- ○ 1. "I'm not as hungry as I used to be."
- ○ 2. "My backaches seem to be relieved."
- ○ 3. "I can breathe so much more easily now."
- ○ 4. "I've noticed slight contractions lately."

97 Which one of the following would be the *best* evidence that rescue breathing is being performed appropriately?
- ○ 1. The chest rises when air is forced in.
- ○ 2. The pupils of both eyes are dilated.
- ○ 3. A carotid pulse is palpated at the neck.
- ○ 4. The rescuer forms a seal over the nose.

98 A rectal tube is ordered for a client who has abdominal distention. The client experiences no relief after the tube has been in place for approximately 20 minutes. The *best* action for the nurse to take at this time is to
- ○ 1. rotate the tube several times within the rectum.
- ○ 2. insert the rectal tube farther into the rectum.
- ○ 3. remove the tube and reinsert it in 2 to 3 hours.
- ○ 4. replace the tube with one with a larger diameter.

99 The nurse observes resuscitation efforts on a 6-month-old infant. Cardiac compressions are being administered *correctly* if the rescuer uses
- ○ 1. both hands.
- ○ 2. two fingers.
- ○ 3. the heel of one hand.
- ○ 4. the palm of one hand.

100 A person reports taking all of the following medications. Which one places the client at risk for thromboembolism?
- ○ 1. Iron supplement
- ○ 2. Oral contraceptive
- ○ 3. Nasal decongestant
- ○ 4. Stomach antacid

101 The best time for the nurse to plan to perform postural drainage is when the client
- ○ 1. has an empty stomach.
- ○ 2. feels short of breath.
- ○ 3. experiences coughing.
- ○ 4. says it is necessary.

102 Which one of the following is the *earliest* indication that a person is hypoxic?
- ○ 1. Cyanosis

○ 2. Disorientation
○ 3. Restlessness
○ 4. Hypotension

103 Following a perineal prostatectomy for cancer of the prostate, which one of the following nursing actions is *essential* to include on the written plan for care?
○ 1. Perform Valsalva's maneuver during defecation.
○ 2. Maintain high Fowler's position postoperatively.
○ 3. Administer laxatives to promote bowel elimination.
○ 4. Provide perineal care following each bowel movement.

104 If a client has obstructive jaundice, which one of the following is the nurse *most* likely to observe?
○ 1. Urine appears dark brown.
○ 2. Saliva is thick and paste-like.
○ 3. Stool is green and watery.
○ 4. Skin is hot, warm, and dry.

105 In the early postoperative period, a client with a cataract extraction should be taught to *avoid* activity that includes
○ 1. turning in bed.
○ 2. breathing deeply.
○ 3. bending over.
○ 4. moving his head.

106 A child with asthma is receiving aminophylline (theophylline) by intravenous infusion. Which one of the following adverse effects is the nurse *likely* to observe?
○ 1. Bradycardia
○ 2. Drowsiness
○ 3. Restlessness
○ 4. Hypotension

107 The *best* position for the client that the nurse should plan to use when assisting with an abdominal paracentesis is
○ 1. sitting up.
○ 2. standing.
○ 3. lying on the back.
○ 4. lying on either side.

108 A nurse collects information to prepare the discharge plan for a client. If the client describes having all of the following items in her home, the one that presents the *greatest* safety hazard is a
○ 1. television set in the bedroom.
○ 2. shower rather than a bathtub.
○ 3. throw rug in front of the bedroom door.
○ 4. grounded electric outlet in the kitchen.

109 When performing a physical assessment on a person with anorexia nervosa, which of the following should the nurse look for to support that the client has an eating disorder?

○ 1. Growth of fine body hair
○ 2. Bruises over the upper torso
○ 3. Hyperactive bowel sounds
○ 4. Club-shaped fingertips

110 Which of the following statements best indicates that a client has understood the instructions concerning a computerized axial tomography (CAT) body scan?
○ 1. "I will be asked to change my position several times."
○ 2. "I will need to drink a quart of water before the test."
○ 3. "I will hear clicking noises as the test is performed."
○ 4. "I will have several blood samples taken during the test."

111 When the nurse performs a physical assessment, which one of the following is *likely* to be associated with lithium carbonate (Lithane) therapy?
○ 1. Hirsutism
○ 2. Striae
○ 3. Hand tremors
○ 4. Coated tongue

112 The nurse must assess the vital signs of an uncooperative 3-year-old child with hemophilia. Which of the following plans for assessing body temperature would be the *safest* technique to use in this case?
○ 1. Use an oral electronic thermometer.
○ 2. Take an axillary temperature.
○ 3. Use a tympanic thermometer.
○ 4. Take the temperature rectally.

113 What effect, if any, would the nurse expect acute congestive heart failure to have on the central venous pressure (CVP) measurement? The measurement would *likely*
○ 1. be above normal.
○ 2. be below normal.
○ 3. fluctuate widely each time it is taken.
○ 4. remain unchanged from normal ranges.

114 A 10-year-old child is admitted with subacute bacterial endocarditis. If this child is typical of most with this condition, the nurse would suspect that it has been caused by
○ 1. a defect that developed prior to birth.
○ 2. an untreated streptococcal infection.
○ 3. inadequate nutrition during childhood.
○ 4. failure to receive proper immunizations.

115 An adult client has experienced a mild allergic reaction to an antibiotic and receives diphenhydramine hydrochloride (Benadryl) to counteract it. Which of the following would *best* indicate that the adverse reaction has been controlled? The client's
○ 1. respirations are 22 per minute and effortless.

○ 2. diastolic blood pressure is stable at 54 mm Hg.

○ 3. pulse rate is 104 per minute and regular.

○ 4. urine is clear, light yellow, and odorless.

116 A person who undergoes a radical prostatectomy for advanced cancer is receiving diethylstilbesterol. Which one of the following is *likely* to be an effect of this drug?

○ 1. Increased facial hair

○ 2. Testicular atrophy

○ 3. Deepening of the voice

○ 4. Weight loss

117 What information is *most* essential for the nurse to report and record when discontinuing the administration of intravenous fluid?

○ 1. The volume of fluid infused

○ 2. The name of the client's physician

○ 3. The time the infusion started

○ 4. The rate of fluid infusion

118 Following the physician's explanation of the risks and benefits of a transurethral resection of the prostate (TURP), the best evidence that the client understands the effect this surgery will have on his sexual function is the statement

○ 1. "I won't ejaculate normally anymore."

○ 2. "I won't have an orgasm anymore."

○ 3. "I won't have an erection anymore."

○ 4. "I won't desire to have sex anymore."

119 The nurse reviews the plan of care for an elderly client. If the client has dry, flaky skin, which of the following instructions on the care plan is *most* appropriate for the identified problem?

○ 1. Offer an evening snack.

○ 2. Bathe every other day.

○ 3. Ambulate twice daily.

○ 4. File fingernails weekly.

120 The nurse finds a diabetic client perspiring, feeling weak, and trembling. After administering orange juice, which of the following is the *best* indication that the nurse's efforts have been successful?

○ 1. The client says he is hungry.

○ 2. The client's skin is cool.

○ 3. The blood sugar is normal.

○ 4. The blood pressure is stable.

Correct Answers and Rationale

Two numbers appear in parentheses following each rationale. The first number identifies the textbook listed in the references, page 451, and the second number identifies the page(s) in that textbook on which the correct answer can be verified. Occasionally, two textbooks are given for verifying the correct answer.

1 3. Typical signs that indicate a tracheostomy needs suctioning include noisy respirations, dyspnea, and increased respiratory and pulse rates. Auscultation of the chest helps most to determine when suctioning of a tracheostomy should be done. (18:718)
Nursing Process—Collecting data
Client Need—Physiological integrity

2 3. Giving oxygen before suctioning prevents hypoxemia and hypoxia while removing air and debris from the upper airway. Before inserting the catheter, saline may be instilled to liquefy thick secretions. The catheter is then inserted. Once the tip is at the desired level, usually 6 to 10 in, the vent is occluded, and the catheter is twisted as it is removed. The client is then reoxygenated a second time. (18:718; 3:417)
Nursing Process—Planning
Client Need—Safe, effective care environment

3 1. A hearing aid only amplifies sound waves that are transmitted by air and bone conduction. If a person currently hears garbled, distorted sound, he will continue to hear these same sounds, only more loudly with a hearing aid. (3:860; 7:694)
Nursing Process—Implementation
Client Need—Health promotion/maintenance

4 2. Owing to local anesthesia, swallowing is impaired until the gag reflex returns. If food or fluids are provided in the absence of a gag reflex, aspiration may occur. Taking the radial pulse and raising the head of the bed are appropriate. Providing a blanket is a comfort measure. (3:377)
Nursing Process—Evaluation
Client Need—Safe, effective care environment

5 2. It is generally the best policy to allow an angry person to express his feelings. By remaining neutral the nurse demonstrates acceptance of the client as a person. The nurse acts as a role model for assisting him to regain control. Using humor, leaving him, or providing an explanation may add to his angry feelings at the moment. (12:358-359)
Nursing Process—Implementation
Client Need—Psychosocial integrity

6 1. Most people with a retinal detachment describe seeing flashes of light. Only the most profoundly blind cannot see light. Photophobia is associated with many primary and secondary disorders, but generally it is not experienced by someone with a retinal detachment. The client with a retinal detachment generally retains vision in a large portion of the retina. The visual defect is evident only in the area of the tear or separation of the sensory layer from the pigmented layer. Therefore, in the intact retina, vision during daylight would be unchanged. (16:500-501; 7:688)
Nursing Process—Collecting data
Client Need—Safe, effective care environment

7 2. This child most likely has "nursing bottle syndrome." It is associated with allowing a child to go to sleep while sucking on a bottle that contains a sugar-sweetened beverage. A 2-year-old child should not be independently responsible for his own oral hygiene. Although an unsweetened vitamin would be preferable, the amount of sugar in a daily vitamin ought not cause severe dental decay at this age. Thumb sucking will not have a detrimental effect as long as it is not prolonged beyond the time that the second set of teeth have erupted. (8:382; 14:647; 19:399)
Nursing Process—Collecting data
Client Need—Health promotion/maintenance

8 3. When a child is in Bryant's traction, the buttocks should just clear the mattress. The ropes that lead to pulleys above the bed keep the child's legs at a 90-degree angle to his trunk. The child should not sit up or use a trapeze. The legs should be pulled toward the ceiling. (3:644; 18:696)
Nursing Process—Evaluation
Client Need—Safe, effective care environment

9 3. During a sickle cell crisis, the nurse should plan to assess, intervene, and evaluate the client's level of discomfort. At this time, severe pain in the chest, joints, and abdomen is common. Analgesics are often administered routinely. The type of analgesic, the dosage, or its administration schedule may need frequent adjustment depending on the response of the client. Activity,

including a client's self-care, is usually limited during sickle cell crisis to prevent tissue hypoxia. Although helping a chronically ill client improve his self-esteem is an appropriate nursing goal, it would not be a priority during the acute phase of the person's illness. (7:420; 16:374)
> Nursing Process—Planning
> Client Need—Physiological integrity

10 4. To avoid additional injury to the skin, the client should use gentle washing with warm water and a soft cloth. Water will not harm the skin, but harsh soaps, lotions, alcohol-based cosmetics, and rubbing the skin should be avoided. Covering the reddened area with clear plastic will not serve any therapeutic purpose. (16:212; 3:280)
> Nursing Process—Implementation
> Client Need—Physiological integrity

11 4. The client should be advised to see her physician promptly, the same day if at all possible. A persistent headache may be insignificant, but it could be an accompanying sign of pregnancy-induced hypertension, formerly known as toxemia or eclampsia. Any of the other suggestions may be appropriate after the client has been assessed further. (8:184; 19:84)
> Nursing Process—Planning
> Client Need—Health promotion/maintenance

12 3. The client's physician should always be consulted before attempting to cut the toenails of a person with peripheral vascular disease. If tissue on the feet and lower extremities is injured, these people are slow to heal. Impaired skin may become infected or necrotic owing to poor circulation. It may be appropriate to refer this type of care to a podiatrist, a person with special training in the care of feet. For people who are essentially healthy, the feet should be soaked first before cutting the nails. The nails can then be trimmed straight across using special toenail clippers. (18:114; 14:991; 3:509)
> Nursing Process—Implementation
> Client Need—Safe, effective care environment

13 1. Children with cystic fibrosis lose abnormally large amounts of salt in their perspiration. Vomiting immediately after eating is a sign of pyloric stenosis, a condition generally manifested shortly after birth. Soft, bright yellow stools are a characteristic of breastfed infants. In cystic fibrosis the stools are large, foamy, and foul-smelling. Dilute urine, as produced in people with diabetes insipidus, is very light colored. (8:697-698; 19:650)
> Nursing Process—Collecting data
> Client Need—Safe, effective care environment

14 3. Corneas are not refused based on the age of the donor. It is not legal to sell organs or tissue in the United States. The demand for donor organs and tissue far exceeds the supply. The nurse should contact the designated organ procurement coordinator whenever there is a potential organ donor available. (18:752, 755)
> Nursing Process—Implementation
> Client Need—Safe, effective care environment

15 1. It can be life-threatening if a person discontinues taking a prescribed corticosteroid abruptly. Acute adrenal insufficiency can occur. This condition also is called Addisonian crisis or adrenal crisis. Death may occur owing to fluid volume depletion, hypotension, and shock. Taking steroid medication should not interfere with a person's reaction time. A dose of medication should never be doubled without consulting a health professional. Although long-term therapy causes many side effects, some people need to take steroid medication for the rest of their lives. (16:208; 3:724)
> Nursing Process—Evaluation
> Client Need—Health promotion/maintenance

16 3. An audible stridor, sometimes described as a croaking, squeaking, or high-pitched wheezing sound, can be heard when there is partial obstruction of the upper air passages. A client's voice may be hoarse from irritation due to passage of the instrument. As long as the client can cough, air can pass through the respiratory passages. Respiratory impairment is manifested by a rapid respiratory rate. (3:395; 14:431)
> Nursing Process—Collecting data
> Client Need—Physiological integrity

17 1. Daily to weekly weights are a way of monitoring the effectiveness or compliance of a client who takes a diuretic at home. Other valuable assessments the nurse could perform would be to measure the client's blood pressure, listen to lung sounds, and inspect the skin for signs of edema. Pulse rate, appetite, and reflexes are not affected by diuretics. (15:127; 16:335)
> Nursing Process—Evaluation
> Client Need—Physiological integrity

18 1. The dosage of nitroglycerin ointment is ordered in inches. The nurse should squeeze a ribbon of the drug onto calibrated application paper. The paper can be placed on the chest, back, or arms, not necessarily over the heart area. Applying it over the heart may interfere with the assessment of heart sounds or in obtaining an apical pulse rate, or it may create hazards if the client must be defibrillated in an emergency. It is covered with plastic wrap and taped to hold it in place.

The nurse must avoid coming into direct skin contact with the ointment while measuring or applying it. Contact will result in the nurse absorbing the medication as well. The drug need not be rubbed into the skin. (5:110; 18:588)
Nursing Process—Implementation
Client Need—Physiological integrity

19 3. An infant should receive controlled, gentle breaths of air from the rescuer. They are sometimes described as "puffs" of air. The volume of air should be just large enough to make the chest rise. The rate of rescue breaths for an infant should be approximately 20 per minute. (8:549; 18:741)
Nursing Process—Implementation
Client Need—Health promotion/maintenance

20 2. Maintaining and improving oxygenation is a priority goal when planning the nursing care of a client with an acute respiratory infection. In some circumstances, such as if there are moist secretions in the airways, it is important to promote coughing rather than relieve it. Nourishment is important in the care of any person with an infection. However, impaired breathing is more life-threatening than a brief reduction in caloric intake. Eventually assuming self-care would be desirable. During the acute phase of illness, however, providing rest and assistance to reduce oxygen requirements would be appropriate. (3:398; 16:253)
Nursing Process—Planning
Client Need—Physiological integrity

21 2. A stable blood pressure is the best evidence that a client who has undergone hemodialysis has adjusted to the alteration in his fluid balance. Warm, dry skin also is a good sign that blood circulation is adequate, but it is not as measurable a criterion. Loss of weight indicates only that dialysis was effective; it is not an indication of how the client has tolerated the procedure. Feeling less fatigued is a subjective evaluative statement that supports that hemodialysis has had a therapeutic outcome; however, more objective evidence should be obtained for evaluation purposes. (3:541; 16:767)
Nursing Process—Evaluation
Client Need—Physiological integrity

22 3. The name of the drug is essential in determining the potential effects and what treatment may be needed. Secondly, determining the approximate number of pills would help assess the potential lethality of the overdose. It would also be important to determine how long ago they were taken. While the client's life is threatened, discussing the reason for the overdose is not a priority. The source of the pills will not affect the client's treatment. (16:182; 3:879)
Nursing Process—Collecting data
Client Need—Physiological integrity

23 3. Custom-made ear plugs are used as a barrier against water entering through the tubes used to equalize pressure within the middle ear. Suppurative (producing pus) otitis media is a potential consequence of introducing water from these activities. There are no dietary restrictions while tympanostomy tubes are in place. The child's hearing should improve as pressure within the middle ear is relieved. Instilling water would be contraindicated for the same reasons that water from swimming and showering is prohibited from entering the ear. (8:707; 14:980)
Nursing Process—Planning
Client Need—Health promotion/maintenance

24 4. Sterile gloves are used to prevent introducing organisms into the client's respiratory tract. The client can be instructed to cough before suctioning and breathe deeply during preoxygenation. Panting breaths promote oxygenation during suctioning. To ease the passage of the catheter, it is premoistened by dipping the end into sterile normal saline. Suction should not be applied until the catheter is situated about 6 to 10 in (15 to 25 cm) into the respiratory passageway for a client with a tracheostomy. (14:818; 18:718)
Nursing Process—Implementation
Client Need—Physiological integrity

25 1. Observing if a client can move the fingers or toes on the extremity within a cast is the best method for assessing neurologic function. Muscles cannot move unless the nervous system is intact. Monitoring capillary refill, feeling the skin temperature, and inspecting the size of exposed fingers or toes are techniques for assessing the vascular status. (18:692)
Nursing Process—Collecting data
Client Need—Physiological integrity

26 2. People who develop anorexia nervosa often are described as being perfect children. They perform above average in school and often participate in a variety of extracurricular activities. Anorectics are not uniquely the middle child or sickly during childhood. No data suggest that a characteristic of this disease is a feeling that others dislike them. (17:380; 4:297)
Nursing Process—Collecting data
Client Need—Psychosocial integrity

27 1. Reasonable weight gain is expected during pregnancy. Poor nutrition owing to poverty or lack of knowledge is a leading contributor to high risk during pregnancy. It is important to the health of the mother and the infant to eat a variety of foods. Many physicians do not restrict sexual activity during pregnancy unless complications, such as uterine bleeding, have occurred or the amniotic sac has ruptured. A certain amount of regular exercise is preferable to sporadic activity. The type and amount of exercise depends on the health, habits, and obstetric history of each person. Pregnancy beyond age 35 is more likely to be considered a risk factor. (8:169; 19:308, 310)

    Nursing Process—Collecting data
    Client Need—Health promotion/maintenance

28 4. A client weighing 88 lb should receive 80 mg of drug prescribed at 2 mg/kg. There are 2.2 lb/kg; therefore, 88 lb divided by 2.2 equals 40 kg. Because the client should receive 2 mg for every kilogram, the nurse would then multiply $2 \times 40 = 80$ mg. Using the ratio–proportion method, the dosage can be calculated as follows: (15:12; 18:574)

Step 1 (known ratio to unknown ratio):
$$\frac{2 \text{ mg}}{1 \text{ kg}} \times \frac{X \text{ kg}}{40 \text{ kg}}$$

Step 2 (across multiply and solve for X):
$1 X = 80$
$X = 80$

    Nursing Process—Implementation
    Client Need—Physiological integrity

29 2. Oxytocin produces uterine contraction, causing the muscle to become firm and hard. This action helps to control postpartum bleeding and hemorrhage. When administered as a nasal spray it stimulates the milk ejection reflex. (8:106; 15:225)

    Nursing Process—Evaluation
    Client Need—Physiological integrity

30 2. Increased physical activity helps sustain an increased elevation in the basal metabolic rate for a prolonged period of time, thus using more calories. Exercise also firms muscle and reduces stress. Appetite suppressants increase cardiac risks and are effective only for short-term use. Fasting is not a nutritionally sound approach to weight loss. Most adults require more than 1000 calories per day to avoid ketoacidosis. Very low calorie diets should be attempted only under the supervision of a physician. Generally, this type of diet is reserved for people who are more than 40% overweight and should not be maintained longer than 2 to 3 months. (4:373-374)

    Nursing Process—Planning
    Client Need—Health promotion/maintenance

31 4. Paraphrasing the content of the client's statement is a therapeutic communication technique. It helps the client know that the message was heard and how it was interpreted. This technique likely will encourage the client to continue verbalizing. Classifying the statement as an exaggeration is belittling. Telling the client that talking will contribute to sadness indirectly is saying that this line of communication should cease. Demanding an explanation by asking "why" also is a block to therapeutic communication. It requires that the client justify a rationale for the statement and puts the client on the defensive. (12:260; 17:69)

    Nursing Process—Implementation
    Client Need—Psychosocial integrity

32 1. It is important to keep the client at rest and his head in a dependent position. It is best to keep the room darkened because bright lights cause discomfort when drugs are used to dilate the pupil. There is no need to restrict fluids following surgery for a detached retina. (7:689-690; 14:972)

    Nursing Process—Planning
    Client Need—Physiological integrity

33 2. Acetylsalicylic acid, also known as aspirin, interferes with platelet aggregation. Salicylates should be avoided preoperatively and postoperatively to reduce the potential for hemorrhage. (15:71)

    Nursing Process—Implementation
    Client Need—Health promotion/maintenance

34 4. If the pubococcygeal muscles are being contracted and relaxed properly during the performance of Kegel exercises, the client should be able to stop and restart the flow of urine during voiding. Kegel exercises are performed to relieve stress incontinence. (18:509; 8:79)

    Nursing Process—Evaluation
    Client Need—Health promotion/maintenance

35 1. The most predominant finding associated with this condition is the characteristic cough, which is described as barking, seal-like, hoarse, or brassy. The child is usually restless owing to anxiety and hypoxia. Although the child may have had an earlier upper respiratory infection, symptoms of croup are localized in the larynx, trachea, and bronchi. There may be occasional, but not severe, vomiting accompanying croup. The vomiting is related to the laryngospasm rather than to gastrointestinal upset. (14:650; 8:702; 19:634)

    Nursing Process—Collecting data
    Client Need—Safe, effective care environment

36 3. The nurse should wear a sturdy latex glove or a double finger cot as a barrier against contact with the shedding virus. Handwashing should follow removal of the protective hand cover. Touching the tube to the lesion would transfer the virus to the tip and mouth of the container. The nurse should select the type of universal precaution garments according to the nursing care that will be provided. Gloves are always essential when there is the potential for direct contact. The entire vesicle should be covered with ointment. (3:785; 14:930)

>   Nursing Process—Implementation
>   Client Need—Health promotion/maintenance

37 3. Apgar scoring involves rating the baby's appearance (skin color), heart rate, response to a catheter inserted in the nostril, activity, and respiratory effort. (8:140; 19:846)

>   Nursing Process—Collecting data
>   Client Need—Health promotion/maintenance

38 3. Charting should be as clear and objective as possible. Quoting the client is always appropriate. Interpreting or labeling what the nurse suspects is occurring is not the best form of documentation. (14:273; 18:65)

>   Nursing Process—Implementation
>   Client Need—Safe, effective care environment

39 4. Adults who are unable to control their elimination are extremely anxious and distressed. The best approach for preserving a client's self-esteem in this situation would be to assist the client immediately in a nonjudgmental manner. Assigning only male personnel to his care, asking the client's wife to assist, and holding the client responsible are likely to communicate nonverbally that this type of care is disgusting. Delegating this form of care is more likely to damage the client's self-esteem. (16:562; 9:75)

>   Nursing Process—Planning
>   Client Need—Psychosocial integrity

40 3. Dried food substances rehydrate in the presence of any liquid substance. Once rehydrated, the enlarged vegetative matter is likely to become impacted within the ear canal. Pounding the side of the head may move liquid trapped within the ear but not an impacted object. Using a blow dryer is likely to be tedious and, most likely, ineffective. (7:695; 14:979)

>   Nursing Process—Planning
>   Client Need—Health promotion/maintenance

41 1. To remove an object from the airway of an unconscious, nonpregnant adult, the rescuer administers six to ten forceful thrusts upward from the abdomen. If the abdominal thrusts do not clear the airway, the rescuer should attempt a finger sweep followed by two breaths. The cycle is repeated until respiration is restored. If the

adult is conscious, the abdominal thrusts are repeated until the object is dislodged or the victim becomes unconscious. Ventilating the client will be ineffective as long as the airway is obstructed. Chest compressions are performed when the victim no longer has a pulse. (18:715; 14:432)

>   Nursing Process—Implementation
>   Client Need—Physiological integrity

42 3. Performing self-care indicates that a client has progressed from denial and anger into a stage of acceptance. Wearing loose-fitting garments can be an attempt to hide the change in body image. Applying cologne heavily indicates that the client is self-conscious about possible fecal odor. There could be many reasons a client could ask to see a clergyman. (16:593; 18:563)

>   Nursing Process—Evaluation
>   Client Need—Psychosocial integrity

43 2. Following any barium procedure the nurse should monitor the client's bowel elimination. Retained barium can cause constipation and even bowel obstruction. A laxative or some other method for promoting the passage of the stool may be needed if elimination is delayed. The color of the stool will likely appear white or chalky. (14:849; 18:312)

>   Nursing Process—Collecting data
>   Client Need—Physiological integrity

44 2. Inhaling moist air will help liquefy secretions. The warm droplets are soothing and may reduce edema by increasing blood flow in the respiratory passages. Milk and milk products tend to increase the production of mucus. Limiting the child's activity will reduce his need for oxygen but will not promote expectoration. Aspirin will reduce a fever. However, unless the fever is dangerously high, the increased temperature may be beneficial in controlling the growth of the infectious agent causing the symptoms. The American Academy of Pediatrics does not recommend giving aspirin to children with symptoms associated with influenza or chickenpox because of the link with Reye's syndrome. (8:702; 19:634, 651)

>   Nursing Process—Implementation
>   Client Need—Health promotion/maintenance

45 2. The female nurse assigned to care for the client with a radioactive implant should be certain that she is not pregnant. Acute or chronic exposure to ionizing radiation can cause gene mutation and birth defects. All nurses are at risk from radiation if they do not follow time, distance, and shielding precautions. The presence of a chronic disease or the last place of employment would not be a factor in making the assignment. (7:202; 14:709)

Nursing Process—Collecting data
Client Need—Safe, effective care environment

46 4. An unplanned pregnancy is a type of situational crisis. Crisis intervention involves assessing a client's access to a network of supportive people. Determining how the family feels about the pregnancy will aid in selecting nursing interventions that either build on the family's support or explore other alternatives with the client. Acquiring facts about the baby's father, the client's knowledge of contraception, or reasons for becoming sexually active are not as pertinent to the emotional impact the pregnancy may be having on the unwed mother. (1:128; 12:91)

Nursing Process—Collecting data
Client Need—Psychosocial integrity

47 3. Wire-cutting scissors should be at the bedside of a client with a repaired fracture of the mandible. The fractured bones are fixated with wire. The nurse should be prepared to cut the wire if there is a potential for aspiration in the case of vomiting or impaired swallowing. Nutrition is maintained by providing the client with a diet consisting of liquid or semiliquid food. A tracheostomy set is not usually needed because the airway is generally patent except in instances where vomiting may occur. There would be no purpose for having a rubber tourniquet or gastric tube at the bedside. (16:782-783)

Nursing Process—Planning
Client Need—Physiological integrity

48 1. To detect the presence of thrombophlebitis, the nurse would have the client dorsiflex each foot separately and note if calf pain is experienced. The presence of calf pain is considered a positive Homan's sign and should be reported immediately. Palpating the pedal pulse is a method of assessing distal arterial blood flow. The client may guard the use of a leg with a thrombophlebitis while walking and may even have a slightly elevated temperature. However, these are not the primary assessment techniques for detecting a thrombophlebitis. (3:511; 14:450)

Nursing Process—Collecting data
Client Need—Physiological integrity

49 1. An enterostomal therapist is a health professional who is certified in the specialized care of people who have ostomies. A gastroenterologist is a physician who has specialized in the diagnosis and treatment of all pathology occurring in the gastrointestinal system. A gastronomer is a person who judges cooking. An entomologist is a person who studies insects. (18:565; 14:856)

Nursing Process—Planning
Client Need—Safe, effective care environment

50 1. Missing a dose of disulfiram will not cause a reaction. The reaction occurs when the client ingests or applies alcohol to his skin. To make sure that a reaction does not occur, the client should abstain from alcohol for at least 2 weeks or more after the drug is discontinued. (1:190; 9:235-236)

Nursing Process—Evaluation
Client Need—Safe, effective care environment

51 2. Universal precautions should be followed whenever there is a potential for direct contact with blood, as in removing a needle from an intravenous site. It would be appropriate to pull the privacy curtain and lower the side rail, but it is not essential. It is not essential to weigh a client after discontinuing fluid therapy. (18:361; 14:318)

Nursing Process—Implementation
Client Need—Safe, effective care environment

52 2. When a client indicates signs or symptoms of anxiety, it is best for the nurse to help him to express his concerns. Belittling his fears by saying "there is no need for fear," using a reassuring cliché such as "trust me" and "you have an excellent surgeon," and giving advice such as "try to relax" are all nontherapeutic communication techniques. (12:260; 18:21-22)

Nursing Process—Implementation
Client Need—Psychosocial integrity

53 3. Topical anesthesia is needed when a tonometer is used to measure the pressure within a client's eyes. The anesthetic, prepared in liquid eye drop form, makes it possible to apply the tonometer on the cornea without the client feeling as if something is touching the eye. A reflex hammer is used to test deep tendon reflexes. A speculum should be available to remove vaginal secretions. An otoscope would be needed for examining the eardrums. None of the latter three involve using topical anesthesia. (18:303; 7:670)

Nursing Process—Planning
Client Need—Safe, effective care environment

54 3. Eric Erikson describes generativity as a concern for leaving something of worth to society. Adults over the age of 40 seek to identify a positive contribution for which they will be most remembered. For some, their legacy is having been a good parent, an upstanding citizen, or a community volunteer or performing more tangible activities, such as writing, painting, and so on. (17:159; 12:112)

Nursing Process—Collecting data
Client Need—Health promotion/maintenance

55 2. It is a common orthodox Jewish practice to refrain from eating pork and to eat only food that has been kosher prepared. Most reformed and orthodox Jewish men wear a *yarmulke*, or skull cap, especially on the Sabbath or when attending synagogue. Hebrew is commonly spoken by people who have immigrated from Israel. Many Christian and Jewish men are circumcised. (4:248-249; 18:123)

> Nursing Process—Collecting data
> Client Need—Safe, effective care environment

56 1. Covering the opening from which a chest tube was pulled would prevent air from entering and totally collapsing the lung. Once the tube is out, its sterility could not be ensured. If replaced, a new one should be used. Applying suction would not be adequate to keep the lung from recollapsing. Holding his breath may help temporarily, but the client could not sustain his effort. (3:414)

> Nursing Process—Implementation
> Client Need—Physiological integrity

57 3. Talking and dealing with an anxiety-provoking experience are healthier than avoiding or suppressing. Failing to deal with the terror is thought to cause the symptoms associated with this disorder. Most people can sense if an individual is acting rather than expressing sincere feelings. Associating with others does not ensure that a person verbally will share their emotional issues. Taking vacations and participating in pleasurable activities are forms of stress management, but they are not the best approaches for processing the impact of a traumatic event. (17:274)

> Nursing Process—Planning
> Client Need—Psychosocial integrity

58 4. Visually checking the position of extremities is a sign that the client is adapting to the loss of sensation and even lack of recognition of the structures on the paralyzed side of the body. The ability to express or understand speech is more often a problem experienced by people with a cerebrovascular accident rather than speaking in a normal tone. Participating in self-care is evidence of physical rehabilitation. Sharing feelings would be a sign of emotional progress. (3:343; 7:645)

> Nursing Process—Evaluation
> Client Need—Health promotion/maintenance

59 3. An increase in urinary output is a sign of therapeutic effectiveness in response to treatment of acute glomerulonephritis with corticosteroids. Blood pressure should decrease from previously hypertensive levels as renal function improves. Long- and short-term high-dose therapy with corticosteroids is likely to create muscle weakness and atrophy. Weight gain is a nontherapeu-

tic effect from altered glucose metabolism and sodium retention. (15:206; 19:727)

> Nursing Process—Evaluation
> Client Need—Physiological integrity

60 1. Oral hygiene should be given promptly because the residual odor and taste of the gastric contents is very offensive. Ordinarily, the client begins taking clear liquid nourishment. If the client tolerates clear liquids, the diet can progress to more solid food. Administering an analgesic is not usually necessary. Intake and output should be continued until the client's fluid balance is validated following the resumption of eating. (18:141; 14:852)

> Nursing Process—Planning
> Client Need—Physiological integrity

61 3. One criterion for evaluating how a person is coping with grief is the ability to discuss future plans. Controlling emotions is not necessarily a healthy behavior. Asking friends to come along to visit shows an effort to maintain a network of support. Researching information may indicate that the client is denying or doubting that the diagnosis is correct or that there may be some unattempted form of treatment. (12:368; 18:769)

> Nursing Process—Evaluation
> Client Need—Psychosocial integrity

62 2. Anxiety is produced when a person feels somehow threatened. This happens commonly among hospitalized clients. One of the best techniques for reducing anxiety is to provide instructions before performing any procedure and to provide explanations when something unexpected, such as an alarm sounding, occurs. Hospitalized clients tend to fantasize and exaggerate the significance of what health personnel know is insignificant. Without an explanation, the client's anxiety is not likely to be relieved by switching the infusion to flow by gravity. Anxiety interferes with attention and concentration; reading is not a realistic option. Medication should not be given until the results of other nursing interventions are evaluated. (9:84; 12:354-355; 18:26)

> Nursing Process—Planning
> Client Need—Psychosocial integrity

63 2. Flaccid muscle tone is the most ominous sign among the choices in the item. A healthy newborn generally is active and displays kicking of the feet and flexion of the arms. It is normal for a healthy newborn to have a pulse rate over 100 and display a loud, vigorous cry. The extremities may appear blue for a short time after delivery while the rest of the body is pink. As the newborn's respirations improve and the baby is warmed, the skin color tends to become pink overall. (8:140; 19:176)

Nursing Process—Collecting data
Client Need—Health promotion/maintenance

64 2. When vaginal bleeding is noted shortly after delivery, the nurse should first massage the uterus. This is often sufficient to cause contraction of the uterus, which may have become relaxed and soft. Normally, with firming of the uterus, bleeding will be controlled. If this conservative care is ineffective, the nurse should then collect more data, such as obtaining a current measurement of vital signs, and inform the physician. Intravenous fluids and drugs may be required if independent nursing measures do not suffice in controlling blood loss through massage. (8:201; 19:118, 121)

Nursing Process—Implementation
Client Need—Physiological integrity

65 2. The main reason people undergoing surgery are taught to perform leg exercises is to prevent the formation of blood clots. Leg exercises aid in circulating venous blood. They are used as a substitute compensating for reduced ambulation and activity. Exercise does maintain muscle strength, reduces dependent edema, and relieves congestion of blood in varicose veins. However, none of these are the primary reason for performing leg exercises postoperatively. (14:450, 806; 18:434)

Nursing Process—Implementation
Client Need—Health promotion/maintenance

66 2. When removing an indwelling catheter, the nurse should first deflate the balloon, retaining it in place. The tubing need not be clamped. It is not a standard of practice to irrigate a catheter prior to its removal. Irrigations are performed only if there is a specific medical order to do so. Hygiene can be provided last. (14:460)

Nursing Process—Implementation
Client Need—Safe, effective care environment

67 3. Giving away treasured possessions is a common sign of potentially suicidal behavior. The client is saying in an indirect way that there will be no need for the possession in the near future. It is unlikely that a depressed client would complain about not getting any rest. It is more common for a depressed client to either have insomnia or sleep excessively. A conflict with a roommate or anticipating discharge is not as strongly indicative of suicidal potentiality as giving away something of value. (17:237)

Nursing Process—Collecting data
Client Need— Psychosocial integrity

68 3. Tetracyclines, of which oxytetracycline is one example, should not be given to children younger than 8 years unless their use is absolutely necessary. This family of antibiotics may cause yellow, gray, or brown discoloration of the teeth, which is permanent. Penicillins, cephalosporins, and aminoglycosides do not discolor the teeth if given to young children. (15:163; 8:330)

Nursing Process—Implementation
Client Need—Physiological integrity

69 4. It would be best to promote reality orientation when any client with dementia becomes confused. Disagreeing with the client interferes with therapeutic effectiveness. Collaborating in the delusion by offering to call the school or indicating that a neighbor will care for the children contributes to the alteration in thought processes. (14:1008; 16:445)

Nursing Process—Implementation
Client Need—Psychosocial integrity

70 3. Milk and milk products are avoided because they increase the production of mucus. Croup is accompanied by a severe cough and often requires expectorants to loosen secretions. Clear liquids, popsicles, gelatin, and other fluids are permitted. (14:651)

Nursing Process—Implementation
Client Need—Safe, effective care environment

71 3. Because it may be difficult to palpate the carotid artery in infants who have short, fat necks, it is now recommended that the brachial artery be used for assessment. The brachial artery is located on the inner side of the upper arm, midway between the elbow and the shoulder. The carotid artery at the side of the neck is used when assessing older victims who have experienced cardiac arrest. (19:385; 18:744)

Nursing Process—Collecting data
Client Need—Physiological integrity

72 4. The nurse's chief concern should be the condition of the client. The first step after any accident is to assess the client. Some injuries may be made worse by movement. Once the nurse has examined the client, adequate help should be obtained to help the person to a safer and more comfortable place. After all the data have been collected and the nurse has provided comfort and reassurance to the client, the accident must be reported to the supervisor. A written description of the accident and its outcome is recorded and kept on file in the agency's administration office. (18:233; 14:413)

Nursing Process—Implementation
Client Need—Physiological integrity

73 4. The best evidence of bonding is that parents hold, touch, and talk to their newborn child. Physical contact tends to stimulate the beginning of parental love and protectiveness. It communicates comfort and security to the infant. Observing others caring for the infant or watching from a distance is not as effective as eye-to-eye and direct skin contact in promoting bonding. Being pleased with the baby's gender is a positive sign, but it is not indicative of the future relationship between parents and an infant. (19:179)

> Nursing Process—Evaluation
> Client Need—Health promotion/maintenance

74 3. Treatment of eating disorders involves dealing with both medical and psychologic issues. However, physiologic needs, such as eating and nutrition, have a higher priority. Once the client's weight is stabilized and weight gain is progressing, the focus can then turn to improving the client's body image and methods of coping. Assertiveness may or may not be a problem among people with anorexia nervosa. (4:298; 18:36)

> Nursing Process—Planning
> Client Need—Physiological integrity

75 3. Gelatin is permitted on a clear-liquid diet. Clear liquid diets include transparent fluids and foods. Milk and items containing milk, such as ice cream and creamed soup, would not be permitted. (4:43; 18:133)

> Nursing Process—Planning
> Client Need—Physiological integrity

76 3. A sign that a client has been able to orient himself is the ability to find his own room without assistance. A nursing measure that may be used to promote orientation is to provide environmental cues, such as putting a name card, a picture, or a ribbon on his room door. Walking with others is not evidence that the client could independently find the dining room. The ability to dress himself is evidence that he is maintaining self-care in relation to activities of daily living. Talking on the telephone indicates that the client has retained the ability to communicate verbally. (1:85; 14:1008)

> Nursing Process—Evaluation
> Client Need—Psychosocial Integrity

77 1. The use of a commode would be an appropriate alternative to reduce the workload of the heart. Shortness of breath may indicate that the heart is unable to adapt to the demands required during ambulation. Oxygen given after elimination and continuing ambulation, even with the assistance of the nurse or a walker, is not likely to prevent or reduce the effort of the heart in response to activity. (8:739; 7:375)

> Nursing Process—Planning
> Client Need—Safe, effective care environment

78 2. To maximally disperse the inhaled drug throughout the lung, it is best to hold the inhaled med-

ication for a few seconds. Immediately exhaling would cause some of the effectiveness of the drug to be diminished. Swallowing the air into the gastrointestinal system would not enhance its therapeutic action. Coughing may cause the aerosolized medication to be displaced into the upper airways. (3:420; 7:321)

> Nursing Process—Implementation
> Client Need—Health promotion/maintenance

79 4. A young child may not be able to verbally indicate the location of discomfort. Pulling at the infected ear is a common indication that the symptoms are related to a middle ear infection. It is normal for a 2-year-old child to want to be held by his mother in a strange environment. Middle ear infections are related to the transmission of pathogens through the eustachian tube to the middle ear. However, teething and swallowing are not directly associated with a primary infectious process in the oropharynx. (19:553; 8:705)

> Nursing Process—Collecting data
> Client Need—Safe, effective care environment

80 2. During an acute attack, clients with Meniere's disease experience severe vertigo accompanied by nausea and vomiting. Meclizine is an antihistamine that is prescribed for motion sickness and vertigo due to vestibular disease. Acetaminophen has antipyretic and analgesic actions. Meperidine is a narcotic analgesic. Triazolam is in the benzodiazepine family of drugs. It is a commonly prescribed drug for promoting sleep. (3:856; 7:699)

> Nursing Process—Implementation
> Client Need—Physiological integrity

81 2. Standing is the natural position men assume when urinating. A male may be psychologically helped to relax his urinary sphincter by simulating normal conditions for urinating as much as possible. Using a bedpan would require that the client stand. This client is already distended. Increasing fluids would add to his discomfort. Perineal exercises help to control stress incontinence. (18:504)

> Nursing Process—Implementation
> Client Need—Physiological integrity

82 3. To maintain the integrity of the skin, the fingernails should be cut short. Some also recommend that the client wear cotton gloves to prevent opening the skin in the event that scratching cannot be controlled. Tepid bathing may relieve the discomfort; warm water may accentuate the itching sensation. Dry cornstarch will absorb perspiration but will not relieve itching. When added to water, starch or oatmeal baths are sometimes prescribed to relieve itching. Some hospitals take special care to launder linen in chemicals that do not contain additional dyes or fragrances, or the linen is rinsed especially well to remove soap residue. This measure would be appropriate if the cause of the client's pruritus was allergy related. (16:603)

Nursing Process—Planning
Client Need—Physiological integrity

83 2. Cocaine is a central nervous system stimulant. It can increase blood pressure, heart rate, and cause cardiac dysrhythmias. Any or all of these cardiovascular side effects can result in chest pain, tachycardia, or palpitations in an otherwise young, healthy person. Opioids, such as heroin, barbiturates, and marijuana, are central nervous system depressants that are more likely to cause bradycardia and hypotension. (15:82-84; 3:470)

Nursing Process—Collecting data
Client Need—Physiological integrity

84 1. A heart rate that remains within 60 to 100 beats per minute is a sign that a client is not suffering hypoxia. Tachycardia and irregular cardiac rhythm are warning signs of oxygen deprivation. The volume of secretions and warm, dry skin are not the best assessments for evaluating the oxygenation status of a client. Loss of consciousness would be a late sign of hypoxia. (3:417; 14:813)

Nursing Process—Evaluation
Client Need—Physiological integrity

85 3. Studies suggest that the use of salicylates, especially aspirin, may be involved in the development of Reye's syndrome in children with chickenpox or influenza. Tylenol could be used safely for the relief of minor symptoms, such as fever and headache associated with this disorder. Ibuprofen and indomethacin are more effective in relieving pain. (8:637; 15:71)

Nursing Process—Implementation
Client Need—Health promotion/maintenance

86 1. Early deceleration described in the stem of this item is a benign condition in which no intervention is indicated. A more ominous sign would be one of late deceleration in which the lowest heart rate occurs after the peak of the contraction and does not return to baseline for at least 20 seconds following the completion of the contraction. If late deceleration occurs, the nurse should turn the client onto her side, elevate the legs, and notify the physician. (7:118-119)

Nursing Process—Implementation
Client Need—Health promotion/maintenance

87 4. The frequency of contractions is the time between the beginning of one contraction and the beginning of the next. The duration of a contraction is the time between the beginning and the end of a single contraction. It is incorrect to calculate the frequency of contractions by timing from the end of one to the beginning of the next or the beginning of one to the end of a second contraction. (7:113; 19:101)

Nursing Process—Collecting data
Client Need—Health promotion/maintenance

88 3. When a client complains of cramping while a colostomy irrigation or enema is being administered, the nurse should stop the instillation temporarily. The cramping is caused by the rapid bowel distention and increased peristalsis. After a brief amount of time, the fluid is redistributed, and the irrigation can be resumed. Bearing down will cause the fluid to be expelled. Increasing the rate will cause more discomfort for the client. (18:564)

Nursing Process—Implementation
Client Need—Physiological integrity

89 4. Buzzing, or tinnitus, is a common side effect experienced by people who take large, frequent doses of aspirin. Neither racing thoughts, polyuria, nor diarrhea are side effects associated with aspirin. (15:257)

Nursing Process—Collecting data
Client Need—Physiological integrity

90 1. Sedative drugs, such as benzodiazepines, should never be mixed with alcohol. When combined, they potentiate the possibility of central nervous system depression. Many people have died accidentally when these two types of drugs have been used in combination. Generally, minor tranquilizers are given in low doses for a short time while a person develops other effective coping techniques. Benzodiazepines cause drowsiness rather than insomnia. Blood levels generally are not indicated to monitor the effectiveness of this particular type of drug therapy. (9:246; 15:85)

Nursing Process—Evaluation
Client Need—Health promotion/maintenance

91 2. The most severe form of separation anxiety is manifested by denial. The child denies the need for his parents by becoming detached and disinterested in their presence. This is a coping mechanism to reduce future feelings of being abandoned. Earlier manifestations of separation anxiety include prolonged crying in the absence of a parent and sadness. It is normal behavior to engage in solitary play and take more than one daytime nap during the toddler years. Weight loss is a concern, but it could be attributed to a number of other circumstances besides depression or anxiety. (8:419-421; 19:469-470)

Nursing Process—Collecting data
Client Need—Psychosocial integrity

92 3. Cold water or crushed ice will promote comfort and relieve swelling. Orange juice is likely to

sting irritated tissue at the back of the throat. Warm or hot liquids can dilate blood vessels and increase bleeding. (3:379; 14:653)
>   Nursing Process—Implementation
>   Client Need—Physiological integrity

93 2. It would be most important to examine the emesis of an overdose client to determine if and how many medications are identifiable. If an antidote is available, the toxic substance must be identified. Mouth care, measuring the emesis, and documenting the effect are important but are not of highest priority. (14:420; 16:182)
>   Nursing Process—Collecting data
>   Client Need—Physiological integrity

94 3. Ice is used immediately following an injury to relieve swelling and control bleeding into the soft tissue. The cold application should be removed after approximately 20 minutes. It may be reapplied again after the skin has returned to a similar temperature of the tissue surrounding it. Intermittent applications of cold can be continued for the first 24 to 36 hours after the injury. In a day or so, when the initial swelling has been controlled, warm applications can provide comfort and promote healing by improving circulation. Binding the area should be done with caution because an injured area may continue to swell. The bandage could act as a tourniquet, impairing circulation even further. (18:490; 7:777)
>   Nursing Process—Implementation
>   Client Need—Physiological integrity

95 2. Turning the client frequently will help to dry the complete circumference of a wet plaster cast. Increasing the heat in the room high enough to have a significant effect on the cast would more than likely make the client feel uncomfortable. Manually fanning the cast would be tedious and time-consuming. There are too many risks to the client's safety in taking him outside in the sun. (18:689; 3:639)
>   Nursing Process—Planning
>   Client Need—Physiological integrity

96 3. When a pregnant client indicates that breathing is eased, it is an indication that lightening has occurred. This means that the fetus has settled into the pelvic inlet. Lay people often remark that "the baby has dropped." Multiparas may not experience this phenomenon until just before or during true labor. Lightening may cause backaches to increase owing to the descent of the fetus and relaxation of the pelvic joints prior to delivery. Braxton Hicks contractions are irregular and weak uterine contractions. When these contractions become more noticeable, they are a sign of impending labor. Changes in the appetite are not related to the phenomenon of lightening. (7:109; 19:111)
>   Nursing Process—Collecting data
>   Client Need—Health promotion/maintenance

97 1. Seeing the chest rise is the best evidence that rescue breathing is being performed appropriately. This indicates that the airway is open, and no air is leaking from the victim's nose or mouth. It also indicates that a sufficient volume of air is being administered by the rescuer. Dilated pupils are a sign that the brain is not receiving adequate oxygenation. A pulse indicates that cardiac compressions are not necessary. The rescuer needs to seal or cover both the nose and the mouth. (3:872; 18:737)
>   Nursing Process—Evaluation
>   Client Need—Physiological integrity

98 3. The rectal tube acts as a foreign body and stimulates peristalsis. As the gas is moved toward the rectum, it escapes through the rectal tube. If the rectal tube has not brought relief after approximately 20 minutes, it is best to remove the tube temporarily and wait a few hours for the gas to travel further down the large intestine. (18:551)
>   Nursing Process—Implementation
>   Client Need—Physiological integrity

99 2. Because of the disproportionate size of an adult's hand in comparison with an infant's heart and chest, the rescuer should use just one or two fingers to perform the chest compressions on an infant who is 1 year old or younger. The rate of compressions for an infant should be 100 per minute. The heel of one hand can be used on children between 1 and 8 years of age. Both hands with the fingers interlocked should be used when performing chest compressions on individuals older than age 8. The palms of the hands should not be used during chest compressions regardless of the age of the victim. (19:384-385; 18:741)
>   Nursing Process—Evaluation
>   Client Need—Physiological integrity

100 2. Oral contraceptives that contain estrogen place people who take them at risk for thromboembolic disease. It has been estimated that taking oral contraceptives increases the risk for blood clot formation from 3 to 11 times greater than that for women who do not use this form of birth control. A history of having formed a blood clot is generally a contraindication to taking oral contraceptive agents. Iron supplements, nasal decongestants, and antacids do not promote the formation of blood clots. (15:216; 8:225)
>   Nursing Process—Collecting data
>   Client Need—Physiological integrity

101 1. Postural drainage should be performed before eating or after consumed food has left the stomach. If done on a full stomach, the positioning, coughing, or expectorating may cause the person to feel nauseated and vomit. Postural drainage should be performed according to a scheduled routine to mobilize secretions, not just when people feel short of breath or are actively coughing. Although the client should be consulted concerning the plan for care, waiting until the client says it is necessary to perform postural drainage may not be appropriate. Some may resist this form of therapy because it is tiring and uncomfortable for them. (14:817; 7:320).
Nursing Process—Planning
Client Need—Physiological integrity

102 3. The earliest signs of hypoxia are manifested by behavioral changes, such as restlessness, apprehension, anxiety, decreased judgment, and drowsiness. As hypoxia progresses, the nurse may observe dyspnea, tachypnea, and tachycardia. The blood pressure may become elevated owing to anxiety. Cyanosis is one of the last signs the nurse is likely to observe in a client who is hypoxic. (7:312; 14:813)
Nursing Process—Collecting data
Client Need—Physiological integrity

103 4. There is a high risk for wound infection from stool organisms because the perineal incision is adjacent to the rectum. Therefore, maintaining cleanliness of this area is of highest priority following a perineal prostatectomy. Straining during defecation is contraindicated; therefore, performing Valsalva's maneuver (bearing down against a closed glottis) would be inappropriate. A high Fowler's position can contribute to discomfort in the perineal incisional area. Laxatives generally are too harsh for prophylactically maintaining comfortable elimination of stool. (3:773; 14:896)
Nursing Process—Planning
Client Need—Physiological integrity

104 1. Bilirubin that is not transformed into bile will be retained in the bloodstream. As the blood is filtered by the kidneys, some of the pigment will be removed, giving urine a very dark brown appearance. The other physical assessments have no relationship to obstructive jaundice. (14:877; 7:477)
Nursing Process—Collecting data
Client Need—Safe, effective care environment

105 3. Any activity that can cause strain on the surgical area is not allowed. For example, straining to have a bowel movement, coughing, bending over, and lifting a heavy object are to be avoided.

The other listed activities are not contraindicated. (16:503; 7:685)
Nursing Process—Implementation
Client Need—Safe, effective care environment

106 3. Aminophylline is likely to produce stimulating effects, such as restlessness, insomnia, irritability, tachycardia, and hypertension. It is sometimes difficult to differentiate between the effects of the drug therapy and the manifestations of hypoxia. Lung sounds and respiratory effort should be monitored frequently, along with vital signs. Blood levels of the drug are monitored to evaluate a person's ability to metabolize the drug. Dosages may need to be adjusted depending on the person's response. (15:266)
Nursing Process—Collecting data
Client Need—Physiological integrity

107 1. The position of choice when an abdominal paracentesis is performed is the sitting position. Fluid leaves the abdominal cavity by gravity. Drainage is promoted when the client is sitting. The standing position would promote drainage, but maintaining this position would be tiring and uncomfortable for an acutely ill person. (18:318; 14:847)
Nursing Process—Planning
Client Need—Safe, effective care environment

108 3. Throw rugs are the greatest potential hazard. Owing to their instability, people tend to slip on them. Falls also occur when a foot trips on a wrinkled portion of rug or a curled edge. Taking a shower is safer than bathing in a tub. Grounded outlets that receive cords with three prongs are safer than the customary two-pronged plug. A television in the bedroom is no more dangerous than in any other room in the house. (18:234)
Nursing Process—Collecting data
Client Need—Safe, effective care environment

109 1. People with anorexia nervosa often have *lanugo*, a growth of fine downy hair covering their body. This same condition is found among infants with low birth weights. It is thought that lanugo aids in maintaining body temperature in people who lack much subcutaneous body fat. The ability to manufacture blood cells may be impaired owing to malnutrition. However, if bruising were noted, it would be widely distributed about the body and not confined to just the upper torso. Club-shaped fingertips are associated with longstanding cardiopulmonary disease. (17:380; 4:297)
Nursing Process—Collecting data
Client Need—Physiological integrity

110 3. As the scanning machine rotates, it makes a clicking or whirring sound. Contrast dye is administered for some types of CAT scans. The dye usually is instilled intravenously. Fluid and food generally are withheld to avoid nausea and vomiting. While the test is being performed the client will need to remain very still. Some require sedation to reduce anxiety and claustrophobia. A CAT scan is noninvasive; no blood samples are required. (3:327; 7:200-201)

Nursing Process—Evaluation
Client Need—Safe, effective care environment

111 3. People who take lithium carbonate often develop fine hand tremors. Some people who take lithium carbonate develop hair thinning rather than increased hair growth, or hirsutism. Striae, purplish or white bands in the skin, generally are caused by rapid weight gain. People who take lithium carbonate are more likely to be underweight. A coated or furry tongue, characterized as having a whitish appearance, often accompanies inflammatory disorders. It is not associated with lithium carbonate therapy. (15:257; 12:425)

Nursing Process—Collecting data
Client Need—Physiological integrity

112 3. A tympanic thermometer would be the safest and most accurate method for assessing the body temperature of an uncooperative child with hemophilia. This type of thermometer measures the body temperature in approximately 2 seconds. An uncooperative child may be injured with a thermometer that must be held in place longer in the mouth, axilla, or rectum. Even the slightest injury can predispose to bleeding in a person with hemophilia. (14:637; 18:251, 253)

Nursing Process—Planning
Client Need—Safe, effective care environment

113 1. Any condition that causes a high volume of fluid in the vascular system, such as congestive heart failure, will cause an elevation in the CVP measurement. Dehydration and fluid loss are reflected in low CVP measurements. Wide fluctuations in CVP are not common. Generally, the changes from one measurement to the next are gradual. The nurse should evaluate the overall trend in the measurements rather than base a judgment on just one assessment reading. If the CVP measurements are low, the physician may administer fluid or increase its rate of administration. If the CVP measurements are high, the physician is likely to slow the rate of fluid administration and prescribe a diuretic. (16:288; 7:368)

Nursing Process—Collecting data
Client Need—Safe, effective care environment

114 2. An untreated or inadequately treated streptococcal infection is the most common cause of heart inflammation in children. To prevent rheumatic heart disease and endocarditis, the American Heart Association recommends that children with streptococcal infections receive antibiotic therapy during their acute illness for at least 10 full days. Poverty and lack of insurance often deter parents from seeking medical treatment for ill children. Endocarditis is an inflammatory process that generally is not associated with birth defects, inadequate nutrition, or failure to receive vaccinations for the usual childhood infectious diseases. (3:490; 8:737)

Nursing Process—Collecting data
Client Need—Safe, effective care environment

115 1. Effortless respirations that are within a normal rate are the best indication from among the options provided that the diphenhydramine hydrochloride has successfully controlled the mild allergic reaction. When histamine is released during an allergic reaction, the airways become narrowed, and breathing is impaired. A diastolic blood pressure above 60 would be expected. The pulse rate should be within 60 to 100 beats per minute. Evaluating the characteristics of urine is not the best assessment data. (14:143; 16:98-99; 15:261)

Nursing Process—Evaluation
Client Need—Physiological integrity

116 2. Testicular atrophy would be an expected effect of administering diethylstilbestrol, a synthetic estrogen, to a male. It is used in the palliative treatment of prostatic cancer. The feminizing effects of this drug would cause a decrease in facial hair, a higher vocal pitch, and weight gain from fluid retention. (15:235; 16:709)

Nursing Process—Collecting data
Client Need—Physiological integrity

117 1. The volume of fluid that has been infused is the most essential information in the list of choices. This information facilitates keeping an accurate intake and output record. The other information should already be documented in the client's record. (18:673)

Nursing Process—Implementation
Client Need—Safe, effective care environment

118 1. Following a TURP, men experience retrograde ejaculation. That is, during orgasm ejaculation is "dry." Semen is deposited into the bladder. The first voiding after intercourse is likely to appear cloudy because it contains the seminal fluid and sperm. Because of this change in physiology, men can expect to be unable to impregnate a sexual partner. Despite retrograde ejaculation following a TURP males maintain normal libidos, achieve erections during sexual excitement, and experience orgasms. (3:776; 7:577)

Nursing Process—Evaluation
Client Need—Safe, effective care environment

119 2. The use of soap and daily bathing tend to dry the skin. Elderly clients often have thin skin that is dry because of a decrease in the secretion of sebum. To counteract this condition, the plan of care can be modified to include less frequent bathing, applying an emollient to the skin, and increasing the client's fluid intake. Providing an evening snack would contribute to the client's nutrition. Ambulating the client provides activity and promotes respiratory, circulatory, and musculoskeletal function. Filing the fingernails would promote skin integrity if the client scratches the skin. (14:345, 347; 18:119)

    Nursing Process—Evaluation

    Client Need—Safe, effective care environment

120 3. A normal blood sugar is the best evidence that hypoglycemia has been corrected. Signs of hypoglycemia include hunger and cool, clammy skin. The blood pressure is generally within normal limits or increased during hypoglycemia because of anxiety and the secretion of adrenalin. Assessing the blood pressure is not as valuable in determining the client's response to the nursing intervention. (14:950-952; 16:649-650)

    Nursing Process—Evaluation

    Client Need—Physiological integrity

Classification of Test Items

Comprehensive Examination Part I

Directions: After each question the correct answer is given as well as a classification of each test question. Compare the correct answer with your answer. If a question has been answered *incorrectly*, draw a line to the end of the four columns. When finished, add up your correct scores and place the results at the bottom of each column.

Score Calculation:

   To determine the percentage of the number of questions you answered correctly, divide the **Number Correct** by the **Number Possible**, as example 100 (the number of questions answered correctly) divided by 120 (the number of questions in the test) = .83 or 83%.

NURSING PROCESS

C = Collecting data
P = Planning
I = Implementation
E = Evaluation

CLIENT NEEDS

S = Safe, effective care environment
P = Physiological integrity
M = Psychosocial integrity
H = Health promotion/maintenance

Question #	Answer #	Nursing Process				Client Needs			
		C	P	I	E	S	P	M	H
1	3	C					P		
2	3		P			S			
3	1			I					H
4	2				E	S			
5	2			I				M	
6	1	C				S			
7	2	C							H
8	3				E	S			
9	3		P				P		
10	4			I			P		
11	4		P						H
12	3			I		S			
13	1	C				S			
14	3			I		S			
15	1				E				H
16	3	C					P		
17	1				E		P		
18	1			I			P		
19	3			I					H
20	2		P				P		
21	2				E		P		
22	3	C					P		

NURSING PROCESS
C = Collecting data
P = Planning
I = Implementation
E = Evaluation

CLIENT NEEDS
S = Safe, effective care environment
P = Physiological integrity
M = Psychosocial integrity
H = Health promotion/maintenance

Question #	Answer #	Nursing Process				Client Needs			
		C	P	I	E	S	P	M	H
23	3		P						H
24	4			I			P		
25	1	C					P		
26	2	C						M	
27	1	C							H
28	4			I			P		
29	2				E		P		
30	2		P						H
31	4			I				M	
32	1		P				P		
33	2			I					H
34	4				E				H
35	1	C				S			
36	3			I					H
37	3	C							H
38	3			I		S			
39	4		P					M	
40	3		P						H
41	1			I			P		
42	3				E			M	
43	2	C					P		
44	2			I					H
45	2	C				S			
46	4	C						M	
47	3		P				P		
48	1	C					P		
49	1		P			S			
50	1				E	S			
51	2			I		S			
52	2			I				M	
53	3		P			S			
54	3	C							H
55	2	C				S			
56	1			I			P		

NURSING PROCESS
C = Collecting data
P = Planning
I = Implementation
E = Evaluation

CLIENT NEEDS
S = Safe, effective care environment
P = Physiological integrity
M = Psychosocial integrity
H = Health promotion/maintenance

Question #	Answer #	Nursing Process				Client Needs			
		C	P	I	E	S	P	M	H
57	3		P					M	
58	4				E				H
59	3				E		P		
60	1		P				P		
61	3				E			M	
62	2		P					M	
63	2	C							H
64	2			I			P		
65	2			I					H
66	2			I		S			
67	3	C						M	
68	3			I			P		
69	4			I				M	
70	3			I		S			
71	3	C					P		
72	4			I			P		
73	4				E				H
74	3		P				P		
75	3		P				P		
76	3				E			M	
77	1		P			S			
78	2			I					H
79	4	C				S			
80	2			I			P		
81	2			I			P		
82	3		P				P		
83	2	C					P		
84	1				E		P		
85	3			I					H
86	1			I					H
87	4	C							H
88	3			I			P		
89	4	C					P		
90	1				E				H
91	2	C						M	

NURSING PROCESS

C = Collecting data
P = Planning
I = Implementation
E = Evaluation

CLIENT NEEDS

S = Safe, effective care environment
P = Physiological integrity
M = Psychosocial integrity
H = Health promotion/maintenance

Question #	Answer #	Nursing Process				Client Needs			
		C	P	I	E	S	P	M	H
92	3			I				M	
93	2	C					P		
94	3			I			P		
95	2		P				P		
96	3	C							H
97	1				E		P		
98	3			I			P		
99	2				E		P		
100	2	C					P		
101	1		P				P		
102	3	C					P		
103	4		P				P		
104	1	C				S			
105	3			I		S			
106	3	C					P		
107	1		P			S			
108	3	C				S			
109	1	C					P		
110	3				E	S			
111	3	C					P		
112	3		P			S			
113	1	C				S			
114	2	C				S			
115	1				E		P		
116	2	C					P		
117	1			I		S			
118	1				E	S			
119	2				E	S			
120	3				E		P		
Number Correct									
Number Possible	120	37	24	36	23	30	51	14	25
Percentage Correct									

PART II OF THE COMPREHENSIVE EXAMINATION

Allow yourself 2 hours to complete Part II. Start this part now.

1 A client who is 3 months pregnant complains of extreme fatigue. What suggestion may the nurse give to help relieve this problem?
○ 1. Do not nap during the day because this disturbs the sleeping pattern at night.
○ 2. Try to do most of your work in midafternoon.
○ 3. Get 8 to 10 hours of sleep at night.
○ 4. Take a 10-minute rest in midmorning.

2 The nurse plans a diet for a client requiring an increased iron intake during pregnancy. Which of the following foods are *high* in iron?
○ 1. Corn and potatoes
○ 2. Red meat and dark green leafy vegetables
○ 3. Rice and chicken
○ 4. Ice cream and cheese

3 At a prenatal clinic a client asks the nurse what can be done to relieve heartburn. Which one of the following suggestions will *most* likely relieve this problem?
○ 1. Take an antacid within 20 minutes after eating.
○ 2. Lie flat for 1 hour after eating.
○ 3. Eat small, frequent meals.
○ 4. Limit coffee to 2 to 3 cups per day.

4 A client who is 4 months pregnant states that she lives on a limited income and is having a problem purchasing meat to supply animal protein for her diet. Which of the following plant proteins can the nurse suggest be added to her diet?
○ 1. Corn, broccoli, and celery
○ 2. Leafy green vegetables, radishes, and cauliflower
○ 3. Soup, tomatoes, and oranges
○ 4. Rice, peanut butter, and beans

5 When testing the urine of a client who is 6 months pregnant, the urine tests positive for albumin. This should alert the nurse to the fact that this may be a sign of
○ 1. preeclampsia.
○ 2. liver failure.
○ 3. amniotic fluid embolism.
○ 4. placenta previa.

6 Routine admission orders for clients admitted to the labor department include an enema. Which one of the following clients should *not* have an enema on admission? The client who is
○ 1. in the first stage of labor.
○ 2. bleeding.
○ 3. older than 35.
○ 4. having contractions every 8 to 10 minutes.

7 The nurse knows that a woman is in the first stage of labor when
○ 1. complete cervical dilatation occurs.
○ 2. the fetus descends into the true pelvis.
○ 3. the heart rate of the fetus slows.
○ 4. contractions begin.

8 The nurse stays with a client during the late stages of labor and encourages the client to push down with each vigorous contraction. The nurse should warn the client to
○ 1. exhale as she pushes down.
○ 2. keep her legs flat on the bed when pushing down.
○ 3. not hold her breath for longer than 5 to 10 seconds while pushing.
○ 4. inhale during the strongest part of the contraction.

9 The physician writes an order for the nurse to give ½ oz of syrup of ipecac stat. The nurse would be *most* correct in administering which one of the following equivalents?
○ 1. 30 mL
○ 2. 15 mL
○ 3. 2 teaspoons
○ 4. 1 teaspoon

10 The nurse observes all of the following when caring for a 4-year-old. Which one indicates regressive behavior? The child who
○ 1. talks with an imaginary playmate.
○ 2. sucks on his sibling's pacifier.
○ 3. plays roughly with a friend.
○ 4. dresses up in adult clothing.

11 Which one of the following would be considered incorrect when positioning a child in the prone position?
○ 1. The arms are abducted and flexed.
○ 2. The feet and toes lie on the bed in an extended position.

426

○ 3. The toes and feet extend over the end of the mattress.

○ 4. A thin pillow is placed under the abdomen.

12 A client is receiving penicillin G. Which one of the following requires withholding the next dose of this drug?

○ 1. Skin rash

○ 2. Increase in appetite

○ 3. Decrease in body temperature

○ 4. Constipation

13 When adjusting a heat cradle that uses a light bulb, the source of heat should be placed no closer to the client than

○ 1. 3 to 5 in.

○ 2. 8 to 10 in.

○ 3. 18 to 24 in.

○ 4. 30 to 40 in.

14 A client complains of constipation. Which one of the following may indicate a cause for constipation? Eating extra amounts or portions of

○ 1. fresh fruits and vegetables.

○ 2. breakfast cereals with skim milk and fruit.

○ 3. fibrous foods with a low daily intake of water.

○ 4. meat.

15 If the nursing interventions used to reduce a client's anxiety are effective, the client will indicate he or she feels less

○ 1. depressed.

○ 2. hopeless.

○ 3. worried.

○ 4. resentful.

16 A colleague comes to the nurse to clarify the directions for administering eye drops. The nurse would be *most* accurate in explaining that the abbreviation for instilling medication in both eyes is

○ 1. O.D.

○ 2. O.S.

○ 3. O.U.

○ 4. O.P.

17 A client asks the nurse to explain the purpose for the open wound drain, called a Penrose drain. The nurse would be *most* correct in telling the client that a wound drain such as this is used to

○ 1. decrease the formation of scar tissue.

○ 2. help fluid escape from the surgical area.

○ 3. provide a means for irrigating the wound.

○ 4. release accumulating intestinal gas.

18 During a home care visit, the nurse asks the client to describe how he gives his oral medication through a nasogastric tube. Which one of the following is *incorrect* and requires reviewing this procedure with the client?

○ 1. The medication is crushed and mixed with 30 mL of warm water.

○ 2. 50 mL of water is instilled into the nasogastric tube prior to instilling the medication.

○ 3. The medication and formula are mixed together and instilled.

○ 4. The nasogastric tube is flushed with 50 mL of water.

19 When preparing to give a cleansing enema, the temperature of the water is checked with a thermometer before administration and should be between

○ 1. 70°F and 85°F (21°C and 30°C).

○ 2. 80°F and 90°F (26°C and 32°C).

○ 3. 105°F and 110°F (40°C and 43°C).

○ 4. 120°F and 130°F (48°C and 54°C).

20 When a client is performing postural drainage, the nurse should

○ 1. place the client in a supine position.

○ 2. encourage the client to cough deeply.

○ 3. encourage the client to swallow the raised sputum.

○ 4. instruct the client to take shallow breaths.

21 When preparing a client for the insertion of a nasogastric tube, the position of choice for introducing the tube into the nostril is to have the neck

○ 1. flexed.

○ 2. rotated.

○ 3. circumducted.

○ 4. hyperextended.

22 A client is seen in the emergency department with severe nausea and vomiting, which occurred shortly after eating in a restaurant. Which one of the following is the *most* important information that should be obtained from this client?

○ 1. "What foods did you eat?"

○ 2. "Do you have a fever?"

○ 3. "What do you think caused this problem?"

○ 4. "Have you ever had food poisoning?"

23 Which one of the following indicates that *incorrect* radiation protection measures are being observed when the client is receiving internal radiation therapy?

○ 1. A sign bearing the radiation symbol and warning is posted on the wall outside the room.

○ 2. Assistive nursing personnel are aware that a client is receiving internal radiation therapy.

○ 3. Adequate reading material for the client is placed in the room before therapy is instituted.

○ 4. One nurse is assigned to care for the client until the internal radiation is removed.

24 Following a perineal prostatectomy for cancer of the prostate, which one of the following nursing actions is *essential* to include on the written plan for care?

    ○ 1. Perform Valsalva's maneuver during defecation.

    ○ 2. Maintain in high Fowler's position postoperatively.

    ○ 3. Administer laxatives to promote bowel elimination.

    ○ 4. Provide perineal care following each bowel movement.

25 A client is scheduled for an intravenous pyelogram (IVP). Which one of the following questions should be asked of this client before this test?

    ○ 1. "Are you afraid of needles?"

    ○ 2. "Have you ever had x-rays taken?"

    ○ 3. "Do you have any allergies?"

    ○ 4. "What types of food have you eaten this week?"

26 Which one of the following should be included in a plan of care to provide diversional activity for the client with a recent loss of sight?

    ○ 1. Provide a radio or tapes.

    ○ 2. Encourage the client to interact with others.

    ○ 3. Encourage listening to the television.

    ○ 4. Provide books set in Braille.

27 Which of the following would the nurse look for if a child has a possible fracture of the femur?

    ○ 1. Lack of pain at the fracture site

    ○ 2. Increased function below the fracture

    ○ 3. A rash around the fracture site

    ○ 4. Deformity in alignment

28 If a child is admitted with symptoms suggesting rheumatic fever, which one of the following laboratory tests is *likely* to be elevated?

    ○ 1. Latex agglutination test

    ○ 2. Antistreptolysin O titer

    ○ 3. Heterophile antibody titer

    ○ 4. Fluorescent antibody test

29 A client is to receive 1000 mL of an intravenous solution in 8 hours. Before the infusion is started the nurse should determine the amount that is infused hourly. How many milliliters of solution should be infused in 1 hour?

    ○ 1. 50 mL

    ○ 2. 125 mL

    ○ 3. 200 mL

    ○ 4. 500 mL

30 Which one of the following may indicate that the application of an ice bag to a sprain should be temporarily discontinued?

    ○ 1. Redness of the skin

    ○ 2. Increased pain in the area

    ○ 3. Itching

    ○ 4. Mottling of the skin

31 Which of the following should be included in a plan of care for the aphasic client?

    ○ 1. Use a louder than normal voice when communicating with the client.

    ○ 2. Write out questions and directions for the client to read and answer.

    ○ 3. Take into consideration that aphasia affects the intelligence.

    ○ 4. Give the client time to respond to questions.

32 Which one of the following may indicate that an underwater-seal drainage system inserted 4 hours ago is *not* functioning properly?

    ○ 1. Failure of the fluid in the drainage bottle to rise and fall with each respiration

    ○ 2. Bubbling in the underwater seal

    ○ 3. Drainage appearing in the drainage bottle

    ○ 4. No drainage in the trap bottle

33 To obtain a femoral pulse the nurse's fingers are placed

    ○ 1. behind the knee.

    ○ 2. on the dorsum of the foot.

    ○ 3. on the inguinal area.

    ○ 4. over the lower tibia.

34 The nurse prepares a drug for parenteral administration, which is the administration of a drug by

    ○ 1. the intravenous route.

    ○ 2. any route other than through the digestive tract.

    ○ 3. the intramuscular route.

    ○ 4. the subcutaneous route.

35 When withdrawing a drug from a vial with a rubber stopper, the nurse should

    ○ 1. not inject air into the vial.

    ○ 2. inject 1 mL more of air than the amount of the drug to be withdrawn.

    ○ 3. refrigerate the vial for 10 minutes before withdrawing the drug from the vial.

    ○ 4. inject the same amount of air into the vial as that of the drug to be withdrawn.

36 Which one of the following indicates that the child with hemophilia should be seen immediately by a physician?

    ○ 1. Anorexia

    ○ 2. Severe joint pain

    ○ 3. Depression

    ○ 4. Nasal congestion

37 A client with leukemia is to be discharged from the hospital. Which one of the following questions should the nurse ask before beginning discharge teaching?

    ○ 1. "Are you glad you are going home?"

    ○ 2. "Have you decided what you will do to keep yourself busy once you are home?"

    ○ 3. "Do you have any questions about the information given to you by the physician?"

    ○ 4. "Is there someone who will drive you home?"

38 The nurse is asked to develop a teaching plan for a prenatal class. Which one of the following signs and symptoms of impending labor is correct?
- ○ 1. Severe fatigue
- ○ 2. Lightening
- ○ 3. A rise of the fetus into the upper abdomen
- ○ 4. Sudden loss of weight

39 Which one of the following indicates the client in labor is ready to deliver?
- ○ 1. Bulging of the perineum
- ○ 2. A decrease in show
- ○ 3. A desire not to push down with each contraction
- ○ 4. Leakage of amniotic fluid

40 Which one of the following responses might indicate that a client may have increased intracranial pressure?
- ○ 1. Eyes open spontaneously
- ○ 2. Uses inappropriate words
- ○ 3. Responds to a painful stimulus
- ○ 4. Obeys commands

41 A client is comatose and on life support. The family wishes to discontinue life-support measures. Which one of the following may help determine if life-support measures can be discontinued?
- ○ 1. The cost of continued life-support measures
- ○ 2. If the client's insurance covers life-support measures
- ○ 3. If all relatives agree that life support should be discontinued
- ○ 4. If the client signed a living will

42 A client is seen in the emergency department following ingestion of a chemical. Which one of the following is the *most* important information that the nurse should try to obtain as soon as possible?
- ○ 1. The age of the client
- ○ 2. Who observed the ingestion
- ○ 3. The substance involved
- ○ 4. If water was swallowed along with the chemical

43 Immediately after a client's membranes have ruptured, the nurse should
- ○ 1. monitor the fetal heart rate to detect any fetal distress.
- ○ 2. decrease the flow of the intravenous solution to keep vein open (KVO).
- ○ 3. apply a waterproof pad to the perineal area.
- ○ 4. raise the client to a sitting position.

44 When evaluating a newborn shortly after birth, which one of the following is considered *abnormal*?
- ○ 1. A bluish color of the hands and feet
- ○ 2. An apical pulse of 88 per minute
- ○ 3. Respirations of 40 per minute
- ○ 4. Small pinpoint white or yellow dots on the skin

45 A hospital worker is seen in the emergency department for a minor burn to a finger. To prepare for treatment of the injury the nurse should know that the treatment of minor burns to a small area involves
- ○ 1. application of petroleum jelly to the area.
- ○ 2. covering the area with nonallergenic tape.
- ○ 3. immersing the part in cool water.
- ○ 4. immersing the part in warm water.

46 The nurse is assigned to obtain an initial history. Which one of the following should alert the nurse that the client is taking a medication for the treatment of glaucoma?
- ○ 1. atropine
- ○ 2. Timoptic (timolol maleate)
- ○ 3. digitalis
- ○ 4. penicillin

47 Which one of the following indicates that therapy for acute angle-closure glaucoma is effective?
- ○ 1. Swelling of the eyelids is decreased.
- ○ 2. Redness of the sclera is reduced.
- ○ 3. Pain is reduced or eliminated.
- ○ 4. Peripheral vision is reduced.

48 Prior to the instillation of ear drops the nurse should
- ○ 1. warm the medication to room temperature.
- ○ 2. place the medication in a refrigerator for 30 minutes.
- ○ 3. remove the label from the bottle.
- ○ 4. open the container for 5 to 10 minutes before the medication is instilled.

49 The nurse is assigned to administer eye drops. Liquid ophthalmic preparations are instilled into the
- ○ 1. inner canthus.
- ○ 2. outer canthus.
- ○ 3. upper conjunctival sac.
- ○ 4. lower conjunctival sac.

50 When using a cotton ball to remove crust from a client's eye, the nurse should use a motion that moves the cotton ball
- ○ 1. from the outer to the inner canthus.
- ○ 2. upward toward the forehead.
- ○ 3. from the inner to the outer canthus.
- ○ 4. downward toward the cheek.

51 Which one of the following might indicate to the nurse that a client seen in the emergency department has recently used cocaine?
- ○ 1. Hypotension
- ○ 2. Marked central nervous system stimulation
- ○ 3. Pinpoint pupils
- ○ 4. Central nervous system depression

52 The nurse plans to discuss with a small group of teenage students the dangers associated with alcohol abuse. Which one of the following regarding alcohol abuse is correct?

○ 1. Alcohol is a potentially physically addicting substance.
○ 2. Those drinking alcohol rarely use other illegal drugs.
○ 3. Alcohol is not physically addicting but tolerance to alcohol can occur.
○ 4. Only those drinking large amounts of alcohol become addicted to this substance.

53 A client has a history of chronic alcoholism. When observing this client for signs of alcohol withdrawal, the nurse might expect these signs to appear in
○ 1. 1 to 2 weeks.
○ 2. 2 to 4 days.
○ 3. 12 to 72 hours.
○ 4. 3 to 7 days.

54 A client is admitted to the emergency department with burns around the face and neck. When performing an initial assessment the nurse should look for
○ 1. hemorrhage.
○ 2. evidence of fluid loss.
○ 3. electrolyte imbalances.
○ 4. signs of respiratory distress.

55 When developing a plan of care for a client with extensive burns, the nurse should include measures to prevent contractures. Which one of the following *may* help prevent this problem?
○ 1. Maintaining hyperextension of the extremities
○ 2. Proper positioning and regular exercises
○ 3. Increasing the fluid intake
○ 4. Checking to see that all pressure dressings are changed weekly

56 When assessing the client with severe burns, which one of the following *may* indicate that an infection is occurring?
○ 1. A change in odor
○ 2. Blackening of the eschar
○ 3. An increase in urine output
○ 4. A decrease in the pulse rate

57 A client has been diagnosed as having manic-depressive illness. Which one of the following symptoms might the nurse observe if this client is in the manic phase of her disorder?
○ 1. Flight of ideas
○ 2. Increased appetite
○ 3. Passiveness
○ 4. Slowed physical activity

58 A client in the manic phase of manic-depressive illness is receiving lithium carbonate. Which one of the following is most important when a client is receiving this drug?
○ 1. Noting the ability of the client to communicate with others

○ 2. Weighing the client daily
○ 3. Accurately charting the client's mental and physical status
○ 4. Monitoring vital signs

59 Which of the following might the nurse identify in a client as symptoms of an obsessive-compulsive disorder (OCD)?
○ 1. An inability to concentrate on all activities of daily living
○ 2. Hallucinations
○ 3. An inability to socialize with others
○ 4. The repetition of a stereotyped act

60 A 2-year-old child has been diagnosed as autistic. When developing a plan of care for this client, the nurse should know that this disorder is characterized by
○ 1. excessive involvement with social interactions.
○ 2. unawareness of external reality.
○ 3. preoccupation with a physical symptom or complaint.
○ 4. increased interest in the actions of others.

61 Which one of the following would the nurse include in a plan of care for an autistic child?
○ 1. Provide play activities.
○ 2. Provide constant supervision.
○ 3. Encourage exercise twice daily.
○ 4. Encourage interaction with peers.

62 When obtaining a health history from the parents of a child with possible rheumatic fever, the nurse should inquire if she was recently ill with
○ 1. chickenpox.
○ 2. a sore throat.
○ 3. measles.
○ 4. mumps.

63 When performing an initial assessment of a 3-year-old child who has rheumatic fever, the nurse may expect to note
○ 1. urticaria.
○ 2. lower than normal body temperature.
○ 3. hypotension.
○ 4. joint tenderness.

64 A 7-year-old client has acute lymphoblastic leukemia. Which one of the following tasks is avoided when giving care to this client?
○ 1. Give frequent oral care.
○ 2. Take the temperature rectally.
○ 3. Assess skin daily for petechiae and bruising.
○ 4. Discourage visitors with an illness from seeing this client.

65 When developing a discharge teaching plan for the parents of a child who has idiopathic thrombocytopenic purpura, the nurse should discuss the importance of not giving salicylates, such as aspirin, because these drugs

    ○ 1. interfere with platelet function and cause spontaneous bleeding.
    ○ 2. decrease the number of white blood cells.
    ○ 3. decrease the size of red blood cells.
    ○ 4. increase the number of platelets.

66 How much fluid is normally used when irrigating a colostomy?
    ○ 1. 50 to 100 mL
    ○ 2. 100 to 150 mL
    ○ 3. 250 to 500 mL
    ○ 4. 500 to 1000 mL

67 The nurse is assigned to collect a urine specimen from a client with an indwelling urethral catheter. Which of the following should the nurse use when collecting the urine from a catheter with a special port?
    ○ 1. A suction machine
    ○ 2. An Asepto syringe
    ○ 3. A 5-mL or larger syringe and needle
    ○ 4. A catheter smaller than the indwelling catheter

68 Which one of the following instruments should the nurse provide for the physician performing a pelvic examination and obtaining a Papanicolaou's smear?
    ○ 1. Needle holder
    ○ 2. Speculum
    ○ 3. Simpson's forceps
    ○ 4. Tenaculum

69 When reviewing a client's record, the term amenorrhea is used to describe her primary complaint. To develop questions asked during a health history, the nurse should know that this term refers to
    ○ 1. an absence of a menstrual flow.
    ○ 2. painful menses.
    ○ 3. excessive bleeding at the time of menstruation.
    ○ 4. vaginal bleeding at a time other than a menstrual period.

70 A client has had surgery for testicular carcinoma, which included a radical lymph node dissection. Which one of the following measures may the nurse plan to use to decrease the discomfort associated with coughing and deep breathing?
    ○ 1. Turn the client on his right side, and flex his right knee.
    ○ 2. Have the client sit in a chair.
    ○ 3. Place a pillow on the abdomen, and apply firm, light pressure.
    ○ 4. Have the client cough and deep breathe before administering an analgesic.

71 To plan postoperative nursing care and develop short- and long-term client-centered goals for the person who has had a mastectomy followed by a bilateral oopherectomy, the nurse should know that removing the ovaries

    ○ 1. enhances the action of antineoplastic drugs.
    ○ 2. may slow tumor growth and metastasis of any remaining tumor cells.
    ○ 3. prevents adverse reactions of antineoplastic drugs.
    ○ 4. increases blood levels of progesterone.

72 Which one of the following symptoms is *directly related* to surgical removal of the ovaries and should be included when planning discharge teaching?
    ○ 1. Hot flashes and a feeling of warmth in the face, neck, and chest are reported to the physician.
    ○ 2. Changes in the appearance of the incision may occur over a period of 3 weeks.
    ○ 3. Leg cramps may occur but can be controlled by wearing warm clothing.
    ○ 4. Fatigue may occur and should be reported to the physician.

73 Two days after an abdominal hysterectomy, a client complains of sudden, moderately severe, abdominal pain. Although her pain may be related to the surgery, the nurse also should look for other problems causing pain. Which one of the following may be causing this client's abdominal pain?
    ○ 1. A sodium imbalance
    ○ 2. Obstruction of the urethral catheter
    ○ 3. Dehydration
    ○ 4. Wrinkled sheets

74 A client is scheduled for outpatient chemotherapy for treatment of endometrial cancer, and three drugs will be injected intravenously by the physician. Which one of the following is the *most* important nursing task when assembling materials for the physician administering these drugs?
    ○ 1. Refrigerate the drug 1 hour before it is prepared for administration.
    ○ 2. Have a 24 French needle available for withdrawing the drug from the vial.
    ○ 3. Premix the drug 1 to 3 hours prior to administration.
    ○ 4. Provide gloves for those preparing the drug for administration.

75 A client has terminal cancer, and the physician recommends hospice care to the family. The family asks the nurse, "What is a hospice?" The *most* correct reply is, "Hospice care
    ○ 1. uses nurses who can give better care than hospital nurses."
    ○ 2. is cheaper than hospital care."
    ○ 3. allows terminally ill clients to be cared for at home."
    ○ 4. includes the use of specialized equipment not available in hospitals."

76 Which one of the following characteristics might the nurse identify as *symptoms* of an attention-deficit disorder in a 4-year-old child?
○ 1. Sleeps frequently during the day
○ 2. Appears disinterested in surroundings
○ 3. Has difficulty concentrating
○ 4. Refuses to play with others

77 A 6-year-old client is diagnosed as having an attention-deficit disorder, which is being treated with the drug methylphenidate (Ritalin). He also has been placed on a special diet. The nurse is assigned to explain dietary restrictions to the parents. Which of the following usually are eliminated from the diet of those with this disorder?
○ 1. Green and yellow vegetables
○ 2. Food additives, artificial food coloring, and preservatives
○ 3. Candy, milk, and yogurt
○ 4. Proteins and other animal fats

78 A client is receiving an anticholinesterase drug, pyridostigmine (Mestinon), for the treatment of myasthenia gravis. The nurse can evaluate a positive response to drug therapy when the client
○ 1. has a normal temperature.
○ 2. no longer has diarrhea.
○ 3. is able to chew and swallow food.
○ 4. verbalizes a desire to go home.

79 A 17-year-old is seen in the dermatology clinic for treatment of acne vulgaris. The nurse should caution this client *not* to squeeze the pimples and blackheads because doing so is most likely to result in
○ 1. spreading the infection.
○ 2. injuring nerves in the skin.
○ 3. interfering with lymph drainage.
○ 4. a decrease in the blood supply to the skin.

80 The nurse obtains a health history from a client who has osteoarthritis. Which one of the following symptoms should the nurse recognize as a symptom of this disorder?
○ 1. Bradycardia
○ 2. Fever
○ 3. Redness of the involved joints
○ 4. Stiffness of the involved joints

81 A client with osteoarthritis tells the nurse that his physician told him to exercise. The nurse can advise the client to
○ 1. exercise for 3 hours once a day.
○ 2. lift weights for 1 hour each day.
○ 3. engage in short periods of moderate exercise.
○ 4. exercise once a week.

82 A client is receiving ibuprofen (Motrin) for osteoarthritis. Which one of the following indicates that drug therapy for this disorder is effective?
○ 1. Pain is lessened or relieved.

○ 2. Joint redness is decreased.
○ 3. Temperature is normal.
○ 4. Joint size is decreased.

83 A client has been taking ibuprofen for the discomfort associated with osteoarthritis. Which one of the following problems should the nurse recognize as most likely to be associated with the use of this drug?
○ 1. Double vision
○ 2. Dizziness
○ 3. Irregular pulse
○ 4. Gastrointestinal disturbances

84 A nurse working in a factory is called to see a worker who has been burned by a chemical. Initial emergency treatment of a chemical burn includes
○ 1. irrigating the area with large amounts of water.
○ 2. using a towel or cloth to soak up the chemical.
○ 3. applying a thick layer of petroleum jelly around the edges of the burned area.
○ 4. rubbing ice on the burned area.

85 A 2-year-old client is admitted to the hospital following a head injury. Which one of the following should the nurse consider *abnormal* and immediately report to the physician?
○ 1. Does not react purposefully to stimuli
○ 2. Crying
○ 3. Small bump on the forehead
○ 4. Scratches on the forehead and face

86 A 7-year-old with an inoperable brain tumor requires complete nursing care. When performing routine morning care, the nurse observes a reddened area on the right hip. When rewriting a plan of care the nurse should include a notation to
○ 1. turn on the right side three times a day.
○ 2. keep supine until the area heals.
○ 3. keep off the right hip until the reddened area disappears.
○ 4. apply a lotion before turning onto the right side.

87 A 5-year-old client has a brain tumor and requires upper airway suctioning at frequent intervals. Which one of the following assessments indicates suctioning is necessary?
○ 1. Assessing the temperature of the extremities
○ 2. Assessing for the ability to cough and raise sputum
○ 3. Measuring the amount of sputum raised
○ 4. Determining the type of cough

88 During a nursing conference the charge nurse states that a 7-year-old girl who has severe brain damage should be placed in a prone position for 1 hour the next time her position is changed. When changing this client's position, the nurse should place her

○ 1. on her back.

○ 2. on her right or left side.

○ 3. face down.

○ 4. in a semisitting position.

89 A 4-year-old is seen in the emergency department because she fell and struck her head. After examination the physician discharges the client to her parent's care. Which one of the following instructions should the nurse plan to include when giving instructions to the parents?

○ 1. Have her drink extra fluids for the next 72 hours, and limit her diet to soft foods.

○ 2. Apply a bandage over the injured area, and change it when necessary.

○ 3. Notify the physician if she suddenly becomes sleepy or drowsy and is difficult to arouse.

○ 4. Keep her in bed for the next 5 or 6 days.

90 Which one of the following nursing assessments should be included in a plan of care for a child who has possible intracranial bleeding?

○ 1. Checking the level of consciousness

○ 2. Measuring intake and output

○ 3. Checking the skin for jaundice

○ 4. Measuring central venous pressure (CVP)

91 The postoperative plan of care for the client having a continent ileostomy (Kock pouch) should include

○ 1. measuring ileostomy output once every 24 hours.

○ 2. removing the rectal packing every 8 hours.

○ 3. using a suction machine capable of low, intermittent suction.

○ 4. sealing the stoma with nonallergenic tape.

92 Which one of the following should alert the nurse that there may be an infection under a client's cast?

○ 1. A crack in the surface of the cast

○ 2. Presence of a foul odor

○ 3. Blood on the surface of the cast

○ 4. An indentation on the surface of the cast

93 A 2-year-old girl is placed in a spica cast. Which one of the following measures may the nurse use to prevent soiling of the cast around the perineal area?

○ 1. Insert cotton wadding or mechanics waste between the cast and the skin.

○ 2. Cover the perineal area of the cast with a waterproof material, such as plastic wrap.

○ 3. Offer the bedpan at more frequent intervals.

○ 4. Keep the head of the bed elevated to prevent backward flow of urine.

94 The nurse knows that traction is effective when the client's

○ 1. body weight is counteracting the pull of the weights.

○ 2. legs are parallel to the bed.

○ 3. comfort is not compromised by traction.

○ 4. feet are resting against the footboard.

95 Which of the following data obtained by the nurse may indicate the development of pulmonary edema?

○ 1. Bradycardia, insomnia, and anxiety

○ 2. Tachycardia, decreased respiratory rate, and weak pulse

○ 3. Orthopnea, sudden dyspnea, and elevated blood pressure

○ 4. Flushed face, hypotension, and thick, tenacious sputum

96 How may the nurse decrease the workload of the heart when a client has severe, left-sided heart failure?

○ 1. Encourage complete bed rest.

○ 2. Eliminate daily morning care.

○ 3. Help the client select a low-cholesterol diet.

○ 4. Force fluids.

97 During an initial assessment, a client complains of diarrhea. Which one of the following questions might identify a possible cause of this problem?

○ 1. "Do you use laxatives frequently?"

○ 2. "Do you drink water with your meals?"

○ 3. "Have you eaten any canned vegetables lately?"

○ 4. "Have you gained weight in the past few months?"

98 Which one of the following suggestions can the nurse give to a client who has postural hypotension?

○ 1. Eat a diet low in saturated fats.

○ 2. Rise from a sitting or lying position slowly.

○ 3. Include bananas and other fresh fruits in your diet.

○ 4. Exercise for 5 minutes two or three times a day.

99 If hyperventilation occurs, the nurse can have the client

○ 1. breathe into a paper or plastic bag for 1 to 2 minutes.

○ 2. take several sips of water.

○ 3. exhale forceably 3 or 4 times.

○ 4. hold his or her breath for 30 to 45 seconds.

100 The nurse can determine a positive reaction to a Tine test by noting if there is

○ 1. a blanching of the skin at the testing site.

○ 2. a red, raised area at the testing site.

○ 3. increased swelling distal to the testing site.

○ 4. pain at the testing site.

101 Which one of the following indicates that a client's position should be changed at more frequent intervals?

○ 1. The client's complaints of stiffness in the legs

○ 2. An increase in blood pressure

○ 3. Pale appearance of skin over bony prominences

○ 4. Fever

102 Which one of the following is *not* necessary when a client is placed on blood and body fluid precautions?
  ○ 1. Gowns are worn by caregivers if there is a danger of being splashed.
  ○ 2. All articles and bed linens must be sterilized before use.
  ○ 3. Masks are worn by caregivers if there is danger of being splashed.
  ○ 4. Contaminated linen is double-bagged or discarded before being sent to other departments.

103 A client has been on complete bed rest for 4 weeks. Which one of the following should the nurse look for when getting the client out of bed for the first time?
  ○ 1. Sudden onset of intestinal cramping
  ○ 2. Bradycardia
  ○ 3. Weakness and lightheadedness
  ○ 4. Mild to moderate increase in blood pressure

104 The nurse performs an initial assessment on a 2-year-old child. Which one of the following is considered a delayed motor development skill for a 2-year-old?
  ○ 1. Cannot hop or skip
  ○ 2. Unable to walk up and down stairs alone
  ○ 3. Cannot button clothes
  ○ 4. Unable to catch a ball

105 When instituting a bladder retraining program for the incontinent client, the nurse should first
  ○ 1. determine the client's voiding pattern.
  ○ 2. limit the client's fluid intake.
  ○ 3. write out a schedule for placing the client on the bedpan or offering the urinal.
  ○ 4. show the client how to use a bedside commode.

106 The nurse demonstrates Credé's maneuver to an incontinent client. This maneuver is performed by
  ○ 1. standing to void.
  ○ 2. taking deep breaths before trying to void.
  ○ 3. exhaling slowly while trying to void.
  ○ 4. applying light pressure with the hands over the bladder.

107 Which one of the following 24-hour total measured urine output is *abnormal*?
  ○ 1. 400 mL
  ○ 2. 650 mL
  ○ 3. 800 mL
  ○ 4. 950 mL

108 The nurse assesses a postoperative thyroidectomy client 8 hours after surgery. Which one of the following indicates a *complication* of thyroid surgery?
  ○ 1. A rectal temperature of 100.8°F.
  ○ 2. The client complains of numbness and tingling in the extremities.

  ○ 3. The client is hoarse when talking.
  ○ 4. The client complains of a sore throat.

109 A client with Alzheimer's disease is confused, has an unsteady gait, and a tendency to wander. Which one of the following could the nurse plan to institute to ensure the safety of this client?
  ○ 1. Lock all exit doors.
  ○ 2. Apply restraints when the client tries to leave the area.
  ○ 3. Remove footstools and small tables from the ambulatory area.
  ○ 4. Keep the bed in a high position to prevent getting out of bed at night.

110 The nurse assesses a newborn, full-term infant. Which one of the following is an abnormal finding?
  ○ 1. Turns head from side to side
  ○ 2. Tearless crying
  ○ 3. Appears hungry in 3 hours
  ○ 4. Absent Moro reflex

111 When collecting urine from a client with a suspected ureteral calculus, the nurse should plan to
  ○ 1. encourage the client to drink fruit juices.
  ○ 2. strain all urine through gauze and inspect for calculi.
  ○ 3. encourage the client to eat a diet high in calcium.
  ○ 4. keep the client on complete bed rest.

112 A client has had difficulty coping with the physical aspects of his severe burns. Which one of the following nursing interventions may help him cope with his problem?
  ○ 1. Encouraging him to talk about what he is experiencing and how he feels
  ○ 2. Asking him if he would like to be with other clients
  ○ 3. Explaining to him that this is a normal reaction to a severe burn
  ○ 4. Letting him have as many visitors as he wishes

113 Which one of the following *objective* characteristics might the nurse observe if a client has moderate to severe anxiety?
  ○ 1. Hypotension, flushed face, and pinpoint pupils
  ○ 2. Sleepiness, increased appetite, and bradycardia
  ○ 3. Dry mouth, increased feelings of tension, and fearfulness
  ○ 4. Increased pulse rate, poor eye contact, and tremors

114 A client has a fasting blood glucose of 95 mg/dL. The nurse should recognize this laboratory test result as being
  ○ 1. within normal limits.
  ○ 2. low.

○ 3. higher than normal.
○ 4. dangerously high.

115 When an oral hypoglycemic agent is prescribed for the treatment of diabetes mellitus, the nurse should tell the client that
○ 1. it is not necessary to follow a diet plan.
○ 2. failure to take the drug will result in decreased blood glucose levels.
○ 3. these drugs are taken ½ hour after each meal.
○ 4. hypoglycemic episodes may occur with this drug.

116 Which of the following statements indicates that a client may be having a hypoglycemic reaction?
○ 1. "I feel very lightheaded and dizzy."
○ 2. "I didn't like the oatmeal on my breakfast tray."
○ 3. "My legs still bother me."
○ 4. "I am upset because my doctor didn't see me today."

117 The nurse is assigned to obtain a capillary blood sample to test a client's blood glucose level using a glucometer. When obtaining a blood sample, the nurse must be sure that
○ 1. at least 1 mL of blood is expressed from the puncture.
○ 2. one drop of blood must be adequate to cover and saturate the test pad.
○ 3. the lancet is inserted at least 10 cm into the tip of the finger.
○ 4. the client's hands are washed with cold water before performing the puncture.

118 Which one of the following procedures should the nurse plan to include in a teaching program for the client with diabetes mellitus?
○ 1. Bathe the feet daily in warm water.
○ 2. Walk barefoot as much as possible.
○ 3. Use a hot water bottle to keep the feet warm when sleeping.
○ 4. Soak the feet daily in tepid water for at least 30 minutes.

119 The physician makes a notation on a client's record that he has type I diabetes mellitus. When developing a care plan, the nurse must take into consideration that this type of diabetes is treated
○ 1. with insulin.
○ 2. with an oral hypoglycemic agent.
○ 3. by dietary restrictions.
○ 4. by following a weight loss program.

120 The nurse is assigned to develop a preoperative plan of care for a client with diabetes mellitus who is undergoing surgery. The client's diabetes is controlled with an oral hypoglycemic agent. Which one of the following should the nurse anticipate when planning preoperative preparations?
○ 1. The oral hypoglycemic agent will be given the morning of surgery.
○ 2. Prior to surgery the oral hypoglycemic agent usually is discontinued, and insulin is ordered.
○ 3. Fasting from midnight is not required.
○ 4. Insulin is administered for 3 days prior to surgery.

Correct Answers and Rationale

Two numbers appear in parentheses following each rationale. The first number identifies the textbook listed in the references, page 451, and the second number identifies the page(s) in that textbook on which the correct answer can be verified. Occasionally, two textbooks are given for verifying the correct answer.

1 3. Getting 8 to 10 hours of sleep each night, taking frequent rest periods between activities, taking daytime naps, and resting whenever fatigue occurs may help relieve the extreme fatigue occurring during pregnancy. (19:64)
   Nursing Process—Implementation
   Client Need—Health promotion/maintenance

2 2. Red meat; dark green, leafy vegetables; shrimp; liver; whole grains; and oysters are higher in iron than the other foods listed in this question. (19:60)
   Nursing Process—Planning
   Client Need—Health promotion/maintenance

3 3. Eating small, frequent meals and avoiding coffee and spicy and fried foods may relieve heartburn. If the client does lie down, the head and shoulders should be elevated to prevent a reflux of gastric acid. Antacids should not be used unless their use is approved by the physician. (19:64-65)
   Nursing Process—Implementation
   Client Need—Health promotion/maintenance

4 4. Rice, peanut butter, beans, potatoes, peanuts, and whole wheat are examples of plant proteins that are cheaper than animal proteins, such as meat, chicken, fish, and dairy products. Plant proteins, taken in a sufficient amount, can satisfy the protein needs of a pregnant woman. (19:59)
   Nursing Process—Implementation
   Client Need—Health promotion/maintenance

5 1. The presence of albumin in the urine is one of the first signs of preeclampsia (toxemia of pregnancy, pregnancy-induced hypertension, or PIH). (14:543)
   Nursing Process—Evaluation
   Client Need—Physiological integrity

6 2. Not all clients admitted to the labor department are given an enema, but some hospitals may have this as part of the routine admission orders. Clients who are bleeding are never given a routine enema unless there is a specific order from the physician. (8:180)
   Nursing Process—Evaluation
   Client Need—Physiological integrity

7 4. The first stage of labor begins with the onset of contractions and effacement and dilatation of the cervix. The first stage ends when the cervix is completely effaced and dilated to 10 cm. (8:102)
   Nursing Process—Evaluation
   Client Need—Health promotion/maintenance

8 3. When vigorous pushing is required, the client is encouraged to hold her breath and push down. The breath should not be held for more than 5 to 10 seconds; holding the breath longer reduces the exchange of gases across the placenta. (8:122)
   Nursing Process—Implementation
   Client Need—Health promotion/maintenance

9 2. One ounce is equal to 30 mL; therefore, there is 15 mL in ½ oz. There is approximately 5 mL per teaspoon. The equivalent of ½ oz would be 3 teaspoons. (15:9; 18:575)
   Nursing Process—Implementation
   Client Need—Physiological Integrity

10 2. Sucking a pacifier is an activity that most preschoolers have abandoned. Resorting to this earlier behavior is evidence that the child feels anxious. Four-year-olds have vivid imaginations. It is common at this age for children to develop an imaginary friend or fantasize about the world and his role in it. Preschoolers are very active. Play may be one mechanism by which a 4-year-old tests the limits of social interaction. It is appropriate at this age to imitate adult role models, especially of the same sex. (8:359-360; 9:47-48, 71)
   Nursing Process—Evaluation
   Client Need—Health promotion/maintenance

11 2. When a client lies in the prone position, the toes and feet must extend over the edge of the mattress. Abduction and flexion of the arms make the client more comfortable. A thin pillow placed under the abdomen reduces the lumbar curve and takes the pressure off the chest. (8:471)
   Nursing Process—Evaluation
   Client Need—Safe, effective care environment

12 1. A skin rash may indicate an allergy to penicillin, so the drug should be withheld and the physician notified. An increase in appetite, decrease in body temperature, and constipation are normally not adverse effects associated with the administration of penicillin. (15:155-159)
Nursing Process—Implementation
Client Need—Physiological integrity

13 3. When using a bed cradle with an electric light bulb to provide dry heat to an extremity, the heat source should be 18 to 24 inches from the client's extremity. Placing the heat source too close to an extremity may result in a burn. Placing the heat source too far from an extremity will be ineffective. (18:497)
Nursing Process—Implementation
Client Need—Physiological integrity

14 3. A diet high in fiber requires an increase in the daily fluid intake to prevent constipation. (18:549)
Nursing Process—Evaluation
Client Need—Physiological integrity

15 3. The nurse can assume that anxiety-relieving interventions have been effective if the client says he is less worried. Most anxious people seem to worry unnecessarily or out of proportion to the reality of situations in which they are involved. Other data that would support a reduction in anxiety include reduced heart rate and blood pressure, the ability to remember instructions, restful sleep, and relaxed posture. (7:51; 12:367)
Nursing Process—Evaluation
Client Need—Psychosocial integrity

16 3. The correct abbreviation for both eyes is O.U. The abbreviation for the right eye is O.D. and for the left eye, O.S. O.P. does not represent a standard medical abbreviation. (18:576)
Nursing Process—Implementation
Client Need—Physiological integrity

17 2. A Penrose and other types of open drains are placed within an operative site to help drainage escape from a surgical wound. Drains in a wound do not decrease scar formation. A drain may remove air if it is in the area of a wound, but it is not used to release intestinal gas. Nasogastric and nasointestinal tubes are used to remove air and secretions from the stomach or intestine. A drain is not used to irrigate a wound. (18:480; 3:239)
Nursing Process—Implementation
Client Need—Safe, effective care environment

18 3. Medications should be instilled into a nasogastric tube separately from the formula because a formula may interact with medications. The client should be told to instill medications at the prescribed time and wait approximately 1 hour before instilling formula. (18:587-589)
Nursing Process—Evaluation
Client Need—Safe, effective care environment

19 3. The solution used in a cleansing enema should be slightly higher than normal body temperature. Using temperatures higher or lower than 105°F to 110°F (40°C to 43°C) can cause unnecessary discomfort. Solutions that are too warm or hot may burn the intestinal lining. (18:554)
Nursing Process—Evaluation
Client Need—Safe, effective care environment

20 2. Postural drainage is performed to drain secretions from the lungs by gravity. The position used by the client depends on which lobe(s) of the lung is to be drained. Lying supine will not encourage drainage from the lungs. The client is encouraged to expectorate the raised sputum and cough and breathe deeply. (7:319)
Nursing Process—Implementation
Client Need—Physiological integrity

21 4. When introducing a nasogastric tube into a nostril, it is best to have the client, who is in a sitting position, hyperextend his neck. This position helps the nurse guide and direct the tip of the tube toward the pharynx. Once the tube is inserted to the first mark, or the distance measured from the tip of the nose to the earlobe, the client should be instructed to flex his neck, resting his chin on his chest while the tube is advanced to the second mark, or the distance from the nose to the xiphoid process. Flexing the neck closes the trachea and opens the esophagus so that the nasogastric tube is more likely to progress toward the stomach rather than the respiratory tract. (18:138; 14:851)
Nursing Process—Planning
Client Need—Safe, effective care environment

22 1. When a client gives a history of having become ill shortly after eating food, it is important to know what food the client ate and the name of the restaurant. If the physician suspects that the cause of this client's nausea and vomiting can be traced to food, the local health department will be notified. (16:531)
Nursing Process—Collecting data
Client Need—Safe, effective care environment

23 4. Nursing personnel coming in contact with a client receiving internal radiation therapy must be aware of time, distance, and shielding. One nurse should not be assigned to give care to the client receiving internal radiation therapy. Instead, nursing tasks should be rotated among all members of the unit so that the time of exposure to radiation is minimized. (3:282-284; 16:201-202)

> Nursing Process—Evaluation
> Client Need—Safe, effective care environment

24   4. There is a high risk for wound infection from stool microorganisms because the perineal incision is adjacent to the rectum. Therefore, maintaining cleanliness of this area is of highest priority following a perineal prostatectomy. Straining during defecation is contraindicated; therefore, performing Valsalva's maneuver (bearing down against a closed glottis) would be inappropriate. A high Fowler's position can contribute to discomfort in the perineal incisional area. Laxatives generally are too harsh for prophylactically maintaining comfortable elimination of stool. (3:773; 14:896)

> Nursing Process—Planning
> Client Need—Physiological integrity

25   3. An iodine-based dye often is used in diagnostic tests, such as an IVP. A history of allergies is most important, especially if the client has a history of an iodine or seafood (which contains iodine) allergy. If the client is allergic to iodine, the physician must be notified before the client has the IVP. (16:725-727)

> Nursing Process—Collecting data
> Client Need—Safe, effective care environment

26   1. Of the four choices in this question, a radio or cassette tapes with recorded books or music provide a newly blind client diversional activities. Reading books set in Braille requires special education and time to practice this technique. The newly blind client may not be ready to interact with others as a means of diversion. Listening to the television may create anxiety because the client can only hear and not see what is happening. (16:490-491)

> Nursing Process—Planning
> Client Need—Physiological integrity

27   4. Deformity in alignment, swelling and pain at the fracture site, decreased function or mobility, and ecchymosis at the fracture site might be seen with a fracture of the femur or other long bones. When the femur (which is the long bone between the knee and hip) is fractured, the leg often appears misaligned. (8:646-647)

> Nursing Process—Collecting data
> Client Need—Physiological integrity

28   1. An antistreptolysin O test is used to diagnose conditions resulting from a streptococcal infection. It is useful in the diagnosis of rheumatic fever. This test detects antibodies to the enzymes of the *Streptococcus* Group A, which is

thought to cause rheumatic fever, glomerulonephritis, bacterial endocarditis, scarlet fever, and other related conditions. A latex agglutination test is a nonspecific test that is elevated in many collagen diseases, such as lupus erythematosus. The heterophile antibody titer is performed to determine if a person has infectious mononucleosis. The fluorescent antibody test is used to diagnose syphilis. (8:739; 5:471-472)

> Nursing Process—Collecting data
> Client Need—Physiological integrity

29   2. To determine the number of milliliters of an intravenous solution to infuse in 1 hour, the total amount of milliliters to be given (in this example 1000 mL) is divided by the total hours of infusion (in this example 8 hours). (18:658)

> Nursing Process—Planning
> Client Need—Physiological integrity

30   4. Ice bags should be removed every 30 to 60 minutes to inspect the area and allow it to return to normal. Usually, the ice bag is left off the area for approximately 1 hour. Numbness and mottling and blanching of the skin indicate vasoconstriction and require temporary removal of the ice bag. (18:491; 8:587)

> Nursing Process—Collecting data
> Client Need—Physiological integrity

31   4. Aphasia is the inability to use or understand the spoken word. There are different types and degrees of aphasia. The nurse must first know what type of aphasia a client has. Communication can be improved in many instances if the nurse gives the client time to use motions or signs, write an answer (if able), or to try and speak. Although the speech may be greatly impaired, some aphasic clients can be understood if patience is taken when listening. These clients usually do not have a hearing problem, and their intelligence is not affected by the aphasia. (3:362)

> Nursing Process—Planning
> Client Need—Physiological integrity

32   1. Failure of the fluid in the drainage bottle to rise and fall with each respiration may indicate an obstruction in the drainage tube or that the lung has reinflated. If the chest tube is obstructed, this must be corrected immediately. (3:414; 16:273)

> Nursing Process—Collecting data
> Client Need—Physiological integrity

33   3. A femoral pulse is obtained by placing the fingers in the inguinal (groin) area. (18:256)

> Nursing Process—Collecting data
> Client Need—Physiological integrity

34   2. Parenteral administration of a drug includes the intravenous (into a vein), intraarterial (into an artery), intraarticular (into a joint), intramuscular (into a muscle), intralesional (into a lesion), intradermal (within the skin), intracardiac (into the heart), and intrathecal (intraspinal) routes. (14:483; 15:17)

>Nursing Process—Implementation
>Client Need—Physiological integrity

35 4. Injecting the same amount of air into the vial as the amount of the drug to be withdrawn makes withdrawal of the drug easier. Not injecting the same amount of air as that of the drug to be withdrawn creates a vacuum in the vial once the drug has been withdrawn. Injecting more air than the amount of the drug to be withdrawn creates excessive pressure in the vial, which may force the plunger out of the syringe. It is not necessary to refrigerate a drug before withdrawing it from a vial unless refrigeration is recommended by the manufacturer. (14:489-490)

>Nursing Process—Implementation
>Client Need—Physiological integrity

36 2. Mild to severe joint pain may indicate bleeding into the joint, which can lead to joint deformities or destruction. Hemophiliacs with symptoms suggestive of bleeding should immediately seek medical treatment. (8:653, 730)

>Nursing Process—Collecting data
>Client Need—Physiological integrity

37 3. To effectively plan discharge teaching the nurse needs to know if the client fully understands all the information given by the physician. Areas that are unclear, such as the medication schedule and follow-up appointments, should be reexplained by the nurse. (16:382)

>Nursing Process—Collecting data
>Client Need—Safe, effective care environment

38 2. Lightening, or the movement of the fetus into the true pelvis, is one of the early signs of impending labor. Additional signs include uterine contractions, rupture or leaking of the membranes, bloody show, and frequent urination. (8:109, 150)

>Nursing Process—Planning
>Client Need—Health promotion/maintenance

39 1. Bulging of the perineum indicates that the head of the fetus is pressing on the perineal area. The fetal head (caput) may be seen at this time. This is called "crowning." This is seen late in labor and this sign, as well as others, usually indicates that the mother is ready for delivery. Other signs indicating that the client is ready to deliver include an increase in show, an involuntary desire to push down with each contraction, and dilatation of the anus. Leakage of amniotic fluid can occur at any time. By the time the client is ready for delivery, her membranes have ruptured. (8:124)

>Nursing Process—Collecting data
>Client Need—Health promotion/maintenance

40 2. The Glasgow Coma Scale may be used to detect an increase in intracranial pressure. The three parts of the scale are the eye opening response, the best verbal response, and the best motor response. Using inappropriate words, which is part of the best verbal response, is abnormal. The remaining responses given in this question are normal. (16:408)

>Nursing Process—Collecting data
>Client Need—Physiological integrity

41 4. A living will is one that is a description of how the client wishes to be treated or not treated if the client, at some future time, is unable to make this decision. The client also may select a spokesperson, such as the physician or a spouse, to act on the client's behalf regarding using or withholding medical treatment. The term "relatives" can include aunts, uncles, cousins, and so on. It is normally not necessary for *all* relatives of the client to agree on discontinuing life support. (18:79)

>Nursing Process—Collecting data
>Client Need—Safe, effective care environment

42 3. Correct treatment of poison ingestion and possibly the administration of an antidote depends on substance identification. The age of the client, the observers, and if water was swallowed may be relevant but are less important than identifying the substance. (16:182)

>Nursing Process—Collecting data
>Client Need—Physiological integrity

43 1. Immediately after the membranes have ruptured, the nurse monitors the fetal heart rate to detect any fetal distress. Natural or artificial rupture of the membranes may result in prolapse of the umbilical cord, followed by compression of the cord and cutting off the oxygen supply to the fetus. (8:128)

>Nursing Process—Implementation
>Client Need—Health promotion/maintenance

44 2. The newborn's normal apical pulse rate is 120 to 160 beats per minute. A pulse of 88 is abnormal. The remaining options are normal findings in the newborn. (8:241)

>Nursing Process—Evaluation
>Client Need—Health promotion/maintenance

45 3. Minor burns over a small area are first treated by immersing the part in cool water. Cool compresses also may be applied. Ointments or salves should not be applied to minor burns. Normally, a dressing is not necessary. When a dressing is

necessary, sterile gauze is first applied over the area and anchored with nonallergenic tape above and below the burn site. (3:807)
Nursing Process—Planning
Client Need—Physiological integrity

46 2. Timolol maleate is a beta-adrenergic drug used in the treatment of glaucoma. This drug appears to act by reducing the production of aqueous humor. Atropine is never given to those with glaucoma because administration may result in an acute attack of glaucoma and permanent blindness. Digitalis and penicillin are not indicated for the treatment of glaucoma. (3:838; 16:497-498)
Nursing Process—Collecting data
Client Need—Safe, effective care environment

47 3. The administration of a drug for the treatment of acute angle-closure glaucoma should reduce or eliminate the pain associated with this type of glaucoma. (16:497-498)
Nursing Process—Evaluation
Client Need—Physiological integrity

48 1. Liquid and ointment otic (ear) preparations should be warmed to room temperature if they have been stored in a cool or cold area. Instilling cold medication into the ear is uncomfortable. Labels are never removed from medication containers. Containers of ear preparations should be opened immediately prior to the instillation of the drug. (18:593-594)
Nursing Process—Implementation
Client Need—Physiological integrity

49 4. Eye drops are instilled into the lower conjunctival sac. Prior to instilling eye drops the client is asked to look up as the lower lid margin is pulled downward by exerting downward pressure over the bony prominence of the cheek. (18:588-592)
Nursing Process—Implementation
Client Need—Physiological integrity

50 3. When removing crust from the eye or cleansing the eye prior to the instillation of an ophthalmic preparation, the cotton ball is moved from the inner to the outer canthus. This maneuver will remove secretions, residual medication from previous instillations, and microorganisms away from the nasal duct. (18:591)
Nursing Process—Implementation
Client Need—Physiological integrity

51 2. Recent use of cocaine may be evidenced by symptoms such as agitation, psychotic behavior, violent behavior, hyperthermia, rapid pulse or cardiac dysrhythmias, and dilated pupils. (15:83)
Nursing Process—Collecting data
Client Need—Physiological integrity

52 1. Alcohol is a potentially physically addicting substance. The person addicted to alcohol will experience withdrawal symptoms. The length of time or amount of alcohol consumed required to produce addiction to alcohol varies. (15:85)
Nursing Process—Planning
Client Need—Psychosocial integrity

53 3. Signs of withdrawal from alcohol usually appear in 12 to 72 hours but may appear sooner in some people. (15:85)
Nursing Process—Collecting data
Client Need—Psychosocial integrity

54 4. Burns around the face and neck may injure the respiratory passages; therefore, the client is closely observed for signs of respiratory difficulty or distress. Hemorrhage does not occur with burns unless there has been an additional injury, such as a wound or fracture. Electrolyte imbalances and fluid loss from the burned area do not occur immediately. (3:808)
Nursing Process—Collecting data
Client Need—Physiological integrity

55 2. Proper positioning and regular exercises, when prescribed by the physician, maintain correct body alignment and normal motion in the extremities and prevent muscle contractures and skeletal deformities. (3:810)
Nursing Process—Planning
Client Need—Physiological integrity

56 1. A change in odor may indicate an infection. The odor of infection is different from that of the odor associated with burn exudate. Eschar normally turns black after a period of time. An increase in urine output is normally not related to infection. Tachycardia might be seen if an infection is present. (16:855-856)
Nursing Process—Collecting data
Client Need—Safe, effective care environment

57 1. The client in the manic phase of manic-depressive (bipolar) disorder has flight of ideas, euphoria, and increased physical activity. The client eats and sleeps little and may rapidly lose weight. (1:220-221)
Nursing Process—Collecting data
Client Need—Psychosical integrity

58 3. Accurate charting of the client's mental and physical status is an important aspect of therapy with lithium. The physician may increase or decrease the dose of the drug according to observed client response to therapy. (1:223)
Nursing Process—Collecting data
Client Need—Psychosocial integrity

59 4. The client with an OCD feels the need to perform a stereotyped act repeatedly, such as washing the hands, following a repetitive thought.

For example, the client may have the repetitive thought of wishing to harm someone. This repetitive, obsessive thought is followed by the performance of an act, such as washing the hands or touching an object. Performance of the compulsive act decreases anxiety. Those with OCD usually are able to concentrate on the activities of daily living. Hallucinations, which normally are not associated with this disorder, are not observable by the nurse. Those with OCD are still able to socialize with others. (1:234)
Nursing Process—Evaluation
Client Need—Psychosocial integrity

60 2. Autism is characterized by unawareness of external reality, limited or no social interactions, abnormal speech patterns and conversational ability, preoccupation with objects, and a low range of interest in self or others. (1:158, 201)
Nursing Process—Planning
Client Need—Psychocial integrity

61 2. Constant supervision is necessary in the management of an autistic client. These clients usually do not engage in play activities or scheduled programs. They may become combative if forced to play, be with others, or follow a schedule of activities. (1:158)
Nursing Process—Planning
Client Need—Psychosocial integrity

62 2. Rheumatic fever may follow a recent streptococcal infection. A history of a sore throat, which may have been due to the *Streptococcus* microorganism, would be important information for the health history. Viral infections, such as measles, chickenpox, and mumps, are not known to be associated with rheumatic fever. (8:737)
Nursing Process—Collecting data
Client Need—Safe, effective care environment

63 4. Joint pain and tenderness, which may involve one or more joints, may be noted during an initial physical assessment. Joint pain or tenderness may migrate from joint to joint. As the disease progresses, the joints may become enlarged, tender, and hot. The remaining signs and symptoms normally are not associated with rheumatic fever. (8:737)
Nursing Process—Collecting data
Client Need—Safe, effective care environment

64 2. Rectal temperatures are avoided when a child has leukemia because of the danger of causing hemorrhage and perirectal abscesses. In addition, rectal temperatures usually are avoided when any client, regardless of age, has a bleeding disorder. (8:734-735)
Nursing Process—Implementation
Client Need—Safe, effective care environment

65 1. Platelets are necessary for the clotting of blood. A decrease in the number of platelets results in spontaneous bleeding episodes. In those with idiopathic thrombocytopenic purpura, the platelet count is reduced. Normal platelet function is necessary for the clotting of blood. The administration of salicylates, such as aspirin, may interfere with platelet function. Aspirin administration may result in episodes of spontaneous bleeding, and its use must be avoided. Aspirin does not decrease the size of white or red blood cells or increase the number of platelets. (8:736)
Nursing Process—Planning
Client Need—Health promotion/maintenance

66 4. Normally, 500 to 1000 mL of water are used to irrigate a colostomy. (7:450)
Nursing Process—Implementation
Client Need—Physiological integrity

67 3. A 5 mL (or larger) syringe and a 20 French needle may be used to collect a urine sample from a catheter with a special collection port. An Asepto syringe, suction machine, or smaller catheter is not appropriate for this task. (18:537)
Nursing Process—Implementation
Client Need—Physiological integrity

68 2. A vaginal speculum is inserted by the physician to visually examine the cervix and obtain a sample (smear) of cervical cells for a Papanicolaou's test. (16:663)
Nursing Process—Implementation
Client Need—Safe, effective care environment

69 1. Amenorrhea is the absence of menstrual flow. Painful menses is dysmenorrhea. Menorrhagia is excessive bleeding at the time of normal menstruation. Metrorrhagia is vaginal bleeding at a time other than a menstrual period. (16:670)
Nursing Process—Collecting data
Client Need—Physiological integrity

70 3. The incision necessary for a radical lymph node dissection for testicular carcinoma often extends from the sternum to the symphysis pubis. Because of the length of the incision, coughing and deep breathing usually are uncomfortable. Placing a pillow on the abdomen and applying firm, light pressure may reduce strain on the incision and reduce discomfort. Turning the client on his side or having him sit in a chair probably will not reduce discomfort. When possible, coughing and deep-breathing exercises are performed after the client has received an analgesic and not before the next dose is due. (16:717)
Nursing Process—Planning
Client Need—Physiological integrity

71 2. When a malignant breast tumor is found to be a hormone-dependent tumor, growth is enhanced by the presence of estrogen, which is a hormone secreted by the ovaries. Removal of both ovaries removes the source of estrogen and thus may slow metastasis and growth of any remaining tumor cells. This procedure does not enhance the action of antineoplastic drugs, prevent adverse reactions associated with the administration of antineoplastic drugs, or increase progesterone levels. (16:699)

Nursing Process—Planning
Client Need—Safe, effective care environment

72 1. When the ovaries are removed, the client experiences symptoms of menopause because estrogen levels decrease. Symptoms may be more severe than those associated with natural menopause. Symptoms related to an estrogen deficiency may include flushing of the skin and a feeling of warmth, especially in the face and neck (hot flashes), and excessive perspiration. Other symptoms of menopause may or may not be related to estrogen deficiency and include fatigue, headache, personality changes, and emotional instability. The remaining items in this question should be reported to the physician but usually are not related to a sudden deficiency in estrogen production. (16:699)

Nursing Process—Implementation
Client Need—Safe, effective care environment

73 2. Obstruction of a urethral catheter results in bladder distention. An overdistended bladder is painful, but when the client has lower abdominal surgery, the enlarged bladder presses on the area of surgery and causes increased pain in the operative area. A sodium imbalance, dehydration, or wrinkled sheets are not likely causes of sudden abdominal pain. (3:752)

Nursing Process—Collecting data
Client Need—Safe, effective care environment

74 4. Antineoplastic drugs are highly toxic, and some of these drugs may be absorbed through the skin of those handling the drug. Disposable plastic gloves should be used when preparing or assembling the materials for administration of any parenteral antineoplastic drug. Do not refrigerate a drug or premix the drug unless these tasks are recommended by the manufacturer. Some antineoplastic drugs must be prepared or reconstituted immediately prior to administration. A large needle (18 to 20 French) usually is used to withdraw the drug from the container. (15:238)

Nursing Process—Implementation
Client Need—Safe, effective care environment

75 3. The primary function of a hospice is to allow terminally ill clients to be at home with their families or to be placed in specialized hospital hospice units. The hospital hospice units differ from standard hospital rooms in that they have a warm, home-like atmosphere. (16:205)

Nursing Process—Implementation
Client Need—Psychosocial integrity

76 3. The child with an attention-deficit disorder may have many symptoms, such as difficulty in concentrating, disruptive behavior, failing to complete tasks, constantly moving or fidgeting, and acting in a loud and noisy manner. Sleeping during the day, disinterest in surroundings, and refusing to play with others are not considered typical characteristics of this disorder. (19:816)

Nursing Process—Evaluation
Client Need—Psychosocial integrity

77 2. Dietary restrictions of food additives, artificial food colorings, and food preservatives have been used by some physicians. Although the dietary restrictions of these and other foods have been controversial, some success has been noted. The other items in this question are normally not included in a special restrictive diet for attention-deficit disorders. When this type of a diet is prescribed, the parents are instructed to read food labels carefully. (19:816-818)

Nursing Process—Implementation
Client Need—Health promotion/maintenance

78 3. Myasthenia gravis affects one or more groups of skeletal muscles. The muscles of the face often are affected, thus interfering with the ability to chew and swallow. A normal temperature, a desire to go home, and a normal bowel movement do not indicate an adequate response to this type of drug. (16:416, 15:52)

Nursing Process—Evaluation
Client Need—Physiological integrity

79 1. Squeezing blackheads and pimples can cause the infection to spread and may cause scarring of the skin. A comedone extractor often is used by experienced caretakers to remove blackheads but should not be used by a lay person unless the person has been well taught and can be depended on to use the comedone extractor properly. (8:601)

Nursing Process—Implementation
Client Need—Health promotion/maintenance

80 4. Stiffness and pain on movement are the usual complaints of those with osteoarthritis. Stiffness may be more noticeable in the morning. Bradycardia and fever are not normally associated with osteoarthritis. Redness of the joints is seen in rheumatoid arthritis. (3:657; 16:802-803)

Nursing Process—Evaluation
Client Need—Physiological integrity

81 3. Short periods of moderate exercise, performed daily, often are beneficial for those with osteoarthritis. Prolonged, heavy exercise or lifting weights may harm affected joints and should not be undertaken except on the advice of a physician. (16:802-803)

Nursing Process—Implementation
Client Need—Physiological integrity

82 1. Motrin (ibuprofen) is a nonsteroidal antiinflammatory drug (NSAID). Administration of this type of drug should reduce the pain and discomfort associated with osteoarthritis. Joint redness and fever usually are not seen with osteoarthritis. These drugs do not decrease the size of the joint because joint changes are permanent. (16:802–803)

Nursing Process—Evaluation
Client Need—Physiological integrity

83 4. Gastrointestinal symptoms, such as diarrhea, constipation, abdominal discomfort, and gastrointestinal bleeding, are the most common adverse reactions associated with an NSAID such as ibuprofen. (15:318)

Nursing Process—Evaluation
Client Need—Physiological integrity

84 1. In an emergency, the substance causing a chemical burn may or may not be known. Emergency treatment is directed at diluting and removing the substance as rapidly as possible by flushing the area with large amounts of water. If the substance is lime or phenol, water is not used. The lime is brushed from the skin and clothes. Phenol burns are treated with the application of alcohol to remove the phenol, followed by rinsing the area with water. (3:878)

Nursing Process—Implementation
Client Need—Physiological integrity

85 1. Not reacting purposefully to a stimulus is a most important observation because it may indicate injury to the brain, such as bleeding within the cranium. Certain symptoms, such as poor response to stimuli, abnormal reactions to stimuli, and failure to follow simple commands, may require the immediate attention of a physician. Crying at this time is not abnormal, but the character of the cry may be abnormal. A small bump on the forehead is less important. Scratches on the forehead and face are less important and may or may not require treatment and further investigation. (8:431-432)

Nursing Process—Evaluation
Client Need—Physiological integrity

86 3. When a reddened area is noted, pressure should not be placed on the area until the skin becomes normal in color. (8:433)

Nursing Process—Implementation
Client Need—Safe, effective care environment

87 2. Suctioning is performed when the client is unable to cough and raise sputum. Ineffective coughing and raising sputum, dyspnea, cyanosis, and moist breath sounds indicate that suctioning is necessary. (18:708)

Nursing Process—Collecting data
Client Need—Physiological integrity

88 3. The prone position is face down, the supine position is on the back, and the lateral position is on the left or right side. When a client is placed in the prone position, the nurse must be sure that the airway is patent and there is no danger of suffocation. The client in this position should be checked at frequent intervals. The prone position may be used to relieve pressure on the back and aid in the treatment of pressure sores (decubitus ulcers). (18:384)

Nursing Process—Implementation
Client Need—Safe, effective care environment

89 3. Even a minor blow to the head may result in intracranial bleeding. The client should be closely observed for several days (or for as long as the physician's instructions indicate). If drowsiness or sleepiness occurs and the client cannot be easily aroused, the physician should be notified immediately. Drinking extra fluids and keeping the client in bed usually are not necessary. If a bandage is necessary because of a cut, it would have been applied in the emergency department. (19:601-604)

Nursing Process—Planning
Client Need—Physiological integrity

90 1. Checking the LOC and noting any changes are the most appropriate assessments when a client has suspected intracranial bleeding. Should a change occur, the physician must be notified immediately. Jaundice is not likely to have occurred. Measuring the intake and output and the CVP (if a CVP line has been inserted) is less important than checking the LOC. (19:601-604)

Nursing Process—Planning
Client Need—Physiological integrity

91 3. The stoma is usually intubated with a catheter at the time of surgery. A suction machine capable of low, intermittent suction should be placed in the room prior to the return of the client from surgery. Usually, the stomal catheter is connected to low suction. Ileostomy output should be measured at least once every 8 hours. The rectal packing is removed by the physician usually about a week after surgery. The nurse may reinforce the rectal packing as needed. Sealing the stoma would prevent the flow of fecal drainage and increase pressure in the newly created pouch. (16:586)

Nursing Process—Planning
Client Need—Safe, effective care environment

92 2. The presence of a foul or unusual odor to a cast may indicate an infection. Blood on the cast surface may indicate bleeding beneath the cast. A crack or indentation in the cast does not indicate infection but may compromise the rigidity of the cast. (3:640)

Nursing Process—Collecting data
Client Need—Safe, effective care environment

93 2. The cast edges should be petaled with waterproof tape to avoid soiling. Covering the perineal area of the cast with a waterproof material, such as plastic wrap, may help prevent soiling of the surface of the cast in this area. Cotton wadding or other materials should never be inserted between the cast and the skin unless ordered by the physician. Offering the bedpan at more frequent intervals to a child who is not toilet-trained or keeping the head of the bed elevated will not prevent soiling to the perineal area of the cast. (3:640)

Nursing Process—Implementation
Client Need—Safe, effective care environment

94 1. The client's body weight must counteract the pull of the weights for traction to be effective. The remaining statements in this question do not demonstrate traction effectiveness. (3:644)

Nursing Process—Evaluation
Client Need—Safe, effective care environment

95 3. The symptoms of pulmonary edema include sudden dyspnea, pink frothy sputum, cyanosis, bounding pulse, elevated blood pressure, severe apprehension, and moist or gurgling respirations. (16:348)

Nursing Process—Collecting data
Client Need—Physiological integrity

96 1. Medical management of left-sided heart failure is directed toward reducing the workload of the heart and improving left ventricular output. The workload of the heart may be reduced by bed rest. Complete bed rest often is necessary when the client has severe left-sided heart failure. Morning care need not be eliminated, but the nurse should make every effort to help the client as much as possible. In some instances the client may require complete help with morning care. Selecting a low-cholesterol diet will not decrease the workload of the heart. Forcing fluids may increase the workload of the heart, especially if the client has some renal impairment. (16:343)

Nursing Process—Implementation
Client Need—Physiological integrity

97 1. Frequent use of laxatives can cause diarrhea. Some people become obsessed with having a daily bowel movement and frequently use laxatives. Those who have an eating disorder may use laxatives following eating binges. Drinking water with meals and eating canned vegetables are not likely causes of diarrhea. Those with persistent diarrhea may have lost weight. (18:550)

Nursing Process—Collecting data
Client Need—Physiological integrity

98 2. Postural hypotension may occur during therapy with certain drugs, such as antihypertensive agents. The client can be instructed to rise slowly from a sitting or lying position. Dietary changes or exercise will not relieve the symptoms of postural hypotension. (16:339)

Nursing Process—Implementation
Client Need—Safe, effective care environment

99 1. Hyperventilation is an increase in the rate or depth of respiration. Rapidly breathing in and out or taking rapid deep breaths results in a decrease in carbon dioxide in the blood (acapnia). Rebreathing expired air will increase the carbon dioxide in the blood. The remaining options in this question would not raise the carbon dioxide level in the blood. (14:812)

Nursing Process—Implementation
Client Need—Physiological integrity

100 2. The Tine test is a tuberculin test. A red, raised area at the testing site indicates a positive reaction. A guideline chart for reading test results accompanies the test. (14:815)

Nursing Process—Evaluation
Client Need—Health promotion/maintenance

101 3. A pale appearance of skin over bony prominences is due to a lack of circulation to the area. This is followed by redness. If the client is not turned frequently, the area may become dark and cyanotic. Ultimately, the skin breaks down and an open ulcer (decubitus ulcer) forms. Stiffness may occur with prolonged bed rest, even when the client's position is changed frequently. A fever may indicate an infection but also may be due to other causes. (18:460-461)

Nursing Process—Evaluation
Client Need—Physiological integrity

102 2. When a client is on protective or reverse isolation, articles and bed linens must be sterilized or disinfected before use. This is done to prevent contact between potentially pathogenic microorganisms and the uninfected immunocompromised client. This type of precaution is not necessary for those on blood and body fluid precautions. (18:360)

Nursing Process—Implementation
Client Need—Safe, effective care environment

103 3. Weakness and lightheadedness may occur when a client has been relatively immobile for a prolonged period. These symptoms are due to a drop in blood pressure when the client assumes a standing position. (3:185)
Nursing Process—Collecting data
Client Need—Physiological integrity

104 2. A 2-year-old child should be able to walk up and down stairs alone. The ability to hop, skip, or catch a ball is seen around 5 years of age, and the ability to button and unbutton clothes is normally seen at age 4 years. (8:356)
Nursing Process—Collecting data
Client Need—Health promotion/maintenance

105 1. The first step in instituting a bladder retraining program is determining the client's voiding pattern. Knowing the voiding pattern will allow for setting up a voiding schedule. Limiting the fluid intake is not recommended because the client needs an adequate fluid intake to keep the urine dilute and prevent a fluid deficit. The client may be shown how to use the commode if the client is allowed out of bed when a voiding pattern has been established. (18:506)
Nursing Process—Collecting data
Client Need—Health promotion/maintenance

106 4. Credé's maneuver increases abdominal pressure on the bladder, thus aiding in emptying the bladder. It is performed by using both hands to apply light pressure over the bladder. (18:509)
Nursing Process—Implementation
Client Need—Health promotion/maintenance

107 1. A urinary output of less than 500 mL in 24 hours is considered abnormal. In addition to measuring the output, the fluid intake also must be known. The nurse also must take into consideration other factors, such as current treatment modalities, illness, or injury. (18:502-503)
Nursing Process—Collecting data
Client Need—Physiological integrity

108 2. Numbness and tingling of the extremities are early signs of possible hypocalcemia, which may have occurred if some or all of the parathyroid glands were inadvertently removed. These symptoms require immediate medical intervention. A rectal temperature of 100.8°F may not be unusual after surgery. Hoarseness is not unusual for several days after thyroid surgery. A sore throat may be seen after a general anesthetic and usually is due to the presence of an endotracheal tube during surgery. The rectal temperature, the client's voice quality, and the complaint of a sore throat should be entered on the client's record and evaluated at periodic intervals. (16:634)
Nursing Process—Collecting data
Client Need—Physiological integrity

109 3. When the client with Alzheimer's disease is confused and has an unsteady gait, all objects that pose a hazard, such as footstools and small tables, should be removed from the ambulatory area. It is against local fire laws in most areas to lock entry and exit doors. Restraints may not be applied without a physician's order. Even when restraints are ordered, they may make the client more confused. Keeping the bed in a high position may result in falls when the confused client tries to get out of bed. At night the bed should be kept in a low position and the side rails raised. (16:444-446)
Nursing Process—Planning
Client Need—Safe, effective care environment

110 4. The Moro reflex is present in the newborn and may be seen up to 3 months of age. This reflex response is elicited by bringing the infant's head forward and then allowing it to fall back suddenly. At this time the examiner will see an abduction of the upper extremities at the shoulder and an extension of the arms and hands. Absence of this reflex is an abnormal finding in the newborn. (8:344)
Nursing Process—Collecting data
Client Need—Health promotion/maintenance

111 2. The urine of a client with suspected calculus (stone) in the genitourinary tract is strained through fine gauze and inspected for stones. The client is encouraged to remain ambulatory to help passage of the calculus. Foods high in calcium are discouraged until the type of stone is identified because some calculi are due to increased levels of calcium in the blood. Fruit juices are not encouraged unless approved by the physician because some fruit juices tend to form crystals in the urine. The client is encouraged to increase his water intake up to 3000 mL per day to aid in the passage of the stone. (7:514)
Nursing Process—Planning
Client Need—Physiological integrity

112 1. Encouraging the client to talk about what he is experiencing and how he feels may provide the nurse with additional information. Some clients need an opening to discuss their fears and anxieties. The nurse should listen to the client and consider whether additional interventions, such as discussing the client's problem at a nursing conference or with the physician, are necessary. (3:811)
Nursing Process—Implementation
Client Need—Psychosocial

113 4. *Objective* characteristics are those that are observed by another person, such as a nurse. Objective characteristics of anxiety include tachycardia, poor eye contact, tremors, hypertension, insomnia, superficial vasoconstriction, increased perspiration, quivering of voice, restlessness, and signs of increased wariness. Subjective characteristics are those symptoms described by the client. Dry mouth, increased feelings of tension, and fearfulness are *subjective* characteristics of anxiety. (1:231)

> Nursing Process—Collecting Data
> Client Need—Psychosocial integrity

114 1. The normal fasting blood glucose is 80 to 120 mg/dL. (16:645)

> Nursing Process—Evaluation
> Client Need—Physiological integrity

115 4. Hypoglycemia can occur with the use of an oral hypoglycemic agent. The client should have the symptoms of hypoglycemia (low blood glucose or sugar) explained, as well as what may be done to terminate the reaction. It will be necessary for the client to follow the diet recommended by the physician. Failure to take the drug will result in an increase, not decrease, in blood glucose levels. Oral hypoglycemic agents are taken once or twice daily. The client should read the label of the prescription container concerning the time of day or relationship to meals. Once-a-day dosage is usually before breakfast. Twice-daily dosage is usually before the morning and evening meals. These drugs are not taken after a meal. (16:648)

> Nursing Process—Implementation
> Client Need—Health promotion/maintenance

116 1. Symptoms of hypoglycemia may vary from one client to another. Examples of the more common symptoms of hypoglycemia include vertigo, lightheadedness, nervousness, excessive hunger, personality changes, tremors, drowsiness, and excessive perspiration. (16:649)

> Nursing Process—Evaluation
> Client Need—Physiological integrity

117 2. A sufficient amount of blood to cover and saturate the test pad is required for an accurate reading with the glucometer. One milliliter of blood is more than is needed. The lancet is inserted into a holder that measures the depth of the

puncture; a depth of 10 cm is too deep. The client's hands are washed with warm water to facilitate dilatation of blood vessels, which usually ensures an adequate sample of blood. (18:318-321)

> Nursing Process—Implementation
> Client Need—Physiological integrity

118 1. The feet should be bathed daily using warm (not hot) water. Shoes or slippers should be worn, and walking barefoot is discouraged. Hot water bottles or heating pads are not used to keep the feet warm when sleeping because the diabetic client may have circulatory problems in the extremities, which in turn could result in tissue damage following the application of heat. Loose-fitting cotton socks or blankets may be used to keep the feet warm. Feet should not be soaked because this may lead to cracking of the skin and infection. (3:708)

> Nursing Process—Planning
> Client Need—Health promotion/maintenance

119 1. Type I diabetes mellitus is also called insulin-dependent diabetes mellitus. By knowing the meaning of the classification type I diabetes mellitus, the nurse can develop a plan of care that includes activities such as checking the client for hypoglycemic reactions to insulin, recognizing the symptoms of ketoacidosis, and noting the amount of food eaten at each meal. (16:645)

> Nursing Process—Planning
> Client Need—Safe, effective care environment

120 2. Clients with type II diabetes mellitus controlled with an oral hypoglycemic agent may have this drug discontinued 48 hours prior to surgery. At this time, insulin may be ordered to achieve control of their diabetes immediately before, during, and after surgery. The administration of insulin during this period of stress and nothing by mouth continues until the client is able to take food, at which time administration of the oral hypoglycemic agent may be resumed. (3:707)

> Nursing Process—Planning
> Client Need—Safe, effective care environment

Classification of Test Items

Comprehensive Examination Part II

Directions: After each question the correct answer is given as well as a classification of each test question. Compare the correct answer with your answer. If a question has been answered *incorrectly*, draw a line to the end of the four columns. When finished, add up your correct scores and place the results at the bottom of each column.

Score Calculation:

To determine the percentage of the number of questions you answered correctly, divide the **Number Correct** by the **Number Possible**, as example 106 (the number of questions answered correctly) divided by 120 (the number of questions in the test) = .88 or 88%.

NURSING PROCESS
C = Collecting data
P = Planning
I = Implementation
E = Evaluation

CLIENT NEEDS
S = Safe, effective care environment
P = Physiological integrity
M = Psychosocial integrity
H = Health promotion/maintenance

Question #	Answer #	\<Nursing Process\> C	P	I	E	\<Client Needs\> S	P	M	H
1	3			I					H
2	2		P						H
3	3			I					H
4	4			I					H
5	1				E		P		
6	2				E		P		
7	4				E				H
8	3			I					H
9	2			I			P		
10	2				E				H
11	2				E	S			
12	1			I			P		
13	3			I			P		
14	3				E		P		
15	3				E			M	
16	3			I			P		
17	2			I		S			
18	3				E	S			
19	3				E	S			
20	2			I			P		
21	4		P			S			
22	1	C				S			

NURSING PROCESS
C = Collecting data
P = Planning
I = Implementation
E = Evaluation

CLIENT NEEDS
S = Safe, effective care environment
P = Physiological integrity
M = Psychosocial integrity
H = Health promotion/maintenance

Question #	Answer #	Nursing Process C	Nursing Process P	Nursing Process I	Nursing Process E	Client Needs S	Client Needs P	Client Needs M	Client Needs H
23	4				E	S			
24	4		P				P		
25	3	C				S			
26	1		P				P		
27	4	C					P		
28	1	C					P		
29	2		P				P		
30	4	C					P		
31	4		P				P		
32	1	C					P		
33	3	C					P		
34	2			I			P		
35	4			I			P		
36	2	C					P		
37	3	C				S			
38	2		P						H
39	1	C							H
40	2	C					P		
41	4	C				S			
42	3	C					P		
43	1			I					H
44	2				E				H
45	3		P				P		
46	2	C				S			
47	3				E		P		
48	1			I			P		
49	4			I			P		
50	3			I			P		
51	2	C					P		
52	1		P					M	
53	3	C						M	
54	4	C					P		
55	2		P				P		
56	1	C				S			

NURSING PROCESS
C = Collecting data
P = Planning
I = Implementation
E = Evaluation

CLIENT NEEDS
S = Safe, effective care environment
P = Physiological integrity
M = Psychosocial integrity
H = Health promotion/maintenance

Question #	Answer #	Nursing Process				Client Needs			
		C	P	I	E	S	P	M	H
57	1	C						M	
58	3	C						M	
59	4				E			M	
60	2		P					M	
61	2		P					M	
62	2	C				S			
63	4	C				S			
64	2			I		S			
65	1		P						H
66	4			I			P		
67	3			I			P		
68	2			I		S			
69	1	C					P		
70	3		P				P		
71	2		P			S			
72	1			I		S			
73	2	C				S			
74	4			I		S			
75	3			I				M	
76	3				E			M	
77	2			I					H
78	3				E		P		
79	1			I					H
80	4				E		P		
81	3			I			P		
82	1				E		P		
83	4				E		P		
84	1			I			P		
85	1				E		P		
86	3			I		S			
87	2	C					P		
88	3			I		S			
89	3		P				P		
90	1		P				P		

NURSING PROCESS
C = Collecting data
P = Planning
I = Implementation
E = Evaluation

CLIENT NEEDS
S = Safe, effective care environment
P = Physiological integrity
M = Psychosocial integrity
H = Health promotion/maintenance

Question #	Answer #	Nursing Process				Client Needs			
		C	P	I	E	S	P	M	H
91	3		P			S			
92	2	C				S			
93	2			I		S			
94	1				E	S			
95	3	C					P		
96	1			I			P		
97	1	C					P		
98	2			I		S			
99	1			I			P		
100	2				E				H
101	3				E		P		
102	2			I		S			
103	3	C					P		
104	2	C							H
105	1	C							H
106	4			I					H
107	1	C					P		
108	2	C					P		
109	3		P			S			
110	4	C							H
111	2		P				P		
112	1			I				M	
113	4	C						M	
114	1				E		P		
115	4			I					H
116	1				E		P		
117	2			I			P		
118	1		P						H
119	1		P			S			
120	2		P			S			
Number Correct									
Number Possible	120	35	23	38	24	31	56	12	21
Percentage Correct									

References

1. Barry, P. D. (1990). *Mental health and mental illness* (4th ed.). Philadelphia: J.B. Lippincott.
2. Carpenito, L. J. (1992). *Nursing diagnosis, application to clinical practice* (4th ed.). Philadelphia: J.B. Lippincott.
3. deWit, S. C. (1992). *Keane's essentials of medical-surgical nursing* (3rd ed.). Philadelphia: W.B. Saunders.
4. Eschleman, M. M. (1991). *Introductory nutrition and diet therapy* (2nd ed.). Philadelphia: J.B. Lippincott.
5. Fischbach, F. T. (1992). *A manual of laboratory diagnostic tests* (4th ed.). Philadelphia: J.B. Lippincott.
6. Fuller, J., Schaller-Ayers, J. (1990). *Health assessment, a nursing approach.* Philadelphia: J.B. Lippincott.
7. Harkness H. G., Dincher, J. R. (1992). *Total patient care* (8th ed.). St. Louis: C.V. Mosby.
8. Ingalls, A. J., Salerno, M. C. (1991). *Maternal and child health nursing* (7th ed.). St. Louis: C.V. Mosby.
9. Kalman, N., Waughfield, C. G. (1987). *Mental health concepts* (2nd ed.). Albany: Delmar.
10. Kurzen, C. R. (1989). *Contemporary practical-vocational nursing.* Philadelphia: J.B. Lippincott.
11. Memmler, R. L., Cohen, B. J., Wood, D. L. (1992). *The human body in health and disease* (7th ed.). Philadelphia: J.B. Lippincott.
12. Perko, J. E., Kreigh, H. Z. (1988). *Psychiatric and mental health nursing* (3rd ed.). Norwalk: Appleton & Lange.
13. Phillips, C. R. (1991). *Family-centered maternity/newborn care: A basic text* (3rd ed.). St. Louis: C.V. Mosby.
14. Rosdahl, C. B. (1991). *Textbook of basic nursing* (5th ed.). Philadelphia: J.B. Lippincott.
15. Scherer, J. C. (1992). *Introductory clinical pharmacology* (4th ed.). Philadelphia: J.B. Lippincott.
16. Scherer, J. C. (1991). *Introductory medical-surgical nursing* (5th ed.). Philadelphia: J.B. Lippincott.
17. Taylor, C. M. (1990). *Mereness' essentials of psychiatric nursing* (13th ed.). St. Louis: C.V. Mosby.
18. Timby, B. K., Lewis, L. W. (1992). *Fundamental skills and concepts in patient care* (5th ed.). Philadelphia: J.B. Lippincott.
19. Thompson, E. D. (1990). *Introduction to maternity and pediatric nursing.* Philadelphia: W.B. Saunders.
20. Williams, S. R. (1992). *Basic nutrition and diet therapy* (9th ed.). Philadelphia: J.B. Lippincott.

Answer Sheet

UNIT ONE
REVIEW TEST 1

With a pencil, blacken the circle below the option you have chosen for your correct answer.

	1 2 3 4		1 2 3 4		1 2 3 4		1 2 3 4
1	○○○○	21	○○○○	41	○○○○	61	○○○○
2	○○○○	22	○○○○	42	○○○○	62	○○○○
3	○○○○	23	○○○○	43	○○○○	63	○○○○
4	○○○○	24	○○○○	44	○○○○	64	○○○○
5	○○○○	25	○○○○	45	○○○○	65	○○○○
6	○○○○	26	○○○○	46	○○○○	66	○○○○
7	○○○○	27	○○○○	47	○○○○	67	○○○○
8	○○○○	28	○○○○	48	○○○○	68	○○○○
9	○○○○	29	○○○○	49	○○○○	69	○○○○
10	○○○○	30	○○○○	50	○○○○	70	○○○○
11	○○○○	31	○○○○	51	○○○○	71	○○○○
12	○○○○	32	○○○○	52	○○○○	72	○○○○
13	○○○○	33	○○○○	53	○○○○	73	○○○○
14	○○○○	34	○○○○	54	○○○○	74	○○○○
15	○○○○	35	○○○○	55	○○○○	75	○○○○
16	○○○○	36	○○○○	56	○○○○	76	○○○○
17	○○○○	37	○○○○	57	○○○○	77	○○○○
18	○○○○	38	○○○○	58	○○○○	78	○○○○
19	○○○○	39	○○○○	59	○○○○	79	○○○○
20	○○○○	40	○○○○	60	○○○○	80	○○○○

	1 2 3 4		1 2 3 4		1 2 3 4		1 2 3 4
81	○○○○	91	○○○○	101	○○○○	111	○○○○
82	○○○○	92	○○○○	102	○○○○	112	○○○○
83	○○○○	93	○○○○	103	○○○○	113	○○○○
84	○○○○	94	○○○○	104	○○○○	114	○○○○
85	○○○○	95	○○○○	105	○○○○	115	○○○○
86	○○○○	96	○○○○	106	○○○○	116	○○○○
87	○○○○	97	○○○○	107	○○○○	117	○○○○
88	○○○○	98	○○○○	108	○○○○	118	○○○○
89	○○○○	99	○○○○	109	○○○○	119	○○○○
90	○○○○	100	○○○○	110	○○○○	120	○○○○

Answer Sheet

UNIT TWO
REVIEW TEST 2

With a pencil, blacken the circle below the option you have chosen for your correct answer.

	1 2 3 4		1 2 3 4		1 2 3 4		1 2 3 4
1	○○○○	21	○○○○	41	○○○○	61	○○○○
2	○○○○	22	○○○○	42	○○○○	62	○○○○
3	○○○○	23	○○○○	43	○○○○	63	○○○○
4	○○○○	24	○○○○	44	○○○○	64	○○○○
5	○○○○	25	○○○○	45	○○○○	65	○○○○
6	○○○○	26	○○○○	46	○○○○	66	○○○○
7	○○○○	27	○○○○	47	○○○○	67	○○○○
8	○○○○	28	○○○○	48	○○○○	68	○○○○
9	○○○○	29	○○○○	49	○○○○	69	○○○○
10	○○○○	30	○○○○	50	○○○○	70	○○○○
11	○○○○	31	○○○○	51	○○○○	71	○○○○
12	○○○○	32	○○○○	52	○○○○	72	○○○○
13	○○○○	33	○○○○	53	○○○○	73	○○○○
14	○○○○	34	○○○○	54	○○○○	74	○○○○
15	○○○○	35	○○○○	55	○○○○	75	○○○○
16	○○○○	36	○○○○	56	○○○○	76	○○○○
17	○○○○	37	○○○○	57	○○○○	77	○○○○
18	○○○○	38	○○○○	58	○○○○	78	○○○○
19	○○○○	39	○○○○	59	○○○○	79	○○○○
20	○○○○	40	○○○○	60	○○○○	80	○○○○

	1 2 3 4		1 2 3 4		1 2 3 4		1 2 3 4
81	○○○○	84	○○○○	87	○○○○	90	○○○○
82	○○○○	85	○○○○	88	○○○○	91	○○○○
83	○○○○	86	○○○○	89	○○○○		

Answer Sheet

UNIT TWO
REVIEW TEST 3

With a pencil, blacken the circle below the option you have chosen for your correct answer.

	1 2 3 4		1 2 3 4		1 2 3 4		1 2 3 4
1	○○○○	21	○○○○	41	○○○○	61	○○○○
2	○○○○	22	○○○○	42	○○○○	62	○○○○
3	○○○○	23	○○○○	43	○○○○	63	○○○○
4	○○○○	24	○○○○	44	○○○○	64	○○○○
5	○○○○	25	○○○○	45	○○○○	65	○○○○
6	○○○○	26	○○○○	46	○○○○	66	○○○○
7	○○○○	27	○○○○	47	○○○○	67	○○○○
8	○○○○	28	○○○○	48	○○○○	68	○○○○
9	○○○○	29	○○○○	49	○○○○	69	○○○○
10	○○○○	30	○○○○	50	○○○○	70	○○○○
11	○○○○	31	○○○○	51	○○○○	71	○○○○
12	○○○○	32	○○○○	52	○○○○	72	○○○○
13	○○○○	33	○○○○	53	○○○○	73	○○○○
14	○○○○	34	○○○○	54	○○○○	74	○○○○
15	○○○○	35	○○○○	55	○○○○	75	○○○○
16	○○○○	36	○○○○	56	○○○○	76	○○○○
17	○○○○	37	○○○○	57	○○○○	77	○○○○
18	○○○○	38	○○○○	58	○○○○	78	○○○○
19	○○○○	39	○○○○	59	○○○○	79	○○○○
20	○○○○	40	○○○○	60	○○○○	80	○○○○

	1 2 3 4		1 2 3 4		1 2 3 4		1 2 3 4
81	○○○○	89	○○○○	97	○○○○	105	○○○○
82	○○○○	90	○○○○	98	○○○○	106	○○○○
83	○○○○	91	○○○○	99	○○○○	107	○○○○
84	○○○○	92	○○○○	100	○○○○	108	○○○○
85	○○○○	93	○○○○	101	○○○○	109	○○○○
86	○○○○	94	○○○○	102	○○○○	110	○○○○
87	○○○○	95	○○○○	103	○○○○	111	○○○○
88	○○○○	96	○○○○	104	○○○○		

Answer Sheet

UNIT THREE
REVIEW TEST 4

With a pencil, blacken the circle below the option you have chosen for your correct answer.

	1 2 3 4		1 2 3 4		1 2 3 4		1 2 3 4
1	○○○○	21	○○○○	41	○○○○	61	○○○○
2	○○○○	22	○○○○	42	○○○○	62	○○○○
3	○○○○	23	○○○○	43	○○○○	63	○○○○
4	○○○○	24	○○○○	44	○○○○	64	○○○○
5	○○○○	25	○○○○	45	○○○○	65	○○○○
6	○○○○	26	○○○○	46	○○○○	66	○○○○
7	○○○○	27	○○○○	47	○○○○	67	○○○○
8	○○○○	28	○○○○	48	○○○○	68	○○○○
9	○○○○	29	○○○○	49	○○○○	69	○○○○
10	○○○○	30	○○○○	50	○○○○	70	○○○○
11	○○○○	31	○○○○	51	○○○○	71	○○○○
12	○○○○	32	○○○○	52	○○○○	72	○○○○
13	○○○○	33	○○○○	53	○○○○	73	○○○○
14	○○○○	34	○○○○	54	○○○○	74	○○○○
15	○○○○	35	○○○○	55	○○○○	75	○○○○
16	○○○○	36	○○○○	56	○○○○	76	○○○○
17	○○○○	37	○○○○	57	○○○○	77	○○○○
18	○○○○	38	○○○○	58	○○○○	78	○○○○
19	○○○○	39	○○○○	59	○○○○	79	○○○○
20	○○○○	40	○○○○	60	○○○○	80	○○○○

	1 2 3 4		1 2 3 4		1 2 3 4		1 2 3 4
81	○○○○	90	○○○○	99	○○○○	108	○○○○
82	○○○○	91	○○○○	100	○○○○	109	○○○○
83	○○○○	92	○○○○	101	○○○○	110	○○○○
84	○○○○	93	○○○○	102	○○○○	111	○○○○
85	○○○○	94	○○○○	103	○○○○	112	○○○○
86	○○○○	95	○○○○	104	○○○○	113	○○○○
87	○○○○	96	○○○○	105	○○○○	114	○○○○
88	○○○○	97	○○○○	106	○○○○		
89	○○○○	98	○○○○	107	○○○○		

Answer Sheet

UNIT THREE
REVIEW TEST 5

With a pencil, blacken the circle below the option you have chosen for your correct answer.

	1 2 3 4		1 2 3 4		1 2 3 4		1 2 3 4
1	○○○○	21	○○○○	41	○○○○	61	○○○○
2	○○○○	22	○○○○	42	○○○○	62	○○○○
3	○○○○	23	○○○○	43	○○○○	63	○○○○
4	○○○○	24	○○○○	44	○○○○	64	○○○○
5	○○○○	25	○○○○	45	○○○○	65	○○○○
6	○○○○	26	○○○○	46	○○○○	66	○○○○
7	○○○○	27	○○○○	47	○○○○	67	○○○○
8	○○○○	28	○○○○	48	○○○○	68	○○○○
9	○○○○	29	○○○○	49	○○○○	69	○○○○
10	○○○○	30	○○○○	50	○○○○	70	○○○○
11	○○○○	31	○○○○	51	○○○○	71	○○○○
12	○○○○	32	○○○○	52	○○○○	72	○○○○
13	○○○○	33	○○○○	53	○○○○	73	○○○○
14	○○○○	34	○○○○	54	○○○○	74	○○○○
15	○○○○	35	○○○○	55	○○○○	75	○○○○
16	○○○○	36	○○○○	56	○○○○	76	○○○○
17	○○○○	37	○○○○	57	○○○○	77	○○○○
18	○○○○	38	○○○○	58	○○○○	78	○○○○
19	○○○○	39	○○○○	59	○○○○	79	○○○○
20	○○○○	40	○○○○	60	○○○○	80	○○○○

	1 2 3 4		1 2 3 4		1 2 3 4		1 2 3 4
81	○○○○	89	○○○○	97	○○○○	105	○○○○
82	○○○○	90	○○○○	98	○○○○	106	○○○○
83	○○○○	91	○○○○	99	○○○○	107	○○○○
84	○○○○	92	○○○○	100	○○○○	108	○○○○
85	○○○○	93	○○○○	101	○○○○	109	○○○○
86	○○○○	94	○○○○	102	○○○○	110	○○○○
87	○○○○	95	○○○○	103	○○○○	111	○○○○
88	○○○○	96	○○○○	104	○○○○		

Answer Sheet

UNIT FOUR
REVIEW TEST 6

With a pencil, blacken the circle below the option you have chosen for your correct answer.

	1 2 3 4		1 2 3 4		1 2 3 4		1 2 3 4
1	○○○○	21	○○○○	41	○○○○	61	○○○○
2	○○○○	22	○○○○	42	○○○○	62	○○○○
3	○○○○	23	○○○○	43	○○○○	63	○○○○
4	○○○○	24	○○○○	44	○○○○	64	○○○○
5	○○○○	25	○○○○	45	○○○○	65	○○○○
6	○○○○	26	○○○○	46	○○○○	66	○○○○
7	○○○○	27	○○○○	47	○○○○	67	○○○○
8	○○○○	28	○○○○	48	○○○○	68	○○○○
9	○○○○	29	○○○○	49	○○○○	69	○○○○
10	○○○○	30	○○○○	50	○○○○	70	○○○○
11	○○○○	31	○○○○	51	○○○○	71	○○○○
12	○○○○	32	○○○○	52	○○○○	72	○○○○
13	○○○○	33	○○○○	53	○○○○	73	○○○○
14	○○○○	34	○○○○	54	○○○○	74	○○○○
15	○○○○	35	○○○○	55	○○○○	75	○○○○
16	○○○○	36	○○○○	56	○○○○	76	○○○○
17	○○○○	37	○○○○	57	○○○○	77	○○○○
18	○○○○	38	○○○○	58	○○○○	78	○○○○
19	○○○○	39	○○○○	59	○○○○	79	○○○○
20	○○○○	40	○○○○	60	○○○○	80	○○○○

	1 2 3 4		1 2 3 4		1 2 3 4		1 2 3 4
81	○○○○	99	○○○○	117	○○○○	135	○○○○
82	○○○○	100	○○○○	118	○○○○	136	○○○○
83	○○○○	101	○○○○	119	○○○○	137	○○○○
84	○○○○	102	○○○○	120	○○○○	138	○○○○
85	○○○○	103	○○○○	121	○○○○	139	○○○○
86	○○○○	104	○○○○	122	○○○○	140	○○○○
87	○○○○	105	○○○○	123	○○○○	141	○○○○
88	○○○○	106	○○○○	124	○○○○	142	○○○○
89	○○○○	107	○○○○	125	○○○○	143	○○○○
90	○○○○	108	○○○○	126	○○○○	144	○○○○
91	○○○○	109	○○○○	127	○○○○	145	○○○○
92	○○○○	110	○○○○	128	○○○○	146	○○○○
93	○○○○	111	○○○○	129	○○○○	147	○○○○
94	○○○○	112	○○○○	130	○○○○	148	○○○○
95	○○○○	113	○○○○	131	○○○○	149	○○○○
96	○○○○	114	○○○○	132	○○○○	150	○○○○
97	○○○○	115	○○○○	133	○○○○		
98	○○○○	116	○○○○	134	○○○○		

Answer Sheet

UNIT FOUR
REVIEW TEST 7

With a pencil, blacken the circle below the option you have chosen for your correct answer.

	1 2 3 4		1 2 3 4		1 2 3 4		1 2 3 4
1	○○○○	21	○○○○	41	○○○○	61	○○○○
2	○○○○	22	○○○○	42	○○○○	62	○○○○
3	○○○○	23	○○○○	43	○○○○	63	○○○○
4	○○○○	24	○○○○	44	○○○○	64	○○○○
5	○○○○	25	○○○○	45	○○○○	65	○○○○
6	○○○○	26	○○○○	46	○○○○	66	○○○○
7	○○○○	27	○○○○	47	○○○○	67	○○○○
8	○○○○	28	○○○○	48	○○○○	68	○○○○
9	○○○○	29	○○○○	49	○○○○	69	○○○○
10	○○○○	30	○○○○	50	○○○○	70	○○○○
11	○○○○	31	○○○○	51	○○○○	71	○○○○
12	○○○○	32	○○○○	52	○○○○	72	○○○○
13	○○○○	33	○○○○	53	○○○○	73	○○○○
14	○○○○	34	○○○○	54	○○○○	74	○○○○
15	○○○○	35	○○○○	55	○○○○	75	○○○○
16	○○○○	36	○○○○	56	○○○○	76	○○○○
17	○○○○	37	○○○○	57	○○○○	77	○○○○
18	○○○○	38	○○○○	58	○○○○	78	○○○○
19	○○○○	39	○○○○	59	○○○○	79	○○○○
20	○○○○	40	○○○○	60	○○○○	80	○○○○

#	1 2 3 4	#	1 2 3 4	#	1 2 3 4	#	1 2 3 4
81	○○○○	97	○○○○	113	○○○○	129	○○○○
82	○○○○	98	○○○○	114	○○○○	130	○○○○
83	○○○○	99	○○○○	115	○○○○	131	○○○○
84	○○○○	100	○○○○	116	○○○○	132	○○○○
85	○○○○	101	○○○○	117	○○○○	133	○○○○
86	○○○○	102	○○○○	118	○○○○	134	○○○○
87	○○○○	103	○○○○	119	○○○○	135	○○○○
88	○○○○	104	○○○○	120	○○○○	136	○○○○
89	○○○○	105	○○○○	121	○○○○	137	○○○○
90	○○○○	106	○○○○	122	○○○○	138	○○○○
91	○○○○	107	○○○○	123	○○○○	139	○○○○
92	○○○○	108	○○○○	124	○○○○	140	○○○○
93	○○○○	109	○○○○	125	○○○○	141	○○○○
94	○○○○	110	○○○○	126	○○○○	142	○○○○
95	○○○○	111	○○○○	127	○○○○	143	○○○○
96	○○○○	112	○○○○	128	○○○○		

UNIT FOUR
REVIEW TEST 8

With a pencil, blacken the circle below the option you have chosen for your correct answer.

	1 2 3 4		1 2 3 4		1 2 3 4		1 2 3 4
1	○○○○	21	○○○○	41	○○○○	61	○○○○
2	○○○○	22	○○○○	42	○○○○	62	○○○○
3	○○○○	23	○○○○	43	○○○○	63	○○○○
4	○○○○	24	○○○○	44	○○○○	64	○○○○
5	○○○○	25	○○○○	45	○○○○	65	○○○○
6	○○○○	26	○○○○	46	○○○○	66	○○○○
7	○○○○	27	○○○○	47	○○○○	67	○○○○
8	○○○○	28	○○○○	48	○○○○	68	○○○○
9	○○○○	29	○○○○	49	○○○○	69	○○○○
10	○○○○	30	○○○○	50	○○○○	70	○○○○
11	○○○○	31	○○○○	51	○○○○	71	○○○○
12	○○○○	32	○○○○	52	○○○○	72	○○○○
13	○○○○	33	○○○○	53	○○○○	73	○○○○
14	○○○○	34	○○○○	54	○○○○	74	○○○○
15	○○○○	35	○○○○	55	○○○○	75	○○○○
16	○○○○	36	○○○○	56	○○○○	76	○○○○
17	○○○○	37	○○○○	57	○○○○	77	○○○○
18	○○○○	38	○○○○	58	○○○○	78	○○○○
19	○○○○	39	○○○○	59	○○○○	79	○○○○
20	○○○○	40	○○○○	60	○○○○	80	○○○○

	1 2 3 4		1 2 3 4		1 2 3 4		1 2 3 4
81	○○○○	91	○○○○	101	○○○○	111	○○○○
82	○○○○	92	○○○○	102	○○○○	112	○○○○
83	○○○○	93	○○○○	103	○○○○	113	○○○○
84	○○○○	94	○○○○	104	○○○○	114	○○○○
85	○○○○	95	○○○○	105	○○○○	115	○○○○
86	○○○○	96	○○○○	106	○○○○	116	○○○○
87	○○○○	97	○○○○	107	○○○○	117	○○○○
88	○○○○	98	○○○○	108	○○○○	118	○○○○
89	○○○○	99	○○○○	109	○○○○	119	○○○○
90	○○○○	100	○○○○	110	○○○○	120	○○○○

Answer Sheet

UNIT FOUR
REVIEW TEST 9

With a pencil, blacken the circle below the option you have chosen for your correct answer.

	1 2 3 4		1 2 3 4		1 2 3 4		1 2 3 4
1	○○○○	21	○○○○	41	○○○○	61	○○○○
2	○○○○	22	○○○○	42	○○○○	62	○○○○
3	○○○○	23	○○○○	43	○○○○	63	○○○○
4	○○○○	24	○○○○	44	○○○○	64	○○○○
5	○○○○	25	○○○○	45	○○○○	65	○○○○
6	○○○○	26	○○○○	46	○○○○	66	○○○○
7	○○○○	27	○○○○	47	○○○○	67	○○○○
8	○○○○	28	○○○○	48	○○○○	68	○○○○
9	○○○○	29	○○○○	49	○○○○	69	○○○○
10	○○○○	30	○○○○	50	○○○○	70	○○○○
11	○○○○	31	○○○○	51	○○○○	71	○○○○
12	○○○○	32	○○○○	52	○○○○	72	○○○○
13	○○○○	33	○○○○	53	○○○○	73	○○○○
14	○○○○	34	○○○○	54	○○○○	74	○○○○
15	○○○○	35	○○○○	55	○○○○	75	○○○○
16	○○○○	36	○○○○	56	○○○○	76	○○○○
17	○○○○	37	○○○○	57	○○○○	77	○○○○
18	○○○○	38	○○○○	58	○○○○	78	○○○○
19	○○○○	39	○○○○	59	○○○○	79	○○○○
20	○○○○	40	○○○○	60	○○○○	80	○○○○

81   1 2 3 4   ○○○○   85   1 2 3 4   ○○○○   89   1 2 3 4   ○○○○   93   1 2 3 4   ○○○○

82   1 2 3 4   ○○○○   86   1 2 3 4   ○○○○   90   1 2 3 4   ○○○○   94   1 2 3 4   ○○○○

83   1 2 3 4   ○○○○   87   1 2 3 4   ○○○○   91   1 2 3 4   ○○○○

84   1 2 3 4   ○○○○   88   1 2 3 4   ○○○○   92   1 2 3 4   ○○○○

UNIT FOUR
REVIEW TEST 10

With a pencil, blacken the circle below the option you have chosen for your correct answer.

	1 2 3 4		1 2 3 4		1 2 3 4		1 2 3 4
1	○○○○	21	○○○○	41	○○○○	61	○○○○
2	○○○○	22	○○○○	42	○○○○	62	○○○○
3	○○○○	23	○○○○	43	○○○○	63	○○○○
4	○○○○	24	○○○○	44	○○○○	64	○○○○
5	○○○○	25	○○○○	45	○○○○	65	○○○○
6	○○○○	26	○○○○	46	○○○○	66	○○○○
7	○○○○	27	○○○○	47	○○○○	67	○○○○
8	○○○○	28	○○○○	48	○○○○	68	○○○○
9	○○○○	29	○○○○	49	○○○○	69	○○○○
10	○○○○	30	○○○○	50	○○○○	70	○○○○
11	○○○○	31	○○○○	51	○○○○	71	○○○○
12	○○○○	32	○○○○	52	○○○○	72	○○○○
13	○○○○	33	○○○○	53	○○○○	73	○○○○
14	○○○○	34	○○○○	54	○○○○	74	○○○○
15	○○○○	35	○○○○	55	○○○○	75	○○○○
16	○○○○	36	○○○○	56	○○○○	76	○○○○
17	○○○○	37	○○○○	57	○○○○	77	○○○○
18	○○○○	38	○○○○	58	○○○○	78	○○○○
19	○○○○	39	○○○○	59	○○○○	79	○○○○
20	○○○○	40	○○○○	60	○○○○	80	○○○○

	1 2 3 4		1 2 3 4		1 2 3 4		1 2 3 4
81	○○○○	96	○○○○	111	○○○○	126	○○○○
82	○○○○	97	○○○○	112	○○○○	127	○○○○
83	○○○○	98	○○○○	113	○○○○	128	○○○○
84	○○○○	99	○○○○	114	○○○○	129	○○○○
85	○○○○	100	○○○○	115	○○○○	130	○○○○
86	○○○○	101	○○○○	116	○○○○	131	○○○○
87	○○○○	102	○○○○	117	○○○○	132	○○○○
88	○○○○	103	○○○○	118	○○○○	133	○○○○
89	○○○○	104	○○○○	119	○○○○	134	○○○○
90	○○○○	105	○○○○	120	○○○○	135	○○○○
91	○○○○	106	○○○○	121	○○○○	136	○○○○
92	○○○○	107	○○○○	122	○○○○	137	○○○○
93	○○○○	108	○○○○	123	○○○○	138	○○○○
94	○○○○	109	○○○○	124	○○○○	139	○○○○
95	○○○○	110	○○○○	125	○○○○	140	○○○○

Answer Sheet

UNIT FOUR
REVIEW TEST 11

With a pencil, blacken the circle below the option you have chosen for your correct answer.

	1 2 3 4		1 2 3 4		1 2 3 4		1 2 3 4
1	○○○○	21	○○○○	41	○○○○	61	○○○○
2	○○○○	22	○○○○	42	○○○○	62	○○○○
3	○○○○	23	○○○○	43	○○○○	63	○○○○
4	○○○○	24	○○○○	44	○○○○	64	○○○○
5	○○○○	25	○○○○	45	○○○○	65	○○○○
6	○○○○	26	○○○○	46	○○○○	66	○○○○
7	○○○○	27	○○○○	47	○○○○	67	○○○○
8	○○○○	28	○○○○	48	○○○○	68	○○○○
9	○○○○	29	○○○○	49	○○○○	69	○○○○
10	○○○○	30	○○○○	50	○○○○	70	○○○○
11	○○○○	31	○○○○	51	○○○○	71	○○○○
12	○○○○	32	○○○○	52	○○○○	72	○○○○
13	○○○○	33	○○○○	53	○○○○	73	○○○○
14	○○○○	34	○○○○	54	○○○○	74	○○○○
15	○○○○	35	○○○○	55	○○○○	75	○○○○
16	○○○○	36	○○○○	56	○○○○	76	○○○○
17	○○○○	37	○○○○	57	○○○○	77	○○○○
18	○○○○	38	○○○○	58	○○○○	78	○○○○
19	○○○○	39	○○○○	59	○○○○	79	○○○○
20	○○○○	40	○○○○	60	○○○○	80	○○○○

	1 2 3 4		1 2 3 4		1 2 3 4		1 2 3 4
81	○○○○	89	○○○○	97	○○○○	105	○○○○
82	○○○○	90	○○○○	98	○○○○	106	○○○○
83	○○○○	91	○○○○	99	○○○○	107	○○○○
84	○○○○	92	○○○○	100	○○○○	108	○○○○
85	○○○○	93	○○○○	101	○○○○	109	○○○○
86	○○○○	94	○○○○	102	○○○○	110	○○○○
87	○○○○	95	○○○○	103	○○○○		
88	○○○○	96	○○○○	104	○○○○		

Answer Sheet

UNIT FOUR
REVIEW TEST 12

With a pencil, blacken the circle below the option you have chosen for your correct answer.

	1 2 3 4		1 2 3 4		1 2 3 4		1 2 3 4
1	○○○○	18	○○○○	35	○○○○	52	○○○○
2	○○○○	19	○○○○	36	○○○○	53	○○○○
3	○○○○	20	○○○○	37	○○○○	54	○○○○
4	○○○○	21	○○○○	38	○○○○	55	○○○○
5	○○○○	22	○○○○	39	○○○○	56	○○○○
6	○○○○	23	○○○○	40	○○○○	57	○○○○
7	○○○○	24	○○○○	41	○○○○	58	○○○○
8	○○○○	25	○○○○	42	○○○○	59	○○○○
9	○○○○	26	○○○○	43	○○○○	60	○○○○
10	○○○○	27	○○○○	44	○○○○	61	○○○○
11	○○○○	28	○○○○	45	○○○○	62	○○○○
12	○○○○	29	○○○○	46	○○○○	63	○○○○
13	○○○○	30	○○○○	47	○○○○	64	○○○○
14	○○○○	31	○○○○	48	○○○○	65	○○○○
15	○○○○	32	○○○○	49	○○○○	66	○○○○
16	○○○○	33	○○○○	50	○○○○	67	○○○○
17	○○○○	34	○○○○	51	○○○○	68	○○○○

Answer Sheet

UNIT FOUR
REVIEW TEST 13

With a pencil, blacken the circle below the option you have chosen for your correct answer.

	1 2 3 4		1 2 3 4		1 2 3 4		1 2 3 4
1	○○○○	20	○○○○	39	○○○○	58	○○○○
2	○○○○	21	○○○○	40	○○○○	59	○○○○
3	○○○○	22	○○○○	41	○○○○	60	○○○○
4	○○○○	23	○○○○	42	○○○○	61	○○○○
5	○○○○	24	○○○○	43	○○○○	62	○○○○
6	○○○○	25	○○○○	44	○○○○	63	○○○○
7	○○○○	26	○○○○	45	○○○○	64	○○○○
8	○○○○	27	○○○○	46	○○○○	65	○○○○
9	○○○○	28	○○○○	47	○○○○	66	○○○○
10	○○○○	29	○○○○	48	○○○○	67	○○○○
11	○○○○	30	○○○○	49	○○○○	68	○○○○
12	○○○○	31	○○○○	50	○○○○	69	○○○○
13	○○○○	32	○○○○	51	○○○○	70	○○○○
14	○○○○	33	○○○○	52	○○○○	71	○○○○
15	○○○○	34	○○○○	53	○○○○	72	○○○○
16	○○○○	35	○○○○	54	○○○○	73	○○○○
17	○○○○	36	○○○○	55	○○○○	74	○○○○
18	○○○○	37	○○○○	56	○○○○	75	○○○○
19	○○○○	38	○○○○	57	○○○○		

Answer Sheet

UNIT FOUR
REVIEW TEST 14

With a pencil, blacken the circle below the option you have chosen for your correct answer.

	1 2 3 4		1 2 3 4		1 2 3 4		1 2 3 4
1	○○○○	21	○○○○	41	○○○○	61	○○○○
2	○○○○	22	○○○○	42	○○○○	62	○○○○
3	○○○○	23	○○○○	43	○○○○	63	○○○○
4	○○○○	24	○○○○	44	○○○○	64	○○○○
5	○○○○	25	○○○○	45	○○○○	65	○○○○
6	○○○○	26	○○○○	46	○○○○	66	○○○○
7	○○○○	27	○○○○	47	○○○○	67	○○○○
8	○○○○	28	○○○○	48	○○○○	68	○○○○
9	○○○○	29	○○○○	49	○○○○	69	○○○○
10	○○○○	30	○○○○	50	○○○○	70	○○○○
11	○○○○	31	○○○○	51	○○○○	71	○○○○
12	○○○○	32	○○○○	52	○○○○	72	○○○○
13	○○○○	33	○○○○	53	○○○○	73	○○○○
14	○○○○	34	○○○○	54	○○○○	74	○○○○
15	○○○○	35	○○○○	55	○○○○	75	○○○○
16	○○○○	36	○○○○	56	○○○○	76	○○○○
17	○○○○	37	○○○○	57	○○○○	77	○○○○
18	○○○○	38	○○○○	58	○○○○	78	○○○○
19	○○○○	39	○○○○	59	○○○○	79	○○○○
20	○○○○	40	○○○○	60	○○○○	80	○○○○

        1 2 3 4   1 2 3 4   1 2 3 4   1 2 3 4
81 ○○○○   86 ○○○○   91 ○○○○   96 ○○○○

        1 2 3 4   1 2 3 4   1 2 3 4   1 2 3 4
82 ○○○○   87 ○○○○   92 ○○○○   97 ○○○○

        1 2 3 4   1 2 3 4   1 2 3 4
83 ○○○○   88 ○○○○   93 ○○○○

        1 2 3 4   1 2 3 4   1 2 3 4
84 ○○○○   89 ○○○○   94 ○○○○

        1 2 3 4   1 2 3 4   1 2 3 4
85 ○○○○   90 ○○○○   95 ○○○○

Answer Sheet

PART ONE
COMPREHENSIVE EXAMINATION

With a pencil, blacken the circle below the option you have chosen for your correct answer.

	1 2 3 4		1 2 3 4		1 2 3 4		1 2 3 4
1	○○○○	21	○○○○	41	○○○○	61	○○○○
2	○○○○	22	○○○○	42	○○○○	62	○○○○
3	○○○○	23	○○○○	43	○○○○	63	○○○○
4	○○○○	24	○○○○	44	○○○○	64	○○○○
5	○○○○	25	○○○○	45	○○○○	65	○○○○
6	○○○○	26	○○○○	46	○○○○	66	○○○○
7	○○○○	27	○○○○	47	○○○○	67	○○○○
8	○○○○	28	○○○○	48	○○○○	68	○○○○
9	○○○○	29	○○○○	49	○○○○	69	○○○○
10	○○○○	30	○○○○	50	○○○○	70	○○○○
11	○○○○	31	○○○○	51	○○○○	71	○○○○
12	○○○○	32	○○○○	52	○○○○	72	○○○○
13	○○○○	33	○○○○	53	○○○○	73	○○○○
14	○○○○	34	○○○○	54	○○○○	74	○○○○
15	○○○○	35	○○○○	55	○○○○	75	○○○○
16	○○○○	36	○○○○	56	○○○○	76	○○○○
17	○○○○	37	○○○○	57	○○○○	77	○○○○
18	○○○○	38	○○○○	58	○○○○	78	○○○○
19	○○○○	39	○○○○	59	○○○○	79	○○○○
20	○○○○	40	○○○○	60	○○○○	80	○○○○

	1 2 3 4		1 2 3 4		1 2 3 4		1 2 3 4
81	○○○○	91	○○○○	101	○○○○	111	○○○○
82	○○○○	92	○○○○	102	○○○○	112	○○○○
83	○○○○	93	○○○○	103	○○○○	113	○○○○
84	○○○○	94	○○○○	104	○○○○	114	○○○○
85	○○○○	95	○○○○	105	○○○○	115	○○○○
86	○○○○	96	○○○○	106	○○○○	116	○○○○
87	○○○○	97	○○○○	107	○○○○	117	○○○○
88	○○○○	98	○○○○	108	○○○○	118	○○○○
89	○○○○	99	○○○○	109	○○○○	119	○○○○
90	○○○○	100	○○○○	110	○○○○	120	○○○○

Answer Sheet

PART TWO
COMPREHENSIVE EXAMINATION

With a pencil, blacken the circle below the option you have chosen for your correct answer.

	1 2 3 4		1 2 3 4		1 2 3 4		1 2 3 4
1	○○○○	21	○○○○	41	○○○○	61	○○○○
2	○○○○	22	○○○○	42	○○○○	62	○○○○
3	○○○○	23	○○○○	43	○○○○	63	○○○○
4	○○○○	24	○○○○	44	○○○○	64	○○○○
5	○○○○	25	○○○○	45	○○○○	65	○○○○
6	○○○○	26	○○○○	46	○○○○	66	○○○○
7	○○○○	27	○○○○	47	○○○○	67	○○○○
8	○○○○	28	○○○○	48	○○○○	68	○○○○
9	○○○○	29	○○○○	49	○○○○	69	○○○○
10	○○○○	30	○○○○	50	○○○○	70	○○○○
11	○○○○	31	○○○○	51	○○○○	71	○○○○
12	○○○○	32	○○○○	52	○○○○	72	○○○○
13	○○○○	33	○○○○	53	○○○○	73	○○○○
14	○○○○	34	○○○○	54	○○○○	74	○○○○
15	○○○○	35	○○○○	55	○○○○	75	○○○○
16	○○○○	36	○○○○	56	○○○○	76	○○○○
17	○○○○	37	○○○○	57	○○○○	77	○○○○
18	○○○○	38	○○○○	58	○○○○	78	○○○○
19	○○○○	39	○○○○	59	○○○○	79	○○○○
20	○○○○	40	○○○○	60	○○○○	80	○○○○

	1 2 3 4		1 2 3 4		1 2 3 4		1 2 3 4
81	○○○○	91	○○○○	101	○○○○	111	○○○○
82	○○○○	92	○○○○	102	○○○○	112	○○○○
83	○○○○	93	○○○○	103	○○○○	113	○○○○
84	○○○○	94	○○○○	104	○○○○	114	○○○○
85	○○○○	95	○○○○	105	○○○○	115	○○○○
86	○○○○	96	○○○○	106	○○○○	116	○○○○
87	○○○○	97	○○○○	107	○○○○	117	○○○○
88	○○○○	98	○○○○	108	○○○○	118	○○○○
89	○○○○	99	○○○○	109	○○○○	119	○○○○
90	○○○○	100	○○○○	110	○○○○	120	○○○○

NCLEX Practice Test Program Instructions

This software program has been designed to be used with an IBM or IBM-compatible computer and requires DOS 3.0 or higher and 512 RAM. To start the program, insert the diskette in the floppy drive and set the default to the floppy drive (eg, Drive A or Drive B). At the prompt (A:\> or B:\>), type GO and press the Enter key.

This program enables you to answer 100 questions on the computer similar to the way in which you will take the NCLEX Examination after the NCLEX–CAT is implemented

As in the NCLEX Examination, all questions on this program are multiple choice. To answer questions, you will need only three computer keys—the up and down Arrows and the Enter key. Use the Arrow keys to highlight the answer you want to select. To enter the highlighted answer as your choice, simply press the Enter key. (The NCLEX Examination requires you to use the Space Bar to move the cursor among the answer choices and to press the Enter key twice to select the answer choice.)

This practice test allows you two testing options and an option to see your test results. Each computer screen has prompts at the bottom of the screen that will provide any needed instructions. The program menu will look like this:

1. Instructions
2. Take the Test
3. Try Again
4. Review Your Results
5. Quit

The "Take the Test" option will allow you to answer all 100 questions and will store your answers in memory. To do this, select number two (2) from the menu. You can choose to have the test timed, the program show you the time remaining, and the program show you the number of questions you have completed. When you have completed the test, you can choose to see the "Review Your Results" screen. You also can choose the "Review Your Results" option, (4) from the menu, which will show you a chart that indicates the following (the chart will look like the Classification of Test Items grids that appear after each review test in the book):

- question number
- whether you answered the questions correctly (a checkmark indicates that you answered the question correctly, an "X" indicates that you answered the question incorrectly, and no mark indicates that you did not answer the question)
- the Attributes for each question
    - Nursing Process Step
    - Client Need
    - Nursing Care Area

This way, you can see how well you did on this sample test.

The "Try Again" option, (3) from the menu, will give you all 100 questions again with a check mark next to each question you answered correctly. All questions without a check mark were either answered incorrectly or not answered. The "Try Again" option allows you to work on those questions that you got wrong or did not answer. This way, you can practice questions that were a problem. This option will give you three tries to answer the question (the screen will say "NO, try again"). If your third answer choice is also incorrect, the program will show you the correct answer. If your second (or third) answer choice is correct, the screen will say "That's right". (As the Preface of this book describes, the NCLEX Examination will not allow you to try a question a second time and will, of course, not provide you with test results.)

Good luck and enjoy practicing on this disk before you take the real examination!